Contemporary Nursing

ISSUES, TRENDS, & MANAGEMENT

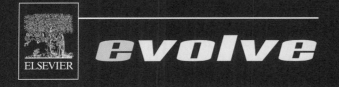

ELSEVIER

evolve

To access your Student Resources, visit the Web address below:

http://evolve.elsevier.com/Cherry/

Evolve Online Resources for *Contemporary Nursing: Issues, Trends, & Management,* edition 3, offers the following features:

- **Student Learning Resources**
  An exciting resource that includes case studies, appendices, additional textbook material, critical thinking activities, internet activities, and suggested readings.

- **WebLinks**
  An exciting resource that lets you link to hundreds of websites carefully chosen to supplement the content of the textbook. The WebLinks are regularly updated, with new ones added as they develop.

Contemporary Nursing

ISSUES, TRENDS, & MANAGEMENT

BARBARA CHERRY, MSN, MBA, RN

Director of Interdisciplinary Programs in Aging
Texas Tech University Health Sciences Center
Lubbock, Texas

SUSAN R. JACOB, PhD, MSN, BSN, RN

Executive Associate Dean and Professor
The University of Tennessee Health Science Center
College of Nursing
Memphis, Tennessee

THIRD EDITION

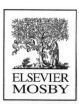

ELSEVIER
MOSBY

ELSEVIER
MOSBY

11830 Westline Industrial Drive
St. Louis, Missouri 63146

CONTEMPORARY NURSING: ISSUES, TRENDS, & MANAGEMENT
Copyright © 2005 Elsevier Inc. All rights reserved.

Previous editions copyrighted 1999, 2002

ISBN-13: 978-0-323-02968-1
ISBN-10: 0-323-02968-X

Acquisitions Editor: Tom Wilhelm
Associate Developmental Editor: Jennifer L. Anderson
Publishing Services Manger: John Rogers
Senior Project Manager: Helen Hudlin
Designer: Teresa McBryan

Printed in the United States of America

Last digit is the print number: 9 8 7 6 5 4 3 2

To all the student nurses whose curiosity and enthusiasm for nursing created the inspiration to develop this text and to all practicing nurses who face serious challenges but reap great rewards for providing high-quality patient care

Being a Nurse Means . . .

You will never be bored,
You will always be frustrated,
You will be surrounded by challenges,
So much to do and so little time.
You will carry immense responsibility
And very little authority.
You will step into people's lives,
And you will make a difference.
Some will bless you.
Some will curse you.
You will see people at their worst,
And at their best.
You will never cease to be amazed at people's capacity
For love, courage, and endurance.
You will see life begin
and end.
You will experience resounding triumphs
And devastating failures.
You will cry a lot.
You will laugh a lot.
You will know what it is to be human
And to be humane.

Melodie Chenevert, RN

Contributors

TONI BARGAGLIOTTI, DNSc, RN
Dean
Loewenberg School of Nursing
The University of Memphis
Memphis, Tennessee

VIRGINIA TROTTER BETTS, MSN, JD, RN, FAAN
Commissioner, Tennessee Department of Mental
   Health and Development Disabilities
Tennessee Department of Mental Health
Nashville, Tennessee

RUTH ANN BRIDGES, MSN, RN, BC
Assistant Professor
School of Nursing
Texas Tech University Health Sciences Center
Lubbock, Texas

M. ELIZABETH CARNEGIE, DPA, RN, FAAN
Editor Emerita, *Nursing Research*
Chevy Chase, Maryland

BARBARA CHERRY, MSN, MBA, RN
Director of Interdisciplinary Programs in Aging
Texas Tech University Health Sciences Center
Lubbock, Texas

GENEVIEVE J. CONLIN, MS, MBA, MEd, RN, CRRN
Department Administrator
Nursing and Patient Care Services
Dana-Farber Cancer Institute
Boston, Massachusetts

LAURA H. DAY, BSN, MS, RN
Nurse Consultant
Federal Dam, Minnesota

CHARLOTTE ELIOPOULOS, PhD, RNC, MPH, ND
Specialist in Holistic, Chronic, and Geriatric Care
Education Director, Health Education Network
Glen Arm, Maryland

MARY LYNN ENGELMANN, MSN, EdD, RN
Professor of Nursing
College of Du Page
Glen Ellyn, Illinois

SANDY FORREST, PhD, RN
Department of Nursing
Mesa State College
Grand Junction, Colorado

ALEXIA GREEN, PhD, RN, FAAN
Dean and Professor
School of Nursing
Robert Wood Johnson Executive Nurse Fellow
Texas Tech University Health Sciences Center
Lubbock, Texas

SUSAN R. JACOB, PhD, MSN, BSN, RN
Executive Associate Dean and Professor
The University of Tennessee Health Science Center
College of Nursing
Memphis, Tennessee

MARYLANE WADE KOCH, MSN, RN
Adjunct Faculty
Loewenberg School of Nursing
The University of Memphis
Memphis, Tennessee

ROBERT W. KOCH, DNS, RN
Associate Professor
Loewenberg School of Nursing
The University of Memphis
Memphis, Tennessee

CARRIE B. LENBURG, EdD, RN, FAAN
President, Creative Learning and Assessment
   Systems, Inc.
Roan Mountain, Tennessee

LAURA R. MAHLMEISTER, PhD, RN
President, Mahlmeister and Associates
Belmont, California
Clinical Professor
School of Nursing
University of California, San Francisco
San Francisco, California

LESLIE H. NICOLL, PhD, MBA, RN
President and Owner
Maine Desk, LLC—Professional Editorial Services
Editor-in-Chief, *CIN: Computers, Informatics, Nursing,* and *The Journal of Hospice and Palliative Nursing*
Portland, Maine

LINDA D. NORMAN, DNS, RN
Senior Associate Dean for Academics
School of Nursing
Vanderbilt University
Nashville, Tennessee

TOMMIE L. NORRIS, DNS, RN
Assistant Professor
Loewenberg School of Nursing
The University of Memphis
Memphis, Tennessee

PATRICIA REID PONTE, DNSc, RN, FAAN
Senior Vice President for Patient Care Services
Chief of Nursing
Dana-Farber Cancer Institute
Boston, Massachusetts

TIM PORTER-O'GRADY, EdD, RN, FAAN
Senior Partner, TPOG Associates, Inc.
Otto, North Carolina

LINDA C. PUGH, PhD, RNC, FAAN
Associate Professor
School of Nursing
Johns Hopkins University
Baltimore, Maryland

ANNA SALLEE, PhD(C), RN, CCRN
Professor of Nursing
San Jacinto College South
Houston, Texas

CARLA D. SANDERSON, PhD, RN
Provost and Professor of Nursing
Union University
Jackson, Tennessee

JANET C. SCHERUBEL, PhD, RN, CCRN
Adjunct Professor
Loewenberg School of Nursing
The University of Memphis
Memphis, Tennessee

KATHRYN S. SKINNER, MS, RN, CS
Psychiatric Mental Health Clinical Nurse Specialist
Clinical Instructor
Baptist Memorial College of Health Sciences
Memphis, Tennessee

MARGARET SODERSTROM, PhD, RN, CS-P, APRN
Assistant Professor
School of Nursing
Johns Hopkins University
Baltimore, Maryland

MARGARET ELIZABETH STRONG, MSN, RN, CNA
Associate Administrator/Chief Nursing Officer
Methodist Extended Care Hospital
Memphis, Tennessee

JILL J. WEBB, PhD, MSN, BSN, RN
Associate Professor
School of Nursing
Union University
Jackson, Tennessee

ELIZABETH E. WEINER, PhD, RN, BC, FAAN
Senior Associate Dean for Educational Informatics
Vanderbilt University
Nashville, Tennessee

KATHLEEN M. WERNER, MS, BSN, RN
Director, Medical/Surgical/Pediatric Nursing
Meriter Hospital
Madison, Wisconsin

K. LYNN WIECK, PhD, RN
President, Texas Nurses Association
CEO, Management Solutions for Healthcare
Katy, Texas

SHIPHRAH A. ALICIA WILLIAMS-EVANS, PhD, APRN, BC
Chief Executive Officer
Dean and Professor
Methodist College of Nursing
Peoria, Illinois

Reviewers

PIER A. BROADNAX, PhD, RN
Assistant Professor
Division of Nursing
Howard University
Washington, DC

KATHY BURLINGAME, PhD(C), MSN
Nursing Faculty
Northland Community and Technical College
Thief River Falls, Minnesota

NANCY BURRUS, MSN, RN, CS, CCRN
Assistant Professor
Bellin College of Nursing
Green Bay, Wisconsin

SEAN CLARKE, PhD, RN, CRNP
Assistant Professor
Associate Director
Center for Health Outcomes and Policy Research
School of Nursing
University of Pennsylvania
Philadelphia, Pennsylvania

DEBRA MARSALA, MS, RN, ANP
Professor of Nursing
Chair of Nursing Department
Jefferson Community College
Watertown, New York

GLENNA C. McMINN, MS, RN
Associate Professor of Nursing
Tompkins Cortland Community College
Dryden, New York

Preface

At no other time in the history of modern nursing have nurses been presented with such tremendous opportunities to improve health care and advance the nursing profession. By understanding and providing leadership to address the very serious issues currently faced by the U.S. health care system, including patient safety and quality care, the nursing shortage, advancing technology, changing legal and ethical concerns, evolving nursing education trends, threats of major terrorist attacks, and working within a multi-cultural society, nurses can contribute to the evolution of an efficient, effective health care system that promotes and protects the health and well-being of each individual in our society. The third edition of *Contemporary Nursing: Issues, Trends, & Management* is an excellent resource for nurses who must understand these very complex issues in order to implement strategies from the direct patient care level to the national legislative level that can significantly advance patient care, the health care system, and the nursing profession.

Every chapter in the third edition has been updated to include the most current and relevant information available. Two new chapters have been added that reflect emerging issues faced by our health care system: *Nursing in the Ever-Evolving Health Care System,* which focuses on numerous issues surrounding rapidly advancing health care technology with recommendations for new nursing practice models for the 21st century, and *Emergency Preparedness and Response for Today's World,* which provides an excellent resource for all nurses who must now be prepared for disaster management.

Additionally, new content in the third edition focuses on the following areas and topics:

- The series of reports in the Institute of Medicine's quality initiative, including *To Err is Human: Building a Safer Healthcare System, Crossing the Quality Chasm: A New Health System for the 21st Century, Keeping Patients Safe: Transforming the Work Environment of Nurses,* and *Health Professions Education: A Bridge to Quality*.
- New case law regarding the roles and responsibilities of charge nurses and how to deal with criminal acts and intentional torts in nursing practice.
- New and emerging bioethical dilemmas such as stem cell research, transplants, and cloning.
- Most current information to date on the nursing shortage and on workplace issues such as mandatory overtime and staffing shortages.
- American Nurses Association's most recently established organizational affiliates—the Center for American Nurses (CAN) and the United American Nurses (UAN).
- Recommendations for culturally and linguistically appropriate services.
- Telehealth nursing standards.
- New case scenarios related to delegation decision-making.
- Model for achieving evidence-based practice.
- Descriptions and examples of the new NCLEX-RN alternate item format questions.

Each chapter in the third edition contains the same features that made the previous editions so successful: opening real-life Vignettes and Questions to Consider, which peak the reader's interest in the chapter content and stimulate critical thinking. Integrated Learning Outcomes, which provide both instructors and students with a clear understanding of what behaviors can be expected after a study of the chapter is completed. **Key Terms,** which contain clear and concise definitions of terms that are critical to enhance the readers' understanding of the topics and expand their vocabulary related to health care issues. Finally, each chapter refers to a set of **On-Line Resources on the Evolve website** that provides a great reference for further exploration of the topic and to **Critical Thinking Activities** that encourage students to reflect on the content and provide instructors with excellent in-class and on-line learning activities.

UNIT ONE: THE DEVELOPMENT OF NURSING

The book opens with a presentation about the exciting evolution of nursing: its very visible public image and its core foundations, which include nursing theory, nursing education, and licensure and certification. These opening chapters provide the reader with a solid background for understanding and studying current and future trends.

UNIT TWO: CURRENT ISSUES IN HEALTH CARE

This unit provides a comprehensive overview of the most current trends and issues occurring today in nursing and health care, including health care financing and economics, the evolving health care system, legal and ethical issues, health policy and politics, cultural and social issues, workplace issues, emergency preparedness, nursing informatics, and alternative healing. Students, faculty, and veteran nurses will be challenged to critically examine each of these significant issues that are currently shaping the practice of professional nursing and the health care delivery system.

UNIT THREE: LEADERSHIP AND MANAGEMENT IN NURSING

This unit offers a primer on nursing leadership and management, with a focus on the basic skills that are necessary for nurses to function effectively in the professional nursing role. Chapters examine leadership roles and management theory, effective communication, delegation and supervision, staffing and nursing care delivery models, quality improvement, and nursing research and evidence-based practice. The updated content in this unit provides the most current information available related to nursing leadership and management and will serve as both a valuable educational tool for students and a very useful resource for practicing nurses.

UNIT FOUR: CAREER MANAGEMENT

The final unit prepares the student to embark on a career in nursing. Making the transition from student to professional, managing time, understanding career opportunities, finding a good match between the nurse and the employer, and passing the NCLEX-RN examination are all presented with practical, useful advice that will serve as an excellent resource for both students and novice nurses as they build their career in professional nursing.

TEACHING AND LEARNING SUPPORT

Featured in this edition of *Contemporary Nursing* is a dedicated website (http://evolve. elsevier.com/Cherry/) with access to hundreds of active sites keyed specifically to each chapter of the text. These WebLinks are continually updated to provide the most current topics related to the content in the text.

   Also new to this edition and available through the Cherry and Jacob website are online resources specifically designed for the instructor. These resources include suggested outlines for lectures, extra credit activities, suggestions for teaching-learning activities, an Instructor's Electronic Resource Manual, a Test Bank, and PowerPoint slides. All of these instructor resources are password protected, so please contact your local sales representative for further details.

About the Authors

BARBARA CHERRY, MSN, MBA, RN

Barbara Cherry received her diploma in nursing from Methodist Hospital School of Nursing in 1973, her BSN from West Texas A&M University in 1980, her MBA from Texas Tech University in 1995, and her MSN from Texas Tech University Health Sciences Center in 1997. Barbara's clinical background is in critical care, medical-surgical, and nephrology nursing. She has over 20 years' clinical and nursing management experience and currently directs two academic programs at Texas Tech University Health Sciences Center: Interdisciplinary Programs in Aging and Business Enterprises for the School of Nursing. Barbara is also a student in the DNSc program at The University of Tennessee Health Science Center, Memphis, Tennessee.

SUSAN R. JACOB, PhD, MSN, BSN, RN

Susan Jacob received her BSN from West Virginia University in 1970, her MSN from San Jose State University in 1975, and her PhD from the University of Tennessee, Memphis in 1993. Her extensive experience as a clinician, educator, and researcher has been focused in the community health arena, specifically home health and hospice. She has taught undergraduate and graduate nursing courses such as Community Health Nursing, Professional Nursing Issues, Nursing Research, Nursing Theory, and Intercultural Issues. Dr. Jacob's research has addressed the bereavement experience of older adults and enhanced models of home health care delivery. Dr. Jacob is Executive Associate Dean and Professor in the College of Nursing at The University of Tennessee Health Science Center, Memphis, Tennessee. She is a leader in professional nursing organizations at the state and national level.

Acknowledgments

Our contributors deserve our most sincere thanks for their high-quality, timely work that demonstrates genuine expertise and professionalism. Their contributions have made this book a truly first-rate text that will be invaluable to nursing students and faculty and will serve as an outstanding resource for practicing nurses. We extend a special thanks to our reviewers who gave us helpful suggestions and insights as we developed the third edition.

We would like to express our grateful appreciation to the Mosby staff—Tom Wilhelm, Senior Editor, and Jennifer Anderson, Associate Developmental Editor, Lisa Newton, and Michael Ledbetter—for their very capable and professional support, guidance, and calm reassurance.

Our deepest appreciation goes to the most important people in our lives—our husbands, Mike and Dick, our children, our families, and our friends. Their enduring support and extreme patience have allowed us to accomplish what sometimes seemed to be the impossible.

Contents

3   **Theories of Nursing Practice, 47**

Margaret Soderstrom, PhD, RN, CS-P, APRN
Linda C. Pugh, PhD, RNC, FAAN

UNIT Two
CURRENT ISSUES IN HEALTH CARE

9   **Ethical and Bioethical Issues in Nursing and Health Care, 189**
Carla D. Sanderson, PhD, RN

13   Emergency Preparedness and Response for Today's World, 292

Linda D. Norman, DNS, RN

Elizabeth E. Weiner, PhD, RN, BC, FAAN

UNIT Three
LEADERSHIP AND MANAGEMENT IN NURSING

20   Nursing's Role in Improving the Quality of Health Care, 467

Kathleen M. Werner, MS, BSN, RN

21   Nursing Research, 492

Jill J. Webb, PhD, MSN, BSN, RN

UNIT Four
CAREER MANAGEMENT

23   Managing Time: The Path to High Self-Performance, 536

Patricia Reid Ponte, DNSc, RN, FAAN
Genevieve J. Conlin, MS, MBA, MEd, RN, CRRN

24   Contemporary Nursing Roles and Career Opportunities, 560

Robert W. Koch, DNS, RN

25   Job Search: Finding Your Match, 582

Kathryn S. Skinner, MS, RN, CS

Laura H. Day, BSN, MS, RN

26   NCLEX-RN Examination, 604

Mary Lynn Engelmann, MSN, EdD, RN

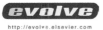

The Evolution of Professional Nursing

Shiphrah A. Alicia Williams-Evans, PhD, APRN, BC; Susan R. Jacob, PhD, MSN, BSN, RN; and M. Elizabeth Carnegie, DPA, RN, FAAN

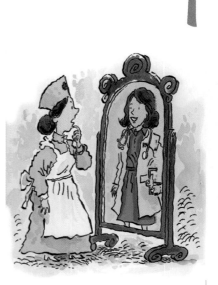

Oh, my, how we've changed.

VIGNETTE

Tabitha Louise Pitts is an 88-year-old nurse who retired from the military 30 years ago and then began a career as an educator at a state university. She was diagnosed with diabetes mellitus 40 years ago. During the past 3 months she began to have difficulty with elevated blood sugar, swelling, and painful urination. Three years ago Mrs. Pitts had her second below-the-knee amputation. She decided to go to the local health clinic to see Dr. Aldora James, who is an advanced practice nurse, as well as a certified family nurse practitioner with a doctorate in nursing science.

After completing the physical examination and analysis of laboratory findings, Dr. James determined that Mrs. Pitts was suffering from end-stage renal disease and brittle uncontrolled diabetes. Dr. James ordered consultations with a nephrologist and endocrinologist to ensure that comprehensive care was provided. Both consulting physicians made a determination that Mrs. Pitts' condition was terminal. Mrs. Pitts is a widow whose only son died 4 years ago in a motor vehicle accident. After reviewing all the possible treatments available, Mrs. Pitts made a decision not to have dialysis.

Dr. James referred Mrs. Pitts to the local hospice. Hospice set up a schedule of twice-a-day home visits to monitor Mrs. Pitts' blood sugar. Juanita Smith was the registered nurse who made these visits. Albee Winthrop, a psychiatric mental health clinical specialist, visited with Mrs. Pitts three times each week to provide support and assist her with grief work. Mrs. Winthrop also contacted Mrs. Pitts' minister to ensure that her spiritual needs were met.

Within 3 weeks Mrs. Pitts' condition worsened. She shared with Mrs. Winthrop that she had feared dying alone ever since her son died. However, because she had hospice care, her line of support expanded to an umbrella of support. Even though the health care that Mrs. Pitts required was affected by capitation, her overall care did not suffer. Parish nurses in her church congregation took turns being with her around the clock. She was never alone, thanks to the services provided by the diversity of nursing care.

Mrs. Pitts reminisced about her experiences in nursing. She recalled that she had seen nursing come full circle. She remembered when it was okay for individuals to die peacefully at home, and she had also seen a time when individuals were rushed to the hospital to die. She marveled at the fact that now an individual could make choices about end-of-life care and "die with dignity, surrounded by caring health professionals."

Questions to consider while reading this chapter:
1. What were the challenges faced by nurses in the 1900s?
2. How has managed care affected professional nursing practice?
3. What are the challenges facing nurses in the twenty-first century?

KEY TERMS

Advanced practice nurse A registered nurse who provides care to patients in the roles of certified nurse midwife, clinical nurse specialist, certified nurse anesthetist, or certified nurse practitioner. Formal knowledge and skill are required above the basic level of nursing (BSN). Since 1994, a master of science degree in nursing is required to obtain national certification in advanced practice roles (Katz et al, 2004).

Doctor of nursing science An advanced clinical doctoral degree in nursing that builds on the master's degree in a clinical specialty area and provides knowledge and ability to create, initiate, develop, implement, and evaluate nursing research in all settings and/or educate nurses of the future. This terminal degree provides the foundation for the nurse scientist to augment clinical, didactic, health policy, and research expertise (Katz et al, 2004).

Florence Nightingale (1820-1910) Considered the founder of organized, professional nursing. She is best known for her contributions to the reforms in the British Army Medical Corps, improved sanitation in India, improved public health in Great Britain, use of statistics, and the development of organized training for nurses.

Professional nursing A specially trained profession that addresses the humanistic and holistic needs of patients, families, and environments and provides responses to patterns/needs of patients, families, and communities to actual and potential health problems. The professional nurse has diverse roles, such as health care provider, client advocate, educator, care coordinator, primary care practitioner, and change agent (Katz et al, 2004).

LEARNING OUTCOMES

After studying this chapter, the reader will be able to:
1. Summarize health practices through the course of history.
2. Analyze the impact of historic, political, social, and economic events on the development of nursing.
3. Describe the evolution of professional challenges experienced by nurses of diverse ethnic backgrounds.

CHAPTER OVERVIEW

Throughout the pages of recorded history, nursing has been integrated into every facet of life. A legacy of human caring was initiated when, according to the Book of Exodus, two midwives, Shiphrah and Puah, rescued the baby Moses and hid him to save his life. This legacy of caring has progressed throughout the years, responding to psychologic, social, environmental, and physiologic needs of society. Nurses of the past and present have struggled for recognition as knowledgeable professionals. The evolution of this struggle is reflected in political, cultural, environmental, and economic events that have sculptured our nation and world history (Katz et al, 2004; Snodgrass, 1999).

In the beginning men were recognized as health healers. Women challenged the status quo and transformed nursing from a mystical phenomenon to a respected profession (Snodgrass, 1999). Florence Nightingale and Mary Seacole played major roles in bringing about changes in nursing. Using the concept of role modeling, these women demonstrated the value of their worth through their work in fighting for the cause of health and healing. During the twentieth century nurses made tremendous advancements in the areas of education, practice, research, and technology. Nursing as a science progressed through education, clinical practice, development of theory, and rigorous research. Today nurses continue to be challenged to expand their roles and explore new areas of practice and leadership. This chapter provides a brief glimpse of health care practices and nursing care in the prehistoric period and early civilization and then describes the evolution of professional nursing practice. Box 1-1 summarizes some of the important events in the evolution of nursing.

BOX 1-1 Important Events in the Evolution of Nursing

1751 The Pennsylvania Hospital is the first hospital established in America.

1798 The U.S. Marine Hospital Service comes into being by an act of Congress on July 16. It is renamed the U.S. Public Health Service in 1912.

1840 Two African-American women, Mary Williams and Frances Rose, are listed as nurses in the City of Baltimore Directory.

1851 Florence Nightingale (1820-1910) attends Kaiserswerth to train as a nurse.

1854 During the Crimean War, Florence Nightingale transforms the image of nursing. Mary Seacole, a black woman from Jamaica, West Indies, nurses during the same time.

1861 The outbreak of the Civil War causes African-American women to volunteer as nurses. Among these women are Harriet Tubman, Sojourner Truth, and Susie King Taylor.

1863 Harriet Newton Phillips graduates from the Women's Hospital in Philadelphia.

1872 Another school of nursing opens in the United States: the New England Hospital for Women and Children in Boston, Mass.

1873 Linda Richards is responsible for designing a written patient record and physician's order system—the first in a hospital.

1879 Mary Mahoney, the first trained African-American nurse, graduates from the New England Hospital for Women and Children in Boston, Mass.

1882 The American Red Cross is established by Clara Barton.

Continued

BOX 1-1 *Important Events in the Evolution of Nursing—cont'd*

1886 The Visiting Nurses Association (VNA) is started in Philadelphia; Spelman College, Atlanta, Ga., establishes the first diploma nursing program for African-Americans.

1893 Lillian Wald and Mary Brewster establish the Henry Street Visiting Nurse Service in New York. The American Society of Superintendents of Training Schools for Nurses is established (becomes the National League of Nursing Education in 1912 and the National League for Nursing [NLN] in 1952). A nursing program (diploma) is established at Howard University, an African-American school in Washington, D.C.—the first in a university setting.

1896 The Nurses' Associated Alumnae of the United States and Canada is established (becomes the American Nurses Association [ANA] in 1911).

1898 Namahyoke Curtis, an untrained African-American nurse, is assigned by the War Department as a contract nurse in the Spanish-American War.

1900 The first issue of the *American Journal of Nursing* is published. Jessie Sleet Scales becomes the first African-American public health nurse.

1901 The Army Nurse Corps is established under the Army Reorganization Act.

1902 School nursing is established in New York City by Linda Rogers.

1903 The first Nursing Practice Acts are passed, and North Carolina is the first state to implement registration of nurses, followed by New Jersey, New York, and Virginia.

1908 The National Association of Colored Graduate Nurses is founded; it is dissolved in 1951.

1909 Ludie Andrews sues the Georgia State Board of Nurse Examiners to secure African-American nurses the right to take the state board examination and become licensed; she wins in 1920.

1912 The U.S. Public Health Service and the National League for Nursing (NLN) are established.

1916 Membership in ANA is derived through the state associations.

1918 Eighteen black nurses are admitted to the Army Nurse Corps after the Armistice is signed ending World War I.

1919 *Public Health Nursing* is written by Mary S. Gardner. A public health nursing program is started at the University of Michigan.

1921 The Sheppard-Towner Act is passed providing federal aid for maternal and child health care.

1922 Sigma Theta Tau is founded (becomes the International Honor Society of Nursing in 1985).

1923 The Goldmark Report criticizes the inadequacies of hospital-based nursing schools and recommends increased educational standards.

1924 The United States Indian Bureau Nursing Service is founded by Eleanor Gregg.

1925 The Frontier Nursing Service is founded by Mary Breckenridge.

1929 The Great Depression begins.

1930 Massive unemployment of nurses occurs.

1931 Estelle Massey Riddle Osborne earns master's degree—the first for an African-American nurse.

1935 The Social Security Act is passed.

1937 Federal appropriations for cancer, venereal diseases, tuberculosis, and mental health are begun.

1939 World War II begins.

1941 The U.S. Army establishes a quota of 56 black nurses for admission to the Army Nurse Corps. The Nurse Training Act is passed.

1943 An amendment to the Nurse Training Bill is passed that bars racial bias.

1945 The U.S. Navy drops the color bar and admits four African-American nurses.

1946 Nurses are classified as professionals by the U.S. Civil Service Commission. The Hospital Survey and Construction Act (Hill-Burton) is passed.

1948 Estelle Osborne is the first African-American nurse elected to the board of the ANA. The ANA votes individual membership to all African-American nurses excluded from any state association.

1949 M. Elizabeth Carnegie is the first African-American nurse to be elected to the board of a state association (Florida).

1950 The Code for Professional Nurses is published by the ANA.

BOX 1-1 — cont'd

1952 National nursing organizations are reorganized from six to two: ANA and NLN.

1954 The Supreme Court decision *Brown v. Board of Education* asserts that "separate educational facilities are inherently unequal."

1955 Elizabeth Lipford Kent is the first African-American nurse to earn a doctoral degree.

1965 The Social Security Amendment includes Medicare and Medicaid.

1967 Warren Hatcher is the first black male nurse to earn a doctoral degree.

1971 The National Black Nurses Association is organized.

1973 The NLN requires conceptual frameworks in nursing education. The Health Maintenance Organization Act (HMO) is passed.

1973 The ANA forms the American Academy of Nursing.

1974 The ANA receives a grant from the National Institute of Mental Health to initiate a fellowship program to help minorities earn PhDs. The First National Transcultural Conference is held at the University of Utah College of Nursing. The first certification examinations are offered by the ANA.

1975 The American Hospital Association publishes the "Patient's Bill of Rights."

1977 This year is declared the "Year of the Nurse" by the ANA to help the public better understand nursing.

1978 Barbara Nichols is the first African-American nurse elected president of the ANA. M. Elizabeth Carnegie, an African-American nurse, is elected president of the American Academy of Nursing.

1979 Brigadier General Hazel Johnson Brown is the first African-American Chief of the Army Nurse Corps.

1980 Nita Barrow, Governor General of Barbados, West Indies, is the first African-American nurse knighted as Dame of St. Andrew Order of Her Majesty Queen Elizabeth II. Colorado passes a new nurse practice act that enables nurses to practice independently in private settings. Nursing diagnosis evolves as a separate component of the nursing process.

1981 Carolyn Davis becomes the first nurse to head the Centers for Medicare and Medicaid Services (CMS), formerly the Health Care Financing Administration (HCFA). AIDS becomes an increasing epidemic in America.

1982 The nurse licensure examination changes to a comprehensive test developed by the National Council of State Boards of Nursing.

1985 Vernice Ferguson, an African-American nurse, is elected president of Sigma Theta Tau International.

1986 The Association of Black Nursing Faculty is founded by Dr. Sally Tucker Allen.

1989 *Promoting Health/Preventing Disease: Year 2000 Objectives for the Nation* is drafted and distributed for public review.

1990 Congress proclaims March 10 as Harriet Tubman Day in the United States, honoring her as a brave African-American freedom fighter and nurse during the Civil War. The Bloodborne Pathogen Standard is established by OSHA—all health care providers are required to use Universal Precautions for body substance isolation when caring for all patients. Computers enter most facets of the health care system. The largest number of nurses participate in the war effort: Operation Desert Shield/Desert Storm.

1991 *Healthy People 2000* is published.

1992 Eddie Bernice Johnson, an African-American nurse from Texas, is elected to the House of Representatives—the first nurse to be elected to Congress. The ANA Congress of Nursing Practice establishes nursing informatics as a distinct area of nursing practice. Hospitals downsize by reducing the number of full-time nurses. Home health nursing is rapidly increasing.

1993 The National Center for Nursing Research is upgraded to the National Institute of Nursing Research within the National Institutes of Health.

1994 Approximately 135 million Americans are enrolled in managed care plans (HMOs and PPOs). NCLEX-RN, a computerized nurse-licensing examination, is introduced.

1996 The Commission on Collegiate Nursing Education is established as an agency devoted exclusively to the accreditation of baccalaureate and graduate degree nursing programs.

Continued

BOX 1-1 *Important Events in the Evolution of Nursing—cont'd*

1997 Rhetaugh Dumas, an African-American nurse, is elected president of the NLN.

1999 The demand for advanced practice nurses increases. New drugs are on trial for the treatment of AIDS. Nursing assistants or unlicensed assistive personnel (UAPs) are used increasingly as nurse extenders. Distance learning becomes more popular in nursing education. Beverly Malone, the second African-American president of the ANA, is named Deputy Assistant Secretary for Health, Department of Health and Human Services, Office of Public Health and Science. The IOM releases its landmark report: "Too Err Is Human: Building a Safer Health System."

2000 M. Elizabeth Carnegie is inducted into the ANA Hall of Fame. The American Nurses Credentialing Center gives its first Psychiatric Mental Health Nurse Practitioner examination. *Healthy People 2010* is published. The National Council of State Boards of Nursing releases a new Test Plan, to begin in April 2001.

2000 AACN reports a faculty vacancy rate of 7.4% among the 220 nursing schools that responded to a survey. According to AACN, the average age of full-time faculty is over 50 years old; average age of doctorally prepared professors is 55.9.

2001 Beverly Malone is appointed General Secretary, Royal College of Nursing, London. Health Care Financing Administration (HCFA) becomes Centers for Medicare and Medicaid Services (CMS).

2002 Johnson and Johnson Health Care Systems, Inc. launches "The Future of Nursing," a national publicity campaign to address the nursing shortage.

2002 Winston-Salem State University School of Nursing becomes the first historically black university to offer a master of science degree in nursing in the state of North Carolina.

2002 To address the shortage of nurses, the U.S. Congress adopts the Nurse Reinvestment Act; President George W. Bush signs the bill into law in August.

2002 National Survey of Minority Nurses and follow-up pilot project provide wealth of data and insights to workplace barriers.

2002 Significant funding is obtained for Geriatric Nursing Initiative.

2003 To develop strategies to deal with current shortage of nurses, The American Nurses Foundation launches an "Invest in Nursing Campaign."

2003 *Online Journal of Nursing* reports 11 categories of clinical errors/clinical incidents: medications (1—not given/wrong time; 2—incorrect medications; 3—incorrect dose); treatment clinical errors (4—not given/wrong time; 5—incorrect administration; 6—incorrect treatment); untoward clinical incidents (7—fall, i.e., patient; 8—pressure ulcer, i.e., stage 2, 3, 4; 9—unplanned admission; 10—restraint, i.e., physical or chemical; 11—nurse injury on the job.)

2003 Medicare Prescription Drug Bill is passed in November. This is a controversial $400-billion plan that may put Medicare in competition with private insurance companies and HMOs.

2003 IOM report "Who Will Keep the Public Healthy?" examines the education of public health professionals. Recommends establishing partnerships between schools of public health and other academic disciplines, local and state health departments, and community organizations; calls for additional training; and suggests medical and nursing school curricula.

2003 IOM report "Keeping Patients Safe: Transforming the Work Environment of Nurses" is released.

2004 National Council of State Boards of Nursing raises the passing standard for NCLEX-RN in the interest of public safety.

Sources: Carnegie, 1995; Deloughery, 1998; Kalisch and Kalisch, 1995; Donahue, 1999; AACN Report, 2003; IOM Report, 2003.

PREHISTORIC PERIOD

Nursing in the prehistoric period was delineated by health practices that were strongly guided by beliefs of magic, religion, and superstition. Individuals who were ill were considered to be cursed by evil spirits and evil gods that entered the human body and caused suffering and death if not cast out. These beliefs dictated the behavior of primitive people, who sought to scare away the evil gods and spirits. Members of tribes participated in rituals, wore masks, and engaged in demonstrative dances to rid the sick of demonic possession of the body. Sacrifices and offerings, sometimes including human sacrifices, were made to rid the body of evil gods, demons, and spirits. Many tribes used special herbs, roots, and vegetables to cast out the "curse" of illness.

EARLY CIVILIZATION

Egypt

Ancient Egyptians are noted for their accomplishments in health care at an early period in civilization. They were the first to use the concept of suture in repairing wounds. They also were the first to be recorded as developing community planning that resulted in a decrease in public health problems. One of the main early public health problems was the spread of disease through contaminated water sources. Specific laws on cleanliness, food use and preservation, drinking, exercise, and sexual relations were developed. Health beliefs of Egyptians determined preventive measures taken and personal health behaviors practiced. These health behaviors were usually carried out to accommodate the gods. Some behaviors were also practiced expressly to appease the spirits of the dead (Ellis and Hartley, 2004). The Egyptians developed the calendar and writing, which initiated recorded history. The oldest records date back to the sixteenth century B.C. in Egypt. A pharmocopia that classified over 700 drugs was written to assist in the care and management of disease (Ellis and Hartley, 2004). As in the case of Shiphrah and Puah, the midwives who saved the baby Moses, nurses were used by kings and other aristocrats to deliver babies and care for the young, the elderly, and those who were sick. Other documentation regarding nurses in Egypt is scant.

Palestine

From 1400 to 1200 B.C. the Hebrews migrated from the Arabian Desert and gradually settled in Palestine, where they became an agricultural society. Under the leadership of Moses, the Hebrews developed a system of laws called the Mosaic Code. This code, one of the first organized methods of disease control and prevention, contained public health laws that dictated personal, family, and public hygiene. For instance, laws were written to prohibit the eating of animals that were dead longer than 3 days and to isolate individuals who were thought to have communicable diseases. Hebrew priests took on the role of health inspectors (Ellis and Hartley, 2004).

Greece

From 1500 to 100 B.C. Greek philosophers sought to understand man and his relationship with the gods, nature, and other men. They believed that the gods and goddesses of Greek mythology controlled health and illness. Temples built to honor Asclepius, the god of medicine, were designated to care for the sick. Asclepius carried a staff that was intertwined with serpents or snakes, representing wisdom and immortality. This staff is believed to be the model of today's medical caduceus. Hippocrates (460-362 B.C.), considered the "father of medicine," paved the way in establishing scientific knowledge in medicine. Hippocrates was the first to attribute disease to natural causes rather than supernatural causes and curses of the gods. Hippocrates' teachings also emphasized the patient-centered approach and use of the scientific method for solving problems (Ellis and Hartley, 2004).

India

Dating from 3000 to 1500 B.C., the earliest cultures of India were Hindu. The sacred book of Brahmanism (also known as Hinduism), the Vedas, was used to guide health care practices. The Vedas, considered by some to be the oldest written material, emphasized hygiene and prevention of sickness and described major and minor surgeries. The Indian practice of surgery was very well developed. The importance of prenatal care to both mother and infant was also well understood. Public hospitals were constructed from 274 to 236 B.C. and were staffed by male nurses with qualifications and duties similar to those of the twentieth-century practical nurse. In rare instances older women were allowed to assume a nursing role outside the home (Ellis and Hartley, 2004).

China

The teachings of the Chinese scholar Confucius (551-479 B.C.) had a powerful impact on the customs and practices of the people of ancient China. Confucius taught a moral philosophy that addressed one's obligation to society. Several hundred years after his death, Confucius' philosophy became the basis for Chinese education and government. Central to his teachings were service to the community and the value of the family as a unit.

The early Chinese also placed great value on solving life's problems. Their belief about health and illness was based on the yin and yang philosophy. The yin represented the feminine forces, which were considered negative and passive. The yang represented the masculine forces, which were positive and active. The Chinese believed that an imbalance between these two forces would result in illness, whereas balance between the yin and yang represented good health (Ellis and Hartley, 2004). The ancient Chinese used a variety of treatments believed to promote health and harmony, including acupuncture. Acupuncture involves insertion of hot and cold needles into the skin and underlying tissues to manage or cure conditions (such as pain, stroke, or breathing difficulty) and ultimately to affect the balance of yin and yang. Hydrotherapy, massage, and exercise were used as preventive health measures (Giger and Davidhizar, 1999). The Chinese also used drug therapy to manage disease conditions; they recorded more than 1000 drugs derived from animals, vegetables, and minerals (Walton, Barondess, and Locke, 1994). Many of the drugs used by the Chinese in ancient times such as ephedrine continue to be used today (Ellis and Hartley, 2004).

Rome

The Roman Empire (27 B.C.-476 A.D.), a military dictatorship, adapted medical practices from the countries they conquered and the physicians they enslaved. The first military hospital in Europe was established in Rome. The physicians were enslaved and forced to provide details about their medical practice. Both male and female attendants assisted in the care of the sick. Galen was a famous Greek physician who worked in Rome and made important contributions to the practice of medicine by expanding his knowledge in anatomy, physiology, pathology, and medical therapeutics (Walton, Barondess, and Locke, 1994).

THE MIDDLE AGES

The Middle Ages (476 B.C.-1450 A.D.) followed the demise of the Roman Empire (Walton, Barondess, and Locke, 1994). Women used herbs and new methods of healing, whereas men continued to use purging, leeching, and mercury. This period also saw the Roman Catholic Church become a central figure in the organization and management of health care. Most of the changes in health care were based on the Christian concepts of charity and the sanctity of human life. Wives of emperors and other women considered noble became nurses. These women devoted themselves to caring for the sick, often carrying a basket of food and medicine as they journeyed from house to house (Bahr and Johnson, 1995). Widowers and unmarried women became nuns and deaconesses. Two of these deaconesses, Dorcas and Phoebe, are mentioned in the Bible as outstanding for the care they provided to the sick (Freedman, 1995).

During the Middle Ages physicians spent most of their time translating medical essays; they actually provided little medical care. Poorly trained barbers, who lacked any formal medical education, performed surgery and medical treatments that were considered "bloody" or "messy." Nurses also provided some medical care, although in most hospitals and monasteries female nurses who were not midwives were forbidden to witness childbirth, help with gynecologic examinations, or even diaper male infants (Kalish and Kalish, 1986). In addition, these nurses were not permitted to have contact with male patients, administer enemas, or care for a man with a venereal disease. Female nurse midwives did, however, provide the bulk of obstetric care within the community (Ellis and Hartley, 2004).

During the Crusades, which lasted for almost 200 years from 1096 to 1291, military nursing orders known as templars and hospitalers were founded. Monks and Christian knights provided nursing care and also defended the hospitals during battle, wearing a suit of armor under their religious habits. The habits were distinguished by the Maltese cross to identify the monks and knights as Christian warriors. The same cross was used years later on a badge designed for the first school of nursing and became a forerunner for the design of nursing pins (Ellis and Hartley, 2004).

THE RENAISSANCE AND THE REFORMATION PERIOD

Following the Middle Ages came the Renaissance and the Reformation, also known as the rebirth of Europe (the fourteenth through the sixteenth centuries, A.D.). Major advancements were made in pharmacology, chemistry, and medical knowledge, including anatomy, physiology, and surgery. During the Renaissance new emphasis was given to medical education, but nursing education was practically nonexistent.

The Reformation was a religious movement that resulted in a dissension between Roman Catholics and Protestants. During this period, religious facilities that provided health care closed. Women were encouraged toward charitable services, but their main duties included bearing and caring for children in their homes. Furthermore, hospital work was no longer appealing to women of high economic status, and the individuals who worked as nurses in hospitals were often female prisoners, prostitutes, and drunks. Nursing was no longer the respected profession it had once been. This period is referred to as the "Dark Ages" of nursing (Ellis and Hartley, 2004).

During the sixteenth and seventeenth centuries, famine, plague, filth, and horrible crimes ravaged Europe. King Henry VII eliminated the organized monastic relief programs that aided the orphans, poor, and other displaced people. It became common to encounter homeless men, women, and children begging in the streets. Beggars were beaten, branded, and chained to the galleys of boats as punishment for their disgraceful behavior (Ellis and Hartley, 2004).

Out of great concern for social welfare, several nursing groups, such as the Order of the Visitation of St. Mary, St. Vincent de Paul, and the Sisters of Charity, were organized to give time, service, and money to the poor and sick. The Sisters of Charity recruited young women for training in nursing, developed educational programs, and cared for abandoned children.

In 1640 St. Vincent de Paul established The Hospital for the Foundling to care for the many orphaned and abandoned children (Ellis and Hartley, 2004).

THE COLONIAL AMERICAN PERIOD

The first hospital and the first medical school in North America were founded in Mexico—the Hospital of the Immaculate in Mexico City and the medical school at the University of Mexico. During this time in the American colonies, individuals with infectious diseases were isolated in almshouses or "pest houses" (Kalisch and Kalisch, 1986). Procedures such as purgatives and bleeding were widely used, leading to shortened life expectancy. Plagues such as yellow fever and smallpox caused thousands of deaths. Benjamin Franklin, who was outspoken regarding the care of the sick, insisted that a hospital be built in the colonies. He believed that the community should be responsible for the management and treatment of those who were ill. Through his efforts the first hospital, called The Pennsylvania Hospital, was built in the United States in Philadelphia in 1751 (Oermann, 1997).

FLORENCE NIGHTINGALE

Florence Nightingale was born in Florence, Italy, on May 12, 1820. The Nightingale family was wealthy, well traveled, and well educated. Nightingale was a highly intelligent, talented, and attractive woman. From an early age she demonstrated a deep concern for the poor and suffering. At the age of 25 she became interested in training as a nurse. However, her family were strongly opposed to this choice and preferred that she marry and take her place in society (Kelly and Joel, 1996). In 1851 her parents finally permitted her to pursue training as a nurse. Nightingale attended a 3-month nursing training program at the Institution of Deaconesses at Kaiserswerth, Germany. In 1854 she began training nurses at the Harley Street Nursing Home and also served as superintendent of nurses at King's College Hospital in London (Small, 1998).

The outbreak of the Crimean War marked a turning point in Nightingale's career. In October 1854 Sidney Herbert, British Secretary of War and an old friend of the Nightingale family, wrote to Nightingale and asked her to lead a group of nurses to the Crimea to work at one of the military hospitals under government authority and expense (Small, 1998). Nightingale accepted his offer and assembled 38 nurses who were sisters and nuns from various Catholic and Anglican orders (Kelly and Joel, 1996; Small, 1998).

Nightingale and her team were assigned to the Barracks Hospital at Scutari. The Barracks Hospital actually was a dilapidated, barnlike building that had been formerly used as artillery barracks. Thousands of cholera victims and hundreds of battle casualties were taken to Scutari. To get to the hospital from the front lines, the wounded and ill soldiers were put aboard hospital ships to cross the long and often tortuous Black Sea (Small, 1998).

When Nightingale arrived at the Barracks Hospital, she found deplorable conditions. Between 3000 and 4000 sick and wounded men were packed into the hospital, which was originally designed to accommodate 1700 patients. There were no beds, blankets, food, or medicine. Many of the wounded soldiers had been placed on the floor, where lice, maggots, vermin, rodents, and blood covered their bodies. There were no candles or lanterns. All medical care had to be rendered during the light of day (Small, 1998).

Despite the distressing conditions at the Barracks Hospital, the army doctors and surgeons at first refused Nightingale's assistance. However, within a week, faced with scurvy, starvation, dysentery, and the eruption of more fighting, the doctors, in desperation, called her to help.

Nightingale immediately purchased medical supplies, food, linen, and hospital equipment, using her own money and that of the Times Relief Fund. Within 10 days she had set up a kitchen for special diets and had rented a house that she converted into a laundry (Small, 1998). The wives of soldiers were hired to manage and operate the laundry service. She assigned soldiers to make repairs and clean up the building. Just weeks later she initiated social services, reading classes, and even coffeehouses, where soldiers could enjoy music and recreation (Small, 1998).

Nightingale worked long, hard hours to care for these soldiers. She spent up to 20 hours each day caring for wounds, comforting soldiers, assisting in surgery, directing staff, and keeping records. Nightingale introduced principles of asepsis and infection control, a system for transcribing doctor's orders, and a procedure to maintain patient records. By the end of the Crimean War, Nightingale had trained as many as 125 nurses to care for the wounded and ill soldiers (Small, 1998).

Nightingale is credited with using public health principles and statistical methods to advocate for improved health conditions for British soldiers. Through carefully recorded statistics, Nightingale was able to document that the soldiers' death rate decreased from 42% to 2% as a result of health care reforms that emphasized sanitary conditions. Because of her remarkable work in using statistics to demonstrate cause and effect and improve the health of British soldiers, Nightingale is recognized for her contributions to nursing research (Nies and McEwen, 2001).

Nightingale also demonstrated the power of political activism to effect health care reform by writing letters of criticism accompanied by constructive recommendations to British army leaders. Nightingale's ability to overthrow the British army management method that had allowed the deplorable conditions to exist in the army hospitals was considered one of her greatest achievements (Nies and McEwen, 2001).

In 1855, after visiting the front lines and hospitals in Balaclava, Nightingale contracted "Crimean Fever" and was taken to the Castle Hospital. There she received intensive care from the doctors and nurses she trained. She remained in poor condition for several weeks. Soldiers wept when they heard of her illness and near death. She eventually recovered, but the illness had taken a heavy toll on her overall health.

In 1860 Nightingale established the first nursing school in England. By 1873 graduates of Nightingale's nurse training program in England migrated to the United States, where they became supervisors in the first of the hospital-based (diploma) nursing schools: Massachusetts General Hospital in Boston, Bellevue Hospital in New York, and the New Haven Hospital in Connecticut.

Florence Nightingale's work, from the Crimean War to the establishment of formal nursing education programs, was a catapult for the reorganization and advancement of professional nursing. Until her death in August 1910 Nightingale demonstrated the powerful impact that well-educated, creative, skilled, and competent individuals have in the provision of health care. She is honored as the founder of professional nursing (Small, 1998).

MARY SEACOLE

Mary Seacole was a Jamaican nurse who learned the art of caring and healing from her mother. In her native land of Jamaica, British West Indies, she was nicknamed "Doctress" because of her administration of care to the sick in a lodging house in Kingston (Carnegie, 1995). Seacole learned of the Crimean War and wrote to the British government requesting to join Nightingale's group of nurses. However, she was denied the right to join because she was black. She was confused about this denial because many of the British soldiers had lived in Jamaica, where she had already provided health care to them.

Seacole had previously served as a nurse in Cuba and Panama during the yellow fever and cholera epidemics. She had also conducted forensic studies on an infant who died of cholera in Panama. She felt that her experience would be valuable in treating disease in the Crimean War, and she sailed to England at her own expense. She provided a letter of introduction to Nightingale, which was blocked because Seacole was black, even though she had been trained by British army doctors (Carnegie, 1995).

After several efforts to join Nightingale's group failed, Seacole, who was not a woman of wealth, purchased her own supplies and traveled over 3000 miles to the Crimea, where she built and opened a lodging house. On the bottom floor of the house was a restaurant, and on the top floor an area was arranged like a hospital to nurse sick soldiers (Carnegie, 1995).

When Seacole finally met Nightingale, the response was still the same: "no vacancies" (Carnegie, 1995). However, being denied enlistment did not deter Seacole; she remained faithful and nursed the sick throughout the Crimean War. Her efforts did not go unnoticed by the English people. Long after the war was over, the British government finally honored Seacole with a medal in recognition of her efforts and the services she provided to the sick and injured soldiers.

NURSING IN THE UNITED STATES
The Civil War Period

During the U.S. Civil War, or the War Between the States (1861 to 1865), health care conditions in the United States were similar to those encountered by Nightingale and Seacole. Numerous epidemics plagued the country, including syphilis, gonorrhea, malaria, smallpox, and typhoid (Nelson, 2001; Oermann, 1997).

The Civil War was initiated by the attack on Fort Sumter, South Carolina, April 17, 1861. At this time there were no nurses formally trained to care for the sick. However, thousands of men and women from the South and North volunteered to care for the wounded. Hospitals were set up in the field, and transports were put in place to carry the wounded to the hospitals (Carnegie, 1995).

The Secretary of War, Simon Cameron, appointed a schoolteacher named Dorothea Lynde Dix to organize military hospitals and provide medical supplies to the Union army soldiers. Dix received no official status and no salary for this position.

Nurses served during the Civil War under primitive working conditions. Maintaining sanitary conditions was often not possible. More than six million patients were admitted to hospitals, with approximately a half million surgical cases. Unfortunately, there were only about 2000 individuals who served as nurses, far less than the number needed to provide adequate care (Fitzpatrick, 1997; Kalisch and Kalisch, 1995). According to records kept at three hospitals, 181 African-American nurses, both men and women, served between July 16, 1863, and June 14, 1864. Caucasian nurses were paid $12 per month; African-American nurses received $10 per month (Carnegie, 1995). Three African-American nurses made particularly important contributions to nursing efforts during the Civil War: Harriet Tubman, Sojourner Truth, and Susie King Taylor.

Harriet Tubman cared for the sick as a nurse in the Sea Islands off the coast of South Carolina and was later known as the "Conductor of the Underground Railroad." It is also reported that she was the first woman to lead American troops into battle (Carnegie, 1995).

Sojourner Truth, known for her abolitionist efforts as well as her nursing efforts, was an advocate of clean and sanitary conditions for patients so they could heal. Susie King Taylor, although hired to work in the laundry, served as a nurse because of the growing number of wounded who needed care. Having learned to read and write, which was against the law for African-Americans at the time, she also taught many of her comrades in Company E to read and write (Carnegie, 1995).

Many other volunteer nurses made important contributions during the Civil War. Clara Barton served on the front line during the Civil War and operated a war relief program to provide supplies to the battlefields and hospitals. Barton also set up a postwar service to find missing soldiers and is credited with founding the American Red Cross (Nelson, 2001; Oermann, 1997). Louisa May Alcott, who served as a nurse for 6 weeks until stopped by ill health, authored detailed accounts of the experiences encountered by nurses during the war for a newspaper publication entitled *Hospital Sketches* (Kalisch and Kalisch, 1995).

When the Civil War ended, the number of nurse training schools increased. These early nursing programs offered little or no classroom education, and on-the-job training occurred in the hospital wards. The students learned routine patient care duties, worked long hours 6 days a week, and were used as supplemental hospital staff. After graduation most of the nurses practiced as private duty nurses or hospital staff (Lindeman and McAthie, 1990). The first nursing textbook, entitled *A Manual of Nursing*, was published in 1876 and was used by the New York Training School for Nurses at Bellevue Hospital (Kalisch and Kalisch, 1995).

During the 1890s the nationwide establishment of African-American hospitals and nursing schools gained momentum as African-American musicians, educators, and community leaders became alarmed at the high rates of African-American morbidity and mortality. Because of segregation and discrimination, African-Americans had to establish their own health care institutions to provide African-American patients with access to quality health care and to provide African-American men and women with opportunities to enter the nursing profession. In 1886 John D. Rockefeller funded the establishment of the first school of nursing for African-American women at the Atlanta Baptist Seminary—now known as Spelman College (Jones, 2004; Salzman, Smith, and West, 1996).

1900 to World War I

In the 1900s states began to require nurses to become registered before entering practice. By 1910 most states had upgraded education requirements to high school, upgraded training, and required registration before practice (Deloughery, 1991; Donahue, 1999).

Lillian Wald, a pioneer in public health nursing, is best known for the development and establishment of a viable practice for public health nurses in the twentieth century. The main location for this practice was the Henry Street Settlement House, located in the Lower East Side of New York City. Its purpose was to provide well-baby care, health education, disease prevention, and treatment of patients with minor illnesses. Nursing practice based at the Henry Street Settlement House formed the basis of public health nursing for the entire country. Instead of relying on patients visiting the clinic, public health nurses made their way to the various tenements located around Henry Street (Snodgrass, 1999; Stanhope and Lancaster, 2004).

Lillian Wald also developed the first nursing service for occupational health. She believed that prevention of disease among workers would improve productivity and was able to convince the Metropolitan Life Insurance Company that her ideas had merit. As a result, nursing agencies such as those in place at the Henry Street Settlement House provided skilled nursing services to employees. Another innovation that emerged from this program was the sliding fee scale, by which patients were billed according to their income or their ability to pay. This innovative nursing service existed for 44 years before it was dissolved by the Metropolitan Life Insurance Company (Stanhope and Lancaster, 2004).

In 1911 Wald chaired a committee formed by members of the Associated Alumnae of Training Schools for Nurses, later to become the American Nurses Association (ANA), and the Society of Superintendents of Training Schools for Nurses, the precursor of the National League for Nursing (NLN). The purpose of the committee was to develop standards for nursing services performed outside of the hospital environment. The committee determined that a new organization was necessary to meet the needs of community health nurses. The result of the committee's recommendation was the formation of the National Organization for Public Health Nursing, whose goals were to establish educational and practice standards for community health nursing (Stanhope and Lancaster, 2004).

The ANA and the NLN are still leading nursing organizations today. The ANA has focused primarily on professional aspects of nursing, and the NLN was the only accrediting body for nursing schools until 1996, when the Commission for Collegiate Nursing Education (CCNE), an autonomous arm of the American Association of Colleges of Nursing (AACN), was established as an agency devoted exclusively to the accreditation of baccalaureate and graduate degree nursing programs (Stanhope and Lancaster, 2004).

World War I and the 1920s

During the early 1900s the world was rapidly changing—and moving toward global conflict. Germany was arming, and the rest of Europe was trying to ignore the threat. "Prosperous" was the word used to describe the U.S. economy. Women were granted the right to vote and were moving into the work force on a regular basis.

Advancements in medical care and public health were being made. The primary site for medical care moved from the home to the hospital, and surgical and diagnostic techniques were improved. Pneumonia management was the focus of scientific study. Insulin was discovered in 1922, and in 1928 Alexander Fleming discovered the precursor of penicillin, which would eventually be used to successfully treat patients with pneumonia and other infections (Kalisch and Kalisch, 1995) (Box 1-2).

Environmental conditions improved, and the serious epidemics of the previous century became nonexistent. Lillian Wald, in *The House on Henry Street,* linked poor environmental and social conditions to prevalent illnesses and poverty and used this information to lead the fight for better sanitation and housing conditions (Stanhope and Lancaster, 2004).

With the outbreak of World War I in 1914, nurses were desperately needed to care for the soldiers who were injured or who suffered from the many illnesses that were a result of trench warfare (Stanhope and Lancaster, 2004). The war offered nurses a chance to advance into new fields of specialization. For example, nurse anesthetists made their first appearance as part of the surgical teams at the front lines. More than 20,000 U.S.-trained nurses served in WWI (Oermann, 1997).

Because many nurses volunteered to provide services during the war, the community health nursing movement in the United States stalled. However, the American Red Cross, founded by Clara Barton in 1882, assisted in efforts to continue public health nursing. The Red Cross nurses originally focused on the rural communities that were not able to access health care services. As the war continued, however, the Red Cross nurses also moved into urban areas to provide health care services (Glass and Murphy, 2002).

BOX 1–2 *Duties of the Hospital Floor Nurse in 1887*

In addition to caring for your 60 patients, each nurse will follow these regulations:

1. Daily sweep and mop the floors of your ward, dust the patient's furniture and windowsill.
2. Maintain an even temperature on your ward by bringing in a scuttle of coal for the day's business.
3. Light is important to observe the patient's condition; therefore, each day fill kerosene lamps, clean chimneys, and trim wicks. Wash the windows once a week.
4. The nurse's notes are important in aiding the physician's work. Make your pens carefully; you may whittle nibs to your individual taste.
5. Each nurse on day duty will report every day at 7 a.m. and will leave at 8 p.m. except on Sabbath, on which day you will be off from 12 noon to 2 p.m.
6. Graduate nurses in good standing with the Director of Nurses will be given an evening off each week if you regularly attend church.
7. Each nurse should lay aside from each payday a good sum of her earning for her benefits during her declining years, so that she will not become a burden. For example, if you earn $20 a month, you should set aside $10.
8. Any nurse who smokes, uses liquor in any form, gets her hair done at a beauty shop, or frequents dance halls will have given the Director of Nurses good reason to suspect her worth, intentions, integrity.
9. The nurse who performs her labors, serves her patients and doctors faithfully and without fault for a period of five years will be given an increase by the hospital administration of five cents per day, providing there are no hospital debts that are outstanding.

From Lois Turley © 1981-2004. Used by permission. All rights reserved. From CareNurse.com.

During WWI the U.S. Public Health Service, founded in 1798 to provide health care services to merchant seamen, was charged with the responsibility to provide health services at the military posts located within the United States. A nurse, "loaned" by The National Organization for Public Health Nursing, established nursing services at U.S. military outposts. The responsibilities of the U.S. Public Health Service continued to grow; eventually it was composed of physicians, nurses, and other allied health professionals, who provided indigent care and practiced in community health programs (Stanhope and Lancaster, 2004).

Further changes were in store for nursing during WWI. In 1918 the Vassar Camp School for Nurses was established. Its purpose was to provide an intensive, 2-year nurses training program for college graduates. Graduates of the program were given an army reserve commission and would be activated during times of war to meet increased nursing needs. Sponsored by the American Red Cross and the Council of National Defense, the school graduated 435 nurses. The Vassar Camp School for Nurses was a short-lived enterprise. When peace was declared in 1919, the program was permanently disbanded (Snodgrass, 1999; Stanhope and Lancaster, 2004).

In 1921 the federal government recognized the need to improve the health of women and children and passed the Sheppard-Towner Act, one of the first pieces of federal legislation passed to provide funds to assist in the care of special populations (Oermann, 1997). This funding provided public health nurses with resources to promote the health and well-being of women, infants, and children.

Following these improvements, the Frontier Nursing Service (FNS) was established in 1925 by Mary Breckenridge of Kentucky. Born into a wealthy family, Breckenridge learned the value of providing care to others from her grandmother. Breckenridge began her career in New York's St. Luke's Hospital School of Nursing. After serving as a nurse during WWI, she returned to Columbia University to learn more about community health nursing. Armed with her new knowledge and a passion to assist disadvantaged women and children, Breckenridge returned to Kentucky and the rural Appalachian Mountains (Oermann, 1997; Stanhope and Lancaster, 2004).

Breckenridge believed that the rural mountain area of Kentucky, cut off from many modern conveniences, was an excellent place to prove the value of community health nursing. She established the FNS in a five-room cabin in Hyden, Kentucky. After overcoming serious obstacles, such as no water supply or sewage disposal, six other nursing outposts were constructed in the rural mountains from 1927 to 1930. The FNS based its hospital in Hyden and eventually attracted physicians and nurses to provide medical, dental, surgical, nursing, and midwifery services to the rural poor. Financial support for the FNS ranged from fees for labor and supplies to funds raised through annual family dues to donations and fundraising efforts. Nurses working for the FNS traveled a 700-square mile area, often on horseback, to provide services to approximately 10,000 patients (Oermann, 1997).

Breckenridge established an important health care service for rural Kentucky communities. Equally important was her documentation of the results of community health nursing in rural communities. Breckenridge followed the advice of a consulting physician and collected mortality data on the communities before nursing services actually were started. The results were startling, mortality was significantly reduced and the need for the nursing services was clearly documented. Breckenridge proved that even in appalling environmental conditions without heat, electricity, or running water, nursing services could make a substantial positive impact on the health of the community (Stanhope and Lancaster, 2004). The FNS is still in operation today and provides vital service to the rural communities of Kentucky.

The Great Depression (1930 to 1940)

The U.S. economy prospered during WWI and well into the 1920s. However, after the stock market crash in October 1929 economic prosperity quickly dissipated. Millions of men and women became unemployed. Before the depression many people had private duty nurses. However, during the depression, many nurses found themselves unemployed because most families could no longer afford private duty nurses.

Franklin D. Roosevelt, elected President of the United States in 1932, faced a country in shambles. He responded with several innovative and necessary interventions and ushered in the first major social legislation that had been enacted in U.S. history. Entitled the "New Deal," the legislation had several social components that affected the provision of medical care and other services for indigent people across the country (Connelly, 2004; Karger and Stoesz, 1994).

The piece of legislation that had the greatest impact on health care in the United States was the Social Security Act of 1935, which set the precedent for the passage of the Medicare and Medicaid Acts that followed in 1965. The main purposes of the 1935 Social Security Act were to provide (1) a national old-age insurance system; (2) federal grants to states for maternal and child welfare services; (3) vocational rehabilitation services for the handicapped; (4) medical care for crippled children and blind people; (5) a plan to strengthen public health services; and (6) a federal-state unemployment system (Karger and Stoesz, 1994).

The passage of the 1935 Social Security Act provided avenues for nursing care, and nursing jobs were created. With funds from the Social Security Act, public health nursing became the major source of health care for dependent mothers and children, the blind, and crippled children. Nurses found employment as public health nurses for county or state health departments (Connelly, 2004). Hospital job opportunities also were created for nurses, and the hospital became the usual employment setting for graduate nurses.

World War II (1940 to 1945)

The United States officially entered World War II after the bombing of Pearl Harbor in December 1941. At that time the nursing divisions of all of the military branches had inadequate numbers of nurses. Congress passed legislation to provide needed funds to expand nursing education. A committee of six national nursing organizations, called the National Nursing Council, received a million dollars to accomplish the needed expansion. The U.S. Public Health Service became the administrator of the funds, which further strengthened the tie between the U.S. Public Health Service and nursing (Sarnecky, 2001; Stanhope and Lancaster, 2004).

The war was considered a global conflict, and nursing became an essential part of the military advance. Nurses were required to function under combat conditions and had to adapt nursing care to meet the challenges of different climates, facilities, and supplies. As a result of their service during WWII, nurses finally were recognized as an integral part of the military and attained the ranks of officers in the army and navy. Colonel Julie O. Flikke was the first army nurse to be promoted to colonel in the U.S. Army and served as superintendent of the Army Nurse Corps from 1937 to 1942 (Deloughery, 1991; Robinson and Perry, 2001).

Post–World War II Period (1945 to 1950)

The period after WWII was a time of prosperity for the average American. The GI Bill enabled returning veterans to complete their interrupted education. The unemployment rate dropped to an all-time low in the United States. In an effort to provide more areas of employment for the returning men, the government mounted a massive campaign to encourage women to return to the more traditional roles of wife and mother. Consequently, numerous women in all professions, including nursing, chose to return to marriage and childrearing rather than continue employment outside the home.

After WWII, Communism demonstrated its strength more than ever before as the Soviet Union began invading and taking over Eastern European countries. With support from China, the North Koreans made a grab for South Korea, resulting in the Korean War. Again, nurses volunteered for the armed services to provide care to patients near the battlefields in Korea. This time, they worked in Medical Army Surgical Units, better known as MASH units, where medical and surgical techniques were further refined.

The two decades after WWII saw the emergence of nursing as a true profession. Minimal national standards for nursing education were established by the National Nursing Accrediting service. In 1945 State Boards of Nurse Examiners in 25 states adopted the State Board Test Pool. By 1950 all state boards were participating in the Test Pool; they continue to do so today. Nursing continued to improve the quality and quantity of educational programs as the number of nursing baccalaureate programs grew and associate degree programs developed in community or junior colleges (Kalisch and Kalisch, 1995; Robinson and Perry, 2001) (Box 1-3).

The end of WWII and the early 1950s marked the beginning of significant federal intervention in health care. The Nurse Training Act of 1943 was the first instance of federal funding being used to support nurse training. The passage of the Hill-Burton Act, or the Hospital Survey and Construction Act of 1946, marked the largest commitment of federal dollars to health care in the country's history. The purpose of the act was to provide funding to construct hospitals and to assist states in planning for other health care facilities based on the needs of the communities. Nearly 40% of the hospitals constructed in the late 1940s and the early 1950s were built with Hill-Burton funds. The hospital construction boom created by the

BOX 1-3 *Qualities of Good Nurses During Post World War II*

1. Tidy and loyal to the hospital and its personnel
2. Compliant with the orders of the doctors and directives of nursing management
3. Always busy
4. If census was low, fold laundry, clean shelves, prepare supplies to be sterilized
5. Ability to get work done no matter how many patients assigned

From Martell LK: Maternity care during the post World War II baby boom: the experience of general duty nurses, *West J Nurs Res* 96(3):387-391, 1999.

Hill-Burton Act led to an increased demand for professional nurses to provide care in hospitals (Connelly, 2004; Williams and Torrens, 1993).

It was also in the early 1950s that the National Association of Colored Graduate Nurses (NACGN) went out of existence. This was the organization that fought for integration of the African-American nurse into the ANA. From 1916 to 1948, African-American nurses in the South were barred from membership in the ANA because of segregation laws in the Southern states. In the 1940s the NACGN began to wage an all-out war against discrimination by the Southern constituents of the ANA. The NACGN chose as its central issue the route to membership in ANA. This issue was raised by the NACGN on the floor at every national convention of the ANA, and it evoked strong opposition from the Southern state constituents. Speaking from the floor of the House of Delegates at the 1946 convention in Atlantic City, a Caucasian nurse from Georgia referred to African-American nurses as "our darkies." Immediately a motion was passed to strike the reference from the record. However, this comment caused an uproar, and the African-American nurses who were barred from membership in the Southern states started the wheels turning to bypass the states and join ANA directly. This arrangement, known as individual membership, was put into effect in 1948. With the establishment of individual membership, African-American nurses in the South could bypass their states and become members of the ANA. This type of individual membership continued until all barriers had been dropped in the early 1960s (Carnegie, 1995).

Nursing in the 1960s

Federal legislation enacted during the 1960s had a major and lasting effect on nursing and health care. The Community Mental Health Centers Act of 1963 provided funds for the construction of community outpatient mental health centers; opportunities for mental health nursing were expanded when funds to staff these centers were appropriated in 1965 with the passage of the Medicare and Medicaid Acts (Boschma, 2003). Medicaid, Title XIX of the Social Security Act, was enacted and replaced all programs previously instituted for medical assistance. The purpose of the Medicaid program, which was jointly sponsored and financed with matching funds from federal and state governments, was to serve as medical insurance for those families, primarily women and children, with an income at or below the federal poverty level. Medicaid quickly became "the largest public assistance program in the nation, covering about 9.7% of the population, including more than 15% of all children" (Baer et al, 2001).

Health departments employed public health nurses to provide the bulk of the care needed by children and pregnant women in the Medicaid population. Services provided by these nurses included family planning, well-child assessments, immunizations, and prenatal care. A physician assigned as the district health officer supervised the nurses. Without the public health nurses and local health departments, many women and children in the inner city areas and rural communities would have been without access to basic health care.

Another important amendment to the Social Security Act was Title XVIII, or Medicare, passed in 1965. The Medicare program provides hospital insurance, Part A, and medical insurance, Part B, to all people age 65 and older who are eligible to receive social security benefits; people with total, permanent disabilities; and people with end-stage renal disease. As a result of Medicare reimbursement, many hospitals began catering to physicians who treated Medicare patients. Medicare patients were attractive to the hospitals because all hospital charges, regardless of amount or appropriateness of services, were reimbursed through the Medicare program (Connelly, 2004; Glass and Murphy, 2002).

As a result of Medicare reimbursement, hospital-bed occupancy increased, which led to increased numbers of nurses needed to staff the hospital. Nursing embraced the hospital setting as the usual practice area and moved away from the community as the preferred practice site. Nursing schools also followed the trend by reducing the number of curriculum hours devoted to community health and concentrated their efforts on hospital-based nursing (Stanhope and Lancaster, 2004).

Another outcome of the Medicare legislation was the home health movement. To receive Medicare reimbursement for home health services, patients had to have (1) home-bound status; (2) a need for part-time or intermittent, skilled nursing care; (3) a medically reasonably and necessary need for treatment; and (4) a plan of care authorized by a physician. Home health agencies were established and began to employ increasing numbers of nurses. The number of home health agencies began to grow in the mid-1960s; and, as a result of Medicare reimbursement and other influences including a growing elderly population, advances in medical technology, and public demand for increased access to health care, the home health industry continued unprecedented growth into the 1990s. Home health was one of the first employment settings that provided nurses the opportunity to work weekdays only.

Nursing in the 1970s

The women's movement of the 1970s greatly influenced nursing. Nurses began to focus not only on providing quality care to patients but also on enhancing the economic benefits of the profession. Hospitals were receiving significant reimbursements for patient care; however, nurses' salaries did not reflect an adequate percentage of that reimbursement. Health care costs soared. This increase in health care costs built the framework for mandated changes in reimbursement. Nursing practice and the educational focus remained in the hospital setting.

During this time nurses played a major role in providing health care to communities and were instrumental in developing hospice programs, birthing centers, and day care centers for the elderly (Buhler-Wilkerson, 2001). Although basic educational programs for nurse practitioners expanded during the 1970s and master's level preparation was developed as the requirement for graduation and practice, certification was also required to practice as a nurse practitioner. Before this time, only certification was required. State Nursing Practice Acts were amended to provide for monitoring and licensing advanced practice nurses.

In 1974 the ANA conducted research in the area of ethnic minorities and submitted a proposal to the National Institute of Mental Health to fund a project to permit minority nurses—African-Americans, Hispanics, Asians, and American Indians—to earn PhDs. Of the graduates of the project, the vast majority serve on faculties of universities and are conducting research on factors in mental health and illness related to ethnicity and cross-cultural conflict, thereby fulfilling their commitment to advance the cause of quality health care for all people of color.

Despite past laxity, the ANA House of Delegates, at its 1972 convention, did pass an affirmative action resolution calling for a task force to develop and implement a program to correct inequities. The House also provided for the position of an ombudsman to evaluate involvement of minorities in leadership roles within the organization and to treat complaints by applicants for membership or by members of the Association who had been discriminated against because of nationality, race, creed, lifestyle, color, age, or sex. It was also in the 1970s that the ANA elected its first African-American president, Barbara Nichols, who served two terms.

Within the structure of many professional organizations is a unit referred to as an *academy,* which is composed of a cadre of scholars who deal with issues that concern the profession and take positions in the name of the Academy. The American Academy of Nursing (AAN) was created by the ANA Board in 1973. An elected group of highly accomplished leaders across all sectors of nursing (education, research, and practice) use the credential FAAN (Fellow, American Academy of Nursing). Through the application of visionary leadership, the intent of the AAN is to transform health care policy through nursing knowledge to optimize the well-being of the American people.

At its convention in Atlantic City in 1976, the ANA launched its Hall of Fame to pay tribute to those nurses who not only had paved the way for others to follow but also had made outstanding contributions to the profession.

Nursing in the 1980s

The types of patients needing health care changed in the 1980s. Homelessness became a common problem in large cities. Unstable economic developments contributed to an increase in indigent populations (Baer et al, 2001). Acquired immune deficiency syndrome (AIDS) emerged as a frightening, fatal epidemic.

Runaway health care costs became a national issue in the 1980s. Medicare was still reimbursing for any and all hospital services provided to recipients. From 1966 to 1981 the federal contribution to hospital care rose from 13% to 41% (Baer et al, 2001). In 1983 in an attempt to restrain hospital costs, Congress passed the diagnosis-related group system for reimbursement, better known as the DRG system.

Before 1983 Medicare payments were made to the hospital after the patient received services. Although there were restrictions, the entire bill generally was paid without question. DRGs were implemented to provide prospective payment for hospital services based on the patient's admitting diagnosis and thereby to reduce the overall cost to Medicare. Hospitals now were to be reimbursed one amount based on the patient's diagnosis, not on hospital charges. The system was developed by physicians at the Yale–New Haven Hospital and addressed approximately 468 diagnoses classified according to length of stay and cost of procedures associated with the diagnosis (Nies and McEwen, 2001).

As a result of the DRG reimbursement system, hospitals were forced to increase efficiency and more closely manage hospital services, including the patient's length of stay, laboratory and radiographic testing, and diagnostic procedures. Case management and critical pathways were developed to more efficiently manage patient care, and case management became a new area of specialization for the professional nurse.

Despite the high cost of health care, medicine prospered. Medical care advanced in areas such as organ transplantation, resuscitation and support of premature infants, and critical care techniques. Physician specialization and advances in medical technology flourished. Medical specialties such as nephrology, cardiology, endocrinology, orthopedics, neurosurgery, cardiovascular surgery, and advanced practices for obstetrics all led to improved health care services—and costs—in the hospital setting. The advanced technology also led to the development of outpatient surgery units.

Outpatient surgery services blossomed and provided a quick and efficient site for surgery that did not require extended hospital stays. Costs were greatly reduced because of fewer staff members needed for coverage, fewer supplies, and reduced facility costs. Nurses were interested in employment opportunities in outpatient facilities because they afforded a chance to work only during the day with no weekend assignments.

As the concern over increasing health care costs heightened, use of ambulatory services increased and enrollment in health maintenance organizations grew. Advanced nurse practitioners increased in popularity as cost-effective providers of primary and preventive health care. A growing number of nurses moved from the hospital setting into the community to practice in programs such as hospice and home health. Consumers began to demand bans on unhealthy activities, such as smoking in public. Health education became more important as consumers were encouraged to take responsibility for their own care (Stanhope and Lancaster, 2004). Even the terminology changed; the individual once known as the *patient* became known as the *client* or *consumer* and was afforded respect as a person who purchases a service.

Public health programs struggled to survive as counties and states cut health department budgets. A landmark study conducted by the Institute of Medicine (IOM) in 1988, entitled *The Future of Public Health,* indicated a dismal picture for public health. The study determined that public health had moved away from its traditional role and core functions and that no strategy was in place to bring public health back to its original purpose (Stanhope and Lancaster, 2004). Inadequate funding for public health continues to be a problem; however, it is hoped that in the near future public health will be restored to its original function and purpose.

Nursing enrollments dropped drastically in the late 1980s. This drop in enrollment occurred as the complexity of health care was rapidly increasing and more nurses were assuming expanded roles. As a result of these trends, a serious national shortage of nurses occurred across all settings (Ellis and Hartley, 2004).

Toward the end of the 1980s the American Medical Association announced its answer to the nursing shortage. It proposed to establish a 9-month program to prepare Registered Care Technologists. This proposal incensed nurses who unified to fight against it. As a result, the proposal was rejected (Schorr and Kennedy, 1999).

Also in the late 1980s several nursing scholars suggested that nursing research be firmly focused on the substantive information required to guide practice, rather than on philosophic and methodologic dilemmas of scientific inquiry. In 1985, the creation of the National Center for Nursing Research at the National Institutes of Health brought with it an increase in federal resources for nursing research and research training (Baer et al, 2001; Hinshaw, 1999).

Nursing in the 1990s

The 1990s began with alarm over the state of the U.S. economy. Government statisticians reported an alarming increase in the national debt complicated by slow economic growth. In the early 1990s average household incomes were stagnating. More women with families entered the workforce to afford the increasing cost of living. More nurses selected jobs in which they could work more hours in fewer days for more money, sometimes sacrificing the fringe benefits, allowing them to work a second job or earn higher pay through shift differential for working evening and night shifts. Creative shifts such as the 10-hour day/4-day work week or the 12-hour day/3-day work week became commonplace in health care facilities. Just as in the 1980s, the cost of health care continued to increase with the technologic advancements in medical care.

There also were growing concerns in the 1990s about the health of the nation, which prompted the Healthy People 2000 initiative. Many diseases associated with preventable causes characterized mortality in the United States. In 1990 more than two million U.S. residents died from diseases such as heart disease, cancer, cerebral vascular disease, accidents, chronic obstructive pulmonary disease, liver cirrhosis, tuberculosis, and human immunodeficiency virus infection. Factors contributing to these common disease states relate to lifestyle patterns, behaviors, and habits (modifiable risk factors). More youth were at risk because of behavior such as smoking cigarettes, using abusive drug substances, eating poorly balanced diets, failing to exercise, having sex with multiple partners, and being subjected to acts of violence. *Healthy People 2000: National Health Promotion and Disease Prevention Objectives* was published in 1991 by the U.S. Department of Health and Human Services as a nationwide effort to help states, cities, and communities identify health promotion and disease prevention strategies to address these health risk problems.

The AIDS epidemic radically changed the process for infection control among health care workers in health care institutions across the nation. Recapping needles, wearing latex gloves, and using isolation precautions were issues that triggered much dialog and debate among health care workers. Health care workers were mandated to use preventive measures in the form of Universal Precautions; all contact with blood and body fluids from all patients was considered potentially infectious.

Exposure to hazardous materials became a major issue of concern not only for health care workers but also for the general public. Chemical and radioactive substances that created dangerous exposure and health risks were increasingly used in the workplace. Employers were held legally accountable for informing their employees of the actual or potential hazards and for reducing their exposure risk through training and the use of protective equipment. The hazardous materials issue was especially important in nursing and medicine, particularly with regard to exposure to carcinogenic chemicals used in drug therapy and in environmental infection control.

In 1990 the increasing costs of Medicaid and Medicare triggered political action for health care reform. Findings of a federal commission appointed to evaluate the American health care system included the following (Connelly, 2004; Kalisch and Kalisch, 1995):

- Fifteen percent of the gross national product was related to health care expenditures (this amounts to approximately 1 trillion dollars annually).
- The United States spent more than twice as much as any industrialized nation for health care services.
- Americans were living longer, which indicated a growing demand for home health and nursing home care, as well as increased Medicare expenditures.

It became apparent that, if health care spending continued to increase, the U.S. economy would be in danger of collapse. Thus the health care system moved toward managed care in an attempt to control health care expenditures. The managed care movement has had a tremendous impact on nursing.

The focus of managed care was on providing more preventive and primary care, using outpatient and home settings when possible, and limiting expensive hospitalizations.

Massive downsizing of hospital nursing staff occurred, with an increased use of unlicensed assistive personnel to provide care in hospitals. There was an increasing demand for community health nurses and advanced practice nurses to provide primary care services. The nurse of the 1990s had to be focused on delivering health care services that (1) encompassed health risk assessment based on family and environmental factors, (2) supported health promotion and disease prevention, and (3) advanced counseling and health education (Jones, 2004).

In June 1993 the National Center for Nursing Research was renamed the National Institute of Nursing Research. Moving nursing research into the National Institutes of Health enhanced the interdisciplinary possibilities for collaborative investigation. As a result, nursing research grew rapidly during the 1990s. Multiple research programs focused on important health issues such as health promotion across the life span. Nursing research began to inform health care policy through federal commissions and agency programs (Hinshaw, 1999; Jones, 2004).

In the 1990s a partnership was forged between mandatory state licensure authorities, which set practice standards at the level of entering associate degree graduates, and national, nongovernmental bodies that certify graduate-prepared specialists. These national certifying agencies were intensely engaged in improving methods for determining the continuous competence of certified nurse practitioners within the swift current of health care change. The consumer's voice in the partnership was heard via collaboration with advocacy organizations and the appointment of more public members to licensing, certifying, and accreditation boards. Voluntary credentialing bodies recognized that, if they were to serve effectively, they had to engage in active public information campaigns to inform consumers about their health care choices (Buhler-Wilkerson, 2001).

Nursing in the Twenty-First Century

Professional nurses in the twenty-first century are faced with many challenges within the dynamic state of health care. In addition to the issues of access, cost, quality, and accountability in health care, nurses today are challenged by an aging population, complex consumer health values, and an increasingly intercultural society. Nurses have identified numerous areas of concern, including insufficient staffing, inadequate salaries, effects of stress and overwork, lack of participation in decision-making, and dissatisfaction with the quality of their own nursing care.

A survey conducted from October 2002 through December 2002 involving 1386 registered nurses and focused on the subject of clinical errors and ethics revealed that these nurses felt that they had compromised their standard of practice because of the nursing shortage. For example, 78% of these RNs reported that they had either not given an ordered medication or had given the medication to the patient at the wrong time. Of these RNs, 69% believed that this error was somewhat related to the nursing shortage, and 73% reported that they felt strong moral distress as a result of their actions (Silva and Ludwick, 2003).

Changing duties, responsibilities, and conflicts amidst nursing shortages and public concern over patient safety and quality of care characterize present-day practice. These changes require professional nurses to have core competency in critical thinking, communication, interdisciplinary team collaboration, assessment, leadership, and technical skills, as well as knowledge of health promotion/disease prevention, information technology, health systems, and public policy.

The American Association of Colleges of Nursing (AACN) reported in 2000 a 7.4% faculty vacancy rate for the 220 nursing schools surveyed. It was also reported that the average age of full-time faculty members was slightly over 50 years and that the average doctorally prepared faculty member's age was 55.9 years. It was suggested that public funding to schools of nursing be increased to attract and retain nursing faculty. In support of the nursing profession, the U.S. Congress adopted the Nurse Reinvestment Act to provide funds for nursing education, recruitment, and retention programs. President George W. Bush signed the bill into law in August 2002.

In addition to the issues of access, cost, quality, and accountability in health care, nurses today are challenged by an aging population, complex consumer health values, and an increasingly intercultural society. The IOM released in May 2003 recommended partnerships of academic institutions, local and state public health departments, community health agencies, and schools of public health to establish training for medical and nursing school curricula. The future of public health in our nation depends on a competent, well-trained public health workforce. A well-trained workforce is in the best interest of all those concerned with maintaining a healthy society (IOM Report, 2003).

With over 2.6 million members, the nursing profession has risen to the challenges of the twenty-first century by uniting efforts to shape health care and the profession. Numerous coalitions have been formed to address the critical nursing shortage; increased political liaisons have influenced health policy; and involvement in evidence-based practice is more prevalent than ever and continues to improve health outcomes for individuals, groups, communities, and the nation (Connelly, 2004).

SUMMARY

Nursing is a dynamic profession that has evolved into a theory and research-based practice. From its unorganized and poorly defined beginnings, a profession based on the framework of competence, autonomy, determination, and human caring has evolved. The challenges and struggles have paralleled the path of world history and have brought about significant changes in the profession. From the men who opened the path, to the women who brought dignity and respect to their philosophy of caring, to the pioneers who brought unity to the profession plagued by a history of racism, sexism, and sometimes disgrace, nursing has become recognized as critical to the health of the nation. Despite a myriad of challenges, the practice of nursing has been distinguished and qualified by the intellect, skill, commitment, and contribution of countless sisters, deaconesses, and individuals such as Seacole, Dix, Barton, Wald, Breckenridge, and Nightingale.

The nursing shortage has forced the nation to focus on a variety of ways to educate and utilize nurses of the future. Nurses play an important role in determining that future and the future of health care in America. Congress will continue to play a major role in providing funding to alleviate the shortage of faculty, clinical practitioners, and advanced practice nurses. As society changes, so does the role of the nurse. The quality of health care provided to our citizens cannot be compromised. Therefore, nurses must continue to play major roles in future health care initiatives (Connelly, 2004; Jones, 2004).

Through periods of war, socioeconomic change, and health care reform, nurses have played a vital role in initiating change to improve the health care arena. Nurses have provided the integrity to maintain the quality of care in all health care settings. The evolution of the practice from the treatment of disease to health promotion and disease prevention has led the way in determining the type of providers needed to care for patients in the future (Connelly, 2004). This evolution will continue to provide the foundation for the scope of practice, educational curricula, scholarship, and research necessary for nurses to lead and manage the health care environment of the future (Catalano, 2003). Nurses will continue to increase knowledge, manage technology, and maintain ethical standards to provide high-quality, patient-centered safe care to individuals, families, communities, and populations throughout the world (Box 1-4).

BOX 1–4 *Helpful Websites*

www.aacn.nche.edu/Publications/issues/96july.htm
www.mtsu.edu/~kmiddlet/history/women/wh-med.html
www.nursingworld.org/pressrel/2002/ltr0726.htm
www4.umdnj.edu/camlbweb/blacknurses.html
www.nursing.upenn.edu/history/default.htm
www.contemporarynurse.com/vol12_1.htm
http://libweb.apu.ac.uk/journals/journals.php
www.mohoman.org/mni/history_of_nursing_education.htm
www.aahn.org/
www.firstaid.about.com/cs/historyofnursing/
www.thoemmes.com/social/nursing_intro.htm
www.umich.edu/~inden/papers/sindhu.html
www.internurse.com/history/
http://womenshistory.about.com/cs/medicine/
www.geocities.com/Athens/Forum/6011/
http://encarta.msn.com/encnet/refpages/refarticle.aspx?refid=751557139
www.nursewebsearch.com/History/Military_Nurses/
http://womenshistory.about.com/cs/nursesandnursing/
http://womenshistory.about.com/cs/nursesandnursing/
www.nurseweek.com/features/98-7/forensic.html
www.aahn.org/resource.html
www.nursingnetwork.com/education.htm
www.enfermundi.com/infoenf/conferen/CF10nursing.htm
http://community.nursingspectrum.com/MagazineArticles/article.cfm?AID=5926
http://ans-info.net/PanelPolicies.htm
www.nursingworld.org/hof/maascl.htm
Women in Medicine—www.med.virginia.edu/hs-library/historica /antiqua/stext.htm
Vincent de Paul and Louise de Marillac, Compassionate Servants and Saints—www.cptryon.org/vdp/vdp-ldm/index.html
Nursing Individuals—web.bu.edu/specco/nursind.htm
Nurses and Human Rights—www.web.amnesty.org/ai.nsf/index/ACT750021997

CRITICAL THINKING ACTIVITIES

1. How have the historical aspects of nursing affected nursing as we know it today?
2. Compare and contrast various contributions made by nurse pioneers. Describe how this affects your philosophy of nursing.
3. What was the historical significance of racial segregation and the impact of racial integration on professional nursing? Explain why this is important.
4. What is your vision for the profession of nursing in the future?
5. What are some of the challenges you see facing the nursing profession in the future?

Additional resources are available on-line at: http://evolve.elsevier.com/Cherry/

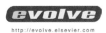

http://evolve.elsevier.com

REFERENCES

Baer E et al: *Enduring issues in American nursing,* New York, 2001, Springer Publishing Company.

Bahr L, Johnson B: *Collier's encyclopedia,* vol 18, New York, 1995, Collier's.

Boschma G: *The rise of mental health nursing: a history of psychiatric care in Dutch asylums 1890-1920,* Chicago, 2003, University of Chicago Press (Amsterdam University Press in US).

Buhler-Wilkerson K: *No place like home: a history of nursing and home care in the United States,* Baltimore, 2001, Johns Hopkins.

Carnegie ME: *The path we tread: blacks in nursing: 1854-1994,* ed 3, New York, 1995, National League for Nursing.

Catalano JT: *Nursing now: today's issues, tomorrow's trends,* ed 3, Philadelphia, 2003, FA Davis.

Connelly CA: Beyond social history: new approaches to understanding the state of and the state in nursing history, *Nurs Hist Rev* 12:5-24, 2004.

Deloughery GL: *Issues and trends in nursing,* St Louis, 1998, Mosby.

Doheny MD, Cook CB, Stopper MC: *The discipline of nursing: an introduction,* ed 4, Stamford, Conn, 1997, Appleton and Lange.

Dolan J: *Nursing in society: a historical perspective,* Philadelphia, 1978, WB Saunders.

Donahue MP: *Nursing: the finest art—an illustrated history,* St Louis, 1999, Mosby.

Ellis JR, Hartley CL: *Nursing in today's world: challenges, issues and trends,* ed 7, Philadelphia, 2001, JB Lippincott.

Ellis JR, Hartley CL: *Nursing in today's world: challenges, issues and trends,* ed 8, Philadelphia, 2004, JB Lippincott.

Fitzpatrick MF: The mercy brigade, *Civil War Times* 36(3):34-40, 1997.

Freedman D: *The Anchor Bible dictionary,* New York, 1995, Doubleday.

Giger J, Davidhizar R: *Transcultural nursing: assessment and intervention,* ed 2, St Louis, 1999, Mosby.

Glass LK, Murphy EK: *AORN emergence and growth,* Denver, 2002, AORN.

Hinshaw AS: Nursing research and the explosion of knowledge. In Schorr TM, Kennedy MS, editors: *One hundred years of American nursing,* New York, 1999, JB Lippincott.

Institute of Medicine: *Who will keep the public healthy?* Workshop Summary. Hernandez I, editor, Committee on Education, Public Health Professionals for the 21st Century, 2003, The National Academy of Sciences Press.

Jones ZO: Knowledge systems in conflict: the regulation of African American midwifery, *Nurs Hist Rev* 12:167-184, 2004.

Kalisch P, Kalisch B: *The advance of American nursing,* ed 2, Philadelphia, 1986, JB Lippincott.

Kalisch P, Kalisch B: *The advance of American nursing,* ed 3, Philadelphia, 1995, JB Lippincott.

Karger HJ, Stoesz D: *American social welfare policy: a pluralist approach,* New York, 1994, Longman.

Katz JR et al: *Keys to nursing success,* ed 2, Columbus, Ohio, 2004, Pearson/Prentice Hall.

Kelly L, Joel L: *The nursing experience: trends, challenges and transition,* ed 3, New York, 1996, McGraw-Hill.

Lindeman C, McAthie M: *Nursing trends and issues,* Springhouse, Pa, 1990, Springhouse Corporation.

Nelson S: *"Say little, do much": nineteenth century religious women and care of the sick,* Philadelphia, 2001, University of Pennsylvania Press.

Nies MA, McEwen M: *Community health nursing: promoting the health of populations,* ed 3, Philadelphia, 2001, WB Saunders.

Oermann MH: *Professional nursing practice,* Stamford, Conn, 1997, Appleton and Lange.

Robinson TM, Perry PM: *Cadet nurse stories: the call for and response of women during World War II,* Indianapolis, Ind, 2001, Center Nursing Press.

Salzman J, Smith D, West C, editors: *Encyclopedia of African-American culture and history,* vol 3, New York, 1996, Macmillan Library Reference USA; Simon and Schuster Macmillan.

Sarnecky M: Nurses at Pearl Harbor: the true story, *Reflect Nurs Leadersh* 27(4):16-21, 2001.

Schorr TM, Kennedy MS: *One hundred years of American nursing,* New York, 1999, JB Lippincott.

Silva M, Ludwick R: Error, the nursing shortage, and ethics: survey results, *Online J Iss Nurs* August 15, 2003 (www.nursingworld.org/ojin).

Small H: *Florence Nightingale: avenging angel,* London, England, 1998, Constable.

Snodgrass ME: *Historical encyclopedia of nursing,* Santa Barbara, 1999, ABC-CLIO.

Stanhope M, Lancaster J: *Community and public health nursing,* St Louis, 2004, Mosby.

Walton J, Barondess J, Locke S: *The Oxford medical companion,* New York, 1994, Oxford University Press.

Williams SJ, Torrens PR: *Introduction to health services,* ed 4, Albany, NY, 1993, Delmar Publishing.

U.S. Department of Health and Human Services, Public Health Service: *Healthy people 2020: national health promotion and disease prevention objectives,* Washington, DC, 1991, USDHHS.

SUGGESTED READINGS

Anteau CM, Williams LA: What we learned from the Oklahoma City bombing, *Nursing* 36(5):52-55, 1998.

Aronitz F: Competition for the education of nurses, *Community College Week* 13(6):2-4, 2000.

Bezyack ME: Advanced practice: is it right for you? *Am J Nurs* 96(1):15-25, 1996.

Carnegie ME: Black nurses at the front, *Am J Nurs* 84(10):1250-1252, 1984.

Carnegie ME: *The path we tread: blacks in nursing: 1854-1984,* Philadelphia, 1986, JB Lippincott.

Carnegie ME: *The path we tread: blacks in nursing worldwide: 1854-1994,* ed 3, New York, 1995, National League for Nursing.

Collins H: Mission for the millennium: choke out remains of polio. *Charlotte Observer,* March 14, 1999, pp 1A, 10A.

Donaldson MS, Vanselow NA: The nature of primary care, *J Fam Pract* 42(2):397-421, 1996.

Shelton K: A brief history of black women in the military, *Precinct Reporter* 3(9):2-4, 1996.

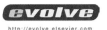
http://evolve.elsevier.com

2

The Contemporary Image of Professional Nursing

Toni Bargagliotti, DNSc, RN

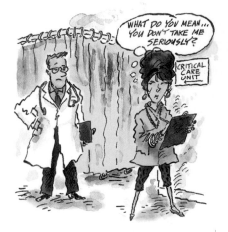

Each nurse forms the
image of nursing every day.

People are always blaming their circumstances for what they are. I don't believe in circumstances.
The people who get on in this world are the people who get up and look for the circumstances they want,
and if they can't find them, make them.

— GEORGE BERNARD SHAW

VIGNETTE

Mary is a senior nursing student who asks a faculty member, "Why can't we wear different scrubs and jewelry to clinical? Have you seen what nurses wear? I don't know what difference it makes anyway. Patients don't care what we're wearing. They care that we know how to take care of them. You know, 2 months after we graduate, we'll be wearing what everyone else does. Yes, I know we look better than everyone else does. But why?"

Questions to consider while reading this chapter:
1. How does the image of a nurse differ from that of a physician?
2. How does the nurse's appearance affect the patient's opinion of the quality of care the nurse provides?

Additional resources are available on-line at: http://evolve.elsevier.com/Cherry/

KEY TERMS

Art Any branch of creative work, especially painting and drawing, that displays form, beauty, and any unusual perception.

Literature All writings in prose or verse.

Media All means of communication, such as newspapers, radio, and television.

Stereotype A fixed or conventional conception of a person or group held by a number of people that allows for no individuality.

LEARNING OUTCOMES

After studying this chapter, the reader will be able to:

1. Explain the contributing factors to the nursing shortage.
2. Describe the image of nursing in art, media, and literature over time.
3. Identify nursing actions that convey a negative image of nursing.
4. Suggest strategies that would enhance the image of nursing.
5. Create an individualized plan to promote a positive image of nursing in practice.

CHAPTER OVERVIEW

This chapter describes how the image of nursing has been shaped and suggests strategies that nurses can use to forge a positive public and professional image of their practice. Because nurses have been the subjects of artists, sculptors, and writers for thousands of years, an historic perspective is used to illustrate the contextual background for the evolving image of this profession. Examples from nursing practice are used to illustrate how different approaches to the same situation continually shape the image of nursing.

IMAGES OF NURSING

When you imagine a nurse, what mental picture comes to mind? Do you think of *Life* magazine's (1942) nurse in a starched white uniform with a cap, the nurses portrayed in Johnson and Johnson's Campaign for Nursing's Future, or your colleagues with whom you practiced yesterday? The contemporary image of professional nursing in the United States is an ever-changing kaleidoscope of the 2.7 million men and women of all ages, races, and religious beliefs who are registered nurses. Adding to this multifaceted collage are the numerous snapshots of nurses and nursing as portrayed in television commercials, bumper stickers, art, poetry, architecture, postage stamps, television shows, movies, newspaper comic strips, stained glass windows, and statues. Second in size to the profession of teaching, nurses have been alternatively described as either saints or sinners, powerless or powerful, admired or ignored, and most recently, those who dare to care. Their practice has captured the attention of historians, economists, and sociologists who have studied this unusual group of people. Although nursing is the profession for which sentimental women need not apply, historians have described nurses as those who were ordered to care.

Since Florence Nightingale reduced mortality rates from 42% to 2% in a Crimean hospital constructed over an open sewer, nurses have been reformers who are expected to use limited resources to address unlimited "wants" for health care. The request for Nightingale's nursing services in the Crimea was born out of newspaper reports about the devastating health care conditions in the Crimean War. Today media reports on the nursing shortage and Gallup poll results indicate the value that the public places on nursing practice.

Although nurses have become concerned with their public image and media portrayal, the extensive work of Kalisch and Kalisch (1995) outlining the image of nursing in film and media over time has permanently etched the image issue into the professional radar screen. While image concerns may appear to be self-serving, deepening national concern about an evolving nursing shortage of unprecedented magnitude is focusing considerable attention on the way that nursing is publicly portrayed. Whether nursing shortages emerge from the public image of nursing or images of nursing emerge from nursing shortages, the two are inextricably related. Understanding the current shortage provides the fundamental basis for a discussion of the image of nurses.

THE NURSING SHORTAGE

The United States Bureau of Labor (2003) reports that registered nurses are one of the top 10 occupations projected to have the largest growth of new jobs in the near future. With an employment rate projected to increase by more than 36% in the next decade, nursing is projected to grow faster than the average of all occupations until 2010. By 2010, the United States is projected to need almost 1 million more registered nurses than will be available. The demand for registered nurses is projected to increase by 40% in 2020, whereas the supply will have increased by only 6% (Projected Supply, Demand, and Shortages of Registered Nurses 2000-2020, 2002). The number of new nurses licensed in 2020 is projected to be 17% lower than in 2002, while, at the same time, the nursing workforce loss from retirement or death is predicted to increase by 128% (Projected Supply, Demand, and Shortages of Registered Nurses 2000-2020, 2002). In 2040, the cohort of women aged 20-54 who could practice as nurses will be in a ratio of 5.4 to every person over the age of 85 (GAO, 2001).

Consider the following data: the average age of a new nursing graduate is 33, the average age of a registered nurse (RN) is 45.2, and the average age of nursing faculty is 51.2 (AACN, 2003; Buerhaus, Staiger, and Auerbach, 2000; HRSA, 2001). By 2015 more than half of U.S. RNs are predicted to retire. The graying of American nurses is occurring because of two factors outside of nursing: (1) the declining birth rate of potential nurses every year following the "baby boomer" generation (1946-1960) and (2) the women's movement in the 1970s that opened new career opportunities for women (Buerhaus, Stagier, and Auerbach, 2000). However, the most serious concern is that between 1995 and 2000, the overall number of students entering nursing declined each successive year (AACN, 2000). Overall, during those years, the number of new graduates declined by 26%. This included a 64% decline in diploma graduates, a 26% decline in associate degree programs, and a 17% decline in baccalaureate graduates (Projected Supply, Demand, and Shortages of Registered Nurses 2000-2020, 2002).

Not surprisingly, work-setting issues parallel enrollment declines. When adjusted for inflation, nursing salaries have remained unchanged since 1991 (Projected Supply, Demand, and Shortages of Registered Nurses 2000-2020, 2002). In comparison with other professions, such as elementary school teachers, the difference of $4,400 between the average salaries of these two groups in 1983, widened to $13,600 in 2000 (Projected Supply, Demand, and Shortages of Registered Nurses 2000-2020, 2002). From 1983 to 1998, the percentage of nurses under the age of 30 declined by more than 41%, although the workforce population under the age of 30 declined by only 1% (GAO, 2001). Almost one in every two nurses (41%) are dissatisfied with their jobs, and 22% plan to leave nursing within a year (Aiken et al, 2001). One-third of those planning to leave the profession are under the age of 30, a group that now constitutes only 9% of the nursing workforce (HRSA, 2001). Nationally, the turnover rate per year of registered nurses in acute care hospitals in 2000 was reported to be 26.2% (GAO, 2001).

To address these issues, President George W. Bush signed the Nurse Reinvestment Act P.L. 107-205 into law in August 2002. This act was funded at $20 million to provide nursing scholarships, public service announcements promoting nursing as a career, faculty loan cancellation programs, geriatric training grants, and nurse retention and safety enhancement grants.

NURSING IN ART AND LITERATURE

Although the portrayal of nursing in art and literature throughout the years may seem to be unrelated to the contemporary image of nursing, the mental image of contemporary nursing is enmeshed with the earliest of these images.

Art and literature have long been the way in which people describe the human condition and cultural values of their time. In the earliest descriptions of nurses and nursing are found the enduring fundamental and essential tensions that exist within the profession today, as well as the eternal question asked by those who know they will one day require nursing care: "Can I trust and entrust my life to this nurse?" Although people hope that nursing is a vocation, a "calling" that requires education, commitment, and dedication, they fear that it is only a job requiring minimal training that the nurse endures for the lack of other opportunities or until something "better" is available.

Antiquity Image of Nursing

The earliest literary reference to nursing chronicles the actions of two nurse midwives in approximately 1900 B.C. In the Old Testament of the Bible, the book of Exodus indicates that the practice of two midwives became the vehicle through which the Israelites, the Jewish race, and the resultant Judeo-Christian heritage survived. From the sixth century until the 1800s, nurses were imaged as either untrained servants, soldiers, women of religious orders, or wealthy people performing acts of Christian charity (Kalisch and Kalisch, 1995; Kampen, 1988). These artistic renderings of nurses convey images that continue to be familiar to contemporary nurses.

Victorian Image of Nursing

In 1844, the same year Florence Nightingale was "called" to become a nurse, Charles Dickens immortalized a different kind of nurse through his character Sairy Gamp, a nurse who endured the profession because of the lack of other opportunities. For Sairy Gamp, a drunken, physically unkempt, uncaring nurse in Dickens' novel *Martin Chuzzlewit*, nursing provided a way to profit from the sick and dying. Reflecting the concern of Victorian England about untrained caregivers, Dickens' narrator advised Sairy of the advantages of " . . . a little less liquor, and a little more humanity, and a little less regard for herself, and a little more regard for her patients, and perhaps a trifle of additional honesty" (p. 894).

Fortunately, Sairy's literary arrival was followed by Longfellow's portrayal of the heroic Nightingale in "Santa Philomena" (1857). As important as Nightingale was to the improved health care of British soldiers and to the development of modern nursing, the increasingly positive images of Nightingale were primarily the result of her ability to succinctly demonstrate the aggregate outcomes of nursing practice. To do so, she became one of the earliest users of the emerging body of knowledge called statistics and developed the pie chart that remains in common use today. Notably, nursing emerged at a time of turbulent social change and reform in Great Britain.

Early Twentieth-Century Nursing

Toward the end of the Nightingale period, at the turn of the nineteenth century, nurses in war settings vividly captured the attention of artists. The most compelling image is Bellows' 1918 canvas entitled *Edith Cavell Directing the Escape of Soldiers from Prison Camp* (Donahue, 1985). During World War I, Germany shocked the world with its 1915 firing squad execution of Edith Cavell, founder of the first nursing school in Belgium, who aided soldiers escaping prison camps. The art of heroic nursing expressed in several famous paintings reflected the reality of WWI nurses who were also the recipients of 3 Distinguished Service Crosses, 23 Distinguished Service Medals, 28 French Croix de Guerre's, 69 British Military Medals, and 4 U.S. Navy Crosses (Donahue, 1985). Notably, although American nurses were not commissioned in the military services during World War I, one of every three nurses served in that war.

The 1930s—Nurse as Angel of Mercy

On a grander scale, Warner Brother's film, *The White Angel* (1936), chronicled the professional life of Florence Nightingale. Endorsed by the American Nurses' Association (ANA), *The White Angel* clearly portrayed Nightingale's persistence and head-to-head confrontation with the medical establishment. Anticipating that the medical staff would deny her nurses rations, she brought provisions for them. When the medical staff locked her out of the hospital, Nightingale sat outside in the snow until patients and soldiers required physicians to admit these nurses. As Jones (1988) notes, *The White Angel* clearly conveyed to the public that nursing was a holy vocation, that nurses had professional credentials, and that their career choice was controversial because of the prevalent belief that women should remain at home. A subtle inference of the film is that Nightingale was smart enough to overcome the obstacles of the medical field.

In 1938 Rich's tall and imposing white limestone statue, the Spirit of Nursing, was placed in Arlington National Cemetery to "honor the compassion and bravery of military nurses" (Donahue, 1985, p. 433). Similarly, Germany's 1936 stamp commemorated nursing with a larger-than-life nurse compassionately viewing people (Donahue, 1985).

The 1940s—Nurse as Heroine

Considered by many to be the most positive movie about nursing, *So Proudly We Hail* is the 1942 story of nurses in Bataan and Corrigedor. The film, starring Claudette Colbert, portrayed a small group of nurses rerouted to the Philippines after the attack on Pearl Harbor. Soon cut off from supplies and replacements as the Japanese took over the Philippines, these nurses, with no staff and few supplies, provided care to the thousands of soldiers in the Philippines. The story of the nurses who served on Bataan is also the subject of Norman's *We Band of Angels: The Story of American Nurses Trapped on Bataan by the Japanese* (1999), in which the gritty, difficult, and heroic struggle of these nurses is chronicled through their diaries and interviews.

Nursing was depicted on a 1940 Australian stamp with a larger-than-life nurse figure looking over a soldier, a sailor, and an aviator; on a 1945 Costa Rica stamp featuring

Florence Nightingale and Edith Cavell; and in the 1945 commissioning of the USS Higbee, a U.S. Navy destroyer named in honor of a Navy nurse (Donahue, 1985).

After nursing's glorious contributions to WWII, nurses returned home to find low salaries, long hours, too few staff, and too many patients. However, nursing continued to be glamorized through numerous romance novels, including the Cherry Ames series and the Sue Barton series.

Nursing in the Antiestablishment Era of the 1960s

In 1962, author Ken Kesey created a modern version of Dickens' Sairy Gamp with his character of Nurse Ratched in *One Flew Over the Cuckoo's Nest*. This best-selling novel later became a play and a motion picture (1975) that won six Oscars, including Best Picture of the Year. Entrusted with the care of the mentally ill, Nurse Ratched, a military nurse in a starched white uniform, was the ultimate power figure who cruelly punished patients to cure their psychoses through conformity to a "system" (Fiedler, 1988).

The reality of the turbulent 1960s is that nursing was one of President Johnson's first salvos in the War on Poverty. The Nurse Training Act of 1964 was funded at $250 million ($1.4 billion in 2002 dollars). Nurses also dramatically shaped the future of health care through the development of coronary care units, intensive care units, hemodialysis, and Silver and Ford's first nurse practitioner program in Colorado. A U.S. Bureau of Labor study indicated that salaries of nurses were woefully inadequate in comparison with other, far less trained American workers (Kalisch and Kalisch, 1995).

Nursing in the Sexual Revolution of the 1970s

Media images of the nurse in the 1970s were formed amidst a sexual revolution and a growing antimilitary stance in American culture. War would again provide the media backdrop. The 1976 postage stamp of Clara Maas ("She Gave Her Life") commemorated the 100th birthday of Maas, a 25-year-old nurse who died after deliberately obtaining two carrier mosquito bites so that she could continue providing care to soldiers with yellow fever in the Spanish-American War (Donahue, 1985). This depiction of a self-sacrificing nurse was in strong contrast to the modern-day portrayal of nurses in the 1970 Robert Altman film *M*A*S*H* and the follow-up hit television series by the same name.

The nursing profession viewed the *M*A*S*H* series, which ran from 1972-1983, as professionally destructive because of its negative portrayal of Margaret "Hot Lips" Hoolihan and the nurses of the 4077th Army MASH (mobile army surgical hospital) unit in Korea. The sexual exploits of nurses and physicians and the often uncaring Margaret provided few positive images. However, for the American public who were receiving a daily dose of what was happening in actual MASH units in the news footage of Vietnam on the nightly news, the television series *M*A*S*H* presented a glimmer of reality. Continuous front-line exposure to the massive trauma of young men did not desensitize these nurses from caring or cause them to run from the horrors of what they were seeing. They coped with the war's horrors with a sense of humor and irreverence toward "the system." Nurses serving in Vietnam would later be imaged in another television series *China Beach*.

Similarly to M*A*S*H, the less popular spin-off series, *Trapper John, MD,* depicted a negative image of nursing while providing at least one strategically important image for the profession: the portrayal of the wise African-American nurse whose "take" on the situation was always accurate. At the time of the series, the profession had fewer than 5% African-American nurses. Historically, it was not until 1964 that the Louisiana State Nurses' Association became the last state to fully admit African-American nurses for membership from all districts of the state (Carnegie, 1995).

Nursing in the 1980s and 1990s

Portraying an actual event, playwright David Feldshuh realistically described the complexities of nursing in his play, *Miss Evers' Boys.* Through the character of Miss Evers, the play tells the true story of Nurse Eunice Rivers, who was hired to recruit young African-American men into the infamous Tuskegee experiment designed to describe the long-term effects of syphilis. When Nurse Rivers' patients asked her to obtain the new treatment of penicillin for them and she sought to do so, the physician investigators required her to discourage them from treatment. Their reasoning, designed to exploit and manipulate her, presented her with several moral dilemmas that she had not been educated to manage. As the narrator of the story, Miss Evers introduces nonnurses to the dilemmas of nursing practice and the consequences of misplaced faith and trust in physicians.

In 1997 three films used war and nursing as a backdrop: *The English Patient, Love and War,* and *Paradise Road.* In all of these films, the nurse character is a knowledgeable, nonjudgmental caregiver.

In contrast to these heroic media portrayals of nursing was the Nicole Miller advertisement in *Golf* (June 1997), a magazine designed to sell golf clothes to men. Four practicing New York physicians were pictured on a golf green with the caption "Playing doctor." Draped around the physicians were young female models in white bikini bathing suits with nursing caps and tennis shoes. As a result of rapid written response from nurses and the American Organization of Nurse Executives (AONE), the company withdrew the advertisement and apologized to Nicole Miller customers and readers of *Golf* magazine (Wood, 1997).

Artistic views of nursing during this period focused on caring. In the Vietnam War Women's Memorial, the central figure is the nurse in battle fatigues cradling the head of a soldier for whom she is providing care. Evident in the bronze statue is the fatigue of the nurse and her care for this dying soldier.

The Image Of Men

Notably absent in these media portrayals of nurses are the men who are entering nursing in increasing numbers. Perhaps one of the most positive film portrayals of men who are nurses occurs in *Meet the Parents,* a comedy released in December 2000. In this film the aspiring son-in-law is Greg Focker, RN, a wonderful character who humorously addresses and rises above the worst of all stereotypes that are endured by men in this profession.

MEDIA CAMPAIGNS FOR NURSING

In 1990 the Tri-Council of Nursing with funding from the Pew Foundation implemented the Nurses of America (NOA) media campaign. Nurses of America was designed to convey to the public that nurses are expert clinicians who are able to interpret technical data in usable ways, as well as coordinate and negotiate health care. This was followed by the Nurses for a Healthier Tomorrow campaign, which led to the Johnson and Johnson $25 million Campaign for Nursing's Future. As a consequence of the Johnson and Johnson campaign, baccalaureate nursing enrollments increased by more than 8% over 2 years and high school sophomores and juniors began to rank nursing more highly as a career choice (Johnson and Johnson, 2003).

A strategically important part of the NOA campaign was raising the consciousness among nurses of the invisibility of nursing in the news media. A study of the sources quoted by journalists in health care–related articles in *The New York Times, LA Times,* and the *Boston Globe* indicated that nurses accounted for only 10 of more than 900 citations (Buresch, Gordon, and Bell, 1991). In fact, nurses ranked last after patients. Sigma Theta Tau International's Woodhull study of 20,000 articles published in 16 newspapers, magazines, and other health care publications (1998) indicated that nurses were cited only 4% of the time in the more than 2000 articles about health care.

THE ENDURING PUBLIC CONCERN WITH NURSING

Against this backdrop of nursing images that extend from antiquity to the latest CNN broadcast is the question of what image will be created by nurses today. Although attention and concern about the professional image of nursing might superficially seem to be a self-serving exercise, the many historical images of nursing indicate otherwise.

People want to believe that the nurse will, as Virginia Henderson indicated, perform nursing care that does for them what they would otherwise do if they had the necessary strength, ability, and knowledge. Perhaps as unnerving as entrusting their lives to someone else is the fear of entrusting knowledge of their most intimate selves to an unkind person. To be seriously ill often means entrusting the most intimate physical functions, fears, and concerns to a nurse (Fagin and Diers, 1983). People know that whatever public facades about their real relationships to "kith and kin" they can maintain when healthy will be immediately stripped bare during illness. They also know that a stranger, the nurse, will soon know their most intimate secrets of "personhood at its worst" when they are ill. Patients hope for a Nightingale who will overcome all obstacles to reduce their mortality from 42% to 2%, but they fear a Sairy Gamp or a Nurse Ratched who will neglect or control them in harmful ways.

What the Public Believes About Nursing

Gallup polls in 2000, 2002, and 2003 indicated that the public ranks nursing as the most ethical of all professions. In December 2001, Chris Matthews of CNBC's *Hardball* was a guest on CBS's *Late Show* with David Letterman. In discussing the changes that occurred following the 2001 World Trade Center attacks, he mentioned the 2001 Gallup poll that ranked nurses second to firemen. He said, "Do you remember when we were 5 or 6 years old and we wanted to be heroes and make a difference? We all wanted to be either firemen or nurses. It's taken 9/11 to remind us of when we had big souls in little bodies."

THE REALITY OF THE CONTEMPORARY STAFF NURSE

The reason for the existence of the modern health care institution—the hospital, the nursing home, the mental hospital, the home care agency—is to deliver nursing. If surgery could be done safely and economically on the kitchen table, and if people could survive it, it would be done that way. If diagnosis and management of serious medical illness could be done in 8.5-minute office visits, it would be. If the chronically mentally ill could be taken care of at home and protected from the world and from themselves, they would be. If the demented, the frail, the paralyzed, the very old could be cared for at home, they would be—and it would be much less expensive because public policy would not contemplate channeling the money to family caregivers since they're supposed to want to do it anyway (Diers, 1988, pp. VIII-2 and VIII-3).

Logically, it could be inferred that nurses' satisfaction with their work setting should be high since their practice settings exist to deliver their services and new practice settings are emerging daily. The public highly values their profession. Nursing's heroic and noble public image has been etched in stone and in stained-glass windows in larger-than-life proportions. Why, then, are there high levels of dissatisfaction?

Clash Between Beliefs and Reality

Mills and Blaesing (2000) found that nurses who were likely to be satisfied with their career over time held three values: (1) a sense of professional status, (2) a belief that they made a difference (patient care rewards), and (3) pride in their profession. Those belief systems, however soon clashed with the health care reform that occurred during the 1990s.

Health care changes in the 1990s shifted practice boundaries and resulted in the widespread marginalization of professional nursing care. Multiskilled unidentifiable workers replaced 20% to 50% of RNs in "downsizing" and "rightsizing" efforts that left nurses doing more and supervising the unskilled with 20% fewer staff than in other industrialized nations (Brannon, 1996; Gordon, 1997; Kitson, 1997). Although these changes were attributed to managed care and the Budget Reconciliation Act of 1997, Grando's historical research (1998) indicates that these same events occurred in the 20-year post-WWII period when the elasticity of nursing was similarly tested with unlicensed persons to avoid increasing salaries.

The megacorporate environments that emerged in the 1990s diminished nursing staffs to increase the margin, while increasing administrative staffs to consume 25% of the hospital dollar. Gordon (1997) cites a 1995 survey that indicated the average compensation for chief executive officers in small hospitals was $188,500; in larger hospitals, $280,900; and in the nation's seven largest for-profit health maintenance organizations (HMOs), $7 million—such salaries far exceeding the average physician income.

Although experiencing significant downsizing, nurses and their employers conveyed and continue to convey to patients that hospitals and other health care settings provide individualized, holistic care. Home health care agencies marketed nursing as "a part of your family," although Coffman's study (1997) indicated that families perceive the home health nurse as a "stranger in the family."

Ironically, although nurses' beliefs about the care they would provide were highly congruent with the marketing claims of the nurse's employer, these claims placed the nurse in direct conflict with a system internally determined to provide essential rather than "nice to have" care. Nurses, expecting to have adequate, competent staff and to be fairly rewarded for providing individualized holistic care, instead faced a quite different reality. The employer asked only one question: How much care was provided for how little to ensure that customers were delighted rather than simply satisfied, healthy, or healthier?

When patients realize that their expectations are not being met, they are rightfully angry. Even when it may be possible for them to understand that the system will only provide minimal care, there remains one additional thorny problem. If the nurse was their advocate, as nursing has claimed, why didn't the nurse or nursing profession fix the system to provide all that was promised (Kelly, 1989)? Patients who believed that their care would be sensitive and individualized were stunned by what actually occurred and angry when they were discharged home requiring skilled nursing care that they must now provide for themselves (Barnum, 1991; Kelly, 1989).

Second, in terms of nursing practice, there was a significant mismatch about the claims of managed care and what actually occurred. Productivity and work redesign literature centered on accountability and identification of core processes. Achieving cost savings through the elimination of "nonvalue–adding" activities such as supervision of recurring tasks, underscored a principle that was advanced by nurses during most of the twentieth century. It was assumed that, since managed care focused on outcomes, the nursing care that prevents hypostatic pneumonia, decubitus ulcers, fractured hips from falls, overmedication of the elderly, and undermedication of pain would be recognized. The nursing care that promotes wound healing, early treatment of dysrhythmias, immediate treatment of chemotherapy reactions, and faster recovery through critical pathways would at last be recognized and rewarded. Since patients would be discharged earlier, patient and family teaching would become central rather than peripheral to nursing practice. However, the outcomes of health care changes that occurred during the 1990s included a mortality rate of 44,000 to 98,000 deaths from medical errors each year (IOM, 2000). Stated differently, more people die each year from medical errors than died in 11 years of combat in Vietnam (48,000 combat deaths) and far more than from alcohol- and drug-related driving deaths (16,653 in 2000) (CDC, 2001).

The fact that nurses are dissatisfied with their practice arena is not surprising (Joint Commission for Accreditation of Healthcare Organizations, 2002). The changing health care system has dramatically increased their workload, devalued their practice, dramatically reduced the margins of error, and resulted in harm to the patient.

WHY IS THIS HAPPENING?

Attributing nursing's high dissatisfaction rates to image or by adding to Rodney Dangerfield's comedic repertoire about lack of respect does not provide an explanatory model. Drucker's (2002) conceptualization of knowledge workers does. Knowledge workers require specialized training to do work that requires judgment. In today's information economy, the work to be done is increasingly "knowledge work."

Drucker suggests that the profession of teaching, which emerged in the late 1700s, and nursing, which followed in the early 1800s, produced the first knowledge workers. Both professions emerged as industrialization began to change an agrarian economy to one that would in the next century be fueled by manufacturing. In a manufacturing economy, workers are highly loyal to the factory that provides them with life-long employment, shift work, and strict policies and procedures that ensure the production line continues. Company loyalty is ensured because without the factory, there is no job. In contrast, knowledge workers are loyal to their profession and freely move to practice in settings that recognize and reward their judgment. As noted by Bargagliotti (2002, 2003), Drucker's description of the motivating forces for knowledge workers mirrors the findings of the Magnet study of hospitals (1983) and the numerous reports on the nursing crisis (AHA, 2002; JCAHO, 2002; Kimball and O'Neil, 2002). Not surprisingly, mandatory overtime that requires nurses to practice beyond their capacity to make safe clinical judgments and "floating" to cover unfamiliar units are management practices that are perhaps suitable for factory workers, but not for knowledge workers. Reframing nursing as knowledge work provides a radically different perspective. Nurses expect to direct nursing care because they are the only knowledgeable people to do so.

Numbers—the Only Language in a Business Model

Nurses are knowledge workers who are in the *business* of health care. In a business environment, cost decisions are based on aggregate, rather than case-by-case, anecdotal data. Nightingale was influential because she reduced mortality rates by 40%. She courted and made the data known. However, when numbers talk, nursing is reduced to a whisper in the absence of data (Hadley, 1996).

A 2001 study by Needleman et al of discharges from 799 hospitals in 11 states indicated that registered nurse staffing was significantly related to lower lengths of stay and reduced rates of nurse-sensitive indicators, such as upper gastrointestinal bleed, pneumonia, urinary tract infections, and "failure to rescue," which resulted in deaths. They found no such relationship between increased staffing levels of licensed practical nurses or nurse's aides and adverse outcomes. In a survey of 831 physicians and 1207 adults, one in three physicians and 42% of the public reported that they or a family member had experienced medical errors when receiving care. More than half of the surveyed physicians and 65% of the public believed increased registered nurse staffing would prevent medical errors (Blendon et al, 2002). Aiken et al (2002) found that for patients undergoing routine surgery (e.g., appendectomies, gall-bladder, and orthopedic surgeries, such as knee and hip replacement) mortality rates increase by 7% for every patient beyond a 1:4 ratio of registered nurses to patients.

Managed care manages health care services from a cost/benefit perspective rather than an altruistic one. Effectively providing care in this climate requires demonstrating the economic benefit of services and the cost of problems.

Nursing's Contribution

Nurses are knowledge workers; yet only one in ten nurses holds an advanced degree in nursing. The way in which nursing students are traditionally taught implies that for nurses, knowledge is a necessary burden. Nursing professors admonish students to learn so that patients will not be harmed or killed, whereas their medical counterparts teach their students that knowledge enables them to *do something* and, subsequently, that knowledge is power (Barnum, 1991; Christman, 1991).

From a different perspective, Aaronson (1989) has contended that nursing fails to understand the basic premise of social exchange theory: societal rewards are in direct relationship to the scarcity of the service provided. By contrast, medicine understands it well. Following the release of the Flexner report (1910), which recommended the closure of 400 medical schools and the retention of only 35 high-quality university-based schools, medicine immediately closed these schools. Within 15 years of making that decision, medicine became the most highly valued occupation in the United States (Christman, 1998). Since that time, medicine has controlled the numbers of physicians and secured a legal monopoly as the sole gatekeeper to health care.

The response to the Flexner report is instructive because in 1910 medicine had a questionable knowledge base at best. On the other hand, in 1910 nursing was the one service that substantially reduced hospital mortality rates. Although nursing was potentially far more powerful because of its demonstrated results, it was unwilling to use this influence. Nursing did not respond to similar reports and recommendations. Medicine is only one example; the teaching profession is another. As Christman (1998) noted, nurses have been "studied more and have responded less" than other professional groups (p. 211).

Although Bowman (1993) has rightfully indicated that individual nurses are not to "blame" for all of the image issues confronting the profession, individual nurses have made and continue to make contributions to the negative image of nursing.

Changing Nurse-Physician Interactions

An enduring mystery and common experience for nurses is how to address a medical problem with the primary customer of the hospital, the physician. Physicians are revenue generators for hospitals, and, in exchange for hospital privileges, agree to be self-governing and to abide by a set of medical staff bylaws. All medical staff bylaws include a disciplinary process that begins with the section chief, who is required to address documented patient care problems.

Consider the following actual clinical situation.

CASE STUDY

In a meeting with a nursing service administrator, the Chief of Medical Staff, and the physician liaison, a nephrologist complains that he is not being notified by nursing about his patients and that nurses do not know how to take care of his dialysis patients.

RESPONSE 1

Nurse 1 tells the nephrologist how well prepared the nursing staff is and says that his is the first complaint of this type that has been received. (The problem is denied.) However, nursing is short-staffed, and there are a lot of agency nurses being used. (Two excuses are provided.) Nurse 1 says she will investigate. (This is the first positive response.) However, without a specific incident and patient, she may not be able to correct the problem. (This is the third excuse.)

RESPONSE 2

Nurse 2 carefully takes notes and limits her comments to clarifying questions while the physician becomes increasingly more derogatory. She concludes with the need to investigate and indicates that a written report will be sent to all parties. The physician is thanked for bringing this matter to the nurse's attention.

The investigation indicates that multiple nurses over time and in different units have all phoned the nephrologist to notify him about patients, but that the nephrologist has loudly announced that they have awakened his baby and has abruptly hung up the phone. Second, this is a difficult physician who never has time to discuss his patients when making rounds. Specific examples of unanswered questions are obtained.

The written findings are prepared, and Nurse 2 poses only one question: "Since the physician is not able to 'take calls' after 5:30 p.m., the patient care issue that concerns nursing is the question of who will be covering his patients."

Outcome: Within 2 weeks this nephrologist's hospital privileges are quietly rescinded.

All too often, when nurses work with a physician whose practice is substandard or who is highly volatile, it is believed that this is a nursing problem, when rather, it is a medical problem that must be addressed by medical staff via their staff bylaws. Only when nurses disengage from emotional responses and the offering of denial and excuses, factually document the problem in patient care terms rather than in personality issues, and forward this in writing to a nurse manager and the appropriate section chief can the problem be resolved.

Just as nursing's involvement with medical problems is confined to appropriate notification, so should medicine's involvement with nursing be so confined. When a physician notifies and informs a nurse about a nursing problem, a positive answer is, "Thank you. Let me investigate the problem and get back to you." Lengthy detailed discussions are seldom useful. When the nurse makes an error, a simple apology and sincere statement of corrective action is sufficient.

Second, ongoing problems between nurses and physicians center on communication and time. Consider how often a physician is paged for a problem and phones the unit but no one on the nursing staff knows the problem or who paged the physician. There may be a need for a change in orders, but the nurse who requested the order is away from the unit or engaged with another patient when the physician makes rounds. In this case, a simple note, such as a post-it note, could prevent the problem.

Effect of Communication Patterns on Image

In observing nurses, Buresch and Gordon (1996) have noted the ongoing subtle self-sabotage of nurses in multiple ways. Nurses refer to other nurses by first name, whereas physicians are "Dr. —." During teaching rounds in hospitals noted for high nurse-physician collaboration, nurses frequently position themselves behind residents and interns, contributing little. Similarly, nurses and physicians differ in the way they approach one another. For example, when a nurse seeks a physician to inquire about a patient issue and finds her in discussion with another physician, the nurse frequently leaves. However, minutes later, the same physician may interrupt the nurse, who may then be in conference with other nurses, and the nurse allows the interruption.

The Look of Nursing

In the 1970s nurses successfully shed the uniform of "authority in gleaming white"—nursing cap, uniform, sensible shoes, and white hose that, according to Curtin (1994a), required pupil accommodation to adjust to the glare. Although this trend has been considered by most to be a positive change, many believe the trend has gone too far. Few other professionals wear pink, purple, or flowered shirts with wrinkled, faded, pajama-style drawstring pants to their professional work setting. In an Emergency Department, a patient told a 28-year-old nurse dressed in a T-shirt and jogging pants that "you're just a kid out of high school telling me what to do" (Zimmerman, 1996).

Meanwhile, as one emergency department staff nurse wrote, staff nurses are in "T-shirts with Mickey Mouse logos, 'Run a Code Naked' and the name of a local bar; college sweatshirts, stretch pants, mismatched jogging suits . . . stained and wrinkled clothes" (Zimmerman, 1996, p. 267), and tennis shoes. Although Zimmerman humorously notes that these nurses appeared to be dressed for a "come as you are party," they were in fact practicing in an emergency department. The clear message nurses are conveying is that nurses should not be taken seriously and have little regard for the seriousness of the situations they encounter.

Molloy (1996) indicated that airlines changed the attire for flight attendants when it was noticed that persons dressed in "cute" designer uniforms could not command the attention of passengers in an emergency. When attire was changed to more businesslike suits, flight attendants were better able to direct passengers and command attention in emergency situations. The current array of nursing attire projects an image that could not be occurring at a less opportune time. Although it is unlikely that nurses will return to gleaming "whites," a far more professional appearance than is currently found in many clinical settings could be achieved by a simple change to conservatively colored "scrubs" with a white laboratory coat monogrammed with "John Smith, RN." Notably, just when professional nursing is being marginalized, the loss of a uniform appearance has resulted in the inability of patients and families to distinguish between the nurse and the housekeeper (Carpenito, 1995).

BELIEVE IN NURSING

Creating a different image and a different reality requires one simple action. Nurses have to believe in who nurses are and in what nurses do. This requires valuing nursing, valuing the name of nursing, and reclaiming the name and the practice.

Valuing Nursing

Everyone employed in a nursing department is not a nurse. Although this is an obvious observation, nurses often behave as if it were not true. Consider how often nursing staff meetings include all staff nurses, assistants, ward clerks, and so on. Nurses need to be the first people to ask why. Discussions of unit problems or directions for the future need to be held first and separately with professional nurses. The dialog would be considerably different and far more useful. Including everyone in a staff meeting indicates to assistive staff that they are expected to offer opinions about professional nursing practice.

Although the initial response to the proposal of separate staff meetings may be that it would be too time-consuming, the alternative is far more likely. The time would be spent far more productively for nurses, as well as for other staff. Although nurse managers periodically meet with other hospital managers, they more frequently have specific nurse manager meetings to discuss care issues that involve nursing.

The devaluing of nursing occurs daily in discussions with patients, families, and physicians. When an intervention occurs with a patient in a hospital or home health care agency, it is almost always the nurse who recognized the problem (Gordon, 1997; Reichstein, 1991).

Reclaiming the Name of Nurse

As the International Congress of Nursing (ICN) determined in 1985, the term "nurse" is reserved for an RN (Holleran, 1991). Referring to anyone else or allowing anyone else to use this title undermines the profession. Nurses should not introduce an aide or multiskilled worker to a patient, family, physician, or anyone else as Mr. Smith's nurse. Nursing practice acts in all 50 states require nursing care to be planned and directed by an RN. Introducing anyone else in the role of THE NURSE is misleading. A patient care assistant should be identified to others as the nurse's assistant. Similarly, health teaching, advice, direction, and progress reports to patients, physicians, or others come only from THE NURSE. When nurses meet patients, they advise them that their questions should be directed to THE NURSE, not to the assistant.

In more and more settings nurses are encountering employers who refer to all employees, including professional nursing staff, as associates. In some settings nurses are being prohibited from including the designation RN on their nametags. Monogrammed scrubs and laboratory coats with first initial, last name, RN, avoids this discussion.

On a daily basis, news stories identify many people as nurses who are not RNs. When this occurs, the public believes that a nurse did whatever is being reported. The image of nursing will improve when all nurses correct inaccurate labeling of nurses and false assumptions.

Reclaiming Personal Identity

Gordon (1994), a journalist intrigued by the image of nursing, made two significant observations about the way in which nurses refer to themselves and to other nurses. The first is the increasingly common use of first names, which is deadly for the profession since "nonpersons have only first names." However, nurses often introduce themselves, for instance, as "Hi. I'm Susie and I'm your nurse." As Curtin (1994b) humorously noted, "The mind boggles at the thought of a physician introducing himself in like manner: 'Hi! I'm Dick, I'm your doctor,' or a lawyer greeting a client with 'Hi! I'm Larry the lawyer'" (p. 10). Second, a common method used to dehumanize people to encourage their conformity is to remove their name. For this reason, prisoners are not referred to by their name. The use of first names, no names, and referral to everyone as "the nurse" has led to professional concerns that patients have no idea who the nurse is (Letters, 1996). More important, information patients may receive from the nursing assistant may well be believed to be from the RN.

The notion that the use of a last name may place the nurse in danger from hostile patients or families is without supporting evidence. Nurses who take pride in their profession and their accountability use their last names in a professional setting.

A Southern California Kaiser hospital emergency department manager noticed that when a nurse instructed a patient to phone if there were any problems, and the patient then asked for the nurse's name and number, the nurse had to sheepishly write on a scrap piece of paper (Bream and Poblador, 1995). Subsequently, the manager insisted that RNs begin using business cards. Implementing this change required that nurses had to become comfortable giving patients, families, or unfamiliar physicians their business card—that is, they had to learn to be comfortable presenting themselves as professionals.

Initially, many nurses resisted because they did not believe "it" was important. "It" was their personal identification as a nurse. Second, some nurses were concerned that if they had no credentials after their name other than RN, they would appear less knowledgeable. Third and most important, some preferred anonymity because they were concerned about being too identifiable and therefore accountable. Ironically, after a year of use, business cards made it possible for patients to proclaim to others the excellence of the nurse's practice.

Reclaiming the Practice

Before anyone else believed that a nurse extender could replace nurses, nurses gave away their role to others through patient assignments. Curtin (1994a) astutely indicated that the place of the nursing assistant, LPN/LVN, multiskilled worker, or whoever else may be invented is not at the bedside. His or her place is at the side of nurses. These roles were designed to *extend,* not to *replace.*

Changing the Song

As Mattera (1999) notes, turning to Ann Landers, a syndicated newspaper columnist, is probably not the best approach to solving the problem of the nurse's image. In her January 27, 1999, column, Landers wrote: "I've had a ton of letters with a litany of complaints (from nurses). The profession is clearly in a state of jeopardy. And now I would like some suggestions on how to fix it." Mattera's frustrated response indicated that "two million creative problem solvers ought to be able to fix the things that are bothering nurses without jeopardizing the hospital bottom line. Because if you can't accept the reality that hospitals need to exist at a certain profit level, and figure that into your problem-solving, then you'll have designed a perfect nursing environment that no one will put into practice" (p. 7).

On a More Positive Note

Notice how often nurses who are widely accepting of patients from different backgrounds, different cultures, and different perspectives are unable to think positively about others in health care. The common thinking is that for nursing to be valued, medical care cannot be valued. For health promotion to be valued, illness care cannot be valued. Valuing critical care practice requires devaluing wellness care. For day nurses to be good at what they do, night nurses are not. For collective bargaining to be useful, those who do not bargain collectively do not care. In short, for any nurse who perceives any other nurse to be different in any way requires that one or the other must be negatively viewed. Instead of collectively going head to head with those who oppose nursing practice, contemporary nurses have gone head to head with each other as they epitomized the sociologic concept of "like against like," termed *horizontal violence,* which is highly indicative of oppressed group behavior (Roberts, 2000).

Often, nurses who disagree with some minor component disagree with the entirety in public and in private. Imagine the difference if nurses told everyone what nurses do well and confined the disagreements to "in-house" discussions. What if nurses thought carefully before disagreeing with one another about minor issues, thus thoughtfully conserving their energy for important issues? What if nurses looked to each other rather than everyone else for consultation and assistance.

Valuing the Future of the Profession

In 1875 Dr. Howard, a Montreal medical professor, suggested that the new nursing profession require the same preliminary education as the medical profession, with the exception that natural science should have a higher place than the classics and professional education should extend over 3 years. Howard was quickly drowned out by numerous medical papers in the late 1800s and early 1900s that argued to "attempt to give nurses instruction as to the reason why . . . would be, in the majority of instances, to inflict a heavy task upon them and to lift them more or less out of their proper sphere . . . to give them more than an insight into it is to demand for them complete education as medical practitioners" (p. 1835). Similarly, Aaronson (1989) cites the president of the Pennsylvania State Board of Medical Examiners, who said in 1909 that "the instruction commonly prevalent in hospital training schools is not only absurdly too comprehensive, but dangerous. It is sufficient to almost entirely result in nurses assuming the right to usurp the functions of physicians" (p. 275).

As health care becomes increasingly more complex, nursing remains the only health profession that claims to require *less* education. Christman (1998) rightfully notes that "knowledge not possessed" cannot be used by even the most highly motivated of nurses. With the expansion of science doubling exponentially every 2 years, the nursing educational issue becomes less understandable (Christman, 1998). The single question for nursing is not entry into practice; it is exit into practice (Bargagliotti, 2002).

Creating a New Image

Envision a new world where nurses value nursing and contribute to its positive image daily. Nurses take themselves seriously and dress the part. Nurses are highly visible to patients, families, and physicians because they have reclaimed their practice. Since nurses are clear about the role boundaries between themselves and those who extend their practice, others are also. Nurses are "stuck like glue" together. Negative comments about a colleague are made to the colleague and to no one else. Professional nurses recognize that their greatest benefit—and one of the most efficient and powerful uses for their money—is the less than 1% of their salary that they spend for membership in the American Nurses Association, the National League for Nursing, Sigma Theta Tau International, and their specialty organizations. They look forward to annual meetings because they provide an excellent opportunity to meet colleagues and discuss issues and practice innovations.

Since all nursing is valued, nurses recognize the value of caring, health promotion, and health teaching, as well as the value of illness care. They celebrate that nurses save lives everyday. In the modern medical climate, nurses supervise assistive personnel and use their authority to ensure that patient care delivery is excellent. Nurses value the use of nursing as a metaphor for mothering, class struggle, equality, and a conscience for medicine (Fagin and Diers, 1983). To this legacy they add astute businessperson, researcher, caregiver for the family, and entrepreneur.

In this new world nurses believe in nursing, in self, and in their colleagues. It is significant to the future of nursing that nurses safeguard the profession's public image in newspapers, television, film, and other media, as well as in daily practice (Box 2-1). Finally, nurses must realize that they themselves play a part in forming the image of nursing on a daily basis.

BOX 2-1 Helpful Websites

American Nurses Association Press Releases
www.nursingworld.org/pressrel/2001/index.htm

American Association of Colleges of Nursing Press Releases
www.aacn.nche.edu/Media/NewsReleases/newslist.htm

National League for Nursing Press Releases
www.nln.org/pressreleases/index.htm

Sigma Theta Tau International Nursing Honor Society—Media
www.nursingsociety.org/

CRITICAL THINKING ACTIVITIES

1. The earliest Western image of nursing is that of patient advocate in 1900 B.C. Four thousand years later, what is nursing's highest priority advocacy role in contemporary society?
2. Recent studies have indicated that nurses are the most highly trusted health professional group. What component of nursing's contemporary image places nurses in this position of trust? What threatens this position?
3. You are a trauma nurse who takes care of a U.S. Senator following a life-threatening car accident. He credits you with saving his life. When he becomes President, he invites you to the White House and asks you to tell him the most important thing he can do to reform the health care system. In one sentence, what would you say?
4. In an ideal health care setting, what would be the most important image of nursing?
5. If you wanted to artistically portray a twenty-first century nurse, what would the nurse be wearing?

Additional resources are available on-line at: http://evolve.elsevier.com/Cherry/

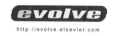

REFERENCES

Aaronson LS: A challenge for nursing: re-viewing a historic competition, *Nurs Outlook* 37(6):274-279, 1989.

Aides relieve nursing shortage, *Life* 12(1):32-34, 36, 1942.

Aiken L et al: Hospital nurse staffing and patient mortality, nurse burnout, and job dissatisfaction, *JAMA* 288(16):1987–1993, 2002.

American Association of Colleges of Nursing: With demand for RNs climbing, and shortening supply, forecasters say what's ahead isn't typical shortage cycle, *AACN Iss Bull*, February, 1998.

American Association of Colleges of Nursing: *2002-2003 salaries of instructional and administrative nursing faculty in baccalaureate and graduate programs in nursing*, Washington, DC, 2003, AACN.

American Association of Colleges of Nursing: *Nursing school enrollments decline as demand for RNs continues to climb*, Washington, DC, 2000, AACN.

American Hospital Association Commission on Workforce for Hospitals and Health Systems: *In our hands: how hospital leaders can build a thriving workforce*, Chicago, 2002, American Hospital Association.

Bargagliotti LA: *Reframing nursing to renew the profession.* Keynote Address at the National League for Nursing Education Summit 2000: Engaging Higher Education in Renewing the Profession. Anaheim, Calif, 2002.

Bargagliotti LA: Reframing nursing to renew the profession, *Nurs Educ Perspect* 24(1):12-16, 2003.

Barnum B: Nursing's image and the future, *Nurs Health Care* 12(1):19-21, 1991.

Blendon RJ et al: Views of practicing physicians and the public on medical errors, *N Engl J Med* 347(24): 1933-1940, 2002.

Bowman AM: Victim blaming in nursing, *Nurs Outlook* 41(6):268-273, 1993.

Brannon RL: Restructuring hospital services: reversing the trend toward a professional work force, *Int J Health Serv* 26(4):642-654, 1996.

Bream TL, Poblador A: Business cards at the bedside, *Am J Nurs* 95(2):71-72, 1995.

Buerhaus PI, Staiger DO, Auerbach DI: Why are shortages of hospital RNs concentrated in specialty care units? *Nurs Econ* 18(3):111-116, 2000.

Bureau of Labor Statistics, U.S. Department of Labor: *Occupational outlook handbook, 2002-03 edition, registered nurses*. Retrieved October 3, 2003, on-line(www.bls.gov/oco/ocos083.htm).

Buresch B, Gordon S: Subtle self-sabotage, *Am J Nurs* 96(4):22-24, 1996.

Buresch B, Gordon S, Bell N: Who counts in news coverage of health care? *Nurs Outlook* 39(5):204-208, 1991.

Burnett, R, executive producer: *Late Show with David Letterman* (Television broadcast), New York, December, 12, 2001, CBSL, Worldwide Pants, Inc.

Carnegie ME: *Paths we tread: blacks in nursing worldwide, 1854-1994*, ed 3, New York, 1995, National League for Nursing Press Pub. No. 14-2678.

Carpento LJ: Bring back the nurse's cap (editorial), *Nurs Forum* 30(4):3-4, 1995.

Center for Disease Control: Notice to readers: national drunk and drugged driving prevention month, December, 2001. *MMWR* 50(47):1063-1064. Retrieved June 12, 2002, on-line (www.cdc.gov/mmwr/preview/mmwrhtml/mm5047a7.htm).

Christman L: Perspectives on role socialization of nurses, *Nurs Outlook* 39(5):209-212, 1991.

Christman L: Who is a nurse? *Image J Nurs Sch* 30(3): 211-215, 1998.

Coffman S: Home-care nurses as strangers in the family, *West J Nurs Res* 19(1):82-96, 1997.

Curtin L: The heart of patient care (editorial opinion), *Nurs Manage* 25(5):7-8, 1994a.

Curtin L: 25 years: a slightly irreverent retrospective, *Nurs Manage* 25(6):9-32, 1994b.

Dickens C: *Martin Chuzzlewit*, New York, 1910, Macmillan Co.

Diers D: *The mystery of nursing: Secretary's Commission on Nursing: support studies and background information*, vol 2, Rockville, Md, 1988, Department of Health and Human Services, pp VIII-1-VIII-10.

Diers D: On waves . . ., *Image J Nurs Sch* 24(1):2, 1992.

Donahue MP: *Nursing: the finest art: an illustrated history*, St Louis, 1985, Mosby.

Drucker P: *Managing in the next society*, New York, 2002, St. Peter's Press.

Fagin C, Diers D: Nursing as metaphor, *N Engl J Med* (2):116-117, 1983.

Fiedler LA: Images of the nurse in fiction and popular culture. In Jones AH, editor: *Images of nurses-perspectives from history, art, and literature*, Philadelphia, 1988, University of Pennsylvania Press.

Flexner A: *Medical education in the United States and Canada*, New York, 1910, Carnegie Foundation.

Gallup Organization: *December 1, 2003*. Retrieved December 2, 2003, on-line (www.gallup.com/poll/releases/pr031201.asp).

Gallup Organization: *Healthcare, September 11-13, 2000*. Retrieved January 26, 2000(a) on-line (www.gallup.com/poll/indicators/ indhealth2.asp).

Gallup Organization: *Honesty/ethics in the professions, November, 2000*. Retrieved January 26, 2000(b) online (www.gallup.com/poll/indicators/indhnsty_ethcs2. asp)

General Accounting Office: *Report to the Chairmen, Subcommittee on Health, Committee on Ways and Means, House of Representatives. Nursing workforce, emerging nursing shortages due to multiple factors*, Washington, DC, 2001, United States General Accounting Office.

Gordon S: What's in a name? (guest editorial) *J Emerg Nurs* 20(3):170, 1994.

Gordon S: What nurses stand for, *Atlantic Monthly* 279(2):31-88, 1997.

Grando V: Making do with fewer nurses in the United States, 1945-1965, *Image J Nurs Sch* 30(2):147-149, 1998.

Hadley EH: Nursing in the political and economic marketplace: challenges for the 21st century, *Nurs Outlook* 44(1):6-10, 1996.

Health Resources and Services Administration (HRSA), Bureau of Health Professions, Division of Nursing: *The registered nurse population,* Washington, DC, 2001, HRSA.

Holleran C: Inside view. Was it a nurse? Why the confusion? *Int Nurs Rev* 38(3):62, 1991.

Institute of Medicine (IOM): *To err is human: building a safer health system,* Washington, DC, 2000, National Academy of Science Press.

Johnson and Johnson: *Program provides nursing student scholarships, nursing faculty fellowships and grants to New Jersey nursing schools to expand their program capacity (news release).* Retrieved October 1, 2003, on-line (www.jnj.com/news/jnj_news/20030924_103747.htm;jsess ionid=PTAXQBBO4XDSICQPCB3SZOYKB2IIWNSC).

Joint Commission for Accreditation of Healthcare Organizations: *Healthcare at the crossroads: strategies for the evolving nursing crisis,* Chicago, 2002, Author.

Jones AH, editor: *Images of nurses: perspectives from history, art, and literature,* Philadelphia, 1988, University of Pennsylvania Press.

Journal of the American Medical Association: Nurses' schools and illegal practice of medicine (editorial), *JAMA* 49 (12):1835, 1906.

Kalisch PA, Kalisch BJ: *The advance of American nursing,* ed 3, Philadelphia, 1995, JB Lippincott.

Kampen MB: Before Florence Nightingale: a prehistory of nursing in painting and sculpture. In Jones AH, editor: *Images of nurses: perspectives from history, art, and literature,* Philadelphia, 1988, University of Pennsylvania Press.

Kelly LS: Editorial. Image, niceness and the illusion of quality, *Nurs Outlook* 37(6):5, 1989.

Kersbergen AL: Managed care shifts health care from an altruistic model to a business framework, *Nurs Health Care Perspect* 21(2):81-86, 2000.

Kesey K: *One flew over the cuckoo's nest,* New York, 1962, New American Library/Signet.

Kimball B, O'Neil, E: *Health care's human crisis: the American nursing shortage,* Princeton, New Jersey, 2002, Robert Wood Johnson Foundation.

Kingsley K: The architecture of nursing. In Jones AH, editor: *Images of nurses: perspectives from history, art, and literature,* Philadelphia, 1988, University of Pennsylvania Press.

Kitson AL: John Hopkins address: does nursing have a future? *Image J Nurs Sch* 29(2):111-115, 1997.

Kohn LJ, Corrigan JM, Donaldson MS, editors: *To err is human: building a safer health system,* Institute of Medicine. Washington, DC, 2000, National Academy Press.

Letters to debates and disputes, *Nursing 96* 16(2):6, 1996.

Lippman DT, Ponton KS: Nursing's image on the university campus, *Nurs Outlook* 37(1):24-27, 1989.

Longfellow HW: Santa Filomena, *Atlantic Monthly* 1(11): 22-23, 1857.

Mattera MD: Ann Landers, again! *RN* 62(3):7, 1999.

Mills A, Blaesing SL: A lesson from the last nursing shortage: the influence of work values on career satisfaction with nursing, *J Nurs Admin* 30(6):309-315, 2000.

Molloy J: *The new woman's dress for success,* New York, 1996, Warner Books.

Morrow H: Nurses, nursing, and women, *Int Nurs Rev* 35(1):22-25, 27, 1988.

Muff J: Of images and ideals: a look at socialization and sexism in nursing. In Jones AH, editor: *Images of nurses: perspectives from history, art, and literature,* Philadelphia, 1988, University of Pennsylvania Press.

Needleman J, Buerhaus P, Mattke S, Steward M, Zelevinsky K: Nurse staffing levels and the quality of care in hospitals, *N Engl J Med* 346(22):1715-1722,2001.

Norman EM: *We band of angels: the untold story of American nurses trapped on Bataan by the Japanese,* New York, 1999, Random House.

Pritchett P: *New work habits for a radically changing world,* Dallas, 1996, Pritchett and Associates.

Projected supply, demand, and shortages of registered nurses 2000-2020, Washington DC, 2002, Department of Health and Human Services Health Resources and Services Administration.

Q and A: *J Emerg Nurs* 21(12):165-166, 1995.

Reichstein J: Let's make nursing the visible profession, *Nursing 91* 11:148-149, 1991.

Roberts SJ: Development of a positive professional identity: liberating oneself from the oppressor within, *Adv Nurs Sci* 224:71-82, 2000.

Sigma Theta Tau International: *The Woodhull study on nursing and the media: health care's invisible partner,* Indianapolis, 1998, Sigma Theta Tau Center Nursing Press.

Wood W: Demeaning portrayal of RNs angers AONE, *Nurseweek* 10(12):3, 1997.

Zimmerman PG: Dressing the part (guest editorial), *J Emerg Nurs* 22(8):267-268, 1996.

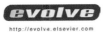
3

Theories of Nursing Practice

Margaret Soderstrom, PhD, RN, CS-P, APRN, and Linda C. Pugh, PhD, RNC, FAAN

Nursing theory provides the direction for nursing practice and research

Science is built up with facts, as a house is with stones. But a collection of facts is no more a science than a heap of stones a house . . .

— **JULES HENRI POINCARE, 1909, FRENCH SCIENTIST AND MATHEMATICIAN**

VIGNETTE

The little boy kicked the stone, using first one shoed foot, then the other. He did not pay much attention until he saw the shiny marks showing through the stone's surface. Only then did he stop and pick it up. Something about its composition fascinated him. It was at that moment that he heard his mother call and ran off in the direction of her voice. The stone sat for weeks as layers of dirt gathered on it. Another stone, swept against it by the wind, comfortably nestled close. Over time the two stones gathered substance as they continued to attract other stones of various sizes and shapes. The pile of stones became larger in height and width. Adjoining stones varied in form and content. Eventually, as one might imagine, quite a mass developed. Years later, a man who was a scientist noticed a large hill composed of stones. Out of the corner of his eye, he observed a shiny surface on one of the stones located near the bottom. It was somehow familiar. Curious, he carefully studied the hill before him. Slowly, he began separating the many stones into piles, organizing and defining what initially appeared to be scattered meaningless objects. Eventually he used scientific equipment to assist in this endeavor. There were occasional setbacks, each assisting in providing feedback and refining the process. Once sorted, the purpose of every item became evident. Each one was carefully laid. He could finally accept the premise. It was the beginning, a scientific foundation for future ideas and the generation of new directions. It remained consistently sturdy, resilient, and withstood the test of time.

MARGARET SODERSTROM, 2001

Additional resources are available on-line at: http://evolve.elsevier.com/Cherry/

Questions to consider while reading this chapter:
1. What is nursing theory?
2. How is nursing theory different from the theory of other disciplines?
3. How does theory relate to nursing practice?
4. Why is it important to understand nursing theory?
5. Why is it important for nurses to develop theory?

KEY TERMS

Concept An idea or a general impression. Concepts are the basic ingredients of theory. Examples of nursing concepts include health, stress, and adaptation.

Conceptual model A group of concepts that are associated because of their relevance to a common theme.

Construct Labels given to ideas, objects, or events.

Nursing science The collection and organization of data related to nursing and its associated components. The purpose of this data collection is to provide a body of scientific knowledge, which provides the basis for nursing practice.

Nursing theory The compilation of data that defines, describes, and logically relates information that will explain past nursing phenomena and predict future trends. Theories provide a foundation for developing models or frameworks for nursing practice development.

Proposition Statement that proposes the relationship between and among concepts.

Schematic model A diagram or visual representation of concepts, conceptual models, or theory.

LEARNING OUTCOMES

After studying this chapter, the reader will be able to:
1. Differentiate between a science and a theory.
2. Identify the criteria necessary for science.
3. Identify the criteria necessary for theory.
4. Explain a nursing theory and a nursing model.
5. Discuss two early and two contemporary nursing theorists and their theories.
6. Explain the impact of nursing theory on the profession of nursing.

CHAPTER OVERVIEW

Explicit, detailed knowledge is the keystone, the foundation, and the carefully laid support that is critical to the classification of a discipline. In a seminal paper *The Discipline of Nursing* (1978), Donaldson and Crowley note, a discipline ". . . is characterized by a unique perspective, a distinct way of viewing all phenomena, which ultimately defines the limits and nature of its inquiry" (p. 113). Nursing, long ranked an art and a science, is actually quite young in its continuing struggle for professional and public recognition as a matchless, expert, and commanding profession. This notion is readily supported as one marks nursing's ongoing effort to define itself as a distinct discipline that is exclusive from other disciplines, particularly the medical practice model. Only when a substantial body of nursing knowledge is collected, organized, and developed will the profession be defined and its scope of practice differentiated. Key in this accomplishment is the development and practice of nursing theory.

It is important for nurses to study the development of nursing theory because without an idea of where you have been, how can you know how, why, when, or where to go? Nursing theory provides nurses with a focus for research and practice. You may consider using a theory as similar to using a map that provides direction while making available a variety of ways to get where you are going. As logical as this seems, the worth of studying nursing theorists and their theories and the role of responsibility these theories contribute toward the evolution of nursing science has been curiously underappreciated. Even more surprising, many of the naysayers are nursing students. Nursing theory is not usually the favorite subject of under-graduates, who would much rather learn technical "hands-on" skills. Whether this is a matu-ration issue or an issue of knowledge and experience remains undetermined by nursing faculty and the profession itself. The philosopher Eden Phillpots said, "The universe is full of things patiently waiting for our wits to get sharper" (Bronowski, 1972). Let us hope they will.

This chapter in no way reflects the breadth and depth of nursing theorists and their the-ories. There are many scholarly works devoted to this topic. Instead, it is a survey, a general overview, a smattering of nursing theories, with chosen segments intended to assist in pro-viding the idea, the notion, and indeed, the semblance of what a theory is and how it is criti-cal to the profession of nursing. Readers interested in examining the theoretic basis for nursing practice will find resources for further exploration at the end of the chapter.

SCIENCE AND THEORY

Science is a method of bringing together facts and giving them coherence and integrity. Science assists us in understanding how the unique yet related parts of a structure fit and become more than the sum of individual parts. In the opening metaphor, the stones represent the facts, the process of laying the stones represents the science, and the future ideas and new directions represent the theory.

Science is both dynamic and static—dynamic in figuring out *how a phenomenon happens,* static in describing *what happens.* Scientific inquiry involves five steps: (1) hypothesis, (2) method, (3) data collection, (4) results, and (5) evaluation. These five steps are described in Box 3-1.

A theory is defined as a group of related concepts that explain existing phenomena and predict future events (Barnum, 2000). Theory development functions in a parallel manner to scientific process, although theory generally applies to a more specific area of the larger scientific process. Even though Freud and Jung each had their individual theories about the psychology of man, their theories were focused on specific ideas taken from the entire knowl-edge base surrounding psychology and psychotherapy and its scientific premise. Similarly, Albert Einstein's theory of relativity was but a fraction of the existing scientific knowledge base of mathematics at the time. Nevertheless, it is an undisputed fact that these theorists changed the thinking of their time and were responsible for the evolution of their philosophic and scientific interests (Anastasi, 1958). For a proposed theory to be accepted as a theory, it must meet the following six criteria: inclusiveness, consistency, accuracy, relevance, fruitfulness, and simplicity. These six criteria are further explained in Box 3-2.

The importance of theories in the evolution of science is unquestioned. Nursing has evolved as a profession and as a science in a similar manner. Nursing theories have explained,

---

BOX 3–1   The Five Steps of the Scientific Process

Hypothesis
Ask the question that is to be the main focus. It usually includes independent and dependent variables.

Method
Decide what data will be collected to answer the question. Decide on and identify the step-by-step procedure that will be used to collect these data. Make sure this process can be easily replicated.

Data Collection
Implement the step-by-step procedure that has been determined to answer the question.

Results
On the conclusion of the data collection, statistically identify the outcomes. Establish parameters (e.g., level of significance) that will determine whether or not the data are relevant.

Evaluation
Examine the results to determine the relevance of outcome data in answering the hypothesis. Determine the significance and identify the potential for future research.

---

explored, defined, and delineated specific areas. Beginning with the work of Florence Nightingale in 1860, nursing theorists have taken the vast pool of scientific information available and focused on precise target areas of interest. In so doing, theoretic models have been conceptualized to guide nursing actions, interventions, and implementation. Specific nursing theories will be discussed later in the chapter.

BOX 3–2   Criteria for Theory Acceptance

Inclusiveness
Does the theory include all concepts related to the area of interest?

Consistency
Can the theory address new entities without having its founding assumptions changed?

Accuracy
Does the theory explain retrospective occurrences? Does the theory maintain its capacity to predict future outcomes?

Relevance
Does the theory relate to the scientific foundation from which it is derived? Is it reflective of the scientific base?

Fruitfulness
Does the theory generate new directions for future research?

Simplicity
Does the theory provide a road map for replication? Is it simple to follow? Does it make sense?

Nursing Science

As might be expected, there are several definitions of nursing science (Abdellah, 1969; Jacox, 1974). Although these definitions differ, they generally support the premise that nursing science is a collection of data related to nursing that may be applied to the practice of nursing. These data encompass a vast array of knowledge that spans all of nursing and its diversity. This knowledge guides the practice of nursing to better serve patients through healing, prevention, education, and health maintenance.

Theories, Models, and Frameworks

"Theories and conceptual models are the primary mechanisms by which researchers organize findings into a broader conceptual context" (Polit, Beck, and Hungler, 2001, p. 144). Different terms are used in relation to conceptual contexts for research. These terms include *theories, models, frameworks, schemes,* and *maps.* Terms are often used differently by different writers, thus resulting in a blurring of distinct terms (Polit, Beck, and Hungler, 2001).

Theory. Theory is generally considered an abstract generalization that presents a systematic explanation about how phenomena are interrelated. Therefore, traditionally, a theory must have at least two concepts that are related in a way that the theory explains (Polit, Beck, and Hungler, 2001).

Conceptual Model. A conceptual model deals with concepts that are assembled because of their relevance to a common theme. The term conceptual framework is used interchangeably with conceptual model. Conceptual models, or frameworks, also provide a conceptual perspective regarding interrelated phenomena, but they are more loosely structured than theories. There are many conceptual models of nursing that offer broad explanations of the nursing process. Four concepts basic to nursing that are included in these models are: (1) nursing, (2) person, (3) health, and (4) environment. The various nursing models define these concepts differently, link the concepts in various ways, and emphasize differently the relationships among the concepts. For example, Roy's Adaptation Model emphasizes the patient's adaptation as a central phenomenon, whereas Martha Rogers emphasizes centrality of the individual as a unified whole. These models are used by nurse researchers to formulate research questions and hypotheses.

The terms *conceptual model* (or *framework*) and *nursing theory* are often used interchangeably. In this chapter the nursing theories described may also be referred to as conceptual models. The term *model* is also used in reference to a diagram depicting the theory. In this chapter the term *model* will refer to a schematic model, which is a diagram or visual representation of the conceptual model or theory.

Nursing Theory

Theory and theoretic thinking guide research and practice. The basic ingredients of theory are concepts. Examples of nursing concepts include health, stress, and adaptation. Propositions are statements that propose the relationship between and among concepts (Polit, Beck, and Hungler, 2001). Theories provide us with a frame of reference, the ability to choose concepts to study, or ideas that are within one's practice. A theory helps guide research, and research helps validate theory.

In the research model the researcher decides what to study and how and why the area of interest is important to the practice of nursing. In the practice model the clinician decides what areas to directly assess, when to assess, and which intervention to implement.

These decisions may or may not be knowingly based on a model or theory. Regardless, often the outcome supports the notion that behavior replicates a theoretic model, even though the nurse may be unaware that he or she is using a theoretic model in the practice process.

Just as in any other discipline, nursing theory has its own unique language. The words of this language identify linkages between the database of scientific nursing knowledge and the extracted information taken from this source for nursing theory. The interpretation of these words translates uniquely to the theory investigated. This application, or language of nursing theory, is the structure, or framework, from which one understands the theory. Table 3-1 presents the language of nursing theory, along with definitions and examples.

Schematic Models

A schematic model is something that demonstrates concepts, usually with a picture. It is a visual representation of ideas. The model depicts concepts and shows how the concepts are related with the use of images such as arrows and dotted lines (Polit, Beck, and Hungler, 2001). For example, a blueprint is a pictorial demonstration of a particular type of house someone might build. A model airplane is a detailed miniature replication of the original full-sized version. Diagramming a sentence outlines the specific parts (adverb, adjective, verb, subject, object, phrases) that make that particular sentence complete. Similarly, a nursing model gives a visual diagram or picture of concepts. Whether that is a critical pathway, decision tree, medication protocol, or other nursing-related practice, the model allows one to view the interrelated parts of the whole in picture form. A model of a nursing theory does the same thing. From the earliest model, offered by Florence Nightingale, nursing theory has been described and explained using this medium. Schematic models are used for clarifying complex concepts. The language of theory is translated into picture form, offering a comprehensive view, or model, of the theory. The schematic model shows how the concepts are related. A model, like a blueprint of a building, allows one to see the layout, including outlines of all features specific to the theory. Although it is not the same as understanding every minute

| **Table 3-1** | **The Language of Nursing Theory** |

LANGUAGE OF NURSING THEORY	DEFINITION	EXAMPLES
Concept	Labels given to ideas, objects, events; a summary of thoughts or a way to categorize thoughts or ideas	Comfort, fatigue, pain, depression, environment
Construct	A group of concepts; they are deliberately invented	Intelligence, motivation, learned helplessness, obesity
Conceptual Model	A structure to organize concepts (ideas)	Roy's *Adaptation Model*
Philosophy	Values and beliefs of the discipline	Watson's *Philosophy and Science of Caring*
Theory	The organization of concepts or constructs that shows the relationship of the ideas with the intention of describing, explaining, or predicting; the purpose is to make scientific findings meaningful and generalizable; our goal in science has been to explain, predict, and CONTROL!	Self-care, adaptation, caring, behavioral system, unitary man, hierarchy of needs, interpersonal relationship, humanistic, nurse-client transactions

detail about the structure, its intent is to provide an overview, which at a glance is informative and descriptive.

Levels of Theory

Many persons refer to the level of a nursing theory, which can range from broad in scope to a smaller, more specific scope. For example, Grand Theory is often broad in scope and may describe and explain large segments of human experience. Rogers' Theory of Unitary Man describes the entire nursing process. Other levels include Middle-Range Theory and Practice Theory, which are smaller in scope and may refer to a specific population such as Jacob's Grief of Older Women (Jacob, 1996) or to a specific situation such as Good and Moore's balance between analgesia and side effects (Good and Moore, 1998). Another example of a middle-range theory is the Theory of Unpleasant Symptoms (Lenz et al, 1997), which examines symptoms that are influenced by physiologic, psychologic, and situational factors as they relate to performance. The model of this theory is presented in Fig. 3-1. Today nurses often use these middle-range theories that are smaller in scope and simpler to understand to guide their daily practice.

To better illustrate the application of theory to nursing practice, Box 3-3 presents a case example of middle-range theory application using Mishel's (1997) Uncertainty in Illness Theory. In examining nursing theories, students may be surprised to discover that they are already using some of the contained concepts in their individual practices. Nursing theories assist with further defining and organizing these concepts into an underpinning that explains, details, and claims nursing practice as a unique discipline.

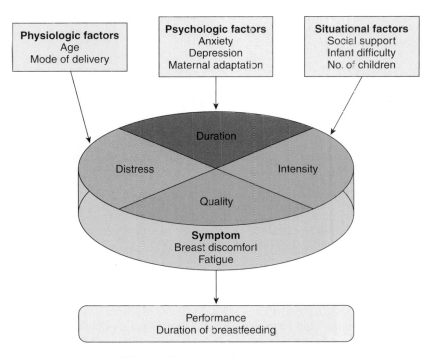

FIG. 3–1 Theory of unpleasant symptoms.

BOX 3–3 *Case Example: Application of Theory to Practice*

Mishel's UNCERTAINTY IN ILLNESS THEORY
Case Presentation
A 9-year-old female, Christine, is admitted to the pediatric unit for evaluation of a new onset of abdominal pain. The admission diagnosis is *intermittent abdominal pain, rule-out appendicitis*. It is her first time as a patient in a hospital. Her father, who is a surgeon, and her mother, who is a nurse, accompany Christine to the unit. Her mother will stay with her. After talking with the parents, you, the nurse, are confident that Christine is well informed, well cared for, and well prepared for her admission. While her parents are speaking with Christine's attending physician in a nearby office, you talk with Christine, who goes from smiling and chatting to bursting into tears. You observe that she is quite upset as she expresses to you that she is afraid because her father told her that if she did need surgery she would not feel anything because she would be asleep. Christine tells you that when she sleeps she wakes up sometimes and that she is sure that if her appendix is "cut out" she will wake up during the operation and it "will hurt a lot." She tells you she has not told her parents she is afraid because they have told her how proud they are that she is so brave. You realize Christine is terrified. Using Mishel's Uncertainty in Illness Theory, you apply the four-stage framework.

1. *Stimuli Frame:* Inadvertently, Christine, who concretely has understood the word "sleep" using her own filter for life experience, has misinterpreted the positive intention of the language used by her father. This misinterpretation has resulted in Christine's negative cognitive schema. Christine notably does not understand "sleep" and its use (or adult misuse, in this case) as a synonym for, or definition of, surgical anesthesia. This is the root cause of Christine's current Uncertainty in illness.

   Nursing intervention: Listen carefully and caringly; explain in simple understandable language what "sleep" means in the context her father presented; initiate, seek, and clarify Christine's concerns and questions; use the term "anesthesia" to differentiate it from "sleep." Inform and involve her parents in the overall process.

2. *Appraisal Stage:* As a result of Christine's concrete experiential interpretation of "sleep," she has applied a negative value to the environmental conditions surrounding her abdominal pain. This is particularly so as it relates to surgical anesthesia.

   Nursing Intervention: Follow up with Christine to make sure she comprehends the newly provided information. Elicit the support of Christine's parents and staff. If there are appropriate postsurgical patients on the unit, have them talk with Christine about their positive anesthesia experience.

3. *Initiation of Coping Mechanisms:* Christine is 9 years old. Her coping skills are limited to those used in her 9 years of life experience.

   Nursing Intervention: Check with Christine and observe verbal and nonverbal cues. Have her verbalize any uncertainties she may be experiencing. Some of this will be influenced by the progress of the illness.

4. *Adaptation:* Dependent on steps 1, 2, and 3.

   Nursing Intervention: As Christine accepts the idea of new information, new schema will follow. Though the outcome of her abdominal pain may initially be uncertain, her acceptance of the new schema will hopefully result in an increased comfort zone and decreased fear.

   Summary: A central tenet of Mishel's theory is the core position that uncertainty in illness must be addressed. If left unheeded, negative perceptions will escalate and clients will suffer. Their quality of life may be affected, and positive outcomes may be compromised. Nursing's responsibility in applying Mishel's theory is to reframe the client's perceived loss of control, or uncertainty and assist the client in developing new skills of assimilation and accommodation. The client will then be able to identify, develop, and master those targets capable of control.

FLORENCE NIGHTINGALE: THE FIRST NURSING THEORIST

If theory means to put concepts in a form in which relationships are described and predictions are made, then Florence Nightingale was the first nursing theorist. Nightingale did not deliberately set out to develop theory; rather her goal was to ease the suffering of soldiers and citizens of England. However, many important influences in her life directed her toward theory development:

- A classic education (philosophy [science], French, Italian, Greek, Latin, the arts, and history)
- Upper-class background, great wealth, and a prominent social life (operas, parties, balls)
- Religion and spirituality (she spent much time daydreaming about how she could serve God and experienced four visions from God)
- Era of reform throughout England (Industrial Revolution and dichotomy among the classes)

Despite her wealth and upper-class status, Nightingale was very dissatisfied with life. In 1852 she wrote a monograph, entitled "Cassandra," in which she pointed out the hopelessness inherent in being a woman in her day. "The family? It is too narrow a field for the development of an immortal spirit . . . . The system dooms some minds to incurable infancy, others to silent misery. Marriage is the only chance (and it is but a chance) offered to women for escape from this death; and how eagerly and how ignorantly it is embraced" (Nightingale, 1992, pp. 37-38). Her diary writings have been interpreted at times to be suicidal. Often depressed, Nightingale resorted to dreams as an escape from her unhappiness and discontent. Her personality and her own individual lifestyle (dogmatic, practical, a critical observer who was fascinated by numbers and recorded everything she saw and experienced) set her apart. She was self-willed, unhappy, and dissatisfied at times in spite of having beauty, a brilliant social career, and an education of which few men of her day could boast. She had enjoyed the best of music and art and the companionship of charming and important people. However, in refusing marriage and the round of social gaiety, she was revolting against the restrictions placed on women of her day, and she struggled to be allowed to work in a serious way.

Florence Nightingale eventually convinced her family to allow her to attend nurses training, and so began her distinguished career in developing professional nursing. Nightingale is well remembered for her significant contributions to professional nursing in the areas of theory of practice, nursing education, scholarship, and statistics. Box 3-4 provides Nightingale's definition of professional nursing.

Nightingale's Theory of Practice

Nightingale's theory of practice was documented for nurses and laypersons alike and served as the foundation for the promotion of health. This theory was referred to by Nightingale as the

---

BOX 3-4   *Nightingale's Definitions of Nursing*

Nursing is an art—and an art requiring an organized practical and scientific training.

Nursing is putting us in the best possible conditions for nature to preserve health—to prevent or restore or to cure disease or injury.

Nursing is therefore to help the patient live.

"Canons of Nursing" and guided the practice of professional nursing. A description of these canons, or standards, follows.

Ventilation and Warming. In the concept of ventilation and warming, Nightingale is very precise to "keep the air he breathes as pure as the external air without chilling him" (Nightingale, 1859, p. 8). Plenty of ventilation is necessary to carry off the noxious elements from a sick person's lungs and skin.

Noise. "Unnecessary noise, or noise that creates an expectation in the mind is that which hurts a patient" (Nightingale, 1859, p. 25). The nurse should guard against sudden noise, thoughtless chatter, and whispering in a patient's room. The effect of music may be beneficial.

Variety. Variety is another concept that helps alleviate suffering. Beautiful objects, brilliant colors, cut flowers, perhaps different things to do (e.g., handwork), and even pets may alleviate the boredom felt by those suffering.

Diet. The fourth concept is diet. "Sick cookery should half do the work of your poor patient's weak digestion" (Nightingale, 1859, p. 38). Nightingale reviews some of the common substances (gruel, arrowroot puddings, and egg flip) given to the sick.

Light. "It is the unqualified result of all my experience with the sick that second only to their need of fresh air is their need of light" (Nightingale, 1859, p. 47). Take the patient outside for direct sunlight. Keep rooms well lighted with no bed curtains or dark windows.

Chattering Hopes and Advices. According to Nightingale, chattering hopes and advices are attempts to cheer the patient by attendants and friends. Nightingale warns against this because she determines this to be false hope and hollow advice. She clearly appeals: "Leave off this practice of attempting to cheer the sick by making light of their danger and by exaggerating their probabilities of recovery" (Nightingale, 1859, p. 54).

Cleanliness (Health of Houses). Nightingale's attention to cleanliness takes up a large portion of her book. She writes that health depends on this. Describing the care of bed and bedding and of rooms and walls, she states the exact steps needed to clean each. In addition, she details how to clean the sick person so as to prevent poisoning by the skin. She describes the patient's feeling of well-being after washing and drying. The nurse needs to wash her own hands with friction as well. Some believe that Nightingale's success was based primarily on cleaning up the hospitals.

Because of these significant contributions to nursing and to improving the health of both soldiers and citizens alike, Nightingale was highly recognized. Her honors, decorations, medals, and citations may be seen in the United Services Museum in Whitehall, London. She was the first woman to ever receive the British Order of Merit by King Edward VII. One of her biographers (Cook, 1942) said "she was not only 'The Lady with a Lamp' throwing light into dark places but also a kind of galvanic battery stirring and sometimes shocking the dull and sluggish public to life and action."

SURVEY OF SELECTED NURSING THEORIES

A brief discussion of selected nursing theories follows. The date identified indicates the year in which the theory was first presented as a theory. However, most theories have continued to be refined and modified. A summary of the major nursing theorists with a brief description of their theory or conceptual model is presented in Table 3-2. This summary table provides the reader with information to guide further exploration of nursing theory. Box 3-5 provides on-line resources to begin further investigation of nursing theories.

Table 3-2 *Summary of Major Nursing Theorists and Theory Description*

DATE AND THEORIST	THEORY DESCRIPTION
1860: Florence Nightingale	Investigated the impact of the environment on healing.
1952: Hildegard E. Peplau	Explored the interpersonal relationship of the nurse and the client and identified the client's *feelings* as a predictor of positive outcomes related to health and wellness.
1960: Faye Abdellah	Client-centered interventions.
1961: Ida Jean Orlando	Nurse-client relationship; deliberate nursing approach using nursing process, which stressed the action of the individual client in determining the action of the nurse; focus is on the present or short-term outcome.
1966: Virginia Henderson	Nursing assists patients with fourteen essential functions toward independence.
1967: Myra Estrin Levine	Four conservation principles of inpatient client resources (energy, structural integrity, personal integrity, and social integrity).
1970: Martha E. Rogers	Science of unitary man: energy fields, openness, pattern, and organization; nurse promotes synchronicity between human beings and their universe/environment.
1971: Dorethea Orem	Nursing facilitates client self-care by measuring the client's deficit relative to self-care needs; the nurse implements appropriate measures to assist the client in meeting these needs by matching them with an appropriate supportive intervention.
1971: Imogene King	Goal attainment using nurse-client transactions; addresses client systems and includes society, groups, and the individual.
1974: Sister Callista Roy	Client's adaptation to condition using environmental stimuli to adjust perception.
1977: Madeline Leininger	Transcultural nursing and caring nursing; concepts are aimed toward caring and the components of a culture care theory, diversity, universality, worldview, and ethnohistory are essential to the four concepts (care, caring, health, and nursing).
1978: Jean Watson	Philosophy and science of caring and humanistic nursing; there are 10 "carative" factors, which are core to nursing; this holistic outlook addresses the impact and importance of altruism, sensitivity, trust, and interpersonal skills.
1979: Margaret Newman	Central components of this model are health and consciousness followed by concepts of movement, time, and space; all components are summative units, described in relationship to health as well as to each other.
1980: Dorothy E. Johnson	Behavioral system model for nursing; separates the psychologic and the physiologic aspects of illness; role of the nurse is to provide support and comfort to attain regulation of the client's behavior.
1981: Rosemarie Rizzo Parse	Man-living-health: man, by existing, actively participates in creating health according to environmental influences; individual is regarded as an open system wherein health is a process
1989: Patricia Benner and Judith Wrubel	Primacy of caring; the practice of nurses depends on the experience absorbed by engaging in five practice areas (novice, advanced beginner, competent, proficient, and expert) in the seven domains of nursing practice (helping, teaching-coaching, diagnostic and patient monitoring, effective management of rapid change, administration and monitoring of therapeutic interventions and regimens, monitoring and ensuring the quality of health care practices, and organizational work-role competencies).
1995: Betty Neuman	Systems model: wellness-illness continuum; promotes the nurse as the agent in assisting the client in adapting to and therefore reducing stressors; supports the notion of prevention through appropriate intervention

Hildegard E. Peplau (1952)—Interpersonal Relations as a Nursing Process: Man as an Organism That Exists in an Unstable Equilibrium

When the client incurs an insult that renders her or him incapable of moving forward because of existing stressful environmental conditions, anxiety increases. This condition creates a situation wherein the option is to either move in a backward direction or to remain on a plateau. Nursing intervention in Peplau's model focuses on reducing the related incapacitating stressors through therapeutic interpersonal interaction. Intervention involves the nurse assisting the client with mutual goal setting. These goals may address exploration of the identified problem, identification of viable options, and implementation of available resources for resolution. Nursing interpersonal process is present and interactive, using associated and appropriate nursing intervention skills, which incorporate the roles of the nurse as resource person, educator, mentor, transfer agent, and counselor. Peplau's model requires that the nurse have a self-awareness and insight regarding her or his own behaviors. This awareness may be applied in identifying and working through those behaviors unique to the client's schema. Fig. 3-2 presents Peplau's Psychodynamic Nursing Model.

Martha E. Rogers (1970)—Science of Unitary Human Beings: Humans as Energy Fields That Interact Constantly With the Environment

When the client/human unit incurs an insult that renders him or her out of balance with the universe, nursing interventions must be geared toward helping the client/human unit attain an increasing complex balance and synchronicity with the universe. Essential to Rogers' theory is the belief that each being is unique and consists of more than the collective sum of parts and that each being is continuously evolving in a forward momentum as he or she interacts continuously with the surrounding environmental field. Rogers theory states that a brain integration is necessary to support the notion of human-environmental synergy, using the right side of the brain to recognize every human unit's capacity for imagery, sensation, and emotion and the left side of the brain for language, abstraction, and thought.

Dorothea Orem (1971)—Self-Care Deficit Model: Self-Care, Self-Care Deficits, and Nursing Systems

When the client incurs an insult that renders him or her incapable of fully functioning, there is a self-care deficit, which makes nursing intervention necessary. The object of Orem's theory is to restore the client's self-care capability to enable him or her to sustain structural reliability, performance, and growth through purposeful nursing intervention. The aim of such intervention is to help the client cope with unmet care needs by acquiring the maximum level of function. This would be to either regain previous function or maximize available function present after the insult, hence restoring a sense of well-being.

Sister Callista Roy (1974)—Adaptation Model: Assistance With the Adaptation to Stressors to Facilitate the Integration Process of the Client

When the client incurs an insult that renders him or her in need of environmental modification, the nurse will be the change agent in assisting the individual with this adaptation. By helping the "biopsychosocial" client modify external stimuli, adaptation will occur. In the case of illness, the outcome will be a diminished or absent integration of the constantly changing setting known as the illness environment, with the constantly changing human, who is interacting with the existing outside surroundings. To attain wellness, adaptation must occur through this integration. The nurse's role is to promote this adaptation by modifying and

Middle-Range Nursing Theory

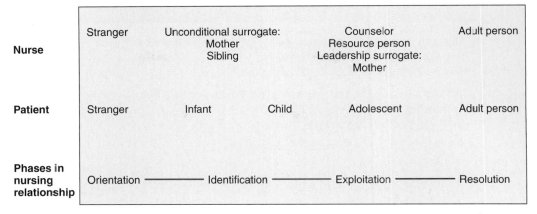

Nurse	Stranger	Unconditional surrogate: Mother Sibling		Counselor Resource person Leadership surrogate: Mother	Adult person
Patient	Stranger	Infant	Child	Adolescent	Adult person
Phases in nursing relationship	Orientation —————— Identification —————— Exploitation —————— Resolution				

FIG. 3–2 Peplau's Psychodynamic Nursing Model. Phases and changing roles in nurse-patient relationships. (From Peplau HE: *Interpersonal relations in nursing*, New York, 1952, GP Putnam and Sons, p. 54.)

regulating peripheral stimuli to enable the client's adaptation and integration with a supportive healing environment. In so doing, the nurse will be instrumental in assisting the client with the areas of health and well-being, life worth and value, and self-respect and dignity. Sister Callista Roy's Adaptation Model is depicted in Fig. 3-3.

Jean Watson (1978)—Model of Human Caring: Transpersonal Caring as the Fulcrum; Philosophy and Science as the Core of Nursing

When the client incurs an insult that renders him or her in need, the transpersonal process between the client and the nurse is considered a healing nursing intervention. An assumption of Watson's theory is that all persons require human caring to quell need. Hence the transpersonal process of "caring," or the caring between nurse, environment, and client, is essential to healing. Caring promotes the notion that every human being strives for interconnectedness with other humans and with nature. The nurse who implements these carative factors is the facilitator in the goal of restoring congruence between client's perceived self and the existent

Grand Nursing Theory

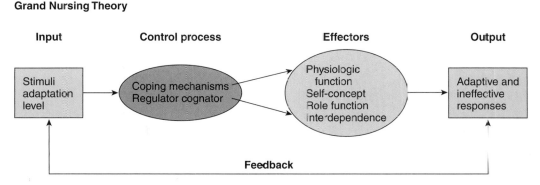

FIG. 3–3 Roy's Adaptation Model. Person as an adaptive system. (From Roy C: *Introduction to nursing: an adaptation model*, ed 2, Englewood Cliffs, NJ, 1984, Prentice Hall, p. 30.)

BOX 3–5 Helpful Websites

These sites provide links to information about several nursing theorists and their work.
www.valdosta.edu/nursing/nursing_theory.html
www.healthsci.clayton.edu/eichelberger/nursing.htm

This site links to theorists: King, Leininger, Levine, Neuman, Newman, Orem, Parse, Peplau, Rogers, Roy, Watson, and others.
www.sandiego.edu/nursing/theory/

This site links to Leininger's Transcultural Nursing model
www.tcns.org/

This site brings together current knowledge and experiences with teaching, practicing, and researching comfort.
www.uakron.edu/comfort/

self through the promotion of health and equilibrium. The expectation is that the client will experience balance and harmony in mind-body-soul. Harmony, or wellness, will prevail, whereas disharmony, or illness, will be altered, eliminated, or circumvented.

Merle Mishel—(1981, revised 1990): Uncertainty of Illness

Uncertainty in illness is frequently a stress-producing incident that is capable of contributing to negative physical and/or psychologic outcomes. Uncertainty exists when the client is unsure about a diagnosed illness. This uncertainty renders the client either incapable of assigning a concrete value to the illness itself or to a predictable outcome. Uncertainty can occur with a client misperceiving a diagnosed illness because of the inadequate information received, the health care provider incorrectly presuming client knowledge, or the health care informant failing to recognize the client's individual unique filtering of provided illness information. Mishel's theory is used in chronic illness and other practice settings. Mishel's model outlines a four-step approach in defining her theory. These include: (1) stimuli frame: antecedents generating client uncertainty, (2) appraisal stage: client assignment of a value, positive or negative, to the uncertainty, (3) initiation of coping mechanisms: client ability to develop, improvise, and implement skills to cope with uncertainty, and (4) adaptation: positive client assimilation and accommodation to uncertainty, resulting from effective coping. Mishel's theory establishes a framework that guides nursing practice by assisting nurses to work with clients in establishing interventions that promote positive outcomes.

Future of Nursing Theories and Theorists

At no time in history have so many health care concerns been the primary focus of federal and state legislative agendas. New questions are being asked in the twenty-first century about how health care is being conducted and managed. It is imperative that nurses be on the front lines to provide testimony in response to these queries.

The nursing shortage, scarce resources, health maintenance organizations, managed care, Medicare, welfare to work plans, confidentiality issues, parity of reimbursement, advanced practice nurses and their scope of practice, mandatory overtime, whistle-blower protection, prescriptive authority, licensure, multistate compacts, telemedicine, and many other policy issues that directly affect nursing practice are coming before the U.S. Congress and individual state legislative bodies for practice-related decisions. The direct impact on nursing cannot be overemphasized.

As nursing continues to operate in an environment of ongoing change, outcome data will be analyzed in an effort to provide quality care and access to that care for all clients in need of health care services. Therefore one may predict that established nursing theories will be reevaluated and modified accordingly. New theories will be created and developed that may help answer the health care questions of the twenty-first century. Simply put, nursing theories in the twenty-first century will embrace complex environmental changes that incorporate new technologies such as genetics, computers, noninvasive surgery, robotics, decreasing energy sources, increasing pollutants under a thinning ozone layer, environmental hazards, new diseases, and antibiotic-resistant illness. These changes have already resulted in client needs that differ from those as recent as 5 years ago.

SUMMARY

Let the reader beware. As stated at the beginning of this chapter, the information provided here is in no manner a substitute for a comprehensive analysis of existing nursing theories and theorists. More exist than are presented here, and, in fact, there are several comprehensive texts that cover these theories in depth. Instead, this chapter offers an overview of theory in the attempt to familiarize readers with the *idea* of theory. Selected theories are described to that end. Readers should identify nursing theories as ideas that have shaped and continue to shape the nursing profession in practice and research. It is our intention to assist students with understanding that practice and research are interdependent entities. In other words, practice and research cannot efficiently or effectively exist one without the other. Like the metaphor at the beginning of this chapter, without the existence of the stones (scientific data), the separation into specific concentrated yet related areas (theory) could not have happened.

CRITICAL THINKING ACTIVITIES

1. Read an article in a recent issue of *Nursing Research* and identify the conceptual or theoretical framework and the major concepts described in the conceptual or theoretical framework.
2. Select a nursing theory that you find most interesting. Then (a) explain the reason for choosing that particular theory and (b) discuss how the theory could guide nursing practice, using relevant examples from your clinical experiences.
3. Interview a master's-prepared and/or doctoral-prepared nurse. Ask the nurse to discuss how a specific theory has influenced her or his nursing practice and has guided her or his nursing research.

Additional resources are available on-line at: http://evolve.elsevier.com/Cherry/

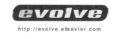

REFERENCES

Abdellah FG: The nature of nursing science, *Nurs Res* 18(5):393, 1969.

Anastasi T: Heredity, environment, and the question "how?" *Psychol Rev* 65:197-208, 1958.

Barnum BS: *Nursing theory: analysis, application, evaluation,* Philadelphia, 2000, JB Lippincott.

Bronowski J: *The origins of knowledge and imagination,* New Haven, Conn, 1972, Yale University Press.

Cook E: *The life of Florence Nightingale,* New York, 1942, MacMillan.

Donaldson SK, Crowley DM: The discipline of nursing, *Nurs Outlook* 26(2):113-120, 1978.

Good M, Moore SM: Clinical practice guidelines as a source of middle range theory: focus on acute pain, *Nurs Outlook* 44:74-79, 1998.

Jacob S: The grief process of older women whose husbands received hospice care, *J Adv Nurs* 24:280-286, 1996.

Jacox AK: Theory construction in nursing: an overview, *Nurs Res* 23(1):4, 1974.

Lenz ER et al: The middle-range theory of unpleasant symptoms: an update, *Adv Nurs Sci* 19(3):14-27, 1997.

Mishel MH: The measurement of uncertainty in illness, *Nurs Res* 30:258-263, 1981.

Mishel MH: Uncertainty in illness, *Image J Nurs Sch* 20: 225-231, 1988.

Mishel MH: Reconceptualization of the uncertainty in illness theory, *Image J Nurs Sch* 22:256-262, 1990.

Mishel MH: Uncertainty in acute illness, *Ann Rev Nurs Res* 15:57-80, 1997.

Nightingale F: *Notes on nursing: what it is, and what it is not* (commemorative edition), Philadelphia, 1992, JB Lippincott.

Nightingale F: *Notes on nursing: what it is, and what it is not,* London, 1859, Harrison and Sons.

Polit D, Beck C, Hungler B: *Essentials of nursing research,* New York, 2001, JB Lippincott.

SUGGESTED READINGS

Benner P: *From novice to expert: excellence in power in clinical nursing practice,* Menlo Park, Calif, 1984, Addison Wesley.

Chinn P, Kramer M: *Theory and nursing: integrated knowledge development,* St Louis, 1999, Mosby.

Johnson BM, Webber PB: *An introduction to theory and reasoning in nursing,* Philadelphia, 2001, JB Lippincott.

King I: *Toward a theory for nursing: general concepts of human behavior,* New York, 1971, John Wiley & Sons.

Leddy S, Pepper J: *Conceptual bases in professional nursing,* Philadelphia, 1998, JB Lippincott.

Leininger MM: *Transcultural nursing: concepts, theories and practices,* New York, 1978, John Wiley & Sons.

Levine M: The four conservation principles of nursing, *Nurs Forum* 6:93, 1967.

Newman MA: *Health as expanding consciousness,* St Louis, 1986, Mosby.

Nicoll L: *Perspectives on nursing theory,* Philadelphia, 1997, JB Lippincott.

Orem DE: *Nursing concepts of practice,* ed 6, New York, 1971, McGraw-Hill.

Parse RR: *Man-living-health: a theory of nursing,* New York, 1981, John Wiley & Sons.

Peplau HE: *International relations in nursing,* New York, 1952, GP Putnam.

Tomey AM, Alligood MR: *Nursing theorists and their work,* ed 5, St Louis, 2002, Mosby.

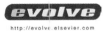
4

The Influence of Contemporary Trends and Issues on Nursing Education

Carrie B. Lenburg, EdD, RN, FAAN

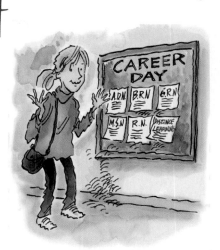

Educational diversity promotes access and career development.

VIGNETTE

John and Rosa met during their first nursing course. John liked the way Rosa spoke up in class and seemed to make the connections the instructor wanted. After class one day he asked her how she had learned so much so quickly, while he was having so much difficulty. As they talked, John learned that Rosa already had a baccalaureate degree in business and was in the second degree program; she wanted to become a nurse administrator. John had recently completed high school and decided that nursing offered good job opportunities in many types of work settings, although he was pretty sure he wanted to work in acute care. They each had searched various websites to find the nursing program right for them. They discovered that the same school could meet their needs, even though their backgrounds and aspirations were very different. After initial courses they would follow different tracks and schedules, but both would earn a BSN degree. Rosa already had plans to continue in the fast track option for a doctoral degree and encouraged John to continue in the MSN program and then earn certification for advanced practice. They both realized that the more challenging positions in nursing, as in other fields, would be available if they had strong educational preparation. Both John and Rosa were ready for this long-term commitment.

Questions to consider while reading this chapter:
1. How have current trends in society, health care, and nursing influenced nursing education?

2. What are the pros and cons of the different types of nurse education programs in term of professional practice?
3. What opportunities exist for you to advance your education beyond the current degree you are seeking, and what factors would influence a decision to pursue them?
4. What local, state, and national resources are available to learn more about the trends and issues that influence nursing education?
5. What are the most compelling reasons the nursing profession advocates ongoing professional development for continued practice and licensure?

KEY TERMS

Community-oriented curriculum Emphasizes health promotion, disease prevention, and health restoration in the context of extended family, community, and populations as clients, throughout the educational program.

Competency outcomes The results, or end-products, of planned study and experience that are focused on specific abilities required for practice.

Contemporary issues The problems, questions, and concerns that are current for the present time, whenever that may be. *Contemporary* always refers to the present time.

Continuing competence The ongoing development and improvement of those abilities and skills required for a given practice or role.

Educational mobility The progressive movement from one type or level of education to another, often based on flexible advanced placement options. Examples are progression from technical or diploma education to academic degree programs, such as RN to BSN or MSN; BSN to doctoral degree; or nonnursing degree to a nursing BSN, MSN, or ND degree.

Initial competence Required beginning knowledge and abilities learned and validated during the education program for a particular level or for certification.

Performance-based assessment Evaluation of abilities based on objective demonstration of specific required competencies rather than on evaluation of knowledge about those abilities. This may include performance in actual or simulated situations and in physical hands-on activities or the observable evidence of thinking skills such as problem solving, planning, writing, or coordination.

LEARNING OUTCOMES

After studying this chapter, the reader will be able to:
1. Integrate knowledge of current trends and issues in society into a more holistic perception of their influence on nursing, nursing education, students, and faculty.
2. Integrate knowledge of current trends and issues into a personal contemporary philosophy of ongoing professional development and practice.
3. Differentiate among various types of conventional and mobility nursing education programs and the issues associated with them.
4. Access pertinent current information resources related to evolving trends and issues as a component of ongoing professional development.

Nursing education (and practice) is influenced by a number of emerging trends and related issues in society; some of which are described in this chapter. Others also are important and are discussed elsewhere in this textbook. The selected trends are presented with related issues to provide students and faculty with a broader view of education. As American society becomes increasingly diverse, each trend precipitates different issues and problems. Trends result from issues in the past, just as these issues will lead to other trends in the future; this is the never-ending process of change. These trends are complex and overlapping, but they are presented here as separate categories to emphasize their importance; all of them influence nursing education and practice. This chapter is a brief overview and a stimulus for more in-depth exploration, using the print and Internet resources suggested in this chapter. The most influential trend in nursing education is the rapid development of knowledge and technology fueled by expanding research, communication, and electronic technology and the widening universe of the Internet. This in turn leads to expectations for nearly instant access and response to almost everything and results in multiple problems for students, faculty, and practitioners. This trend also is revolutionizing nursing and health care delivery on a national and global level. A related trend is the increasing urgency for competence, focused on specified standards and best practice and outcomes that are validated through objective performance assessment methods. Competency outcomes and performance-based evaluation now are required and are more stringent to safeguard consumers, nurses, and employers; therefore they are essential in all aspects of nursing education.

Other trends focus on ethics, bioethical developments, and personal choice. Expanding scientific research and innovations continue to lead to new treatment modalities but also to a multitude of complex issues. Expectations of personal freedom of choice raise ethical issues related to abortion, the right to die, and lifestyle preferences. Several highly interrelated trends include the changing characteristics of the population and the political and economic influences on health and health care. Collectively, they have influenced the trends of community- and consumer-oriented health care, interdisciplinary health care, use of alternative and complementary health practices, and increased collaboration among various agencies and institutions. Two other trends that affect nursing education are the increasing shortage of qualified nurses, faculty, and nursing students and the increasing stress related to the demands of personal and professional responsibilities.

These trends influence the number and types of nursing programs for basic and experienced students at the undergraduate and graduate levels. Students and the effective contemporary practicing nurse need to understand these trends and issues to cope with them and help change them into more positive trends.

TRENDS AND ISSUES IN CONTEMPORARY NURSING EDUCATION

In many ways nursing education is the same as it always has been: focused on preparation of nurses with enough knowledge and skill to safely and compassionately meet the health care needs of consumers and the community. The trends and related issues discussed here influence the content, expected outcomes, learning processes, and assessment methods in nursing education today.

Lenburg (2002) identified ten trends and summarized key issues related to students and faculty; they are described in this chapter and outlined in Table 4-1. These trends and issues

Table 4-1	Summary of Trends and Issues That Influence Nursing Education

MAJOR CONTEMPORARY TRENDS	RELATED ISSUES FOR STUDENTS	RELATED ISSUES FOR FACULTY AND THE PROFESSION
1. Knowledge expansion; use of technology and Internet	• Information overload; virtually unlimited global content via technology, Internet; identifying current and accurate information; outdated textbooks • High faculty expectations; limited time • Achieve core practice competencies	• Constant change of content and curriculum • Limited time to learn, integrate, help students • Changing technology, health care; expanding web of contacts; expected rapid response • Students in multiple locations simultaneously; concern about instruction, assessment by preceptors; varied expectations, goals • Limited time for reflection and creativity
2. Practice-based competency outcomes and evidence-based content	• Learning experiences focused on core practice competency outcomes, professional skills beyond technical psychomotor skills • Integration of "best practices," evidence-based standards, research findings into practice.	• Curriculum and faculty development time, work; focused outcomes and core competencies • Different conceptual model, more practice-specific; evidence-based standards of care • Initial and continuing competence; linked to licensure, multistate regulations, accreditation
3. Performance-based competency learning and assessment methods	• Multiple teaching-learning methods: interactive group work, collaboration, in-class and out-of-class projects, problem-based learning, self-responsibility, accountability for competence; interdisciplinary learning; using computers to access resources • Competency assessment based on performance examinations, licensure requirements	• Major changes for teacher and students regarding roles, methods, content; less lecture; more learner responsibility, interactive learning strategies • Different kind of preparation, focus on specific outcomes, core competencies • Assessment of competence using specific outcomes, core competencies
4. Sociodemographic, cultural diversity, economic and political changes	• Increased aging and ethnic diversity require respect for differences, preferences, customs • Community, congregation groups, service-learning projects; global community • Economic and political change influence health care delivery and access to clinical experiences • Violence in society, workplace; safety concerns • Different content, client care, clinical sites	• Changes in student and consumer populations require respect for diversity, changes in content and clinical experiences; emphasis on geriatrics, cultural diversity; health promotion; violence in society • Changing relationships among teachers, students, nurses, clients; impact on programs • Changes in time, effort, expertise on care delivery • Political, economic influence on care delivery
5. Community-focused, collaborative, interdisciplinary, alternative approaches	• Interdisciplinary collaborative learning • Alternative health practices; diversity • Broad scope of nursing; clinical experiences throughout community; continuum from acute care to health promotion; change from hospitals to home settings, rural to global settings • Requires more planning, travel time, expenses, arrangements; different skills, communications	• Alternative health practices; diversity • Need more time and planning to learn, implement different focus, content, methods, settings; interdisciplinary collaboration • Community concepts integrated throughout program; work with multiple agencies, community groups, congregations to promote health; service-learning; rural to global issues

Table 4-1—cont'd

	• Multiple teachers, preceptors, varying abilities	
6. Consumer-oriented society	• All expect value, quality, individual consideration, attention	• More concern about individual consumer's needs; shared authority, responsibility for health
	• Consumer initiatives for involvement and protection; balance standards and preferences	• Litigation; errors in medical, nursing practice; expectation for safe competent care
	• Increased litigation, medical/nursing errors; focus on safe, competent care	• Need to balance standards and preferences of students and faculty
	• Increased individual responsibility, accountability for learning and health	
7. Ethics and bioethical concerns	• Alternative solutions to ethical dilemmas; issues regarding diverse beliefs, gray zones instead of black-and-white absolutes; separate personal opinions and professional practice consequences for competence	• Teach ethics, bioethical concepts, changes; diverse interpretations and actions
		• Teach alternative solutions to ethical dilemmas; focus on competencies of assessment, reflective judgment, communication, caring
	• Integrate into professional practice acceptance of the individual's right of choice regarding life and death issues, health care methods	• Accountability for ethical competence; separate personal and professional practice
8. Increasing shortage of nurses, students, faculty, and support personnel	• Shortage of staff results in limitations in clinical learning; heavy workload, fewer preceptors with less time to help students	• Too few qualified teachers and preceptors
		• Fewer and less academically able students with economic problems need more help
	• Fewer qualified faculty results in higher ratio	• Aging and retention of nurses results in issues for future of profession
	• Students need more, not less, clinical learning; have more responsibility with less individual help	• Issues regarding recruitment, teaching, counseling
9. Increasing professional and personal responsibilities	• Required to validate initial and continuing competence, lifelong learning, preparation to meet professional expectations	• High stress from changes in curriculum, teaching methods, technology, rapid change in clinical settings and regulations; fewer resources
	• High stress from competing demands of school, home, meeting competency outcome and completing programs; affects nurse's own health	• Required clinical practice, research, publications, service; increasing demands on professional and personal life increase stress
10. Diversity, flexibility, mobility, and delivery of education programs	• Pros and cons of mediated/Internet courses and programs; self-directed learning	• Issues regarding philosophy, curriculum development, and implementation for diverse students; entry into practice debates, conflicts
	• Expenses and time regarding education, care of dependents; conflict of work and study	• Diverse mobility options take more time, energy, resources; students at a distance
	• Increased adult responsibilities influence learning and completion; need multiple-entry, multiple-exit mobility or other flexible options	• Problems regarding use of Internet and other mediated courses; issues of instruction, assessment, quality, and accountability for education, practice; legal, ethical concerns

illustrate nursing's complex environment and help to explain how and why nursing education needs to change and function in contemporary society. The final trend focuses on nursing education itself and on its continuing and emerging issues. The trends actually form a constellation of factors that simultaneously influence nursing education and practice. Box 4-1 lists major organizations concerned with nursing education; they are resources for more data.

Knowledge Expansion and Use of Technology and the Internet

With ever-expanding developments in information technology, the volume of knowledge is growing exponentially on a global level. From e-mails to complex research documents and video images, nurses and students, like everyone else, are communicating more frequently, with more contacts and at the speed of the Internet. This ability to access and disseminate unlimited information almost instantly has enormous benefits but also presents major issues and concerns. Computer-accessible knowledge provides essential content for nursing and other courses. Many textbooks and journal articles are nearly obsolete by the time they are published, thus an expanding array of websites and online journals have become major learning resources. Websites are more interactive than texts and link to multitudes of other

---

BOX 4-1 *Selected Organizations Relevant to Nursing Education: General Description and Purpose*

American Academy of Nursing—The organization of top leaders in all facets of nursing: practice, education, administration, research, organizations, and government; the think tank of the profession; promotes advancement of all aspects of nursing; publishes position papers, conference proceedings, and documents to advance nursing.

American Association of Colleges of Nursing—The organization of deans and directors of baccalaureate and higher degree nursing programs; establishes standards for programs, concerned with legislative issues that pertain to professional nursing education; publishes the *Journal of Professional Nursing, The Essentials of Baccalaureate Education* (1998), and other related documents pertaining to the BSN and higher degree education.

American Nurses Association—The major national nursing organization concerned with broad scope of practice issues; standard of practice, scope of practice, ethics, legal, employment; a federation of state nurses associations; publications related to array of practice issues and standards.

Commission on Collegiate Nursing Education (CCNE)—A subsidiary of AACN with responsibility for establishing and implementing standards for the accreditation of baccalaureate and graduate degree programs in nursing.

National Council of State Boards of Nursing—Organization of all state boards; coordinates licensure activities on national level; conducts studies as basis for creating licensure examination; developed computerized licensure examinations; works with other organizations to promote nursing standards and regulation.

National League for Nursing (NLN)—The national organization of nurse educators, with councils for four types of programs (LPN, diploma, ADN, and BSN); only nursing organization that includes lay citizen concerned with nursing and health care. NLN also has councils for nursing informatics, research in nursing education, wellness centers, and other focused concerns; accredits home health care agencies (CHAPS); multiple types of print and visual publications.

NLN Accreditation Commission—Formed in 1997 as a subsidiary of NLN with responsibility for establishing and implementing standards for the accreditation of all types of schools of nursing; follows guidelines from the U.S. Department of Education.

National Student Nurses Association—Organization of statewide student nurse associations; concerned with education and career issues; provides student perspectives to other national nursing organizations. Internet address to locate many other organizations: www.lib.umich.edu/hw/nursing/organ.html

helpful resources (Nicoll, 2000; Skiba, 1997). Even though updated frequently, websites also become outdated quickly.

Students can easily become distracted by the intriguing web of links they encounter while they search websites to complete assignments and communicate with others in class or around the world. Thus using the Internet actually may take *more* time to find and learn content, although it usually provides broader, more specific, and more current information. With global use of the Internet, students living in other states, or even other countries, now can participate in team projects and research, even though they have never met. To prepare for clinical practice, students must learn the competencies required for information-intensive health care delivery. Mobile computers and software, like the Nightingale Tracker, help nurses manage complex patient data and thus reduce stress and errors (Sloan and Delahoussaye, 2003).

These technology and Internet trends generate several issues. Almost unlimited information is available, but it requires more time and skill to navigate the Web, at a time when most students seem to have less time for study (Focus, 1999; Mallow and Gilje, 1999). Learning from the Internet and using technology in practice requires disciplined focus, clear guidelines, and expected outcomes related to assignments to minimize overload and frustration. Learning from the Internet also helps students develop skills in analytic thinking, decision making, and reflective judgment, all of which are essential competencies but are not easily learned. Other issues related to Internet learning include time management, the integration of information, identifying reputable sources, learning and keeping up with ever-changing technology, and meeting the expectations for immediate responses to a widening network of contacts.

Practice-Based Competency Outcomes

Trends in business and commerce often find their way into higher education and nursing education. One of these trends is the emphasis on using competency outcomes to set directions and goals related to real-world practice. To focus on outcomes is to focus on preferred results. What really matters is that students (nurses) achieve the competency outcomes that specify the skills actually needed in practice. Competency outcomes are the measurable results of time and efforts spent in learning. Achieving competence in realistic practice-based abilities is the preferred outcome; it is the target, the goal to be reached, the purpose of study and of education.

However, for most teachers and students, this outcomes approach is very different from past teaching and learning methods and evaluation. Outcomes are not the same as objectives and are not merely terminology changes. The outcomes approach requires significant revisions in thinking, in course syllabi and learning methods focused on the competencies nurses need for practice and changes in complex contemporary health care environments. For students it means a change from memorizing class notes and readings (the "tell me what I need to know" attitude) to actually learning to integrate knowledge in making complex decisions and to be competent and confident in applying the designated abilities.

Practice-based competency outcomes specify the destination students need to reach. The interactive learning strategies are the directions and guidelines for getting there, and performance-based assessment confirms they have arrived at the right place. The process is important, but achieving final competency outcomes is the bottom line.

Nursing organizations continue to revise standards to focus on competencies. Explore the websites in Table 4-2 for the most current information for groups such as the American Association of Colleges of Nursing (AACN), the American Nurses Association (ANA), the Joint

Table 4-2 Online References Related to Nursing Education

The list below represents *examples* of Internet resources as beginning points. It is not a complete or "best" list; it is a suggested sampling. At the time of this writing addresses are operational, but be aware that they may change, become obsolete, or be discontinued; others are added frequently. Most addresses listed below begin with "http://www." unless otherwise indicated. Note that some have hyphens, or other symbols, and some are case-sensitive, meaning that the capital letters MUST be used exactly as specified. Search engines to use to find sites on the Internet include Google, Yahoo, Teoma, and others (all of these end with ".com").

NAME OF SOURCE	ADDRESS	COMMENTS
Nursing organizations and associations directly or indirectly concerned with nursing education		
American Association of Colleges of Nursing	aacn.nche.edu	BSN and higher degree schools
American Association for History of Nursing	aahn.org	Membership, contacts, publication
American Holistic Nurses Association	ahna.org	Publications, certificate program, and CE course listings
American Nurses Association	nursingworld.org	Links to organizations, publications (*American Nurse*), career, job lists
American Nurses Credentialing Center	nursingworld.org/ancc/	Information regarding certification programs, requirements, etc.
American Nursing Informatics Association	ania.org	Links to multiple informatics sites
American Organization of Nurse Executives	aone.org (ahaonlinestore.com)	Information; publications regarding nursing leadership, administration
Commission on Collegiate Nursing Education	aacn.nche.edu/accreditation/index.htm	Accreditation of BSN and higher degrees
International Congress of Nurses	icn.ch	ICN resources and links
International Parish Nursing Resource Center	ipnrc.parishnurses.org	Information, links to congregational, parish resources
National Council of State Boards of Nursing	ncsbn.org	Information regarding NCLEX and regulations
National League for Nursing (NLN)	nln.org	Information regarding schools, testing
National League for Nursing Accrediting Commission	nlnac.org	Information regarding accreditation of all types of nursing schools
National Student Nurses Association	nsna.org	Information for students (see www.toledolink.com/~ornrsg/)
Nursing Alliance	nursing-alliance.org	Consortium of nursing organizations (specialty and others)
Sigma Theta Tau International	nursingsociety.org	Honor society information; research directory; case studies
Southern Nursing Research Society	snrs.org	Example: regional organization; research; new on-line journal
Midwest Nursing Research Society	mnrs.org	Example: regional organization; links to resources
Examples of on-line journals		
Online Journal of Nursing Informatics	hhdev.psu.edu/nurse/ojni/index/htm	Hosted by Pennsylvania State University, Health and Human Development
Online Journal of Issues in Nursing	nursingworld.org/ojin/	Hosted by American Nurses Association at Kent State University
Southern Online Journal of Nursing Research	snrs.org/sojnr/	Southern Nursing Research Society (began 2000)
Resources concerned with health, nursing, and/or education		
Agency for HealthCare Research and Quality	ahrq.org	U.S. Dept of HHS; proceedings (working conditions, safety, etc.)

Table 4-2—cont'd

All Star Directories, Inc.	allnursingschools.com	Resource links to schools of nursing and on-line guide to nursing education
Alternative Health Care	wholenurse.com	Resource links, information regarding alternative health practices
American Hospital Association	hospitalconnect.com	Hospital links; nursing shortage, and workforce issues
Electronic College Guide	ecollege.com	Links to colleges by type, state; resources
Discover Nursing	discovernursing.com	Listing of programs, scholarships in nursing
Distance Learning Channel	ed-x.com	Listing of about 3000 courses, schools, programs
Fuld Institute of Technology in Nursing	fitne.net	For educators; publications, links; Nightingale Tracker system
Health and Environment Resource	noharm.org	Patient safety, products; coalition of 429 nursing and other organizations
Health (multiple links to resources)	healthweb.org/index.cfm	Links to multiple health resources
Healthy People 2010	health.gov/healthypeople	Publication; other links
Institute of Medicine	iom.edu	Publications, other links via National Academy of Sciences
Lippincott Publisher (multiple links)	nursingcenter.com	Links to journals, schools, organizations, publications
Martindale's Health Science Guide	maartindalecenter.com	Link: HSG/Nursing/Martindale Virtual Nurse Center
National Library of Medicine	nlm.nih.gov/locatorplus/	National Library locator, databases; information retrieval
Nightingale Institute for Health and Environment	nihe.org	Resource to promote health and environment
Nursing Ethics Network	bc.edu/nursing/ethics	New resource (Boston College); RN ethics survey; helpful links
Nursing Informatics	nursing-informatics.net	Links to international resources
Nursing (multiple links to resources)	nursingnet.org	Links to resources, allied health, continuing education, jobs
Nursing (multiple links; alpha listings)	inurse.com	Links to institutions, organizations, continuing education, jobs
Nursing (multiple web resources)	ublib.buffalo.edu/libraries/units/ hsl/internet/nsgsites (very informative)	
Nursing: University of Michigan (multiple resources)	lib.umich.edu/hw/nursing/organ	Organizations, practice, education
Pew Health Professions Commission	futurehealth.ucsf.edu/	Publications regarding health care changes, service learning projects
Robert Wood Johnson Foundation	rwjf.org	Colleagues in Caring project, multiple others, grants
Slack Publisher (multiple links)	slackinc.com	Link: nursing-related journals, organizations, etc.
Southern Regional Electronic Campus	srec.sreb.org	Links to online resources, courses, college programs in South
U.S. Government Resources	firstgov.gov	Excellent links to multiple official resources, documents
U.S. Government (major links to resources)	medlineplus.gov	Links regarding disease, health, DHHS, clinical trials, etc.

Continued

Table 4-2   *Online References Related to Nursing Education—cont'd*

U.S. Government consumer gateway	healthfinder.gov	Links to health; consumer-focused support groups; one for kids
U.S. Government Division of Nursing	bhpr.hrsa.gov/	Nurse survey; databases available by state
Virtual Nurse	virtualnurse.com	Links to career, education, resources, health, alternative resources

Online nursing education resources

Most colleges and universities offer some form of distance learning and/or on-line courses; some offer entire degrees. Some examples of these educational institutions located throughout the country are cited below with website addresses; use these as a format guide to locate others of interest. Please note: Specific addresses, names, and/or offerings may change subsequent to this publication. (In most instances the address follows " http://www. ".)

California State University, Dominguez Hills	csudh.edu	State-wide mobility program; distance learning
Case Western Reserve University	cwru.edu	Multi-option; international; research; nursing informatics
Excelsior College (Regents College)	excelsior.edu	External degrees: AND, BSN, master's programs
George Mason University	gmu.edu	Campus and mobility programs; WANRR (research resource)
Indiana University/Purdue University	iupui.edu	Multiple programs and sites; nursing informatics
University of Alabama, Birmingham	uab.edu	Campus and distance programs
University of Colorado Health Sci Center	uchsc.edu	Undergraduate and graduate Internet courses, programs
University of Kansas	kumc.edu	Campus and distance programs
University of Maryland	umd.edu	Multiple programs; mobility; nursing informatics
University of Phoenix	phoenix.edu	Multiple on-line Internet programs; courses
University of Texas, Austin	utexas.edu	Campus; multiple options; nursing informatics
University of Washington	son.washington.edu	Campus; research focus; multiple programs

Commission on Accreditation of Healthcare Organizations (JCAHO), the Nursing Alliance (an alliance of many specialty organizations), the National League for Nursing Accrediting Commission (NLNAC), and the Pew Commission (Bellack and O'Neil, 2000). These emerging trends and issues related to competency outcomes have a direct impact on all types of nursing education and practice.

Performance-Based Learning and Assessment Methods

A change in methods used to promote learning and evaluate competence is another trend closely linked to competency outcomes. In the era of cost containment and risk management, finding the most effective and efficient ways for students to become competent is paramount and challenging. An important related issue is the need for students and teachers to change their roles and accountability in this learning process. Instead of being passive senders and receivers of information (giving lectures and taking notes during class), students and instructors need to engage in more interactive and collaborative roles to promote competence in the eight core practice-based competencies and related course content.

In actual clinical practice nurses must be competent in creative and effective problem solving, communication, teaching, caring, and management. These skills are learned more effectively through participation in interactive exercises such as problem-based learning, case study analysis, and diverse projects that require engagement and integration of relevant content. In addition to hospitals and extended care facilities, clinical learning settings include community agencies, congregational health, parish nursing, hospice care, homeless clinics, rural migrant clinics, schools, and prisons (Brendtro and Leuning, 2000; Mathews-Smith et al, 2001; Mundt, 1997; Palmer, 2001; Solari-Twadell and McDermott, 1999).

The concept of clinical evaluation also is changing to focus on documented actual competence in the most realistic circumstances possible, rather than just paper-and-pencil tests and informal observations by instructors or preceptors. Objective validation of competence requires performance examinations that specify the critical elements (the application of mandatory principles) that must be met according to established practice standards (Lenburg, 1999; Luttrell et al, 1999; Scanlon, Care, and Gessler, 2001; Tracy et al, 2000). In addition to "hands-on" basic skills, the development of a structured portfolio is another method to document some competencies of students and nurses (Lenburg, 2001; Serembus, 2000; Trossman, 1999). The rapid expansion of knowledge and technology and related changes in competency outcomes require major changes in teaching-learning process and evaluation of actual performance abilities.

These trends precipitate issues for students and teachers. Sometimes students think it is easier just to figure out "what the teacher wants" and "study for the test" rather than engage in interactive exercises in and out of class. Through such exercises, however, students learn to make realistic decisions, collaborate in group process, and manage time and resources. It is easier to take written tests than to demonstrate actual competence through performance examinations that require 100% accuracy of specified critical elements. Yet this kind of competence is what consumers need, employers expect, and practitioners must deliver. Memorization is ineffective for complex problem solving and collaborative communication. The increase in reported medical-related errors vividly emphasizes the need for more effective validation of performance competence in school and the workplace (Bellack and O'Neil, 2000; IOM, 2000).

Sociodemographic, Cultural Diversity, and Economic and Political Changes

From rural to metropolitan areas throughout the United States the population is undergoing significant transformation (Baer et al, 2000). More people are living longer and experiencing the chronic consequences. The number of diverse ethnic minorities is expanding in rural as well as in urban areas, and more families survive in poverty, become homeless, or are uninsured. Other significant changes include differences in lifestyle choices and personal living arrangements. The definition of "family" is radically different today, as evident in the number of single individuals living with other singles, single-parent households, and same-sex couples (with and without children). Other economic and political trends pertain to health care policy and delivery, Medicare, social security, immigrants, and education. These changes present many issues for nursing and education, as described in such references as Lutz, Herrick, and Lehman, 2001, and Lenburg et al, 1995. Increasing violence, abuse, intolerance, and terrorism in society and the workplace are other concerns faced by health care providers and educators (Melamed, 2000; ANA, 1999, 2002).

Some relevant issues for students are the distinct differences among patients in their responses to illness, treatments, and caregivers, which are based on differences in age, culture, religion, and life experiences in family and community (Ryan et al, 2000). Additional factors pertain to the heritage of patients' ethnic and geographic location. For example, issues related to nursing care may differ considerably among those in areas that are rural or urban, mountains or plains, north, south, east, or west. Ways of healing and caring may include many alternative, nonmedical, natural remedies and embrace the benefits of religion, rituals, and traditions (LaSala et al, 1997; Moylan, 2000). How the nurse responds to these modalities may make all the difference in the therapeutic relationship and outcome of care.

Effective and thoughtful nursing care is individualized according to client characteristics and circumstances, which is why students need to learn as much as possible from sociology, cultural diversity, psychology, ethics, religion, economics, history, and literature, as well as basic and nursing sciences. Learning the stories of diverse peoples, their customs, life experiences, and expectations not only is interesting but also expands human understanding and creativity essential in professional practice.

Community-Focused Interdisciplinary Approaches

The societal trends described above, along with the large-scale economic and political influences to reduce health care costs, helped foster community-focused health care with an interdisciplinary emphasis. The extraordinary expansion of knowledge and innovative treatment technologies make it common practice for surgical procedures to be performed in ambulatory outpatient settings or for drugs to be used instead of surgery. In addition, diverse health-conscious groups are making progress to change the national orientation from "illness care" to promoting more efficient and effective health care. Another contributing factor is the increasing emphasis on health of the family as a whole and on entire communities and populations (Kiehl and Wink, 2000; Lutz, Herrick, and Lehman, 2001).

The concept of community is perceived as groups of individuals who share particular characteristics that shape their collective relationships, regardless of where they are located—for example, religious communities, ethnic or cultural communities, and homeless communities. The concept of community agencies also has changed, with hospitals seen as one of many community resources. These changes require a very different philosophy of care that embraces interdisciplinary and interagency collaboration. This health care culture incorporates concepts of shared responsibility for health promotion among individuals, family, community, and multiple care providers. More than ever, family members (and even neighbors) become caregivers and members of the health care team and thus need to learn caregiving skills.

One issue that results from these changes is the role change from "nursing as illness care in hospitals" to "nursing as health promotion and care management for individuals in the context of family, and family within the community." This requires a different perception and integration of core practice competencies. Care delivery is more complex as general hospitals have become extended critical care units, and patients with less acute conditions receive care in ambulatory settings or at home. Thus many acutely ill and postsurgical patients now need acute nursing care, as well as health maintenance and promotion, in their homes or other settings (Mathews-Smith et al, 2001; Mitty and Mezey, 1998; Ryan et al, 2000). Regardless of the setting, care management involves an interdisciplinary team usually coordinated by nurses.

This reality poses the bipolar challenge of how to prepare nurses who are competent to manage illness and preventive health care for diverse clients dispersed throughout the community, as well as to prepare them to provide critical care to hospital patients who are sicker and go home quicker. Students benefit from different clinical experiences dispersed throughout the community and under the supervision of preceptors and nursing staff, they gain the competence and confidence they need to meet these diverse roles. Toward this end, many schools have developed service-learning partnerships with communities and changed the curriculum to promote more competent and effective community-based health care (Green and Adderley-Kelly, 1999; Kiehl and Wink, 2000; Lutz, Herrick, and Lehman, 2001; Miller and Swanson, 2002; Narsavage et al, 2003; White and Henry, 1999).

Like a row of dominoes falling, these changes pose yet more issues. For example, where will new graduates work (institutions or community)? What kinds of patients will they care for (young or old, with acute or chronic conditions)? What skills will they need to provide competent care? This diversity requires more knowledge about the art and science of nursing and essential skill in all core practice competencies, especially creative problem solving, interdisciplinary collaboration, and ability to use electronic information technology and emerging mobile communication technology effectively and independently (Engelke and Britton, 2000).

Other issues include working with preceptors and staff in many locations with less one-to-one clinical instructor interaction. This requires planning, time, and resources for travel to multiple clinical settings and out-of-class peer group work and projects, but it promotes opportunities for students to learn collaboration and different approaches to care in multiple settings and to develop confidence and competence. In addition to acute care, useful experiences may include projects in congregational health, parish nursing, rural health, and alternative health care (Brendtro and Leuning, 2000; Palmer, 2001).

Consumer-Oriented Care: Engagement, Safety, and Privacy

As consumers have become more knowledgeable about illness care, health promotion, and the consequences of errors in care, they also have become more assertive about their right to competent and prudent care and their right to privacy of information. The economics and politics of health care and access to comprehensive information via the Internet have promoted more consumer involvement in setting health care standards and policies. Consumers are more active on health-related boards and committees and consumer advocacy groups. For example, AARP, with its millions of senior citizen members, promotes political action to influence improved health care and encourages members to use Internet resources. (See Internet resources in Table 4-2.)

Informed and engaged patients are better able to make effective decisions and promote their well-being; thus, patient-teaching is a core practice competence. Interactive learning and service-learning projects are valuable ways for students to learn to work with consumers in planning projects that promote safety, health, and community responsibility for health (Hurst and Osban, 2000; White and Henry, 1999). Nurses need to change their approach from "giving patient care" to "working with" the patient and family as members of the health care team. These changes require a different emphasis on interpersonal communication, making decisions for care outcomes, safety, and privacy. The new HIPAA law passed in 2002 protects patient privacy and dignity and requires new levels of scrutiny by providers (HIPAA, 2002).

Another major issue affecting nursing education is the increasing number and consequences of serious medical errors. These errors have led to an astonishing number of deaths and an increased number of lawsuits with high associated costs, which further increase the cost of health care and tarnish the belief in the quality of health care in this country (Institute of Medicine, 2000). Unfortunately, a large percentage of errors are attributed to nurses. Therefore, nursing faculty and administrators are increasingly concerned with ensuring the competence of students and nurses (Bellack and O'Neil, 2000). This serious problem is exacerbated by the increasing shortage of nurses and other personnel as well as by the preparation of nurses, as reported in a recent study by Aiken (2003).

The medical-error issues have in large part supported the need to require competency-based education and performance assessment in schools of nursing and as part of employer annual evaluations and accreditation (JCAHO, 2000). Another important study submitted to the US Department of Health and Human Services in 2000 was conduced jointly by the Advisory Council on Nursing Education and Practice and the Council on Graduate Medical Education (USDHHS, 2000). Its primary focus is the collaboration between nurses and physicians to promote patient safety and reduce errors (see http://bhpr.hrsa.gov/nursing/nacnep/patientsafety.htm).

Ethics and Bioethical Concerns

Another trend affecting nursing education is the growing number of patients who have different ways of responding to illness, treatment, and care providers, which raises ethical issues of who is right and who has the right to prevail. This is particularly relevant for end-of-life issues (Matzo et al, 2003; Rushton and Sabatier, 2001) and freedom of choice issues. Some issues are based on the separation of professional practice behaviors from personal beliefs and preferences; this often means acceptance of the concept of "a gray continuum" instead of simplistic black-and-white interpretations.

Diversity of backgrounds also usually means diversity in interpretation of behaviors, events, and language (Lenburg, et al, 1995; Riley and Fry, 2000). Some of the most controversial issues include the right of individual choice regarding abortion, artificial insemination, organ transplant, human tissue cloning, preference in sexual partners, and euthanasia or the right to die a dignified death. Other issues emerge from the growing use of alternative health remedies outside the mainstream of traditional Western medicine such as herbs, acupressure, magnets, or touch.

Increasing Shortage of Nurses, Students, and Faculty

A recurring trend over many decades is the shortage of qualified nurses and, more recently, of nurse teachers and students. In addition to other chapters in this book, the following references provide historical and current details regarding the numbers and causes of the shortage: Baer, 2000; Heller, Oros, and Durney-Crowley, 2000; and Nursing Shortage, 2001. The shortage and its consequences are also explored on several websites such as AACN (2000b), ANA (1999), and specialty organizations (see Table 4-2). As previously discussed, one of the most serious consequences of the nursing shortage is the increasing number of errors in patient care (Bellack and O'Neil, 2000; IOM, 2000). Two primary aspects of the trend include the predicted short- and long-term shortage and the increased aging of those already in the profession (Buerhaus, 2001; Buerhaus, Staiger, and Auerbach, 2000).

The shortage and the aging of nurses have additional consequences and pose further issues for students, teachers, and the profession. Inadequate clinical staff results in lower quality of care, as well as fewer staff preceptors who are under increased stress and do not have enough time to work with students. More nurses work part-time and for staffing agencies, which means that some students may be in clinical settings without adequate instruction and supervision or may have fewer opportunities to learn specific clinical skills. Another consequence is that students may be assigned to multiple and diverse community clinical settings, which also may be short-staffed, making it difficult for a student to find a willing preceptor or role model. Students also may work with nurses who have inadequate educational or clinical background to help them integrate classroom content with clinical practice, which could lead to undesirable nursing care. In such frustrating circumstances students need to take more

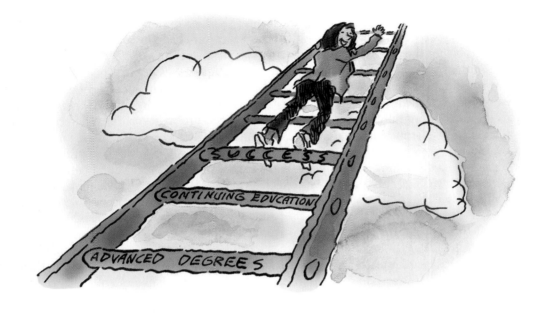

Education is the ladder
to success

individual responsibility and initiative to gain core competencies. These conditions present special concerns for students in distance learning and Internet-based programs who are even more dependent on qualified nurses as preceptors.

The number of qualified applicants to nursing programs declined especially between 1998 and 2003. Enrollments increased slightly in 2003-2404 but not enough to relieve the shortage (AACN, 2000b). Many students are older and/or have prior education in nursing or in other fields (Frik, Speed, and Pollock, 1996). Such students often seek kinds of learning experiences that are different from those of young students; they may find available courses and experiences too restrictive and thus frustrating. Nursing programs also are faced with shortage of qualified teachers because of the declining number of students in master of science in nursing (MSN) and doctoral programs that focus on education. This in turn may lead to a ratio of more students per teacher—at a time when one-to-one supervision is more important than ever because of the complexity of the clinical learning experience.

These trends and issues precipitated a national drive in 2001-2003 by nursing leaders and organizations to recruit and retain nurses, students, and teachers (AACN, 2001; Newell-Withrow and Slusher, 2001; NLN, 2003; Tanner, 2003). Their efforts also resulted in the U.S. Congress passing legislation to increase funding to help resolve the shortage (AACN, 2003b).

Increasing Professional and Personal Responsibilities

In this context another trend with multiple related issues has become increasingly evident. Students, teachers, and nurses confront increasing life responsibilities and associated stressful demands on time and resources. Many cope simultaneously with the explosion of new information and technology; changing health care systems; more precise expectations for learning outcomes; more interactive and out-of-class methods of learning; multiple care settings; higher expectations for competent performance; shortage of nurse preceptors and teachers; and multiple cultural, ethical, and legal aspects of an ever-changing society. Many may also be responsible for the care of dependent children and aging parents.

At the same time, contemporary conditions require nurses to keep their skills and training current through planned ongoing professional development. Complexities in practice, emphasis on reducing errors, and increasing consumer activism increase the need for nurses to document continuing competence for initial licensure, relicensure, and recertification. Changes in state and multistate regulations increasingly focus on the need for initial and continuing competence (Gaffney, 1999; NCSBN, 2001-2003). Many states require continuing education, and some mandate a portfolio approach to validate continuing competence (see websites for NCSBN and specific states, such as California, Kentucky, Oklahoma, Tennessee). ANA has cited the continuing competence of nurses as one of its focus issues of concern since the late 1990s (ANA 1999, 2000; also see issues of *The American Nurse*, 2000-2003).

At this writing, the New York State Board of Nursing has proposed a significant change for ADN graduates. If the proposal becomes a regulation, future ADN graduates in New York must earn a baccalaureate or higher degree within 10 years after graduation or their RN license will revert to an LPN license (Zittel, 2003). This proposal follows a model already established to require advanced education for teachers and other disciplines and is designed as an incentive for lesser-prepared nurses to continue formal preparation for professional practice. The model would also serve as an incentive for future students to seek BSN and higher degrees for entry into practice.

The high stress levels associated with these professional and personal demands have consequences for nurses' individual health, as well as the heath and well-being of those around them. These issues illustrate how important it is for all individuals involved in the educational process to be more caring, understanding, respectful, and helpful to one another. Teachers, students, administrators, staff nurses, employers, family, and friends need to learn anew the meaning of "caring community" in the context of rapid and complex change.

DIVERSITY IN NURSING EDUCATION PROGRAMS

A brief review of the major types of education programs that prepare nurses for licensure sets the stage for summarizing some contemporary issues related to diversity, flexibility, and distance delivery of education programs. Details about numbers and types of programs, students, and graduates are provided by the National League for Nursing (NLN; 1997), and also by the AACN (see websites listed in Table 4-2 for publications and reports). Table 4-3 provides a concise overview of program types.

Licensed Practical Nurse Programs

Practical nurse programs provide the shortest and most restricted option for individuals seeking a nursing license. Typically, licensed practical nurse (LPN) programs are 9 to 12 months in length and may be offered by high schools, adult education and vocational technical schools, or hospitals. In California and Texas the term *vocational nurse* is used, and graduates who are licensed are called *LVNs*. Each state board of nursing sets responsibilities and scopes of practice. The LPN/LVN usually is required to work under the supervision of a registered nurse (RN) or other licensed person, and scope of practice focuses on technical nursing procedures and treatments. LPNs/LVNs typically are employed in hospitals, nursing homes, offices, and other

Table 4-3	Types of Nursing Education Programs		
TYPE OF PROGRAM AND CREDENTIAL	**TYPE OF INSTITUTION**	**LENGTH OF PROGRAM**	**PURPOSE AND SCOPE**
Practical/vocational nurse program: prepares for LVN/LPN license	High school, hospitals, vocational-technical schools	9-12 mo	Basic technical bedside care hospitals, nursing homes, home care, offices in LPN positions
Diploma program: prepares for RN license	Hospitals, some in conjunction with colleges	2-3 yr	Basic RN positions; hospitals and agency care
Associate degree nursing: prepares for RN license	Community and junior colleges	2 yr	Basic technical care in RN positions, primarily in institutions
Bachelor's degree in nursing (BSN): prepares for RN license	Colleges and universities	2-4 yr (depends on type option)	Basic professional practice as RN; management, community and public health settings; prepares for graduate school and certification; basic programs are 4 yr; mobility options may be only 2 yr
Master's degree in nursing (MSN)	Universities	1-2 yr beyond BSN degree	Advanced clinical practice, management, education, leadership positions
Doctoral degree in nursing (PhD, DSN, DNSc, ND, DNP)	Universities	Varies	Advanced nursing for research, clinical practice, and leadership positions

structured settings. In 1995 more than 1100 LPN/LVN programs produced approximately 44,000 graduates, although the number was 2% less than the previous reporting period (NLN, 1997).

For many reasons, some individuals want or need to begin a career in nursing in these short programs. Once licensed, they can obtain employment and subsequently many continue education by enrolling in programs that prepare for registration as a professional nurse (RN). Many associate degree nursing programs (ADN) offer mobility options for LPNs. Although they are currently employed in many settings, LPN preparation is considered inadequate for the complexities of contemporary nursing care except in structured, stable environments.

Hospital Diploma Programs

The oldest and most traditional of nursing education programs that prepare for RN licensure are hospital-based diploma programs. These programs were initially developed in the United States in the late 1800s in general hospitals in cities such as Boston, New York, Hartford, and Philadelphia and subsequently spread across the country. They began as training programs taught by physicians and were only a few weeks in length. Soon the nurse graduates began developing and teaching courses from the nursing perspective, although many still were taught by physicians. Gradually, programs were extended to several months, then to 1 year, then to 2 years, and by the latter half of the 1900s, most programs were 3 years in length and had fairly uniform courses of study and clinical hours. Linda Richard and other early graduates wrote initial nursing textbooks and began offering specialty training to staff hospitals and clinics (Kalisch and Kalisch, 1995). Richards also became a nurse consultant to help develop other schools in the United States and later in Japan.

As the number of hospitals expanded, the need for nurses likewise increased, and essentially every hospital developed its own training program, which was the main source for nursing staff. At their peak in the 1950s and 1960s, approximately 1300 diploma programs were in operation. Many changes in society related to education and health care also influenced nursing education, and by 2000 the NLN reported only 86 diploma schools still operating. These remaining programs now are more similar to associate degree programs and typically are 2 years in length and follow an academic calendar, even though they include considerably more hands-on clinical experience. Many diploma programs have arrangements with colleges to offer arts and sciences courses and in some cases lead to students earning dual credentials, a hospital diploma and an associate degree.

Associate Degree Programs

In the late 1950s a different trend in nursing education emerged in response to social, political, and educational changes in society and to a growing shortage of RNs. During World War II the need for RNs prepared in a much shorter time was critical. The Cadet Nurse Corp was developed and proved to be very successful during the war. From this necessity, came the realization that nurses could be prepared in less time and still meet RN licensure and practice requirements. This new program evolved in the context of the developing community college movement that offered 2-year associate degree programs in many technical fields. These 2-year programs (AA/AS) reinforced the ideas of shorter college study for any citizen, the integration of content into fewer but more integrated courses, and the differentiation of technical education in a college setting (versus trade schools) from the more conventional 4-year academic degree programs that prepared students for graduate study and higher level positions.

After WWII cities all over the country rapidly acquired new federal funding to develop community colleges and public and private junior colleges. They prepared many more citizens for new emerging technical jobs required for the era of expansion and industrialization. This was an era in which the idea of a college education for the ordinary person was not just a remote dream. Military benefits for college tuition and funds to develop institutions allowed thousands of men and women to rise above the heritage of their parents to earn a college degree within their economic means and to fill jobs needed by burgeoning business and industry.

At the same time the increasing complexity and expansion of medical care required more and better prepared RNs. A few educators began to create a new 2-year nursing program for the community college, which required courses in arts and sciences and a more integrated approach to nursing content and clinical learning (Kalisch and Kalisch, 1995; Montag, 1959). These pioneers reasoned that nursing belonged in college settings along with other disciplines to provide a better education for nurses and women and to establish more respect and recognition for nursing's contribution to the community's health. As the number of community colleges grew and the need for nurses increased, associate degree nursing (ADN) programs became a logical program for development and expansion. Baer and colleagues (2000), Dillon (1997), and Kalisch and Kalisch (1995) provide brief and interesting historical accounts of ADN education.

Associate degree nursing education is a vivid example of how changes in society influence the evolution of nursing education; it was another significant "first" in nursing and an important part of the evolving professionalization of nursing as a discipline. For the first time it was possible for all RN education programs to be offered in college settings and for all graduates to earn a college degree. The original concept was that technical RNs (ADN) would work with professional RNs (nurses with a bachelor of science in nursing [BSN]) as a team. ADN programs were so successful that they became the new career pathway for thousands of students, and today the majority of practicing RNs are ADN graduates. By 2000 approximately 885 ADN programs were listed by the NLNAC. During the same time the number of 4-year BSN programs slowly but steadily increased. Thus the combination of 2-year ADN and 4-year BSN programs became the undergraduate backbone of the profession and a progressive model for students, educators, and employers.

Baccalaureate Degree Nursing Programs

In 1909 the efforts of progressive physicians and nurses resulted in a nursing program offered by the University of Minnesota; however, it was a diploma model and did not offer a college degree. During the next decade more than 15 similar programs were developed by other universities. It was not until 1924 that Yale University offered the first separate department of nursing whose graduates earned the baccalaureate degree. The 28-month program required scientific studies and clinical work and had the prestige and authority of other departments, with its own dean and budget (Kalisch and Kalisch, 1995). About the same time, (1923-24) a true 4-year nursing (BSN) degree program was opened at Western Reserve University (later named Case Western Reserve University). The nursing school later was named after its main benefactor, Frances Payne Bolton, and is a leading school today. This early beginning of BSN programs was another first in the history of nursing education.

Nurse leaders of the day envisioned nursing as a professional discipline far exceeding the technical hands-on care provided by less educated nurses. They believed that nurses could provide more comprehensive and compassionate care and be more effective if they had a solid foundation in the arts and sciences before or during the 4-year nursing program offered by colleges and universities. To a large extent this debate continues today. The number of colleges and universities offering the BSN degree slowly continued to increase, and by 2003 the AACN reported 569 basic BSN programs, 620 offering a BSN mobility option for RNs from associate degree or diploma programs (Berlin, Stennett, and Bednash, 2003).

BSN degree programs typically require 2 years of arts and sciences as the foundation for 2 years of nursing courses. Nursing courses include typical content related to the care of patients with medical, surgical, pediatric, obstetric, and psychiatric conditions, although course sequencing differs considerably. BSN programs also include courses in community and public health, beginning research, management, and leadership. The broader scope of professional practice also emphasizes the need for courses such as epidemiology, statistics, and pathophysiology. Additionally, the BSN program has an expanded focus on the family and community and an emphasis on health promotion and illness prevention, with an increasing part of clinical experiences in diverse community settings. Graduates of BSN programs take the same NCLEX-RN licensure examination as diploma and ADN graduates. An increasing number of specialty areas require the BSN degree for practice and as part of the certification process. Admission into master's programs usually requires the BSN degree.

Master's Degree Nursing Programs

In the 1960s and 1970s the increasing complexity of health care, along with the need for qualified nurse educators, administrators, and clinicians and the increasing number of

BSN graduates stimulated the federal government to provide support for the development of a master of science in nursing (MSN) degree and other types of programs. In 1977 most nurse administrators were diploma graduates (46%); only 28% had MSN or doctoral degrees (Kalisch and Kalisch, 1995). Efforts of lobbyist and nurse leaders resulted in federal funding for building construction, nursing program development, and student tuition. Traineeship and fellowship grants enabled thousands of RNs to return to school to earn BSN and advanced degrees to prepare for positions in education, administration, practice, and research. Until the late 1970s MSN programs primarily focused on preparing educators and administrators, but in the next decade the curriculum trend shifted to an overwhelming emphasis on clinical practice, with little attention to these functional areas. By the 1990s, both the negative and the positive consequences of these decisions became apparent with more competent clinicians but less well prepared educators and administrators.

Currently most MSN programs are designed to prepare advanced nurse practitioners and clinical specialists in a wide array of specialty areas. The extraordinary and rapid changes in health care during the 1990s highlighted the cost-effective and quality care benefits of using advanced practice nurses to provide primary health care. In the past two decades nurses have waged intensive and persistent legal battles to change state laws to permit nurse practitioners to write prescriptions, receive reimbursement for care, and operate independent nurse practices and health centers. The resulting recognition and expanded scope of practice changed the definition and roles of advanced practice nurses and increased the number of MSN students. Most nurse educators, managers, and administrators now are required to have a master's or doctoral degree. These factors have had a marked influence on the MSN curriculum and the number of programs available. In 2003 the AACN listed 398 master's degree nursing programs (Berlin, Stennett, and Bednash, 2003).

Different MSN programs are available, the most common being for graduates of BSN programs; other options are designed for graduates of nonnursing degree programs. A growing number of universities offer multiple options and clinical specialty majors in response to changes in health care needs. Financial constraints, changes in education philosophy, and information technology have provided incentives for universities to develop more programs that offer flexible distance learning and mobility options, especially for part-time working students.

One of the current trends is MSN programs that can be completed almost entirely through Internet courses. Some programs use computerized online courses and other mediated arrangements such as audio and/or video teleconferencing, closed statewide computer and/or video networking, correspondence courses, and various types of cognitive and performance examinations (Skiba, 1997; Wambach et al, 1999). Some require short periods of intensive on-campus classes or assigned clinical experiences with designated preceptors. Technology has made it possible for nurses to meet requirements for higher degrees and still meet other obligations and constraints.

Doctoral Programs

Nurse pioneers developed the first doctoral programs for nurses at the end of the nineteenth century at Teachers College, Columbia University. The first nurse graduated in 1932 with a doctor of education degree (EdD) in nursing education; in 1934, New York University offered a PhD program for nurses. More than 30 years elapsed before doctoral programs in nursing were offered, for example, the doctor of nursing science degree (DNS, or DNSc). By 2003 the AACN survey reported 83 nursing doctoral programs (Berlin, Stennett, and Bednash, 2003).

Currently four types of doctoral degrees are available in nursing: (1) the doctor of philosophy (PhD) for those interested in research; (2) the doctor of nursing science (DNS or DNSc) for those interested in advanced clinical nursing practice; (3) the doctor of nursing (ND) for those with BS or higher degrees in nonnursing fields who want to pursue a career in leadership; and (4) the doctorate in clinical nursing practice (DNP), designed to prepare graduates for advanced clinical practice and clinical leadership with the credential that corresponds with the complexity and demands of contemporary clinical practice. The ND degree, which prepares nurses for basic licensure (NCLEX-RN), was first offered at Case Western Reserve University in 1979. Shortly after, Rush University and the University of Colorado Health Science Center offered ND programs, and a few others followed later. Some schools offer options combined with another majors in areas such as business, law, informatics, or social sciences.

FLEXIBLE EDUCATION, MOBILITY, AND DISTANCE LEARNING PROGRAMS

Nursing literature over the past 30 years substantiates the need for, and the effectiveness of, various mobility and distance delivery programs (AACN, 1998, 1999a, 2002a, 2003a [websites]; Baer et al, 2000; Kalisch and Kalisch, 1995; Lenburg and Johnson, 1974; Lenburg, 1975). During the 1990s mobility and distance learning programs proliferated and became more accepted. Organizations such as the AACN, the NLN, the National Council of State Boards of Nursing (NCSBN), and others have published position statements related to mobility options, even though they were initially resistant to them (AACN 1998; NLN, 1993). By the year 2000 most BSN programs had flexible options for RN students, and many ADN programs had options for LPNs (Frik, Speed, and Pollock, 1996; Redmond, 1997).

The oldest and most controversial distance mobility program in nursing is the external degree program headquartered in New York. Initially named Regents External Degree Program, it was renamed Regents College and then Excelsior College in 2001. Its ADN program was initiated in 1972 and the BSN in 1976, both of which were fully accredited by NLN shortly thereafter, albeit with considerable controversy (Lenburg, 1975, 1990). Nearly all Excelsior College students are LPNs or RNs, although a prior license is not required; many students with health-related certificates or degrees have completed the programs. A master's degree program in nursing informatics was added in 2000. These options offer the most extensive national and international mobility programs, because they are based entirely on assessment of knowledge through standardized written examinations, clinical competence through extensive nursing performance examinations, and the evaluation of arts and sciences either through prior college credit or college proficiency examinations. Thousands of nurses have completed degrees this way and have continued through graduate school and into leadership positions in nursing, substantiating their success (Lenburg, 1990). Other nursing programs have adopted these ideas and, with the rapid expansion of computer and communications technology, have expanded opportunities further. Explore websites for Excelsior College, University of Phoenix Online, and others in Table 4-2.

Career ladder programs designed as "1-plus-1" or "2-plus-2" options have been offered for many years by some schools and through several statewide programs. Examples of statewide programs are those offered by Georgia (Kish et al, 1997), Iowa (McClelland et al, 1997), and Maryland (Rapson, 2000); also see websites for Colorado and Kentucky (see Table 4-2). The consortium of 25 nursing programs in northeast Ohio illustrates a different model. Cooperating leaders from these schools named the project the Nursing Education Mobility

Action Group (NEMAG) and successfully developed the ACCESS model in the early 1990s. The consortium continues to assist LPNs and RNs in that region to earn ADN and BSN degrees using options such as the transition course or the escrow/bypass methods. The 5-year evaluation of the project supported its effectiveness and efficiency (Nichols, Lenburg, Soehnlen, 2000; Rolince et al, 2001). Project LINC is another innovative mobility program for working adults; it was initiated in New York City and was so successful that it subsequently has been implemented in several other states (Westmoreland et al, 1998). Benjamin-Coleman and colleagues (2001) provide a review of a decade of distance learning programs.

Changes in the social, political, financial, and philosophical climates; the knowledge and technology explosion; research from past experiences; and the continuing shortage of nurses have combined to make education mobility and distance learning opportunities a necessity and a reality throughout the country. The long-standing debate over "entry into practice" continues as nursing pursues its professionalization destiny (AACN, 1999b, 2000a, 2002b, 2002c, 2003a; NLN, 1993). Many nurse leaders have long considered mobility programs a method to achieve this goal. A review of websites for universities and colleges (see Table 4-2) illustrates how widespread distance learning options have become, including some schools that offer entire degree programs or a number of courses via the Internet. For example, see websites for the offerings in California, Colorado, Florida, Kansas, and Maryland.

With the escalating nursing shortage and aging of nurses, students, and nurse educators, more schools have initiated one or more mobility options. Some of these programs target potentially underrepresented groups, such as males, minority groups, and those with existing academic degrees. Different models appeal to different groups; those that are growing fastest, however, target second-degree students for the BSN degree or the generic master's degree. Other options include the ND or generic doctoral programs. These students must have already earned a bachelor's or higher-level degree and meet certain other criteria. These fast-track programs also make it possible for students to complete doctoral degrees more quickly. Other accelerated programs are designed for RNs seeking a BSN, MSN, or doctoral degree; each option focuses on the needs of different students, and details vary from school to school. Many of these mobility programs or "nontraditional" accelerated programs are described in an article on the AACN (2002a) website (www.aacn.nche.edu/publications/issues/Aug02.htm), accessed by clicking on the website's *Issues* icon. This article describes various BSN and higher degree models with links to many schools for specific information. Mobility models for LPN to AD, LPN to BSN, or diploma to BSN are widely available. NLN lists these mobility options in its directories.

Trends and issues that influence nursing education make it even more important to comply with quality standards and accreditation and to emphasize competency outcomes for students and graduates. Changes in number and qualifications of students and shortage of faculty and finances make it necessary to develop effective learning strategies for remote, off-campus students. This includes advisement, tutoring, peer mentoring, and mediated learning programs to promote competence especially among older, rural, or minority students (Griffiths and Tagliareni, 1999; Ramsey et al, 2000). Although distance programs and Internet courses are often more convenient, they also present challenges for students. Some difficult factors relate to access to current hardware and software technology and the time, ability, and money to use it. Students also need discipline and determination to pursue courses and clinical learning when a teacher is not physically present and learning is the responsibility of learners, most of whom work full-time and manage multiple other responsibilities.

APPROVAL AND ACCREDITATION OF NURSING PROGRAMS

All nursing programs must meet the rules and regulations of the State Board of Nursing for the particular state involved. A program must go through a rigorous process before it is officially approved to enroll students; thereafter it is reviewed periodically to ensure that it continues to meet the specified criteria. A newly developing trend that has implications for schools of nursing is multistate licensure, which is not yet approved by all states. This is a legal arrangement (contract) to allow nurses licensed in one state to practice in other states as well. Schools and their graduates, however, must be prepared to meet certain standards of those other states (see the NCSBN website, 1997-2003, at ncsbn.org).

All colleges and universities must meet additional regulations and standards established by regional accrediting bodies to ensure that the academic institutions actually offer the programs, courses, and resources they proclaim. Accreditation by regional education agencies requires that the faculty undertake a serious self-study process and respond in a written report to multiple specific criteria that define a school worthy of accreditation status. After submitting the self-study report, trained evaluators visit the school to verify the contents of the report. The final decision ultimately is made by or approved by a final peer review board.

Professional schools, like nursing, also undergo additional voluntary accreditation by a professional association approved by the U.S. Department of Education. The NLN accredits all types of basic nursing programs, currently through its accrediting commission, the NLNAC. The AACN accredits baccalaureate and graduate degree nursing programs through its subsidiary, the Commission on Collegiate Nursing Education (CCNE).

NURSING EDUCATION FOR THE FUTURE

The American Association of Colleges of Nursing (AACN) in collaboration with a broad array of leaders from practice environments, is calling for the creation of a new nursing role to better meet client care needs within the health care delivery system. The New Nurse is envisioned as a leader in the health care delivery system across all settings in which health care is delivered, not just the acute care setting. The new role will not be one of administration or management, but one who assumes accountability for client care outcomes through the assimilation and application of research-based information to design, implement, and evaluate client plans of care. This clinician will be a provider and manager of care who will design, implement, and evaluate client care by coordinating, delegating, and supervising the care provided by the health care team, including licensed nurses, technicians, and other health professionals. Dialogue between leaders of academic institutions and practice arenas is taking place to explore the optimum level of education and strategies for integrating this new role into the practice setting.

In 2002 AACN submitted reports and a draft of several education models to differentiate a new role requiring a clinical doctoral degree and substantially change existing BSN and higher degrees for nursing. They outlined changes needed in educational preparation, licensure, titles and scope of practice for the proposed roles, as distinguished from the existing roles and license for RNs from ADN, diploma, and BSN programs. The several proposed education models can be accessed via the AACN website and various other sources (2002b, 2000c).

Subsequently, another group was appointed to continue to study the issues, draft potential responses, and begin to identify the roles and associated required competencies and content that should be included in the curriculum and actual practice for the newly identified programs and practice roles. They affirmed the central need for more competent and compelling clinical nurse leadership and named the new role "Clinical Nurse Leader" (CNL). In 2003 their draft white paper "The Role of the Clinical Nurse Leader" was published by AACN (2003a).

Details of this "new nurse project" and the draft white paper can be accessed through the AACN website (www.aacn.nche.edu) and its embedded links. Briefly summarized, the models proposed by the Task Force suggest leaving the LPN/LVN and ADN levels essentially as they are to function as a means to a smoother transition to newly differentiated roles. The levels most affected are the BSN, master's, advanced practice, and doctoral options, which are conceived differently in the six new draft models. All of the new models propose the DNP as the clinical doctoral pathway, and most require a period of residency to improve clinical competency. The Task Force emphasized the need to markedly increase academic and clinical preparation and to enhance role performance of advanced practice nurses; to fulfill that role they need credentials equivalent to those in other health care disciplines (e.g., physical therapist and pharmacist). Other doctoral options still available would include the PhD, DNS, and ND as preparation for research, scholarship, education, administration, and other leadership roles. The new DNP, however, is designed to prepare graduates for advanced clinical practice and clinical leadership with the credential that corresponds with the complexity and demands of contemporary clinical practice. As of this writing, the University of Kentucky offers the DNP degree (see www.mc.uky.edu/nursing).

As nurses examine ideal ways to educate the nurse of the future, they must take into account recent reports of the Institute of Medicine (IOM). The IOM study *Crossing the Quality Chasm* (2001) recommended that an interdisciplinary summit be held to further the reform of health professions education in order to enhance quality and patient safety. *Health Professions Education: A Bridge to Quality* (2003) is the follow-up to that summit, held in June 2002, where 150 participants across disciplines and occupations discussed strategies for restructuring clinical education to be consistent with the principles of the twenty-first–century health system. This report says that doctors, nurses, pharmacists, and other health professionals are not being adequately prepared to provide the highest quality and safest medical care possible and that there is insufficient assessment of their ongoing proficiency. Educators and accreditation, licensing, and certification organizations have been challenged to ensure that students and working health care professionals develop and maintain proficiency in five core areas: delivering patient-centered care, working as part of interdisciplinary teams, implementing evidence-based practice, focusing on quality improvement, and using information technology.

S U M M A R Y

This chapter has presented 10 major trends and related issues for students and faculty in education programs and an overview of multiple types of nursing education programs. To a large extent the trends and issues reviewed influence the content, learning process, and evaluation methods used in all types of programs. They also influence the persistence of multiple types and levels of programs for entry into practice and the acceptance of diverse mobility and distance learning programs, all of which are increasingly using the Internet and electronic databases and resources in learning and practice. As students integrate current trends and attempt to resolve issues, they are learning to create the trends for the next generation; they are participating in nursing history in the making. As active learners, they integrate the words of Oliver Wendell Holmes, who said, "The mind once stretched with a new idea never regains its original dimensions."

CRITICAL THINKING ACTIVITIES RELATED TO EACH LEARNING OUTCOME

NOTE: Learning Outcomes that were presented at the beginning of this chapter are listed again here, each followed by activities specifically designed to address that particular outcome.

Learning Outcome 1: Integrate knowledge of current trends and issues in society into a more holistic perception of their influence on nursing, nursing education, students, and faculty.

Critical Thinking Activities

a. List the major trends and associated issues in rank order of importance (relevance) to you from (1) most important to (10) least important. Offer rationales for your top three selections.
b. Create a chart with three columns, reflecting your sense of the importance of these trends in nursing before and after studying this chapter. List the trends in the far left column. Then label the second column as "Before" and the third column as "After." Use a rating scale of 1 to 5, with 5 being the most important, to reflect your perceptions of each trend on nursing.
c. Write a reflective analysis of at least three issues you have experienced in nursing education and how they relate to the broader trends described in the chapter.
d. Write a one-page reflective summary of your perception of the nursing profession and nursing education that incorporates four or five of the trends described in the chapter.

Learning Outcome 2: Integrate knowledge of current trends and issues into a personal contemporary philosophy of ongoing professional development and practice.

Critical Thinking Activities

a. In a small work group, discuss changes in philosophy of nursing among group members related to the major trends and issues presented in the chapter.
b. Summarize key points that support the need for ongoing professional development by group members.
c. Write a personal philosophy of nursing (one to two paragraphs) that integrates elements of four or five trends presented in this chapter.
d. Outline a plan for continuing professional development that incorporates elements of at least five trends presented.

Learning Outcome 3: Differentiate among various types of conventional and mobility nursing education programs and the issues associated with them.

Critical Thinking Activities

a. Create a defining features matrix that identifies the major characteristics and differences among programs that prepare individuals for registered nurse licensure.
b. Create a pro and con grid to summarize issues related to various flexible and educational mobility options.
c. List at least three issues presented by major nursing organizations, with their positive or negative positions related to diverse entry points into the profession.
d. Critique the major issues related to Internet-based nursing degree programs (or clinical courses) and the corresponding justification for having them.

Learning Outcome 4: Access pertinent information resources related to evolving trends and issues as a component of ongoing professional development.

Critical Thinking Activities

a.   In a small group, analyze several issues that are particularly relevant to members of the group and classify them under one or more of the trend headings.

b   Submit a list of questions that could be used as guidelines to analyze issues and their merit within the context of broader trends and the goals of nursing education. (Include questions regarding what, who, why, when, where, and how.)

c.   Access three additional websites not listed in this chapter and describe their usefulness for ongoing professional development in the context of trends and issues.

Additional resources are available on-line at: http://evolve.elsevier.com/Cherry/

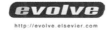

http://evolve.elsevier.com

REFERENCES

Aiken L: Educational levels of hospital nurses and surgical patient mortality, *JAMA* 290(12):1617–1623, 2003.

American Association of Colleges of Nursing: *Position statement: education mobility*, Washington, DC, 1998, AACN (www.aacn.nche.edu).

American Association of Colleges of Nursing: *Position statement: education mobility*, Washington, DC, 1998, AACN (www.aacn.nche.edu).

American Association of Colleges of Nursing: *White paper: distance technology in nursing education*, Washington, DC, 1999a, AACN (www.aacn.nche.edu).

American Association of Colleges of Nursing: *Position statement: nursing education's agenda for the 21st century*, Washington, DC, 1999b, 2002b, AACN (www.aacn.nche.edu).

American Association of Colleges of Nursing: *Position statement: baccalaureate degree in nursing as minimal preparation for professional practice*, Washington, DC, 2000a, AACN, (www.aacn.nche.edu).

American Association of Colleges of Nursing: *Nursing school enrollments decline as demand continues to climb*, Washington, DC, 2000b, AACN (www.aacn.nche.edu).

American Association of Colleges of Nursing: *Strategies to reverse the nursing shortage*, Washington, DC, 2001, AACN (www.aacn.nche.edu/education/position statements/).

American Association of Colleges of Nursing: *Accelerated programs: the fast-track to careers in nursing*, Washington, DC, 2002a, AACN (www.aacn.nche.edu/Issue/Aug02).

American Association of Colleges of Nursing: *Report of the Task Force on Education and Regulation*, Washington, DC, 2002b, AACN (www.aacn.nche.edu/education/report/Apr02).

American Association of Colleges of Nursing: *Report of the Task Force on Education and Regulation: Models*, Washington, DC, 2002c, AACN (www.aacn.nche.edu/education/models).

American Association of Colleges of Nursing: *The clinical nurse leader: developing a new nurse*, Washington, DC, 2003a, AACN (www.aacn.nche.edu/projects/newnurse/index).

American Association of Colleges of Nursing: *Thousands of students turned away from the nation's nursing schools despite sharp increase in enrollment*, Dec 2003b, AACN (www.aacn.nche.edu/homepage/listing).

American Nurses Association: *One strong voice*, Kansas City, Mo, 1976, ANA.

American Nurses Association: ANA to focus on core issues, *Am Nurs*, Nov/Dec 1999, pp 17, 19. (See www.nursingworld.org/tan for multiple other articles concerning profession issues: adequate staffing, continuing competence, patient safety, advocacy, and workplace health and safety; also regarding organization unity.)

American Nurses Association: Articles about competencies, continuing education, *Am Nurs* (multiple issues), 2000-2003, ANA (www.nursingworld.org/tan).

American Nurses Association: *Report on bioterrorism; several reports, 2002*, ANA (www.nursingworld.org/homepage/menu/).

Baer ED et al: *Enduring issues in American nursing*, New York, 2000, Springer.

Bellack JP, O'Neil EH: Recreating nursing practice for a new century: recommendations and implications of the Pew Health Professions Commission's final report, *Nurs Health Care Perspect* 21:14-21, 2000.

Benjamin-Coleman R et al: Distance education: a decade of distance education: RN to BSN, *Nurs Educator* 26:9-12, 2001.

Berlin LE, Stennett J, Bednash, G: *2002-2003 Enrollment and graduations in baccalaureate and graduate programs in nursing,* Washington, DC, 2003, American Association of Colleges of Nursing.

Brendtro MJ, Leuning C: Nurses in churches: a population-focused clinical option, *J Nurs Educ* 39:285-288, 2000.

Buerhaus PI: Aging nurses in an aging society: long-term implications, *Reflect Nurs Leadersh* 27(1):35-36, 2001 (www.nursingsociety.org).

Buerhaus PI, Staiger DO, Auerbach DI: Implications of an aging registered nurse workforce, *JAMA* 283(22): 2948-2954, 2000.

Dillon P: Changing directions: the future of associate degree nursing, *Nurs Health Care Perspect* 18:20-24, 1997.

Engelke MK, Britton BP: From black bags to interactive workstations, *Reflect Nurs Leadersh* 26(4):30-32, 2000.

Focus on technology (special issue), *J Nurs Educ* 38:entire issue, Sept 1999.

Frik SM, Speed DJ, Pollock SE: A special pathway for registered nurses with baccalaureate degrees in fields other than nursing, *J Nurs Educ* 35:152-156, 1996.

Gaffney T: The regulatory dilemma surrounding interstate practice, *Online J Iss Nurs,* May 1999 (www.nursingworld.org/ojin). (See other articles on same focused issue.)

Green PM, Adderley-Kelly B: Partnership for health promotion in an urban community, *Nurs Health Care Perspect* 20:76-81, 1999.

Griffiths MJ, Tagliareni E: Challenging traditional assumptions about minority students in nursing education: outcomes from Project IMPART, *Nurs Health Care Perspect* 20:290-295, 1999.

Heller BR, Oros MT, Durney-Crowley J: The future of nursing education: 10 trends to watch, *Nurs Health Care Perspect* 21:9-13, 2000.

HIPAA: 2002 (www.hhs.gov/ocr/hippaa and www.hipaa.org).

Hurst CP, Osban LB: Service learning on wheels: the Nightingale mobile clinic, *Nurs Health Care Perspect* 21:184-187, 2000.

Institute of Medicine (IOM): *To err is human: building a safer health system,* National Academy of Science Press, 2000 (www.iom.edu/). See nursing response (www.aacn.nche.edu and www.nursingworld.org).

Institute of Medicine (IOM): *Crossing the quality chasm,* 2001, National Academy Press.

Institute of Medicine (IOM): Committee on the Health Professions Education Summit, Greiner A, Knebel E, editors: *Health professions education: a bridge to quality,* Washington, DC, 2003, The National Academies Press.

Joint Commission on Accreditation of Healthcare Organizations: *Criteria, journals, news, 2000,* on-line (www. jcaho.org).

Kalisch PA, Kalisch BJ: *The advance of American nursing,* ed 3, Philadelphia, 1995, JB Lippincott.

Kiehl EM, Wink DM: Nursing students as change agents in the community: community-based nursing education in practice, *Nurs Health Care Perspect* 21:293-297, 2000.

Kish C et al: Georgia's RN-BSN articulation model, *Nurs Health Care Perspect* 18:26-30, 1997.

LaSala KB et al: Rural health care and interdisciplinary education, *Nurs Health Care Perspect* 18:292-298, 1997.

Lenburg CB: *Open learning and career mobility in nursing,* St Louis, 1975, Mosby.

Lenburg CB: Do external degree programs really work? *Nurs Outlook* 36:234-238, 1990.

Lenburg CB: The framework, concepts and methods of the Competency Outcomes and Performance Assessment (COPA) model, *Online J Issu Nurs* Sept 1999 (www.nursingworld.org/ojin).

Lenburg CB: The Competency Outcomes and Performance Assessment model applied to nursing case management systems. In Cohen E, Cesta T: *Nursing case management: from concept to evaluation,* ed 3, St Louis, 2001, Mosby, pp 269-279.

Lenburg CB: Changes that challenge nursing education, *The Tennessee Nurse,* on-line, pp 10-13, 2002 (www.tnaonline.org/TNNurse).

Lenburg CB, Johnson W: Career mobility through nursing education, *Nurs Outlook* 32:250-254, 1974.

Lenburg CB et al: *Promoting cultural competence in nursing education,* Washington, DC, 1995, American Academy of Nursing.

Luttrell MF, Lenburg CB, Scherubel JC, Jacob SR, Koch RW: Redesigning a BSN curriculum: competency outcomes for learning and performance assessment, *Nurs Health Care Perspect* 20:134-141, 1999.

Lutz J, Herrick CA, Lehman BB: Community partnership: a school of nursing creates nursing centers for older adults, *Nurs Health Care Perspect* 22:26-29, 2001.

Mallow GE, Gilje F: Technology-based nursing education: overview and call for further dialogue, *J Nurs Educ* 38:248-251, 1999.

Mathews-Smith G et al: A new module in caring for older adults: problem-based learning and practice portfolios, *J Nurs Educ* 40:73-78, 2001.

Matzo ML et al: Communication skills for end of life nursing care: teaching strategies from the ELNEC curriculum, *Nurs Educ Perspect* 24:176-183, 2003.

McClelland E et al: The Iowa articulation story: collaboration works, *Nurs Educ* 22(2):19-24, 1997.

Melamed A: Nurses attack hidden dangers of health care, *Am Nurse,* on-line, Nov/Dec 1999, p 17 (www.nursingworld.org/tan/).

Miller MP, Swanson E: Service learning and community health nursing: a natural fit, *Nurs Educ Perspect* 23:30-33, 2002.

Mitty E, Mezey M: Integrating advanced practice nurses in home care: recommendations for a teaching home care program, *Nurs Health Care Perspect* 19:264-270, 1998.

Montag ML: *Community college education for nursing,* New York, 1959, McGraw-Hill.

Moylan LB: Alternative treatment modalities: the need for a rational response by the nursing profession, *Nurs Outlook* 48:259-261, 2000.

Mundt MH: A model for clinical learning experiences in integrated healthcare networks, *J Nurs Educ* 36:309-316, 1997.

Narsavage GL et al: Developing personal and community learning in graduate nursing education through community engagement, *Nurs Educ Perspect* 24:300-305, 2003.

National Council of State Boards of Nursing (NCSBN): National Council studies continued competence: committee develops personal accountability profile, *Issues* 18(2):1, 1997 (see www.ncsbn.org/ 2001-2003 for updates).

National League for Nursing: *A vision for nursing education,* New York, 1993, Author (www.nln.org).

National League for Nursing: Nursing datasource 1997, vol 1, *Trends in contemporary nursing education,* New York, 1997, Author.

National League for Nursing: *NLN 2002-2003 survey of RN nursing programs indicates positive upward trend,* Dec 2003 (nln.org/press release).

Newell-Withrow C, Slusher IL: Diversity: an answer to the nursing shortage, *Nurs Outlook* 49:270-271, 2001.

Nichols EF, Lenburg CB, Soehnlen JJ: Evaluation of a collaborative articulation mobility project using escrow and transition course methods, *Nurs Health Care Perspect* 21:188-195, 2000.

Nicoll LH: *Nurses' guide to the Internet,* ed 3, Philadelphia, 2000, JB Lippincott (www.lww.com).

Nursing: bridging worlds (special issue on cultural diversity and health issues), *Nurs Health Care* 15:227-261, 1994.

Nursing shortage (feature issue): *J Iss Nurs,* on-line, Feb 2001, entire issue (www.nursingworld.org/ojin/topic/14).

Palmer J: Parish nursing connecting faith and health, *Reflect Nurs Leadersh* 27(1):17-18, 2001.

Ramsey P et al: The NURSE center: a peer mentor-tutor project for disadvantaged nursing students in Appalachia, *Nurs Educ* 25:277-281, 2000.

Rapson MF: Statewide nursing articulation model design: politics or academics? *J Nurs Educ* 39:294-301, 2000.

Redmond GM: LPN-BSN: education for a reformed healthcare system, *J Nurs Educ* 36:121-127, 1997.

Riley JM, Fry ST: Nurses report widespread ethical conflicts, *Reflect Nurs Leadersh* 26(2):35-36, 2000 (www.bc.edu/ nursing/ethics).

Rolince P et al: A regional collaboration for educational and career mobility: the nursing education mobility action group, *Nurs Health Care Perspect* 22:75-80, 2001.

Rushton CH, Sabatier KH: The nursing leadership consortium on end-of-life care: the response of the nursing profession to the need for improvement in palliative care, *Nurs Outlook* 49:58-60, 2001.

Ryan M et al: Learning to care for clients in their world, not mine, *J Nurs Educ* 39:401-408, 2000.

Scanlon JM, Care WD, Gessler S: Dealing with the unsafe student in clinical practice, *Nurs Educ* 26:23-27, 2001.

Serembus JF: Teaching the process of developing a professional portfolio, *Nurs Educ* 25:282-287, 2000 (see references cited in this article).

Simmons J, editor: *Perspectives–celebrating 40 years of associate degree nursing education,* New York, 1993, National League for Nursing.

Skiba DJ: Transforming nursing education to celebrate learning, *Nurs Health Care Perspect* 18:124-129ff, 1997.

Sloan HL, Delahoussaye CP: Clinical application of the Omaha system with the Nightingale Tracker: a community health nursing student home visit program, *Nurs Educ* 28:15-17, 2003.

Solari-Twadell PA, McDermott MA, editors: *Parish nursing— promoting whole person health within faith communities,* Thousand Oaks, Calif, 1999, Sage.

Tanner CA (moderator): Nursing shortage update: effects on education and specialty areas, *J Nurs Educ* 42:529-534, 2003.

Tracy SM et al: The clinical achievement portfolio: an outcomes-based assessment project in nursing education, *Nurs Educ* 25:241-246, 2000.

Trossman S: The professional portfolio: documenting who you are, what you do, *Am Nurse* March/April 1999 (see www.nursingworld.org/tan/ for this and later articles).

U.S. Department of Health and Human Services, Bureau of Health Professions: *Nursing: collaborative education to ensure patient safety,* 2000 (http://bhpr.hrsa.gov/nursing/ nacnep/patientsafety.htm).

Wambach K et al: Beyond correspondence, video conferencing, and voice mail: Internet based master's degree courses in nursing, *J Nurs Educ* 38:267-271, 1999.

Westmoreland D et al: Replicating Project LINC in two Midwestern states: implications for policy development, *Nurs Health Care Perspect* 19:166-174, 1998.

White SG, Henry JK: Incorporation of service-learning into a baccalaureate nursing education curriculum, *Nurs Outlook* 47:257-261, 1999.

Zittel B: *Memo to Council of Chairs of Associate Degree Nursing Programs,* The University of the State of New York, State Education Department, State Board for Nursing, Oct 31, 2003.

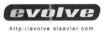

http://evolve.elsevier.com

Nursing Licensure and Certification

Janet C. Scherubel, PhD, RN, CCRN

5

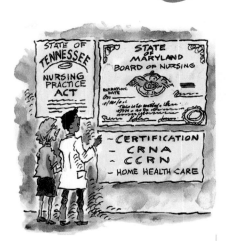

Legal regulations and certification ensure safe, competent nursing care.

VIGNETTE

Three nurses are discussing their nursing practice licenses. Joe Branch, a senior nursing student, is preparing to take the NCLEX exam. Mary Stone's license is due for renewal. Carmella Larkin has just moved into the state. As the three are talking about these changes in their practice, Georgio Gonzales, a nurse practitioner, joins the group. Georgio recently completed a certification examination and is interested in becoming certified for advanced practice. All these nurses have a general knowledge of the requirements for licensure and certification but lack the specific information needed to legally practice within the state. Mary suggests contacting the State Board of Nursing. The nurses agree that this is a sensible idea, and Mary leaves to phone the Board. On returning, Mary informs the group that the answers to all their questions may be found in the state's Nursing Practice Act and accompanying Rules and Regulations. Furthermore, the State Board of Nursing office will send free copies of both documents to each nurse.

The situation described here is not uncommon. Nurses need specific, current information on licensure and renewal of licensure. The most comprehensive sources for this information are the state Nursing Practice Act and the State Board of Nursing. These resources provide accurate advice on the relevant provisions for practicing nursing within each state, as well as the U.S. territories. All nurses and nursing students should obtain copies of their state's practice act and become familiar with its contents.

Questions to consider while reading this chapter:
1. Who establishes the "rules" for nursing practice—the state or the employer?
2. Do graduates from different types of nursing education programs require different types of licenses?

Additional resources are available on-line at: http://evolve.elsevier.com/Cherry/

3.   If a nurse graduate passes the NCLEX-RN, does that person still need a license?
4.   What happens if a nurse's license expires? Can the nurse still practice?
5.   Must a nurse complete graduate school and take an examination to be an advanced practice nurse?
6.   Are the regulations governing advanced nursing practice the same in all states?

KEY TERMS

Accreditation Process by which schools of nursing are approved to conduct nursing education programs.

Advanced practice nurse Legal title for nurses prepared by education and competence to perform independent practice.

American Nurses Association Professional organization that represents all registered nurses.

American Nurses Credentialing Center Independent agency of the American Nurses Association (ANA) that conducts certification examinations and certifies advanced practice nurses.

Certification Process by which nurses are recognized for advanced education and competence.

Commission on Collegiate Nursing Education (CCNE) A subsidiary of the American Association of Colleges of Nursing (AACN) with responsibility for accrediting baccalaureate and higher-degree nursing programs.

Compact state A term of law. In the context of the Mutual Recognition Model, refers to a state that has established an agreement with other states allowing nurses to practice within the state without an additional license. The interstate compacts have been enacted by the state legislatures.

Continued competency Program initiatives to ensure nurses' knowledge, skills, and expertise beyond initial licensure.

Grandfathered Statutory process by which previously licensed persons are incorporated into revisions or additions in nursing practice acts.

International Council of Nursing Professional organization that represents nurses in 119 countries around the world.

Licensure by endorsement Process by which nurses licensed in one state may seek licensure in another without repeat examinations. The requirements are included in state nursing practice acts or accompanying rules and regulations.

Mandatory continuing education State-level educational requirements for renewal of license.

Mutual recognition of nursing Program developed by the State Boards of Nursing, Inc. The model proposes interstate compacts so that nurses licensed in one jurisdiction may practice in other compact states without duplicate licensure.

National Council of State Boards of Nursing, Inc. Organization whose membership consists of the board of nursing of each state or territory.

National League for Nursing Professional organization whose members represent multiple disciplines. The National League for Nursing conducts many types of programs, including accrediting nursing education programs.

Nursing practice act Statute in each state and territory that regulates the practice of nursing.

State Board of Nursing Appointed board within each state charged with responsibility to administer the nursing practice act of that state.

Sunset legislation Statutes that provide for revocation of laws if not reviewed and renewed within a specified time period.

LEARNING OUTCOMES

After studying this chapter, the reader will be able to:

1. Explain the development of licensure requirements in the United States.
2. Summarize current licensure requirements in the context of historical developments.
3. Analyze the various components of a nursing practice act.
4. Discuss mutual recognition of nursing practice and identify compact states.
5. Differentiate among requirements for certification for advanced practice in different specialties.
6. Use appropriate resources to obtain current information on licensure and certification.
7. Describe the development of certification requirements for advanced practice in the United States.

CHAPTER OVERVIEW

To be a registered nurse! That is the goal of almost every student nurse. It is a worthy goal reached through study, clinical practice, and successful completion of the NCLEX-RN, the National Council Licensure Examination–Registered Nurse. This chapter discusses how and why nursing licensure developed, the steps necessary to becoming licensed, licensure regulations, and the responsibilities of a registered nurse (RN).

After licensure as an RN, nurses still must maintain and increase their knowledge and skills. Some may wish to specialize in a particular area of nursing or expand their practice. Nurses with these goals may seek certification in a specialty field. This chapter describes certification, the means to achieve certification, and the organizations that administer certifying examinations. Whether it is licensure or certification, the nursing profession is continually progressing. Legal requirements to practice are continually revised to ensure the protection of the public. Just as in the past, nurses today face issues and challenges as they seek to increase their competence and the nursing services they provide to patients and clients. This chapter explores issues related to licensure and certification. Finally, future challenges emerging on the horizon are identified.

THE HISTORY OF NURSING LICENSURE
Recognition: Pins and Registries

The aim of caregivers since early times has been to be identified and recognized for one's skills and achievements. Early caregivers, particularly in the monasteries and convents of the medieval period, were identified by the habits they wore. Frequently, special insignia designated health personnel. During the Crusades, a large Maltese cross adorned the black habits of the Knights Hospitalers of St. John of Jerusalem on the battlefield (Kalisch and Kalisch, 1995). These forms of identification allowed others to recognize their particular skills in caregiving and healing. More recently, nurses wore a readily identifiable symbol of their school of nursing, the nursing cap.

Today, as in the past, the school of nursing pin identifies graduates from a particular school of nursing. Early in each school's history, students and faculty members crafted the pin. The pin's emblems and text symbolize the philosophy, beliefs, and aspirations of the nursing program. Students receive it at graduation in a "pinning ceremony." Nurses wear their pins proudly as evidence of their achievement, learning, and skill. It is one way in which they distinguish themselves as distinct health care providers with a special body of knowledge and clinical skills.

Nursing programs also maintain a record of all graduates. Florence Nightingale started this practice by creating a list of graduates in 1860 at the St. Thomas' School of Nursing in England. This list became known as the "registry" of graduate nurses. The registry of nurses initiated by Nightingale provided institutions and clients with the means to identify graduates of nursing programs and ascertain the skills and knowledge of graduates. Today nursing programs around the world continue the tradition started by Nightingale and maintain a registry or listing of all graduates of the nursing program.

Purpose of Licensure

As nursing programs proliferated, variations developed among the programs. Entry criteria differed, and educational programs were structured to meet specific employer needs. A simple registry of graduates was not sufficient to ensure minimal levels of competency in all graduates, regardless of the training program. Another process was necessary to distinguish those sufficiently trained to provide nursing care from untrained or lesser-trained individuals. Graduate nurses, physicians, and hospitals joined to resolve the issue. The outcome was the development of criteria for licensure of nurses. Then, as now, the primary purpose of licensure is the protection of the public.

Early Licensure Activities

As early as 1867, Dr. Henry Wentworth Acland suggested licensure of English nurses. However, it was not until 1896 that licensing nurses was first attempted in the United States. Nursing programs in the United States developed in much the same manner as in England. Before the late 1800s many hospitals began training programs to prepare nursing staff for their own institutions. The programs varied based on the needs of the hospital, the availability of physicians and nurses for training students, and resources devoted to the training. To develop a standard for nurses and to improve the mobility of nurses between institutions, the Nurses Associated Alumnae of the United States and Canada, which in 1911 became the American Nurses Association (ANA), advocated licensure of nursing program graduates. However, the group met with much resistance from hospitals, physicians, and nurses. These first attempts at licensure failed for lack of support (Kelly and Joel, 1996).

Nurses worldwide mounted an extensive educational campaign explaining the purposes and safeguards inherent in licensure, and in 1901 the International Council of Nurses passed a resolution that each nation and state examine and license its nurses. In 1903, North Carolina, New Jersey, New York, and Virginia were the first states to institute permissive licensure. The licensure rules were voluntary. These permissive licenses permitted but did not require nurses to become registered.

Under permissive licensure, educational standards were set at a minimum of 2 years of training for nurses. State boards of nursing were established with rules for examinations and revocation of the license. Nurses not passing the examination could not use the title of RN. Therefore, in addition to protecting the public from unskilled practitioners, these rules were an early move to protect the title of RN. The New York State Board of Regents began a registry of nurses successfully completing all requirements. In 20 years, by 1923, all states had instituted examinations for permissive licensure. Each state's licensure examinations varied in content, length, and format and included written, oral, and practice components. The early work in examinations for licensure was the forerunner of today's licensure and certification requirements (Kalisch and Kalisch, 1995).

The early state efforts in licensing nurses were commendable. Nonetheless, there was considerable variability among states in nursing education requirements, the licensure examinations, and the nursing practice acts themselves. The widespread variability in nursing practice acts prompted the ANA and later the National Council of State Boards of Nursing to design model nursing practice acts. The model acts provided a template for states to follow. The first was published in 1915. These model practice acts have been revised and updated as nursing practice advanced (Kelly and Joel, 1996). For example, the National Council of State Boards of Nursing approved the most recent revision of the Model Practice Act in 2002. The administrative rules are to be approved in 2004 (National Council of State Boards of Nursing, 2004). The model nursing practice act proposes a definition of nursing, the scope of practice for the RN, information on renewal of licenses, descriptions of advanced practice nursing, requirements for prescriptive authority of nurses, and guidelines for disciplinary actions against nurses who violate sections of the act. Separate sections of the model act provide guidelines for State Boards of Nursing and the necessary requirements for entry into practice. From these model acts, each state or jurisdiction developed a unique practice act. Although the individual act addresses the needs of that jurisdiction, each includes these basic sections. The nursing practice act for any state or territory may be obtained by contacting that state's or territory's board of nursing. A listing of state boards of nursing addresses and Internet addresses is provided in Appendix B, which can be found on the Evolve website.

Mandatory Licensure

Once each state had established permissive licensure, the next movement was toward a requirement that all nurses must be licensed. This practice is termed *mandatory licensure.* Likewise, efforts were made to standardize nursing testing procedures. In the mid-1930s, New York was the first state to require mandatory licensure, although this requirement was not effective until 1947. After World War II the ANA formed the National Council of State Boards of Nursing. The council was composed of a representative of each state and jurisdiction in the United States. As part of its original activities, the Council advocated a standardized examination for licensure. This sponsorship led to the National League for Nursing administering the first State Board Test Pool Examination in 1950. The written examination included separate sections on medical-surgical nursing, maternity nursing, nursing of children, and psychiatric nursing. This format for examination continued for over 30 years, and many of today's nurses took these examinations.

The next major event in licensure efforts occurred in 1982 with the development of the first NCLEX examination. The test was revised to include all nursing content within one section of the examination. In addition the format was changed to present questions in a nursing process format. Just as with previous versions of licensing examinations, the NCLEX has evolved over time. Paper-and-pencil testing was replaced with computerized adaptive testing in 1994. Extensive information on the NCLEX can be found in Chapter 26 of this text.

COMPONENTS OF NURSING PRACTICE ACTS

As discussed previously, each state develops rules and regulations to govern the practice of nursing within that state. These rules are in the state's nursing practice act or its accompanying rules and regulations to administer the act. Many nursing practice acts are patterned after the ANA or the National Council of State Boards of Nursing model practice acts, and all contain comparable information.

Purpose of Act

Each act begins with a purpose. All nursing practice acts include two essential purposes. First, each includes statements that refer to protecting the health and safety of the citizens of the jurisdiction. The act describes the qualifications and responsibilities of those individuals covered by the regulations. Likewise, the act delineates those excluded from the practice of nursing. These provisions ensure the protection of the public. The second purpose is to protect the title of *registered nurse (RN)*. The legal title *RN* is reserved for those who have met the requirements to practice nursing and who have attained licensure. Thus unlicensed personnel are prevented from using the title of registered nurse.

Definition of Nursing and Scope of Practice

In each state or jurisdictional nursing practice act the practice of professional nursing is defined. The definition of nursing is of utmost importance because it delineates the scope of practice for nurses within the state. That is, each act outlines the activities of nurses may legally perform within the jurisdiction. Many states follow the guidelines incorporated in the model practice act, although each is specific and delineates practice within that state or jurisdiction. For example, some states describe nursing as a process that includes nursing diagnosis, whereas other states list broad areas of nursing activities. To prevent the acts from becoming outdated, lists of skills or procedures are not included in the acts. As nursing knowledge and practices advance, new techniques are frequently allowable because of the generalized nature of the definition of nursing.

Many jurisdictions incorporate definitions of advanced practice nursing within one definition of nursing. In other states the definitions of advanced nursing practice and the scope of practice for advanced practice nurses are defined separately.

Each state or jurisdiction establishes laws regulating practice within its borders. Therefore it is imperative for the nurse to know and understand the definition of nursing in the states in which he or she practices. Furthermore, jurisdictions retain the rights to govern practice within the jurisdiction, even in the presence of a mutual recognition agreement with other compact states. This retention of states' rights is an essential component in the Mutual Recognition Model.

There are other important reasons for becoming familiar with the definition of nursing practice. Frequently, nurses are asked to perform in ways that are beyond the legal definition of nursing. This is illegal, and if the nurse complies, he or she could lose the privilege of practicing nursing. In other situations, labor laws or other statutes affect nurses. Definitions may include or exclude nurses based on their legal definitions of nursing practice. As nursing practice becomes more complex and sophisticated, states may revise their nursing practice acts. Nurses are accountable for knowing the definition and scope of practice within their jurisdictions and practicing accordingly. Therefore, nurses should obtain copies of and become familiar with nursing practice acts for the states or jurisdictions in which they plan to practice.

Licensure Requirements

A section of each nursing practice act describes the requirements and procedures necessary for initial entry into nursing practice, or nursing licensure. An initial requirement in all jurisdictions is graduation from high school and an accredited nursing program. Candidates for licensure must submit evidence of graduation as defined by each state.

At present North Dakota is the only state requiring a baccalaureate degree for licensure as a professional nurse. This requirement was initiated in 1987. In North Dakota the nurse graduating from an associate degree program may be licensed as a technical nurse. In all other states, graduates of diploma, associate degree, or baccalaureate nursing programs may be licensed as RNs.

Additional requirements for licensure may include the mental and physical health status of the applicant. In addition, jurisdictions may conduct a review of prior legal convictions. This is especially important in reference to felony convictions. Some states have appended provisions related to recreational drug abuse. Finally, most states require statements from the school of nursing attesting the eligibility of the candidate for licensure. Frequently a transcript of coursework, a diploma, or a letter from the dean of the program attesting to the graduation of the applicant is necessary. Once again, as the laws are continually being revised to reflect the current practice of nursing, it is incumbent on the individual to be cognizant of the current licensure requirements in all states in which he or she intends to practice.

Regardless of individual state requirements, all nursing practice acts require candidates for practice to successfully complete the NCLEX-RN licensure examination. In some states it is possible to obtain a temporary permit to practice, pending receipt of success on the licensure examination. This practice was especially prevalent in past years, because in some states it took several months for results of the licensure examinations to be reported. Now, however, with the prompt response from the testing services, the need for temporary permits to practice is becoming less frequent.

A temporary permit is still available for nurses moving from one state to another. To obtain a license to practice in another state, the nurse applies for licensure by endorsement. Nurses licensed in one jurisdiction may apply for licensure in a second jurisdiction by submitting a letter to the second State Board of Nursing. Typically, evidence for the new license is similar to that for initial licensure. In addition, proof of the nurse's current license to practice, as well as any restrictions imposed on the license by the first state, is required. These procedures will continue for all states not participating in the Mutual Recognition Model. For those states designated as "compact states," the nurse should contact the State Board of Nursing to determine the appropriate procedures for nursing practice. Regardless of the type of nursing practice act, the nurse is still responsible for ascertaining the requirements to practice within each jurisdiction.

Renewal of Licensure

In addition to outlining requirements for initial licensure, each nursing practice act includes the requirements and information necessary to renew one's nursing license. These regulations define the length of time a license is valid, generally from 2 to 3 years. In addition, any specific requirements for renewal of licensure are stated.

Mandatory Continuing Education

The nurse will find information on mandatory continuing education for renewal of licensure in the section on license renewal. All nurses are expected to remain competent to practice through various means of continuing education. In 1976 California was the first state to institute mandatory continuing education for renewal of licensure. Since that time a number of states have instituted requirements of continuing education for renewal of licensure.

The number of hours necessary varies, depending on the jurisdiction, ranging from 20 to 40 hours over a 2- to 3-year period. A few jurisdictions require specific course content such as health care ethics or the state nursing practice act. Clinical course content may be designated for specific health problems such as sexually transmitted infections, human immunodeficiency virus, acquired immunodeficiency syndrome, and family violence (Yoder-Wise, 2003). In other states the Board of Nursing allows the nurse wide latitude in meeting the requirements for renewal of licensure.

ROLE OF REGULATORY BOARDS TO ENSURE SAFE PRACTICE
Membership of the Board of Nursing

An important section of every nursing practice act is the designation of a regulatory board of nurses and consumers to administer the nursing practice act. Frequently, this responsibility is assigned to a State Board of Nursing. The practice act outlines guidelines for membership on the board. In addition, procedures by which members are appointed to the Board of Nursing are designated. In most cases, the members are appointed by the Governor's office. Interested individuals or organizations, such as the state nurses association may submit names to the Governor for consideration.

Duties of the Board of Nursing

The responsibilities and duties of the Board of Nursing are delineated in detail. Specific duties of the board may be outlined in the act itself or in the enabling laws. These enabling administrative statutes are frequently designated as Rules and Regulations for the Practice of Nursing. It is through the work of the Board of Nursing that nursing licenses are granted and renewed and disciplinary action taken when provisions of the act are violated. Just as all nurses need to be cognizant of their nursing practice acts, nurses should also become familiar with the role of the State Board of Nursing.

A major responsibility of the Board of Nursing is responding to concerns about a nurse's practice. The review of a nurse's potential malfeasance, violation of the act, or other state and federal laws are within the responsibilities of the Board of Nursing. The nursing practice act describes the due process and procedures for this review. The Board of Nursing will then assign appropriate disciplinary action. These activities are a key responsibility of the Board of Nursing. Actions may include restrictions on the license or suspension or revocation of a nurse's license when provisions of the act are violated. Just as all nurses need to be cognizant of their nursing practice acts, nurses should become familiar with the role of the State Board of Nursing.

SPECIAL CASES OF LICENSURE
Military and Government Nurses

There are many nurses whose practice takes them throughout the country on a regular basis. For example, many nurses are members of the military or join the military nursing services after graduation. The Veterans Administration or Public Health Service employs thousands of nurses. These nurses serve in many jurisdictions, as well as outside U.S. boundaries. It is not necessary for these nursing personnel to obtain a nursing license in each jurisdiction in which they practice. The graduate takes the NCLEX-RN examination in one state. On successful completion, as an employee of the U.S. government, the nurse may practice in other jurisdictions without additional licensure requirements.

Foreign Nurse Graduates

Over 100,000 nurses practicing in the United States completed their nursing education in another country. These nurses met the requirements for practice in those other jurisdictions. When these nurses move to the United States, they take a special examination administered by the Commission on Graduates of Foreign Nursing Schools. The examination is given in English and tests the knowledge required to practice in this country. On successful completion, the foreign nurse graduate may apply for a license to practice in this country. Under new (2003) federal regulations, more stringent screening processes of these nurses have been enacted. The new guidelines call for a review of English competency, preliminary testing to predict success on the NCLEX-RN, review of original nursing education, and any restrictions on the nurse's practice in the home country (Protecting the Public, 2003). The intent of these regulations is not to be punitive or obstructive to the nurse. The regulations are yet the most recent example of two key principles: first, the protection of the public and second, the evolution of nursing laws to mirror current nursing practice.

International Practice

In a similar manner, nurses licensed in the United States may want to practice in other countries. Nurses interested in these opportunities may contact either the International Council of Nurses or the nursing regulatory board of the country in which they wish to practice. The International Council of Nurses is composed of representatives of organized nursing worldwide. A function of the Council is to assist nurses in obtaining licensure in other countries.

Just as a U.S. nurse interested in practice in another state should contact the state board of nursing in that state, the nurse interested in international nursing should contact the nursing regulatory agency in the country of interest. Each country has specific laws and regulations governing nursing practice that must guide the practice of the U.S. nurse. The nurse should be prepared to submit documentation on education, NCLEX-RN results and proof of licensure and practice in the United States to officials in the foreign country. Advance planning and contact with the appropriate regulatory agency will ease the transition for the nurse.

REVISION OF NURSING PRACTICE ACTS

Nursing practice acts, just as other sections of states codes, are written and passed by legislators. Just as in any legislative endeavor, many governmental agencies, administrators, consumers, and special interest groups seek to influence the legislation. These groups become actively involved in developing the accompanying rules and regulations. For example, physicians, dentists, pharmacists, licensed practical nurses, certified nursing assistants, emergency personnel and physician's assistants are just a few of the health care providers who are directly affected by the scope and definition of nursing practice. Likewise, organizations such as schools, hospitals, home health agencies, and extended care facilities are vitally concerned with the role of nurses today. Because of these multiple interest groups, the nursing practice act as finally passed or amended by the state legislature represents the aims and concerns of many individuals and groups, not only nurses. Review of a state's practice act reveals the influential parties involved in creating the act. Each group participates in defining the scope and practice of nursing and regulations affecting nursing practice within the jurisdiction. Because of these varied interests, it is essential for nurses to understand the practice act and the additional legislation that influences and controls their practice. Furthermore, as proposals to amend the nursing practice act are promulgated at the state level, it is imperative for nurses to be involved in this process. The resulting laws affect your profession, your practice, and your livelihood.

Sunset Legislation

One example of legislative activity affecting nursing practice acts is sunset legislation. "Sunset laws" are found in many states. These laws are intended to ensure that legislation is current and reflects the needs of the public. When sunset provisions are included in nursing practice acts, the act must be reviewed by a specific date. If the act is not renewed, it is automatically rescinded. This review process allows for revisions to update practice acts to be consistent with current nursing practice. Many nursing practice acts contain provisions of sunset legislation. It is through these activities that the scope of nursing practice is updated and the diagnosis of nursing problems has been incorporated into many definitions of nursing. Other changes include requirements for mandatory continuing education for renewal of licensure. Equally important, sunset laws have provided the means to define advanced practice nursing and incorporate prescriptive authority for advanced practice nurses. Nurses should determine whether sunset regulations affect the nursing practice act in the state in which they practice. Likewise, nurses should be aware of, and involved in, activities to amend the nursing practice act.

DELEGATION OF AUTHORITY TO OTHERS

The rapid expansion of health care providers, changes in health care delivery systems, and efforts to control health care costs have led to participation of many types of unlicensed personnel in the provision of health care. These personnel present a challenge to RNs working with them. Questions arise as to who can delegate what activities to which unlicensed provider groups. Guidelines for delegation have been developed by many nursing organizations, including the ANA and the National Council of State Boards of Nursing. However, the most current regulations may be found in the nursing practice acts of individual states. Because regulations differ among states, each nurse must identify and understand the regulations for the state in which he or she practices. Chapter 18 presents a detailed discussion of delegation and supervision.

CURRENT LICENSURE ACTIVITIES
Mutual Recognition Model

Efforts to provide common definitions of nursing practice, standards of education, and testing for entry into practice across state boundaries have been very successful. Nonetheless, most nurses are still required to apply for licensure in each state in which they practice. With the increased mobility of nurses, the telecommunications movement, and the necessity of caring for clients across long distances, state boards of nursing have recognized the need to provide practicing nurses with more than procedures of endorsement of their initial license. This need has led to further changes in nursing licensure. In 1997 the Delegate Assembly of the National Council of State Boards of Nursing moved to a new level of nursing regulation. The assembly approved a resolution endorsing a Mutual Recognition Model of nursing regulation. Through this model individual state boards will develop an interstate compact allowing nurses licensed in one state to practice in all other states and territories. Nurses will be responsible for following the laws and regulations of those states, although they will not be required to apply for multiple individual state licenses. Each year more states are developing compact laws. A listing of current compact states may be found on the website of the National Council of State Boards of Nursing, Inc. (2004).

A number of issues associated with mutual recognition concern nurses. On one hand, mutual recognition greatly facilitates interstate practice and movement of nurses to areas of shortage. A national database will provide information on individual nurses' practice and tracking mechanisms. On the other hand, concerns relate to monitoring nurses who practice in multiple jurisdictions, nurse privacy, and due process rights. Differences in practice requirements in different states may cause nurses confusion as to their rights and responsibilities.

The results of mutual recognition compacts will affect all nurses. Nursing students and graduates must remain apprised of changing conditions. The most comprehensive and current sources of information are the websites for the American Nurses Association, the National Council of State Boards of Nursing, Inc., and the State Boards of Nursing for individual jurisdictions.

Continued Competency

As discussed in preceding paragraphs, the primary purpose of nurse licensure is protection of the public. Thus mandatory continuing education was instituted as a strategy to ensure that nurses were competent to remain in practice. These programs have continued for a number of years. However, a growing number of nurses believe that more is required than just attending seminars to demonstrate the degree of competence. Consortiums of nurses in a number of states are examining other alternatives for renewal of licensure. These requirements may include clinical practice hours, portfolios, and other exemplars of practice.

There is increasing concern for patient safety and treatment in today's health care system. Models of continued competency are but one attempt by professional nurses to ensure that patients receive safe, effective nursing care. Another strategy in this quest is establishing programs of certification of advanced practice nurses.

CERTIFICATION

History of Certification

There are distinct differences between licensure and certification. At the most basic level, licensure establishes minimal levels of practice, whereas certification recognizes excellence in practice. Because of this difference, the background, requirements, and practice opportunities for licensure and certification differ markedly.

Just as with the development of nursing licensure, at its inception certification was not legally required; rather it was voluntary. In an effort to recognize nurses who had completed additional education and demonstrated competency in clinical practice, a number of nursing graduate schools and nursing specialty organizations offered certification programs. In the 1970s and later, advanced clinical courses were designed for nurses as a certificate program. The programs varied in length and content and did not offer a full master's course of study in nursing.

A second distinct difference in licensure and certification pertains to the organizations that grant certification. Whereas licensure is granted and governed by legislation and administered through the State Boards of Nursing, certification is awarded by nongovernmental agencies. Typically, these agencies are professional nursing specialty organizations. These organizations have created certification boards that are separate from the parent organization to conform to Department of Education requirements. There are over forty nursing certifying agencies, many of which offer certification in multiple specialties (Yoder-Wise, 2003).

The first field of nursing practice to certify practitioners was nurse anesthesia in 1946. Since that time the National Association of Nurse Anesthetists has maintained strict standards for education, certification, and practice of practicing nurse anesthetists. The policies and procedures established by nurse anesthetists provided a model for subsequently certifying advanced practitioners in nursing. Similarly in 1961 the American College of Nurse Midwives, founded in 1955, began certifying nurse midwives.

As certificate programs developed, it became apparent that standardization in programs was a necessity. In 1975 the ANA convened a national study group at the University of Wisconsin–Milwaukee to explore the issue. This meeting was attended by 75 nursing specialty organizations. The report of the group recommended the formation of a central organization for certification of nurses. This report, in conjunction with efforts of many nurses, resulted in the formation of the American Nurses Credentialing Center (ANCC). At present the ANCC (2003) has certified more than 200,000 nurses in over 40 areas of specialty practice (Box 5-1). In addition to the ANCC, many professional specialty nursing organizations offer certification examinations. A listing of these is provided in Box 5-2 (Yoder-Wise, 2003).

Subsequently in 1991 the American Board of Nursing Specialties organized with eight members: the ANA and the certifying boards of occupational health nurses, neuroscience nurses, rehabilitation nurses, nurse anesthetists, nutritional support nurses, nephrology nurses, and orthopedic nurses. This specialty board represents the majority of nursing organizations that certify nurses. Their mission is to ensure high standards and quality in education, evaluation, and practice of certified nurses. These efforts are further indication of nurses' commitment to protection of the public and the patients that nurses serve.

Certification began as a voluntary effort controlled by nursing organizations. State agencies were not involved in the credentialing process. This is still the case, although state nursing practice acts now include requirements for nurses to practice in advanced roles. Thus state practice acts first contained provisions requiring certification for nurse anesthetists and nurse midwives. With the development of additional advanced practice roles, all states have included requirements of certification in their regulations for advanced practice nurses in all specialty roles.

Purpose of Certification

The purpose of advanced practice laws is first and foremost protection of the public. Within the acts are definitions of advanced practice nursing. A number of states further differentiate the advanced practice of nursing by including separate titles for nurse practitioners and clinical nurse specialists. The scope of practice of the advanced practice nurse is well defined. States describe supervisory or collaborative practice with physicians, with differences existing among states as to the regulations governing these relationships. Requirements for practice vary among states. Although many states require a master's degree in the specialty area for practice, this is not the case in all jurisdictions. All states require evidence of certification in the specialty area. Many states require periods of practice in the specialty prior to awarding certification status. Typically the period of practice is 2 years. Finally, all states incorporate specific provisions for prescribing medications (Pearson, 2003).

BOX 5-1 *American Nurses Credentialing Center, 2003*

Advanced Practice Certification

Acute Care Nurse Practitioner
Adult Nurse Practitioner
Family Nurse Practitioner
Gerontologic Nurse Practitioner
Pediatric Nurse Practitioner
Adult Psychiatric and Mental Health Nurse Practitioner
Family Psychiatric and Mental Health Nurse Practitioner
Clinical Nurse Specialist in Gerontologic Nursing
Clinical Nurse Specialist in Medical-Surgical Nursing
Clinical Nurse Specialist in Pediatric Nursing
Clinical Nurse Specialist in Adult Psychiatric and
  Mental Health Nursing
Clinical Nurse Specialist in Child and Adolescent
  Psychiatric and Mental Health Nursing
Clinical Nurse Specialist in Community Health Nursing
Clinical Nurse Specialist in Home Health Nursing
Advanced Diabetes Management—Clinical Specialist
Advanced Diabetes Management—Nurse Practitioner
Advanced Practice Palliative Nurse

Credentials

Advanced Practice Registered Nurse, Board-Certified
  (APRN,BC)

Baccalaureate-Level Certification

Cardiac/Vascular Nurse
College Health Nurse
Community Health Nurse
General Nursing Practice
Gerontologic Nurse
Home Health Nurse
Informatics Nurse: Baccalaureate degree in nursing
Informatics Nurse: Baccalaureate degree in other
  relevant field of study
Medical-Surgical Nurse
Nursing Professional Development
Pediatric Nurse
Perinatal Nurse
Psychiatric and Mental Health Nurse
Nursing Administration

Nursing Administration, Advanced

Credentials

Registered Nurse, Board-Certified (RN,BC)

Registered Nurse, Certified in Nursing Administration,
  Board-Certified (RN, CNA, BC)
Registered Nurse, Certified in Nursing Administration,
  Advanced, Board-Certified (RN, CNAA, BC)

Associate Degree/Diploma Level Certification

Cardiac/Vascular Nurse
Gerontologic Nurse
Medical-Surgical Nurse
Pediatric Nurse
Perinatal Nurse
Psychiatric and Mental Health Nurse

Credentials

Registered Nurse, Certified (RN,C)

BOX 5–2	Specialty Nursing Certifying Boards

Critical Care Nurses	Nurse Anesthetists
Addictions Nursing	Dermatology Nurses
Diabetes Educators	Infusion Nurses
Spinal Cord Injury Nurses	Lamaze International
Occupational Health Nurses	Neonatal Nurses
Neuroscience Nursing	Nurse Practitioners
Perianesthesia Nursing	School Nurses
Nurse Midwives	Nutritional Support Nurses
Holistic Nurses	Otorhinolaryngology and Head Neck Nurses
Legal Nurse Consultants	Pediatric Nurse Practitioners
Nurse Executives	Obstetric, Gynecologic, and Neonatal Nurses
Psychiatric Nurses	Ophthalmic Nurses
Psychoprophylaxis Nurses	Nephrology Nurses
Camp Nurses	Oncology Nurses
Pediatric Oncology Nurses	Orthopaedic Nurses
Barometric Nurses	Plastic Surgical Nurses
Emergency Nurses	Rehabilitation Nurses
Urologic Nurses	Vascular Nurses
Perioperative Nurses	Wound, Ostomy and Continence Nurses
Gastroenterology Nurses	

Steps to Certification

The best strategy for nurses wishing to practice in an expanded role is to become informed of specific requirements in their chosen field. The nurse should examine carefully the roles and responsibilities inherent in advanced practice nursing; many resources exist to assist nurses (AJN, 2003; O'Malley, 2002). First the nurse should contact both the ANCC and the specialty organization in his or her area of practice to determine the education, experience, and examination requirements necessary to become certified. Concurrently every nurse should contact the state boards of nursing in the state(s) in which he or she wishes to practice and obtain information on legal requirements to practice in those jurisdictions. After gathering the requirements to practice, the nurse should develop a plan of action to complete the necessary advanced course work, clinical practice requirements, and examinations. By completing the requirements of these agencies, the advanced practice nurse may practice in an expanded role. In addition to the certifying agencies, the nurse may wish to contact other advanced practice nurses. These nurses will serve as valuable colleagues to the new advanced practice nurse.

Current Issues in Certification

Despite tremendous strides in development, certification as an advanced practice nurse is still a recent achievement. As with any new endeavor, advances are made in small steps and great leaps. Nurses in advanced practice face professional and legal issues of scope of practice, independence of practice, and their legal relationships with physician practitioners. These issues are not uncommon to nurses in any practice setting; however the advanced practice nurse is charting new territory. A unique challenge of advanced practice nurses is reimbursement for

BOX 5-3 Helpful Websites

American Nurses Association (ANA)—www.nursingworld.org
International Council of Nurses (ICN)—www.nursingworld.org/icn
National League of Nursing (NLN)—www.nln.org
American Nurses Credentialing Center (ANCC)—www.nursingworld.org/ancc
National Council of State Boards of Nursing—www.ncsbn.org

nursing services. There are ongoing efforts at the state and national levels to resolve these issues. Advance practice nurses are in constant communication with their peers and professional organizations. They look to all nurses to become involved in issues facing the advanced practice nurse.

SUMMARY

Nursing practice acts provide protection of the public and protection of the title of *RN*. This is accomplished through the development of specific regulations regarding education and examination of competence to practice. Each act contains guidelines for disciplinary action to protect both the public and professional nursing. The nursing practice act of each jurisdiction addresses the needs of the state and the responsibilities of nurses practicing within that state. It is important for all nurses and students of nursing to become familiar with the regulations guiding their own practice. Box 5-3 contains Internet addresses for nursing organizations with which RNs should become familiar.

As health care delivery evolves and nursing practice advances, it is necessary to make changes in the nursing practice act so that it remains responsive to the needs of all. Nurses must be part of this process. Collaboration with professional nursing organizations, the State Board of Nursing, and individual nurses will enable nursing to continually meet the needs of patients.

CRITICAL THINKING ACTIVITIES

1. Obtain a picture and description of your school/college nursing pin. Examine each aspect of the pin and learn the meaning ascribed to it. Reflect on how the nursing program exemplifies the symbolism of its pin. Think about your own nursing practice and in what manner it represents the meaning of your nursing school pin.
2. Contact the board of nursing in your home state or jurisdiction and obtain a copy of your nurse practice act with the accompanying rules and regulations. Read the act carefully and identify (a) the definition of nursing, (b) the scope of nursing practice, (c) requirements for licensure, and (d) renewal of licensure. Are statements regarding mandatory continuing education or other activities required?
3. Using the State Board of Nursing or the National Council of State Boards of Nursing, Inc. websites, determine whether or not your state is a member of the Mutual Recognition Model. If so, what are the implications for your practice in a neighboring state? If not, what must you do to practice in a neighboring state?

4. With the growth of telehealth and telenursing, nursing is practicing across state lines without nurses ever leaving home. What are the implications of practicing in another state? How does your state regulate telehealth?

5. Use texts, journals, or the Internet to identify current issues related to nursing licensure. Determine how these issues will affect the nursing practice act and nursing practice within your state or jurisdiction. Select and investigate one issue and formulate a position statement on the issue. Identify key nursing organizations (e.g., the state nursing association and a nursing specialty organization). Contact the organizations and determine their position on the issue. In collaboration with other students, faculty, and nursing organizations, develop strategies to become involved in and influence the outcome of your chosen nursing issue.

6. Select a clinical area that interests you. Contact the American Nurses Credentialing Center and the clinical specialty nursing organization to determine whether the specialty offers certification at an advanced practice level. Obtain information and requirements for certification in your chosen field. Identify strategies to prepare for certification.

7. Use the nurse practice act of your state to identify the scope of practice, regulations, and requirements for certified advanced nurse practice.

8. Seek out nurses certified in advanced practice. Learn from them about their roles and the professional practice issues they confront in their practice. Select and investigate one issue and determine strategies to influence the outcome of this issue.

Additional resources are available on-line at: http://evolve.elsevier.com/Cherry/

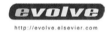

http://evolve.elsevier.com

REFERENCES

American Nurses Credentialing Center: *Certifications available from ANCC, 2003*. Retrieved on-line (www.nursingworld.org/ ancc/certifications/).

Kalisch PA, Kalish BJ: *The advance of American nursing*, ed 3, Philadelphia, 1995, JB Lippincott.

Kelly LA, Joel LA: *The nursing experience: trends, challenges, and transitions*, ed 3, New York, 1996, McGraw-Hill.

National Council of State Boards of Nursing, Inc: *Model nurse practice act*, Chicago, 2004, National Council.

O'Malley P: Update on prescriptive authority for the clinical specialist, *Clin Nurse Specialist* 17(4):191-193, 2002.

Pearson L: Fifteenth annual legislative update, *Nurse Pract* 28(1):26-58, 2003.

Protecting the public, *Am J Nurs* 103(11):69, 71, 2003.

What do credentials mean to you? *Am J Nurs* 102(5):71-73, 2003.

Yoder-Wise PS: State and association/certifying boards: CE requirements, *J Cont Ed Nurs* 34(1):5-13, 2003.

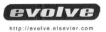

6

Financing Health Care and Economic Issues

Marylane Wade Koch, MSN, RN

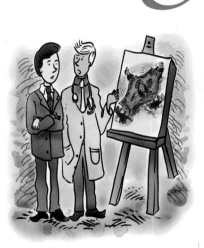

There is a tug-of-war for the shrinking health care dollar.

VIGNETTE

As a home care nurse for many years, my patients primarily have been older adults. Knowledge of Medicare coverage guidelines for service was critical to the financial success of the home care agency. Today in the home care agency, I am caring for patients of all ages with varying reimbursement guidelines for services. These guidelines differ among managed care organizations (MCOs) and insurance companies. When I first took this job, understanding Medicare coverage guidelines was a new challenge. Now even more is required. Today's nurse needs extensive knowledge of managed care and the economic influences on professional practice to provide patient care.

Questions to consider while reading this chapter:

1. Often the role of the professional nurse is influenced by the employer's ability to pay for the costs associated with staffing and providing quality health care services. Is this a passing trend, or is this likely to continue to be a normal part of doing business today in the evolving health care environment?
2. What does health care economics have to do with me as I provide patient care?
3. Why do I need to understand health care economics and its implications for my practice? Isn't that the role of the finance department or business office at my workplace?
4. With so many variations in health care insurance, I have a hard time understanding my own policy coverage. What role do I have in assisting my patients/clients in understanding their insurance or coverage options? Can being a more informed consumer add value to my practice?

Additional resources are available on-line at: http://evolve.elsevier.com/Cherry/

KEY TERMS

Capitation A method of reimbursing providers (usually physicians) with a fixed payment typically expressed as a per-member-per-month payment that is made in advance for future anticipated contracted health services.

Centers for Medicare and Medicaid Services (CMS) The federal government agency that administers Medicare and Medicaid. Formerly known as the Health Care Financing Administration (HCFA).

DRGs (diagnosis-related groups) Refers to reimbursement based on a predetermined fixed price per case or diagnosis for clients in 468 categories.

GDP (gross domestic product) The total output of all goods and services in the country.

Health Care Financing Administration (HCFA) The federal government agency that administered Medicare and Medicaid until 2001.

Marginal An economic term that refers to the change in some variable (e.g., the number of tests performed).

Medicaid A jointly sponsored state and federal program that pays for medical services for persons who are elderly, poor, blind, or disabled and for families with dependent children.

Medicare A federally funded health insurance program for the disabled, persons with end-stage renal disease, and persons 65 years of age and older who qualify for social security benefits.

Prospective payment system A method of reimbursing health care providers (i.e., physicians, hospitals) in which the total amount of payment for care is predetermined based on the patient's diagnosis; provides for a "set price per diagnosis" payment system in contrast to the retrospective or "fee-for-service" system; encourages increased efficiency in the use of health care services since providers are reimbursed at a set level regardless of how many services are rendered or procedures performed to treat a particular diagnostic category; predominant method of payment in today's health care system.

Retrospective payment system A method of reimbursing health care providers (i.e., physicians, hospitals) in which professional services are rendered and charges are billed based on each individual service provided; also known as the "fee-for-service" payment system. This system encourages overuse of health care services because the more services rendered or procedures performed, the more revenue received by providers.

Third party An organization other than the patient and the supplier (hospital or physician), such as an insurance company, that assumes responsibility for payment of health care charges.

LEARNING OUTCOMES

After studying this chapter, the reader will be able to:
1. Analyze major factors that have influenced health care access and financing since the middle of the twentieth century.
2. Analyze the relationship between market issues and health care resource allocation.
3. Integrate knowledge of health care resources, access, and financing into managing professional nursing care.
4. Critique the relationship between contemporary economic issues and trends and professional nursing practice.

CHAPTER OVERVIEW

In the past several decades the costs of health care have continued to increase, with economic issues taking a central role in health care decision making. Hospital managers know that for many patients the hospital will receive a predetermined payment, regardless of length of stay and specific treatments. Physicians recognize that the prescribed course of treatment for their patients may be analyzed by a peer review committee. The costs their patients incur may be compared with those of other physicians or against cost benchmarks. Businesses require employees to cover larger amounts of their health insurance premiums or pay larger deductibles and co-payments. Health insurance companies "manage" care, sometimes placing limits on medical care coverage or on the site of care delivery. These dramatic and relatively new developments are the result of the evolving economics of health care.

The objective of this chapter is to describe and explain the major economic issues and trends driving the critical changes in health care delivery and financing. The chapter has five sections. The first section reviews trends and major changes in health care financing. The second area of discussion is an analysis of the allocation of medical care resources, with emphasis on the dominant issues of access and cost containment. The third section is a discussion of the general approaches available for making health care allocation and delivery decisions. The fourth section explores the mix of health financing methods, distinguishing the varied roles of government and private funding. The final section discusses the major issues of the health care world of managed care and its impact on nursing.

HISTORY OF HEALTH CARE FINANCING

Historically, several underlying themes have driven health care financing in the United States. Among these are:

- The physician's role as being primarily responsible for health care decision making
- The broad objective of providing the "best" possible care to everyone
- The rapidly increasing sophistication and cost of medical technology
- Economic incentives and the fee-for-service payment method that encouraged overuse of health care services

For many years two of these factors—physician domination in decision making and the fee-for-service payment method—were intertwined and contributed to the lack of cost consciousness in health care.

The simultaneous occurrence of the physician's decision-making role and fee-for-service payments was combined with the driving motivation in the health care system to provide the best possible care for all patients, regardless of cost. Physicians made all decisions about what health care services were needed and costs were rarely discussed between physician and patient, so the cost of care almost appeared to be an afterthought until bill-paying time. Medical tests or procedures were provided if the physician determined that additional care might offer any marginal aid or diagnostic information.

Beginning in the 1960s, the approach of "if it *might* help, do it" was furthered by the rapid pace of technologic change. New and sophisticated technologies significantly enhanced physicians' abilities to provide treatment. The more tests or procedures performed, the greater the earnings because physician income was tied to the number of procedures performed. Instead of attempting to allocate medical resources to the highest medical need, there was a financial incentive to provide as much care as possible using the most technically advanced methods of care in all cases. However, as medical technology advanced and medical revenues increased, overuse of health services and rapid cost inflation resulted.

Although health care was overused in many cases and costs were increasing, patients as consumers of health care remained largely insulated from cost inflation. Most patients were covered by some form of insurance or "third-party payment" mechanism, not paying the "full cost" for their care or even for their health insurance premiums. The "full cost" of care generally remained hidden from consumers since the costs were subsidized by their employers or by taxpayers through such programs as Medicare and Medicaid. Because patients were not aware of the costs of their health care, providers had little incentive to be concerned about costs. The lack of cost consciousness in the demand for medical care generated "perverse economic incentives." Providers received more income for using more services with no financial risk for their use of additional resources. Providers were often motivated to provide additional services, because they earned more income from each procedure performed or service provided.

These "perverse economic incentives" had a drastic effect on the Medicare program, which was implemented in 1965 to provide health insurance coverage for people age 65 and older who are eligible for social security benefits, people with end-stage renal disease, and the eligible disabled population. By the early 1980s increased medical usage (increased intensity of care) and high inflation, as well as a growing elderly population and high overall inflation, generated large increases in the total Medicare bill. The rapid growth of Medicare expenditures became a major factor in the federal budget deficit, which caused the Centers for Medicare and Medicaid Services (CMS) (formerly the Health Care Financing Administration [HCFA]) to rethink the entire Medicare payment system. This led to a revolution in health insurance reimbursement.

Health Care Financing Revolution

In 1965, the health care expenditures in the U.S. were $202 per capita; in 2002 health care expenditures were $5,400 per capita. During this same time period, national health expenditures as a percentage of gross domestic product (GDP) rose from 6% to 14.5% (National Health Statistics, 1999). This statistic became 14.9% in 2002. The significance of this growth is that for every dollar a person spends buying products or services in the United States, 14.9¢ goes to pay for health care. Health care spending increased from $1.3 trillion in 2000 to $1.6 trillion in 2002 (CMS, 2004).

To gain control over the rapidly rising health care costs identified in the early 1980s, a health care financing revolution was initiated in 1983, when Medicare moved from a retrospective or fee-for-service reimbursement approach to a new prospective payment system (PPS) based on diagnosis-related groups (DRGs). This shift was critical for hospitals because Medicare is the largest single payer of hospital charges. Under DRGs each Medicare patient is assigned to a diagnostic grouping based on the primary diagnosis when admitted to the hospital. For that patient's care, Medicare limits its total payment to the hospital to the amount preestablished for that DRG. This contrasts sharply with the previous approach under which hospital patients incurred costs for all prescribed therapies and Medicare subsequently reimbursed these charges according to its fairly generous payment schedules.

Since 1983 if hospital costs are greater than the DRG payment for a patient's treatment, the hospital incurs a loss, but if costs are less than the DRG amount, the hospital makes a profit. Thus, hospitals face a strong financial incentive to reduce the length of stay and minimize procedures performed. Although DRGs originally applied only to hospital payments for Medicare patients, once this reimbursement revolution began, similar or comparable reimbursement arrangements were initiated by private insurance companies.

DRG reimbursement also had a profound effect on hospital administration and cost accounting. Implementation of the DRG system substantially expanded the role of hospital management, including nurse administrators. First, it was apparent that gains were made primarily from the careful diagnosis of patients according to their highest potential DRG classification. This initiated new roles for hospital-based nurses in utilization management to assist in determining the appropriate DRG for patients. Utilization nurses play a pivotal role in determining the appropriate DRG, with its resulting length of stay for patients. Second, hospital record keeping and accounting methodologies also were revolutionized. It became necessary for hospitals to adapt new and highly specific Medicare cost accounting procedures. These procedures mandate that all internal hospital costs be carefully allocated to each of the DRG categories. Experienced nurses with business knowledge brought needed technical background and skills to these new accounting and utilization management tasks, expanding opportunities for nurse managers or administrators.

By the early 1990s, based on the success of DRGs in reducing the rate of growth of Medicare payments, the financing revolution extended with a new approach to physician reimbursement. The previous Medicare fee system for physician payments was replaced with a new one determined by an innovative Resource-Based Relative Value Scale (RBRVS). The objective was to bring the payments for different types of medical services more in line with the physician skills required and the actual time spent on specific procedures. For example, when Medicare initially covered cataract surgery, it was a relatively rare and lengthy procedure. However, over time cataract correction has become one of the most frequently performed Medicare surgical procedures. The procedure became so rapid and relatively easy to perform that it was viewed by CMS as overpaid. The RBRVS system sought to correct the disparity between Medicare's high payments for this type of procedure and relatively low payments for more hands-on primary care. Payments to primary care and internal medicine physicians were increased, whereas fees for many specialists were reduced.

Managed Care

As the shift to prospective payment occurred under Medicare, private insurance companies also developed alternate health care financing methods, which generally are termed *managed care*. Managed care organizations (MCOs) encompass several different approaches, such as health maintenance organizations (HMOs), preferred provider organizations (PPOs), and point of service (POS) plans. A commonality of these forms of payment is a method for review and oversight of the medical goods and services used. Under managed care the insurance company, a peer review organization, or another review mechanism is used to bring cost consciousness to bear on medical decision making. In this process a reviewer evaluates the patient's medical options, keeping the concept of cost effectiveness in mind. Coverage may be denied for procedures that are considered unnecessary, excessive, or experimental, which is in strong contrast to the previously pervasive "if it *might* help, do it" approach.

Managed care goals are the same as those sought by Medicare DRGs: to overcome some of the problems of retrospective payment of charges such as inefficiency, overuse, and excess charges. By the late 1980s, costs for businesses to provide health insurance for their employees were increasing 20% a year. These increases in health insurance costs were passed on to consumers in the form of price increases for the products or services sold by the business.

As health care costs became an increasingly significant proportion of the overall cost of products or services, U.S. businesses had more difficulty competing in an international market. Insurance companies were pushed by their largest business customers, such as automobile manufactures, to decrease the rapid rise of insurance premiums and health care costs. In addition to demanding lower premiums from the health insurance companies, some firms began to "self-insure" their workers, establishing reserves and managing their own health benefits program rather than paying premiums to an external insurance company. This resulted in substantial savings as businesses managed their own health plans

The widespread and rapid expansion of managed care in the 1990s was a response to numerous factors, including cost inflation, overuse, an increasing number of persons who are uninsured ("uncompensated" care), and the effects of health costs on business profits and international competitiveness. Therefore employer health insurance markets moved rapidly from conventional insurance plans to MCOs. About 85% of commercially insured people participated in managed care by the late 1990s.

The Employer Health Benefits 2000 Annual Survey conducted by the Kaiser Family Foundation and the Health Research and Educational Trust demonstrates a move by businesses to limit the availability of plan types offered to workers. About 65% of workers are still given a choice of more than one plan. However, survey results showed significant change in the availability of different types of plans; for example, the percentage of workers offered a PPO option increased from 45% in 1996 to 66% in 2000 (News Briefs, 2001). Fewer workers were offered conventional and HMO plans. With managed care, the private insurance market initially accomplished one of the goals sought by national health insurance proposals—slowing the rate of growth in health care costs. Unfortunately, this accomplishment in the 1990s has been short-lived as health care costs have once again begun to rise.

Inflation and Cost Containment

Cost containment was "*the* health issue" from the mid-1970s through the 1980s because health care costs increased much more rapidly than prices of most other goods and services. Health care inflation is measured by the medical care component of the overall Consumer Price Index (CPI), which is the primary measure of U.S. price changes. In the early 1990s health care inflation began to slow considerably, decreasing from 9% in 1993 to 4% in 2003 (U.S. Department of Labor, 2003). Several factors influenced this positive trend of slower health care inflation. Inflation in general declined. General inflation affects health care because hospitals, clinics, and other providers have to hire workers and purchase supplies, energy, and all other inputs at higher prices or wages.

The largest share of health expenditures is for hospital-based care. DRGs led to decreases in hospital admission rates and patients' average lengths of stay. Patients are discharged from hospitals "quicker and sicker." Therefore outpatient procedures and the use of home health and primary care clinics have increased. These changes helped reduce inflation. Hospitals are also using cost-cutting techniques such as decreasing inventories, joining purchasing groups, and using physician review. Drug companies offer more generic alternatives that can be effectively prescribed for patients at lower costs. In addition, cost containment and utilization control strategies under managed care, as well as increased cost sharing by patients, have been used in an attempt to help slow inflation. Despite these measures taken in recent years to reduce inflation in health care to more manageable levels, hospital spending once again increased in 2002 by 9.5%, the fourth consecutive year of growth (CMS, 2004).

Access Issues

Because health care cost inflation significantly slowed in the 1990s, the dominant health issue became access to health care, particularly for the uninsured or underinsured. Lack of access to health care today primarily reflects a lack of insurance coverage, so access is an issue of financial access. Before the passage of Medicare and Medicaid legislation in 1965, few Americans had health insurance, but since then the percentage of persons having health care coverage has increased. In 2002, the population without insurance coverage rose to 15.2% or 43 million people with no health insurance (U.S. Census Bureau, 2002). They include the working poor who are employed by small firms without insurance coverage and part-time workers, as well as indigents, some acquired immune deficiency syndrome patients (who have lost coverage), and other groups.

Medicaid is intended to improve access to health care for the poor, covering 40.4 million people. These include 4.3% elderly, 7.7% blind and disabled, 19.6% children, and 8.8% adults (NGA, 2003). Even though Medicaid recipients have improved access when compared with the uninsured, Medicaid recipients are not as likely to obtain needed health services. The poor are more likely to lack a usual source of care, less likely to use preventive services, and more likely to be hospitalized for avoidable conditions than those who are not poor (U.S. Department of Health and Human Services, 2000).

Although lack of insurance is a serious problem for households, it also presents problems for providers and for all insurers. The uninsured and underinsured populations generate uncompensated or indigent care costs and bad debt for health care providers. These unpaid costs must be covered by those who do pay so that the hospital can continue operating, a process known as "cost-shifting." Providers increase their charges against households and public and private insurers, who pay for their own care plus some contribution for the care of the uninsured population. This in turn increases insurance premiums, which makes it even more difficult for many households and businesses to afford coverage. However, in the new era of managed care and with the growth of HMOs and PPOs, the ability of providers to shift costs has decreased dramatically. The problem of uncompensated care and cost-shifting is a major reason that many people advocate some form of national health insurance coverage.

In addition to the problem of the uninsured population, there are several other barriers to health care access. For those living in rural or inner-city areas, there may be location or geographic problems of access. These may be straightforward transportation issues or may involve the lack of specialists, new technology, or specialized facilities in many regions of the country and in some inner cities. Access to health care may be hampered by long waiting periods that require patients or their families to miss extended periods of work, with lost wages representing an added financial cost to obtaining care. One unique access problem is related to the nature of transplantation technology. In this case, the access issue is how to allocate the limited number of organs available.

The next sections look closer at the issues of financing and access to examine what generates health care costs. Questions regarding the allocation of resources to health care and the production of medical goods and services are examined.

ALLOCATION OF HEALTH CARE RESOURCES
Health Resources

The health care system of any society consists of its entire package of health care delivery and financing mechanisms, combined with its health and medical institutions and any additional institutional framework that affects health. Although the health care systems of various countries may appear to be different, there actually are only a limited number of ways in which health care resources can be allocated for the production and distribution of medical care.

Health care resources include all the inputs devoted to producing medical care and health care: (1) "labor" such as nurses, physicians, technicians, pharmacists, and administrators, including their education, skills, and training; (2) "capital," including all the medical facilities and equipment available; (3) "land," the actual land area for hospitals and other facilities; and (4) "entrepreneurship," which encompasses the skills and risk taking that business persons bring to health businesses, especially to starting new ventures. Because all these resources are "scarce" or limited in the amounts available at any given time, decisions have to be made that involve choices about how to best use them. Basic decisions (choices) must be made in the production and provision of health care (i.e., in the allocation of scarce resources to health and medical care).

Resource Allocation Questions

Each society has to answer several basic underlying questions to decide how to allocate its resources to health care. First, what combination of medical goods and all other goods do we want to produce in the economy using our scarce resources? How much or what share of the total production of all goods and services should be devoted to health care? In 2002, 14.9% of the Gross Domestic Product (GDP) was allocated to health care, with a value of more than $1.6 trillion. The Office of the Actuary at the Centers for Medicare & Medicaid Services projects national health expenditures will reach $2.8 trillion by 2011, with health care expenditures being 17% of the GDP (CMS, 2003). If the share of total expenditures devoted to health increases, then some non-health goods and services will need to be eliminated, transferring the resources or inputs from the things given up to medical care.

The second resource question to be answered is this: What combination of specific medical goods and services do we want to produce in the health care sector of the economy? Or what types of health and medical care do we choose to produce? Do we prefer a high-tech, institution-based mix of health services emphasizing therapeutic (crisis-oriented) medical care, or do we choose a prevention-oriented health system emphasizing primary care and wellness? Such choices are made either explicitly or implicitly. For example, if it is decided to allocate more scarce health resources to hip replacements for elderly osteoporosis patients, then there may be fewer health care resources to allocate to other areas such as prenatal care or child health screenings.

Finally, who should receive the medical goods and services? This is a distribution question, and the answer may depend largely on who has the health insurance coverage to finance the purchase of health care. If the society has some form of national health insurance, it has decided that all of its citizens should have financial access to medical care. In contrast, in the U.S. federal or state funding is only provided for defined groups that have eligibility for specific programs such as Medicare and Medicaid. Some defined groups such as veterans have established (or legislated) "rights" to medical care, but the overall entire population does not.

The way a society answers these basic questions defines that society's type of health care system. Although there are many variations, there are a fairly limited number of approaches to economic decision making and allocating resources in health care. These resource allocation issues are further discussed in the following sections.

ECONOMIC APPROACHES TO ALLOCATING HEALTH CARE

Economic approaches to allocating health care in any society can fall into four basic categories, which are (1) a market system with some government regulation (regulated market system),

(2) a competitive market system, (3) centralized government planning and/or a single-payer financing system, or (4) some combination of the first three options. There is no advanced industrial country with a purely competitive market system for the allocation of health care resources. The United States and South Africa are the only industrialized Western countries that do not have a national health insurance system covering all of their citizens. Most of the European countries have a substantial amount of central government planning in their health systems, with Great Britain being a primary example of a fully centralized or nationalized system. Almost all of the health care resources in the British National Health Service (e.g., hospitals, clinics, nursing homes) are owned and run by the government.

Regulated Market System

In contrast to other countries, the health care system in the United States predominantly relies on decision making through the market system of the U.S. economy, although most U.S. health care markets are regulated to some extent by federal or state legislation. To describe our health care system, first consider exactly what is meant by a market. A market is simply a means by which a buyer and a seller come together. It may be a place such as a pharmacy or a clinic, but market transactions also can be accomplished by telephone (a prescription can be called in, charged, and delivered) or even by computer (prescription can be emailed with the payment information). However, a question arises: Do health services received from a Veterans Administration (VA) hospital involve a market transaction if there are no charges? The answer to this question is no, because this transaction implies a transfer of in-kind services from taxpayers to the VA patient and is a nonmarket transaction or an entitlement given to veterans.

In a regulated market system examples of regulation include requirements of minimum nurse staffing in long-term care facilities, laws regarding the disposal of medical waste products, and regulations affecting the conduct of medical laboratories. In addition, all licensure and certification laws or qualifying examinations represent regulation of medical professionals. Thus we have a market system for most health care goods and services, but virtually no area escapes regulation.

Competitive Market System

A market system implies private ownership of resources and private decision making by consumers about their purchases and by businesses about producing and selling. These decisions are made largely on the basis of the prices of goods and services. For a market system to function effectively and efficiently, it needs to be competitive. Competition implies that (1) there are numerous buyers and sellers in the market, so no single seller or group of sellers can manipulate the price; (2) the products of all suppliers in the market are similar; (3) consumers and sellers are well informed about market conditions and prices; and (4) new resources are free to enter or leave this market.

Although we have a regulated market system for producing health care, there are numerous reasons why these markets are not really competitive. Consumers cannot be well informed about what health care to purchase without a doctor's diagnosis. Also it may be difficult for consumers to get information about the prices of services until after the services are provided. Once the patient visits the physician, the physician is likely to be in charge of numerous subsequent decisions, so the doctor in effect becomes an "agent" for the patient. Furthermore, the physician's income may be affected by what is ordered for the patient. In other words, the physician's reimbursement incentives may encourage overuse or underuse of treatment options.

Another issue in considering whether health care markets can be competitive is "third-party payments" or insurance payments for medical care. A competitive market system assumes that people make their decisions to purchase something on the basis of its price, but health care consumers often pay less than the "full price" because their insurance pays some or all of the cost. Consider the following scenario: If an employer bought "shoe insurance" for employees so they only had to pay a coinsurance payment of perhaps $10 (or possibly only 20% of the full price) for shoes, how many pairs would an employee buy? And would the employee buy more expensive or cheaper shoes? This is exactly the issue that insurance coverage, or third-party payment, adds to the confusion of health care markets. What is important to remember in this scenario is that the cost of the "shoe insurance"—or health insurance—is passed on to the consumer in the form of price increases for the products or services. Because of these "hidden" health care costs, the consumer perceives health care as much cheaper than it actually is and may be motivated to purchase more and possibly overconsume.

Job Growth and the Health Care Industry

An additional resource issue relates to health care as a driving force of new job growth throughout the economy. Between 1988 and 1992 the health services industry created 1.4 million jobs, or half of all the new jobs produced in the United States. Since the long economic expansion of the 1990s began in March 1991, two-thirds of all the new jobs created were in health care.

The Department of Labor predicts that between now and 2010, there will be a 25% increase in health care related jobs, with 13% of all jobs being in this field. The Bureau of Labor Statistics predicts continued fast growth of health care related jobs, with 13.6 million jobs available in 2010 and over 2.8 million of these being newly created jobs. These jobs include traditional health care roles, as well as opportunities for accountants, auditors, personnel specialists, attorneys, computer programmers, operators and support specialists, chemists, engineers, file and purchasing clerks, secretaries, and food service helpers. The increased demand for health care services associated with the aging population will promote new health care job opportunities for the next 50 years. (Healthcare Services and Jobs, 2003)

SOURCES OF HEALTH CARE FINANCING

The $1.6 trillion (more than $5400 per capita) spent on health care in the United States in 2002 was financed by combinations of private and public sources. These expenditures were primarily to pay for health services and supplies for individuals. Other health expenditures are for areas such as health-related research, health professional education, and medical facilities construction. Most individual health care is paid either by households through direct out-of-pocket payments or by third-party public or private insurers. Third-party payers include private insurance companies, independent health plans, and government health programs. Following is a summary of the sources of health insurance coverage for residents of the United States (please note that the total of these percentages is greater than 100% because some people may be covered by more than one type of insurance) (U.S. Census, 2002):

- 61.3% of people are covered by employment-based health insurance.
- 13.4% of people are covered by Medicare.
- 11.6% of people are covered by Medicaid.

- 9.3% of people are covered by direct-purchase health care plans.
- 3.5% of people are covered by military health care.
- 15.2% of people have no health care insurance coverage.

Private Insurance

Although private insurance accounts for the largest percentage of coverage for health care, it is important to remember that the cost of providing health insurance to employees is passed on by the employer to the consumer in the pricing of goods and services. Thus all people pay a part of health care costs in every purchase they make. Additionally, even when covered by insurance, individuals must still pay a portion of their health care costs directly from their own pockets through payments for insurance premiums, deductibles, and co-payments.

In the 1990s private insurance companies increasingly followed the lead of Medicare in implementing the medical reimbursement revolution. Payment mechanisms moved to capitated payments or prospective reimbursement under an array of HMOs, PPOs, and POS arrangements. An HMO is a way of organizing and delivering health care that combines delivery with the payment mechanism (insurance), usually by prepayment or capitation. HMOs reduce costs by constraining use, particularly by encouraging reduced inpatient hospital use and encouraging the use of more preventive services. A PPO is based on contractual arrangements between the insurer and provider, under which the provider agrees to lower prices and the insurer agrees to motivate its entire group of insured members to use that particular facility or physician group. PPOs give a list of providers to consumers and offer them a financial incentive to use these specific providers. POS arrangements give consumers somewhat more flexibility in selection of providers but also involve contracts between medical providers and insurers.

Tax Subsidies of Private Payments

Private sources of health expenditures are subsidized by the government if they represent tax deductions or nontaxable income. The income tax code allows households to deduct health expenditures that total more than a certain percentage of their income and also contributions to health philanthropy. Furthermore, private insurance premiums paid by employers also are subsidized as a fringe benefit that is not a taxable income. The deductibility of these health expenditures represents tax revenue losses to the federal government. In addition, cities subsidize health care real estate through property tax exemptions for nonprofit and public hospitals.

Public Insurance

Government is the biggest influence in the health insurance market, generating half of hospital revenues and more than one-fourth of physician incomes. The largest health insurance program is Medicare. Since enactment of the program in 1965, the population covered by Medicare has doubled, and it is projected to increase to 55 million within 20 years. Medicare is an entitlement program based on age or disability criteria rather than on need. Medicare Part A covers inpatient hospital services, skilled nursing facilities (SNFs), and home health benefits. Hospital coverage has deductible and coinsurance requirements and some coverage limitations. Payments to home health and SNFs are increasing rapidly.

In contrast to Medicare, a federal program with national eligibility criteria, Medicaid is a joint federal-state program for which states establish some of the eligibility criteria based on their Aid to Families with Dependent Children (AFDC) income eligibility levels. The federal government establishes minimum coverage that states may supplement. Medicaid covers primarily disabled persons, AFDC households, and those in nursing homes who qualify based on their low-income level. Thus a program designed to provide health care access to impoverished families, particularly children, has become the primary payer of long-term care nationwide, covering almost half of all nursing home costs. In addition Medicaid is required to cover the deductibles and co-payments for Medicare beneficiaries who are impoverished and thus termed *dual eligible* (that is, dual eligible for both Medicare and Medicaid). For most states Medicaid represents the fastest growing component in the state budget.

Impacts of Payment Modes

As a result of the Medicare prospective payment mechanism (DRGs) and the various versions of managed care that have been implemented by private health insurance companies, there have been clear increases in efficiency in the delivery of care, such as more efficient use of medical services and some decreased prices of services. Other attempts to increase efficiency include the growth of free-standing clinics, more outpatient use, cuts in programs and eligibility, and new options for patients. Because patients are being discharged earlier and sometimes in less stable condition, patient care is shifting from acute care to more community-based sites such as community mental health centers, home health agencies, and multiple other community sites. The economic incentives in medical settings have shifted toward more cost-effective care. Managed care and utilization reviews are shifting the health care system toward increased preventive care and away from its long-standing emphasis on acute care. Nonetheless, after all the efficiency changes, health costs remain the fastest increasing element in federal and state budgets.

IMPLICATIONS FOR NURSING: MANAGING COST-EFFECTIVE, HIGH QUALITY CARE

Nurses represent a major professional force in the delivery of health care services in the U.S. today. Never has there been greater opportunity to advance the practice of professional nursing. Innovation and excellence in all nursing practice is needed to contain costs while attaining positive, measurable outcomes. All professional nurses have a role in managing care in the setting where they work. Practitioners are needed to provide cost-effective care for wellness, acute care, and chronic illness. Educators are necessary to inform the public of ways to improve health, practice prevention, and manage chronic disease. Administrators are necessary to organize health care services for optimal resource management with high-quality outcomes at reasonable costs. Professional nursing practice spans a variety of settings from acute, institutional, or hospital care to outpatient care to community-based clinics, physician offices, home care agencies, and insurance companies. Each setting holds practice challenges in providing and managing care that is efficient, affordable, and of high quality. Box 6-1 summarizes the trends occurring in health care that affect professional nurses. These trends mandate that nurses have a clear understanding of the economic and financing issues underlying the continuously developing roles of nurses.

Many opportunities for nurses in today's health care environment are economically and politically driven. Changes in the financing of health care services directly affect professional nursing practice. Markus (1990) outlined several reasons why payment reform is important to nursing:

1. The rules of payment are important as a reflection of the value and worth society places on health care services for the public.

BOX 6-1   *Economic Issues and Trends*

From		To
Illness emphasis	→	Preventive emphasis
Acute care	→	Preventive, home care
Hospital/institution-based	→	Noninstitution-based (clinic/home)
Fee-for-service (cost-based)	→	Prospective payment and managed care
Physician-directed	→	Diverse decision-makers and managed care
If it helps (at all), use it (regardless of cost)	→	Outcomes measurement and cost-effectiveness
Independent decisions (practice variation)	→	Protocols/guidelines (best practice)
Local perspective (practice variation, standards/benchmarking)	→	Global perspective (protocols/guidelines/practice)
Introduce new technologies (regardless of cost)	→	Outcomes measurement and cost-effectiveness
Paper records, medical charts	→	Information systems, computer records

Change in Orientation

From		To
Illness, crisis	→	Prevention
Specific, specialist	→	Holistic
Quantity of care	→	Quality of care

Location of Service

Inpatient	→	Outpatient, clinic, home

Payment Mode

Retrospective	→	Prospective
Fee-for-service	→	Managed care

Outlook

Just do it	→	Outcomes measurement; evidence-based
Just do it	→	Quality of care; quality of life

2. Government policy influences the public's openness to secure services from various professionals such as nurse practitioners.

3. Financing impacts salaried employees because health care providers build job opportunities based on payment sources. For instance, if a professional service is covered under reimbursed allowances, jobs in that service will be offered by the provider.

4. Payment modes will determine whether a particular nursing role will be reimbursed, affecting specialties and professional autonomy.

As national health care concerns change, the financing rules will reflect the concerns and attitudes of policy makers and hopefully the public at large. In particular, Medicare payment changes will increasingly impact nursing practice as the number of elderly persons, who depend on Medicare for their primary health insurance, increases. Nurses must learn how to proactively position themselves educationally and professionally to work with the new economic challenges of health care.

Efficiency and Effectiveness of Care

Health care financing has progressed from physician-dominated decision making in a fee-for-service mode with third-party and retrospective payment to prospective and capitated payment. Nurses provide services as a resource or input into the health care delivery system to produce patient care and care management. Nurses can affect care management in many ways, including coordinating care, case management, disease management, and outcomes management. Because resources are limited and decisions are based on service costs, administrators may combine non-nursing resources with limited nursing resources to decrease the total costs of services. Thus, professional nurses are pressured to demonstrate excellent clinical resource management and to design care delivery that provides a less costly service that satisfies the customer requirements.

Coordinated Care. Integrated or coordinated care is one way to decrease duplication of services and reduce wasted health care resources. This type of care has brought about the use of more case management and integration of services for cost-efficient care. More care is being delivered in the community through home care, outpatient clinics, and ambulatory care centers at less costly rates as inpatient hospital-based care decreases. These changes in the health care environment require professional nurses to understand basic principles of financial and resource management and take a leadership role to ensure the effective and efficient use of resources.

Case Management. Case management is a role in which nurses can demonstrate cost effectiveness in managing care by ensuring that patients get the most effective treatment in the most appropriate level of care across the continuum of care. Opportunities exist for nurses who understand the overall structure and processes of the health care industry and who bring skills of critical thinking, as well as patient advocacy. Understanding current health care economics is critical to this role. The American Association of Managed Care Nurses has as its mission (1) to be recognized as the "expert" in managed care nursing, (2) to establish standards for managed care practice, (3) to positively impact public policy regarding managed health care delivery, and (4) to assist in educating the public on managed care (American Association of Managed Care Nurses, 2004). To learn more about the American Association of Managed Care Nurses, visit their website (www.aamcn.org).

Disease Management. Disease management programs provide another opportunity for professional nurses to impact effectiveness and efficiency of health care services. Although there is controversy over whether or not these programs consistently deliver improved care in a cost effective way, reports continue to be positive. For example, a coronary artery disease (CAD) management program targets the treatment of heart disease, the disease that consumes the largest percentage of U.S. health expenditures. At Universal Healthcare in Buffalo, New York, results were measured after just 1 year of implementation of a CAD management program, increasing the rate of annual lipid profile testing from 76% to 81%. In the years 1996 to 1999 the rate of Medicare patients taking beta blockers following a myocardial infarction increased from 54% to 98% (Shaw, 2001). Cedar-Sinai Medical Center in Los Angeles is addressing uncontrolled hypertension through a disease management program, which has resulted in statistically significant lower blood pressures and reduced provider visits and provider costs (Hatcher, 2001).

Outcomes Management. Nurses are most successful when they can demonstrate efficiency of care with measurable, effective outcomes. Nurses should know how much their services cost and at what price services can be offered. They must be innovative in minimizing resource use, demonstrating the resulting decrease in costs and responding to the economic incentives of prospective payment and capitation. Rewards will come to those health care professionals who can manage the costs of disease and teach the value of good health. Practitioner value and accountability will be found in clinical and financial management.

Population Diversity and Aging

In the U.S. today more than 13% of Americans are 65 years of age or older. The average life expectancy is 77 years, with women living on the average beyond 80 years. The fastest growing segment of the U.S. population is persons 85 years and older. This trend translates to an increase of health care expenditures consumed by older adults. Management of health expenditures for the elderly will be paramount for a successful financial model for health care services in the U.S..

The aging population means a renewed emphasis on care for chronic disease. In fact, 78% of total medical costs can be attributed to chronic disease conditions; this also applies to 80% of Medicaid costs (NGA, 2003). Nurses can add value to their practice with an ability to delay the onset of chronic illness through education and prevention. Nurses have opportunities to develop and implement disease management programs and measure their effectiveness. The increasing number of elderly in the United States brings many economic and professional challenges as nurses bring value to their care through special education in geriatrics and care of the older adult. Opportunities will be available for nurses to participate in care management in various long-term care settings.

The U.S. population also is becoming more ethnically and racially diverse, with the number of minorities growing at a rate double that of whites. Diversity brings new cultural practices and disease patterns with economic and care implications, and the increase in minority populations brings a new labor source to health care. Increased diversity in professional and nonprofessional health care workers could change the current availability and cost for the services of professional nurses.

Expansion of Technology

Improved technology for diagnostic and therapeutic practice is under examination for cost efficiency versus outcome delivery. Leaders, including professional nurses, in the U.S. health care system must balance the health contributions of the improved technology with the accompanying costs along with issues of quality of life, access to care, risk-benefit analysis, and individual consumer choice.

U.S. consumers have long lived with access to high levels of technology with little concern for costs. Nurses will be key players in educating patients and families about the cost-to-benefit ratio of certain technologies and will assist in selecting alternatives. One example is found in the increased use of pharmaceuticals; more advanced drugs are marketed with varying degrees of actual documented benefit over existing, less-expensive drugs. Many patients are afraid to trust generic drugs, although they are less expensive. The nurse can be a link to educating the public regarding the potential gain in use of a more expensive drug versus a less costly alternative. This is most important to older adults and others on fixed incomes who may already be spending a large portion of their income on health care.

BOX 6–2 *Online Health Care Financing Resources*

American Association of Managed Care Nurses
www.aamcn.org

American Case Management Association
www.acmaweb.org

Centers for Disease Control and Prevention
www.fedstats.gov

Centers for Medicare and Medicaid
www.cms.hhs.gov
www.healthierUS.gov

Managed Care Magazine Online
www.managedcaremag.com

Medicare
www.medicare.gov

U.S. Census Bureau
www.census.gov

The technology of the Internet offers promise for innovative programs (Box 6-2). The e-Case Management program at Wilson Medical Center in North Carolina uses a web-based approach to case management and claims dramatic improvement in quality of care and decreased costs as information can be accessed by providers through the Internet at any location, which promotes continuity of care (Durrer and Wright, 2001).

Information technology is of utmost importance to the professional nurse. The ability to gather and analyze health-related information and data for improved care is critical. Health care information systems are expensive, but they offer many opportunities in managing health care costs. Combining clinical skills with information technology skills can provide significant advantage to the success of professional nurses and new avenues for professional nurses to demonstrate their ability to provide cost-effective outcomes measurement.

Consumer Empowerment

Consumers or patients are health care customers demanding quality health care services at affordable rates. To be selected for services and products, providers are challenged to assess and meet customer requirements. The health care marketplace generates choices among services and products and alternative prices. Nurses must respond to marketplace opportunities and provide customer-focused care, which means putting the customer or patient first—a philosophy that nurses can totally support.

Economic forces are motivating the shift toward a model of health promotion and preventive care to achieve cost-effectiveness. This brings a new relationship with the consumer, emphasizing cost-sharing through individual choices in health practices. For instance, the insurance rate may be higher, or benefits may vary, based on the presence of unhealthy individual practices such as smoking, drinking, or taking drugs. Again, customer choice has economic implications in the health care marketplace of the future.

As managed care grows, legislation is in place to protect Americans enrolled in managed care plans. This protects individuals with special health care needs to ensure continued access to care as they transition from fee-for-service to a managed care plan and assess quality and appropriateness of care. Information for beneficiaries about the managed care plan must be comprehensive and easy to understand. Other aspects of the legislation include access to services, patient-provider communication, network adequacy, marketing activities, and a grievance system. These changes encourage empowerment and protection of the health care consumer (New Patient Protections, 2001).

Nurses have many opportunities in a consumer-empowered marketplace. Nurse practitioners can demonstrate their ability and skills to deliver customer-focused primary care at reasonable costs as a cost-effective alternative to physician services. Opportunities for advanced practice nurses include primary care, case management, utilization management, quality improvement, patient advocacy, triage, education, and resource management. Nurses can take the lead in demonstrating the value of wellness and teaching health consciousness. Written materials for all levels of education will be needed, providing yet another opportunity for nurses who publish.

S U M M A R Y

Changes in the focus of the U.S. health care delivery system have brought new challenges for professional nurses. Health care has moved from emphasis on illness to emphasis on wellness and prevention, including the shift from acute care services to preventive and community-based services such as ambulatory care and home care. This shift mirrors the change in focus from hospital or institutional-based services to noninstitutional services such as home care.

Financing of health care services has gone from retrospective, fee-for-service payment systems to prospective payment and managed care. In the past, health care services were primarily directed by the physician, whereas today there are more diverse decision makers through managed care. The concept of "if it might help, do it" regardless of cost is yielding to practice based on research evidence, outcomes measurement, and cost-effectiveness.

In the past, state-of-the-art technology was introduced and used regardless of price. Today technology is more frequently being used and respected as important to health care delivery but only with demonstrated outcomes, for the appropriate service, and at the right price. Information technology is critical in the move toward data-driven decision making. The "hard-copy" paper patient records are being encompassed by computerized, integrated information systems.

What does this mean to professional nursing? Nursing faces many challenges in professional practice in the twenty-first century. Many of these are directly related to the changing political and economic marketplace of health care. One is demonstrating that nurses provide measurable cost-effective, high-quality care. Practice in a cost-conscious environment is here to stay. Nurses will constantly challenge the current way of practice and examine each process for improvement and cost effectiveness. Accurate data must be collected to show cost containment and positive patient outcomes.

Nurses need to assume the professional self-confidence necessary for leadership in the ever-changing economic and political environment that determines payment for services. Roles on clinical teams, in administration, with insurance companies, and with the government hold promise for empowered change.

Nurses can accept that the job market is changing and that there will be job insecurity. However, changes in the health care marketplace will create new opportunities for health care professionals and eliminate the need for others. Professional nurses can prepare for these changes by recognizing health care trends and shifts in financing care and by educating themselves for evolving careers. This demands a commitment to lifelong learning.

Malone (1997), former president of the American Nurses Association, wrote about the "new order of health care" of the twenty-first century resulting from the many changes in the health care environment. Many of these changes are the result of economic forces, managed care, and technologic innovations. Malone describes the presence of "twin sisters of excitement and anxiety" as this new order evolves. Her positive attitude is shown as she describes the twenty-first century as the "century of opportunity" for nurses.

As new systems are being designed for health care delivery models in managed care, professional nurses are uniquely qualified to play an integral role in this transformation process. The success of managed care will depend on creating healthier and better-informed consumers. The outcomes can be reduced health care costs with increased worker productivity. Nurses can position themselves to take a lead in educating consumers and encouraging personal responsibility for improved health practices. A managed care philosophy is congruent with that of professional nursing practice, bringing nurses back to the basics as society recognizes that healthy people are good business.

CRITICAL THINKING ACTIVITIES

1. The health care financing revolution motivated important changes in the delivery of care across all health care settings. Describe the ways in which these changes are creating new or expanded opportunities for nurses. How do you expect these financing changes to affect your career?
2. Define ways that you, as a professional nurse, can obtain current health care economic information and trends. Why is this important? How can this knowledge add value to the practice of nursing?
3. Describe nursing actions that can increase and actions that can decrease the patient's cost of care.

Additional resources are available on-line at: http://evolve.elsevier.com/Cherry/

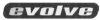

http://evolve.elsevier.com

REFERENCES

American Association of Managed Care Nurses, Inc: *Mission.* Retrieved on-line January, 2004 (www.aamcn.org).

Centers for Medicare and Medicaid (CMS): *Health care spending reaches $1.6 trillion in 2002.* Retrieved on-line Jan, 2004 (www.cms.hhs/gov.media/press/release).

Centers for Medicare and Medicaid (CMS): *Projections of national health expenditures: methodology and model specifications, 2003* (www.cms.hhs/gov).

Durrer C, Wright S: Case management over the Internet, *Managed Healthcare News* 17(2):35, 2001.

Hatcher CE: Cedar-Sinai hypertension program reaches a new high in lows, *Managed Healthcare Executive* 1(2):38-41, 2001.

Health Care Services and Jobs, 2003. In Damp DV: Health care job explosion: high growth health care careers and JOB LOCATOR. Retrieved on-line (http://healthcarejobs.org).

Malone B: President's perspective, *Nurse* 28(8):6, 1997.

Markus G: Medicare payment reform: implications or the nursing specialties, *Spec Nurs Forum* 2(2):2-7, 1990.

National Health Statistics Group: *Office of Actuary, National Health Expenditures, 1998, Health Care Financing Review,* vol 24, no 2, HCFA Publication 03420, Health Care Financing Administration, Washington, DC, 1999, U.S. Government Printing Office.

New patient protections in managed care rule, *Tenn Hosp Health Systems Newsletter* 6(2):5, 2001.

News Briefs: Employee choice, *Managed Healthcare News* 17(2):1, 2001.

NGA Center for Best Practices: *Medicaid fact sheet.* Retrieved on-line, 2003 (http://www.nga.org/center/divisions/1,1188,C_ISSUE_BRIEF^D_5951,00.html).

NGA Center for Best Practices: *Disease management: the new tool for cost containment and quality care.* Retrieved on-line, 2003 (http://www.nga.org/center/divisions/1,1188,C_ISSUE_BRIEF^D_5177,00.html).

Shaw G: Coronary artery disease: practicing prevention, *Managed Healthcare News* 11(2):18, 2001.

U.S. Census Bureau: *Health insurance coverage 2002.* Retrieved on-line (www.census.gov/hhes/www/hlthins.html).

U.S. Department of Health and Human Services, Centers for Disease Control and Prevention, National Center for Health Statistics. *Health insurance coverage, Nov 7, 2000.* Retrieved on-line (www.cdc.gov/nchs/fastats/hinsure.htm).

U.S. Department of Labor, Bureau of Labor Statistics: *Consumer price index, 2003.* Retrieved on-line (www.bls.gov/cpi/home.htm).

SUGGESTED READINGS

Chang CF, Price SA, Pfoutz SK: *Economics and nursing: critical professional issues,* Philadelphia, 2001, FA Davis.

Feldstein PJ: *Health care economics,* ed 4, Albany, NY, 1993, Delmar Publishers.

Phelps CE: *Health economics,* New York, 1992, Harper-Collins.

Santerre RE, Neun SP: *Health economics: theories, insights, and industry studies,* New York, 1996, Irwin Publisher.

Starr, P: *The social transformation of American medicine: the rise of a sovereign profession and the making of a vast industry,* New York, 1982, Basic Books.

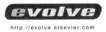
7

Nursing in the Ever-Evolving Health Care System

Tim Porter-O'Grady, EdD, RN, FAAN

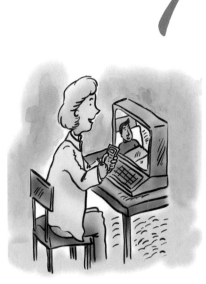

Technologic advancements are requiring nurses to develop new models of nursing care delivery.

VIGNETTE

On her way to work, Nancy Barker, RN, BSN, pushed the communication button on her in-car data center. The screen came up on her data dashboard showing her patient assignment for the day and listing the coded reference containing all of her patients' health care information. Included with Nancy's daily assignments were time estimates for completing each assignment and suggested patient priorities. The voice-accessible system allowed her to open the portal to begin voice-activated documentation. At the first stoplight, Nancy noted a red flashing flag on the data screen next to the name of one of the patients she was scheduled to see during the morning. She voice-dialed the clinical center, accessed the central database to determine the source of the red flag, and learned that the red flag reflected a potentially serious clinical circumstance related to the patient's current vital signs, which had just been assessed through the clinical center's telemedicine system. Nancy voice commanded the data center to connect with the physician's data center and was immediately connected to the physician. The physician's picture appeared on the data screen. Nancy and the physician discussed the patient's current condition and agreed upon a change in the patient's medication regimen and care plan. As Nancy proceeded to the next intersection, the database automatically adjusted the clinical information in the patient record, recalibrated the care plan, and incorporated it into Nancy's clinical schedule for the specific patient. On Nancy's command for directions to the first patient on her schedule, her satellite moderated GPS (global positioning system) created a map and voice-moderated directions.

Additional resources are available on-line at: http://evolve.elsevier.com/Cherry/

Questions to consider while reading this chapter:

1. How does information technology affect the delivery of nursing care in any setting?
2. How has technology transformed Nancy's role in planning for patient care, organizing her work, and documenting care?
3. In what way does Nancy's experience foreshadow the implementation of new models of nursing practice?

KEY TERMS

Cross-platform A programming language, software application or hardware device that works on more than one system platform (e.g., Unix, Windows, Macintosh). Examples of cross-platform languages are Java, JavaScript, HTML, Perl, Python, and REALbasic.

Evidence-based nursing The process of systematically, finding, appraising, and using research findings as the basis for clinical practice.

Information system The network of all communication channels used among people within an organization.

Payer A public or private entity, such as an insurance company, that underwrites or renders payment for health care services provided.

Technology The discipline and processes dealing with the art or science of applying scientific knowledge to practical problems.

Therapeutics Clinical processes concerned with addressing and/or treatment of disease.

Value-driven The quality (positive or negative) that renders something desirable or valuable and sustains that value across work and time measures.

LEARNING OUTCOMES

After studying this chapter, the reader will be able to:

1. Analyze current factors that are forcing significant changes in the health care delivery system.
2. Compare and contrast historical models of nursing with nursing practice models required in the twenty-first century.
3. Explain the impact of current health care payment mechanisms on rapidly evolving technologic innovations.
4. Articulate a new vision of nursing practice based on changing technology.

CHAPTER OVERVIEW

The arrival of the twenty-first century has brought with it a transformation in the delivery of health care services (Fukuyama, 2002). The advent of quantum mechanics and the fast-paced transformation led by technologic innovation have created social and human conditions unparalleled in the history of humankind (Brown and Duguid, 2002). The challenge we are currently facing is that much of this new technologic innovation brought with it a change in the human experience unanticipated by the very people who enthusiastically embraced the conveniences those technologies produced. As a result, the changes and challenges have been somewhat surprising to those people who can now no longer live without these technologies. This reality shift has had no greater impact on anyone than it has had on nurses (Porter-O'Grady, 1997). The following sections of this chapter further explain how technologic innovations and other major factors are forcing an evolution in the U.S. health care system and will require the nursing profession to embrace a new vision of nursing practice for the twenty-first century.

THE HISTORICAL GROUNDING OF NURSING PRACTICE

Nursing practice has historically been grounded in principles of patient care (Ulrich, 1992). Primarily, these principles have been founded in the management of sickness and the treatment of illness. Although nurses have practiced in a wide variety of settings such as clinics, public health settings, government institutions and schools, most nursing practice during the past 75 years has been associated with hospital care (Alcott and Parsons, 1984; American Hospital Association et al, 1942; Baer, 2001; Buerhaus et al, 2002; Johnson, 1964). Indeed, much of basic nursing education is predicated on the hospital-based role of the nurse. Though there have been progressive changes in the hospital management of patients, the basic principles and tenets of nursing care have remained relatively unchanged. It is only in the last two decades that a beginning transformation in the foundations of nursing practice has initiated a trend in nursing that has radically affected the ability of nurses to practice as they always have (Chaska, 2001).

Impact of Technology

Considerable advances in medical technology, especially in the area of minimally invasive medical applications and pharmacologic therapeutics, have radically altered the processes associated with delivering health care (Box 7-1). Health care services have become increasingly portable, less invasive, shorter-term, and faster, thus requiring less institutional time (i.e., shorter length of stays) (Frankel, Quill, and McDaniel, 2003). Medical advances have resulted in an unparalleled growth in noninstitutional and outpatient based delivery of therapeutic services (Kalow, Meyer, and Tyndale, 2001). As a result, the number of inpatient hospital beds in the United States has declined appreciably while the number of outpatient clinical services has radically accelerated (Schappert and National Center for Health Statistics, 1998).

This shift from inpatient care to outpatient clinical services has deeply affected the structure and delivery of nursing care (Hein, 2001). Nurses who once managed inpatient-based longer-term increments of patient care are now managing fast-paced patient turnover. In the past,

BOX 7-1 *Health Service Delivery Changes*	
20th Century	**21st Century**
Fixed service	Fluid service
Functional	Flexible
Institutional	Mobile
Late stage	Early-engagement
Process-driven	Outcomes-driven

nurses were focused on providing excellent care over a relatively long patient stay, and now they are primarily involved in managing increasingly shorter lengths of stay and moving patients out of the acute care setting as quickly as possible. Primary nursing activity has made a drastic transition from fixed models of patient care to emerging models of patient turnover—and this change has become a major source of nursing conflict.

A Conflict Between the Old and the Emerging

The vast majority of nurses in practice today have spent most of their practice lives in the traditional hospital environment. It is in the hospital setting that most of the radical changes in the health care system are more intensely felt. Because the average age of the nurse is 47 years, it is not surprising that those nurses are having difficulty confronting a significantly altered health care system with new therapeutic foundations that are significantly different from those that have been present during most of their careers (Box 7-2). As a result, there is much anger, role confusion, uncertainty, and lack of clarity and consensus over the future direction of nursing practice. In many of the publications and public forums where these issues are explored, the anger and unhappiness is palpable.

Further driving this level of discomfort and unhappiness is the comparison of current issues of nursing practice with past practices. This, of course, is an inadequate perspective. Rather than comparing today's nursing practice issues with yesterday's practice experiences, it would be more viable and beneficial for nurses to begin to assess the meaning of today's changing demands on practice and the growing future obligation for different parameters of practice (Porter-O'Grady, 2001).

SHIFTING REQUIREMENTS FOR NURSING CARE

Today's world is considerably different from the one that most practicing nurses entered into 20 to 30 years ago. Therefore it is imperative that we begin to look at the future of nursing practice within the context of current unfolding and transformational events. The expectation that patients should receive the full range of possibilities in nursing services, which nurses have become accustomed to rendering, is now unrealistic. As lengths of stay become shorter and intervention becomes less invasive, the requirements for nursing care are different. No longer can nurses provide all of those activities of patient care that once were considered fundamental to nursing, such as backrubs and bed baths. Time and circumstances no longer permit this level and extent of care. The problem that emerges in this scenario is that both nurses and patients still carry traditional service expectations that can no longer be fulfilled

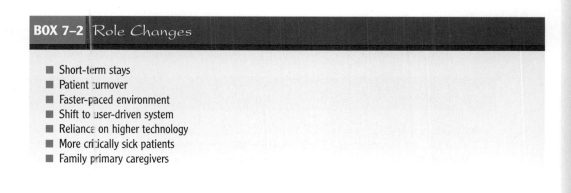

BOX 7-2 *Role Changes*

- Short-term stays
- Patient turnover
- Faster-paced environment
- Shift to user-driven system
- Reliance on higher technology
- More critically sick patients
- Family primary caregivers

within the current context of care (Geisler et al, 2003). With both nurses and patients confronting these circumstances without changed expectations of what should occur, dissatisfaction and unhappiness can be the only expected outcome.

Patients and nurses must now be significantly reoriented to a different reality for their service relationship and for care expectations. Indeed, part of the clinical relationship between patient and nurse is the reorientation and reeducation of the patient in light of changing service obligations and clinical outcomes. An increasing part of the nurse's role is this reconceptualization of the patient to a different set of clinical and outcome expectations. The difficulty in this effort, however, is that the nurse's expectations must first change. Before patients can change *their* expectations for what they receive in the health care system, nurses must communicate the legitimacy and appropriateness of a different set of expectations. Perhaps more difficult to accomplish, the reeducation of patients will include altering or denying the patients' satisfaction with previous expectations, which were validated by patients' historic perceptions and experiences. Indeed, the nurse must see this reeducation of the patient as a fundamental practice obligation of the time. To help patients achieve effective changes in their expectations, nurses must have engaged the reality shift in their own practice perceptions, roles, and performance (Box 7-3) (Frampton et al, 2003).

A reorientation of the perceptions of the nurse requires a considerably different understanding of the shifts in health care delivery and what they mean for nursing practice. It is important that the factors causing the shifts in the health care system are accurately discerned so that their impact on nursing practice can be better understood. Some of the major factors causing shifts in the health care system are listed below:

1. Health care is quickly moving into mobility-based approaches and out of residency-based (inpatient) models as medical therapeutics become more portable and less invasive, requiring less treatment and recovery time.
2. Emerging models of medical interventions no longer require patients to stay for long periods of time to obtain an appropriate service; however, much of nursing education is still based on patient care, teaching, and learning about practices that require patients to stay around long enough to receive what nurses have traditionally had to offer (Osborne, 2002).
3. There continues to be an accelerated movement from an inpatient service structure to a faster growing outpatient care service marketplace, again with service that is nimble, fast, with short lengths of stay.
4. Much of the care traditionally given by nurses following medical procedures and therapeutics in the hospital environment is now provided in the patient's own home; shifting accountability for subsequent care, procedures, and patient activity from the professional caregiver to the patient and his or her significant other, who is now the primary caregiver (McAlearney, 2002).

BOX 7–3   *Primary Role of the Nurse*

The primary role of the nurse in this health care transformation is to change the service expectations of the user. The only template the patient has for service is a twentieth century model of service that is no longer present, nor is it currently relevant.

5. Payment structures for health care services are challenged to respond to the shifting health care system. Transitions to new technologically advanced medical treatments create a challenge for health care payers to determine appropriate payment structures for these new technologies. This creates considerable confusion and uncertainty for both payer and provider.

6. Changes in the locus of control, service environment, clinical processes, and work context are creating staff shortages, which challenge the appropriate distribution and use of professional services, including nursing. The two major contests arising from these circumstances are (1) sufficient and appropriately trained staff and (2) adequately configured practice activities and models of utilization.

7. The behavioral demands of work are now changing from institutional models of service to worker mobility models of service. This creates conflict between mature workers oriented to a more traditional model of work, increasing demands for changing the work itself, and the emergence of new workers with different loyalties and priorities than the traditional majority in the contemporary work place (Lancaster and Stillman, 2002).

8. The pace of innovation and new technology applications creates a growing demand for new processes and procedures that arise faster than providers can accommodate. When a new technology emerges and is applied, within a brief period of time an even newer technology arises, sometimes making the recently acquired technology and its associated practices immediately obsolete. This occurs at a rate beyond the ability of the nurse and other interdisciplinary team members to engage and accommodate previous intermediate technology demands. As a result, the individual is consistently overwhelmed and always attempting to simply keep up (Maysys, 2002).

Portability and Practice

Perhaps the greatest challenge to nursing practice for the future is the increasing portability of health care. This notion of portability changes the very foundations of clinical activity and, therefore, of nursing practice. For the entire latter half of the twentieth century, the vast majority of nurses have practiced in hospitals and other health care institutions. This institutional framework created the locus of control for both the delivery and the experience of health care that defined its application. The schools of nursing preparing nurses and the institutions that employ them created a contextual framework for practice that was definitive and prescribed. This partnership between what was learned and what was practiced provided the contextual framework for all nursing activity (Joel and Kelly, 2002).

Over the past decade the foundations for clinical practice have been quickly shifting. The emergence of digital technology and its application to medical therapeutics has completely changed the processes of treatment and intervention, as well as effecting significant shifts in the payment system (Box 7-4). These new technologic innovations have created a different context for the delivery of service. As previously mentioned, the impact on the system has been significant.

For nursing and nurses, this change is dramatic. In the emerging environment, the predominant issue for nursing practice is no longer the delivery of extended patient care services. It is, instead, the transitioning of patients quickly and efficiently through the system in a way that is both cost- and service-effective. As patients are discharged more quickly, nurses experience conflict about their professional roles because they can no longer provide the same services to patients that they once provided. Now that length of stay is no longer the major element of the delivery of service, lost to both the nurse and the patient are those

BOX 7–4 *Impact of Technology on Health Care Delivery*

- Noninvasive
- Portable
- Flexible
- Convenient
- Fast
- Fewer complications
- Fewer side effects

myriad activities once associated with excellent nursing care. As a result of this major shift, the following newer priorities for nursing practice must now emerge:

- Codifying nursing practice
- Creating easy access
- Building the information infrastructure

Codifying Nursing Practice

Since many of the practices once provided by nurses to patients in the institutional environment are now being provided by others outside of the hospital and health service environment, these traditional nursing practices must now be more clearly enumerated. As more direct patient care is provided by significant others in settings other than the hospital, it is important and appropriate for nurses to undertake a process of skills transfer. Through the creation of service and unit-based websites that are easily accessible and user-friendly, new opportunities for access are provided for these emerging caregivers. In preparation for skills set transfer, nurses must now be creating CDs and DVDs, as well as streaming videos to educate the emerging caregivers.

Creating Easy Access

Access skills are now an important part of the management of patient care. As technology becomes more proficient and generalized to the population, its use must be considered a critical part of the service equation. At all levels, making access easy for the user (i.e., patients and family caregivers) is a fundamental obligation of the provider. Computers and Internet technology make it possible for the user to be continuously linked to the provider of health care services in a way that allows for access of important information and interactive communication between provider and user. In fact, it is now the obligation of nurses and other providers to create ways to keep the user of health care services in constant contact with the health care system. Through this synthesis of activity and constancy of connection, both provider and user can now interact in a more effective and continuous way. In this manner, a stronger and lifelong relationship is established between health care systems, providers, and the users of their services. Increasing attention to this reality by health system providers will be the major focus of health communications systems over the next two decades.

Building the Information Infrastructure

Perhaps the most significant financial and resource allocation issue now and for the next decade is creating a well-linked and integrated clinical information infrastructure. Health providers are now able to collect, collate, and integrate huge amounts of clinical, service, and financial information. In fact, so much information can now be accessed that information management alone overwhelms the delivery of health care services. The increasing complexity of clinical services results in complexity of information related to that service. Because of its importance, this information must be collected, interpreted, applied, and evaluated. In order to do this adequately, huge amounts of information and the tools and devices necessary to manage the information must be obtained and incorporated into the ongoing process of care delivery (Androwich et al, 2003).

In the coming years, well over half of the resources invested to improve health care will likely be devoted to building this information infrastructure—hardware, software, and other technology designed to link and integrate dissimilar systems and manage huge amounts of data. The demand for integrated accessible information is so great that the current information systems cannot adequately collect, integrate, and generate information in a usable fashion. Indeed, many of the resource problems existing today can be tied directly to the inadequacy of the information management systems in most health care organizations. Manual and non-linked information processes increase both workload and intensity for health professionals who need to access and use the very information that the current infrastructure does not yet provide. In fact, most of the emerging focus on quality measures, evidence-based practice, outcome driven processes, and care evaluation mechanisms now demand a better clinical information system than exists in most places where health care is offered (Quaglini et al, 2001).

The three major initiatives that make up the information priorities in our health care delivery system are:

- Integrating the continuum of information
- Building cross-platform information services
- Developing an information-specific mental model for practitioners

Integrating the Continuum of Information. Perhaps one of the most difficult activities associated with the management of information is the interface between elements of information. The most significant work to be accomplished for effective information management in health care is to create linkages between components of the information infrastructure (Box 7-5). Other service arenas such as commercial retail companies (e.g., Visa©, MasterCard©) have mastered the integration of financial, purchase, warrantee, service, and billing information. Many of the techniques used by credit card companies to manage their customers' use of services could be transferred directly to the management of health care information. Unfortunately, much of this transfer has not yet occurred in any significant way across the health care system.

BOX 7-5 *Creating the Information Infrastructure*

- Wired charting
- Virtual records of care
- Integrated information
- Portability of data
- Information access facility
- Cross-platform hardware/software
- Ability to readily upgrade systems

The linkage between clinical, administrative, financial, billing, and service information remains tenuous in most health care services. This lack of integration among key health-related services can no longer continue without immeasurably affecting the kind and quality of health services provided in a technologically driven world. To be successful, both health care providers and health care business administrators need a well-articulated mechanism for information processing and management. Indeed, the success of health systems in the twenty-first century directly relates to their capacity to link and integrate the various functions and activities associated with health care delivery.

Building Cross-Platform Information Services. Perhaps there is no greater challenge than the interface between existing information hardware and software and emerging technology. One of the greatest significant problems in information management is the linkage between past and current hardware and software and emerging enhancements in both arenas. Clearly, a developmental process and approach to linking and integrating current mechanisms and processes with future and emerging technology is a serious and important undertaking in the process of information management. Like other components of the information industry, health care applications must reflect a standard of practice and utility that is industry-wide and can be replicated across systems. Without this approach, the necessary articulation of structure and process in information management will be delayed; more important, the proper and appropriate management of increasingly complex patient care and clinical services and the business processes that support them will be affected.

Developing an Information-Specific Mental Model for Practitioners. The transition to an information-driven clinical practice model is certainly difficult. Moving from a health system whose framework was predominantly manual and mechanical to one that is, today, predominantly high-tech calls for a major reorientation of provider practices and behaviors (Westwood, 2002). Although it is obvious that the health care system has embraced clinically specific technology for the treatment of a wide variety of diseases, it is equally apparent that the transition to a higher use of technology-driven equipment and processes has been slower. Complicating this fast-paced systems shift to increasing use of technology-based approaches is the aging demographics of the health care provider and of this generation's typically slower adaptation to the personal application of technology. Critical work of the time includes establishing mechanisms for both education and adaptation of the provider's clinical role and functions into relationships and proficiencies that better complement the available technology.

EMERGING TECHNOLOGIES AND THE IMPACT ON PAYMENT

Perhaps one of the most difficult political and economic issues in health care today is the matching of payment strategies with the increasing evolution of health care technologies (Dorf, 2001). Through the emergence of the technology age, the structures of payment, essentially grounded in a twentieth century model of health care delivery, are no longer adequate for the growing number of technology applications in health care services. New technology is now emerging at a rate greater than the payment systems both private and public can accommodate (Davis, 2001). Establishing new payment models for health care services will be a priority if the health care system is to continue improving clinical care and health outcomes (Box 7-6).

A current case in point is the emergence of drug-eluting stents (Serruys, 2002) used to treat coronary artery disease. Ultimately meant to replace or reduce coronary artery bypass

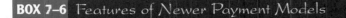

BOX 7–6 *Features of Newer Payment Models*

- Outcome-driven
- Quality-related
- Flexible algorithms
- Evaluated often
- Imbedded in the information system
- Web-based reporting
- Real-time payments

grafts, these newer stents are evolving at a rate greater than the health system and payment structure can accommodate in a timely fashion. As a result, availability and use of the stents that offer less invasive treatment at a considerably lower cost than more traditional and invasive treatments (i.e., coronary artery bypass surgery) has been somewhat slowed and even, in some cases, limited. This dynamic can easily be multiplied across the various disciplines and modalities of clinical care and intervention. Indeed, the issue has risen to such importance in health care delivery that the negative influences driven by inadequate payment structures is having a deleterious effect on the pace of innovation and application in health care.

Furthermore, the payment issue is affecting market conditions in both access to and delivery of health care as the current crisis in drug related pricing clearly indicates. The number of American citizens bypassing currently high-priced drugs in the United States to purchase lower-priced drugs from Canada is a case in point. Here again, the impact is acutely felt because of the growing dependence on pharmacotherapeutics as a part of the ongoing treatment regimen for many patients. In 1965 less than 1% of the public's health care bill was related to paying for drugs; today, that number is 17% (Committee on Health, Education, Labor, and Pensions, 2000).

The relationship of drug therapy to the total cost of health care over the next decade will increase as new drug therapies become more readily available and affordable. Legislation making drugs more available and affordable and more often covered by insurance has already passed through Congress and now forms the foundation for further refinements and enhancements in the payment for drug therapies over the next decade. As a model emerges for the payment of drug therapies over time, such an approach will be replicated for handling other innovations and technologies as they emerge.

THE COOLING OF MANAGED CARE

Managed care is a concept that grew considerably in the United States over the decade between 1990 and 2000 (Andersen et al, 2001). Because employers demanded lower health care costs for their employees, managed care programs emerged and thrived for a short time. At one point, more than 80% of all employed health care workers were enrolled in managed care programs (i.e., health maintenance organizations, point of service plans, preferred provider organizations). These were primarily restrictive-access programs designed to make health service delivery more efficient. For example, managed care plans required primary care providers to control patients' access to specialists. In addition, providers were required to obtain authorization from the managed care company before proceeding with certain medical procedures.

While managed care plans did slow the rate of increase in health care costs, these plans and programs did not lower the overall cost of service, nor did they satisfy the user of these products. In fact, almost no one was satisfied. As a result, interest in managed care programs declined considerably from late 1998 through early 2003. Pressured by a variety of marketplace forces related to dissatisfaction, managed care plans now are making important shifts in their business models because users are seeking opportunities for less restrictive approaches for health care coverage and access. Consumers demand choice and personal control while the managed care plan places a strong emphasis on efficiency and cost control.

A return to greater choice and variability within health payment plans is leading to new models of payment and access (Box 7-7). Managed care companies are adding less restrictive products to their services and adjusting existing services to offer easier access to health care. Managed care companies hope that by providing greater flexibility in choices and services, they will improve consumers' satisfaction. Associated with this approach is managed care companies' attempt to establish stronger relationships with their consumers in order to play a more direct role in consumer health practices. These new approaches serve to change the dynamics of managed care, broaden the availability of services, make access and utilization of care easier for the user and create a more equitable practice environment for the clinical provider (Balkin, 2003).

Health plans, already profitable in 2001 and 2002, are now eager to protect their profitability. Clearly, consumers' demand for more choice over health plan benefits can drive up costs. In the interest of protecting profitability, the plans have begun to pass on a greater share of the burden of paying for services to the user. Therefore, across the board, subscribers to health plans are paying an increasingly larger proportion of the cost of health care services out of their own pockets. As more choices are introduced into the health plan, the burden of paying for those choices will rest with the consumer. Until a definitive national policy is generated or an agreed-upon standard health plan format is determined, cost shifting to consumers will continue to accelerate.

EVIDENCE AND VALUE AS A FOUNDATION FOR PRACTICE AND PAYMENT

In the past few years there has been a subtle yet critical shift in the foundations of practice and payment. Since Boeing engineers developed a methodology and algorithm for the computer-based design, prototyping, modeling, and testing of its new 777 airplane designed for global travel, virtual models have now become the foundation for both conceptualizing quality and for measuring the value. So confident were the engineers of their virtual design process that the Boeing 777 went directly from design to construction (IEEE Computer

BOX 7-7 *Changing Health Plans*

- Less employer-paid
- Stronger occupational role
- Greater script for health practices
- Quality factors for payment
- Renegotiated regularly
- More control over expectations and deliverables

Society, 2002). The process used by Boeing became a model for demonstrating the viability of virtual methodologies in the design and construction of successful new products. The Boeing model has created for all industries a richer understanding of the relationship between process and product and the use of product-based methodologies to define the essential processes that will lead directly to the construction of new products.

As a result of these new product-development models, there is now a growing belief in health care that providers initially should focus on the *outcomes* of service followed by an assessment and determination of what would most effectively ensure that such outcomes would actually be achieved. The health care system's considerable attachment to good process is now seriously questioned. In nursing, as with virtually all other disciplines, there has been a strong historical focus on process. In essence, this focus on process has kept the nursing profession from adjusting its vision of doing good work to a vision of obtaining value for the work that is done. A focus on evidence and outcomes indicates a notable shift from an emphasis on the quality of the work itself to an emphasis on determining whether the work has any impact or makes any difference in the lives of those persons whom nurses serve. In short, this shift to evidence and outcomes is a reflection on the emphasis for obtaining value.

Value determination as a driving force for evidence and outcomes is a critical shift in the foundations of health practices (Institute of Medicine, 2001). From prevention through primary services to highly specialized intervention, the demand is for evidence of the relationship between what is desired, what is done, and what is achieved (Box 7-8). Such a recalibration of focus and service in health care results in a serious shift of emphasis in the provision of health services. This adjustment in focus on value and outcome now calls providers to rethink their actions and processes and place them clearly within the context of value (Soukup and Beason, 2000). Efficiency, effectiveness, and efficacy (E_3) must be related to the *product* of work rather than the *process* of work (Antony et al, 2002). The questions now are:

- What difference did clinical activity make?
- What change occurred?
- What outcome was produced?
- Did any of the work activities through intent or forethought relate directly to the results produced?

Now, the goodness of fit between process and product becomes a central indicator of effectiveness and sustainability. This emerging emphasis on outcomes, driven by the technologic facility necessary to support outcomes management, calls for greater clarity between performance, productivity, and value. As this effort matures, it will serve to establish a new foundation for both evaluating and valuing health care delivery. More directly implied is

---

BOX 7–8 *Value-Driven Nursing Features*

- Focus on product more than process
- Evidence-based practices
- Outcomes-driven measures
- Financial and service value-determined

the growing emphasis on tying payment strategies to the achievement of clearly delineated quality and value outcomes.

Transitions in Public and Private Payment

Perhaps one of the most significant transformations occurring in the delivery of health care services is related to how services will be paid for in the future. As previously discussed, one of the significant challenges of the time is matching payment response with the accelerated rate of technology application. Often, before a payment formula can be generated for an existing technology, the replacement technology is already on the horizon (Box 7-9). Increasingly, the impact of technology transformation and the rate of that change must become a part of the algorithm for determining payment (Andersen et al, 2001).

A part of the formula for addressing future payment relates to how emerging technology influences extinguishing technology (U.S. House of Representatives, 2001). Increasingly, purveyors of new technology must become critically aware of the impact such technology has on the cost of delivering real-time service. A stronger relationship between the price of technology innovation and the cost of extinguishing older technology must be established. As computerized, linked, and integrated financial and clinical databases merge, a more current and accurate fit can be established between the use of technology and the mechanisms for paying for it.

Nursing is dramatically affected by the dynamics of technology transformation (Locsin, 2001). As nursing becomes better able to establish a relationship between nursing process and its impact on the health and clinical outcomes, a value equation emerges. When the relationship between process and outcomes can be established, a financial value can be enumerated. Once that intersection between process and value is established, nursing as a practice moves from a resource user to a value generator. As this occurs, both the role and language of nursing care will necessarily change. For nurses, this means a stronger focus on relevant and evidence-based processes that can be definitively aligned with the products of work. Once that alignment has been achieved, attaching economic value to the work of nursing will become a normative process.

Value Determination in Nursing

The "noise" of this inexorable shift in real-time payment algorithms and formulas is the requirement that value be defined. This means that the slavish attachments to ritual and routine, policy and procedure, function and task will have to be forced out of nursing practice in favor of outcome-defined actions and the creation of a good fit between the *products* of work and its related antecedent, the *process* of work. For the professional nurse, the shift to outcome-defined actions must not only become a new work ethic but also become an essential cornerstone of value-based nursing. When value-based nursing becomes a fundamental

---

BOX 7-9 *Keeping Up With Technology*

- Rescripting the payment algorithm for technology
- Using technology as an economic driver
- Determining the rates of extinguishing and emerging technologies
- Evaluating effective technology before paying for it
- Determining the application and use cost of technology turnover

mechanism of nursing service delivery, the information infrastructure and the documentation and reporting processes will need to facilitate the aggregation of clinical practice data in a manner that establishes the relationship among price, costs, margin of effectiveness, and financial value added.

In addition, the value activities of nursing must be integrated into the other interdisciplinary and organizational value determinants and must be done in a way that indicates quality enhancements, best practice utilization, or other comparative quality indicators to maximize both private and public sources of financial payment. The move to a quality-based, outcome-defined mechanism for payment, while in its earliest stages, is an inevitable byproduct of the aggregation, consolidation, and integration capacity for linking financial and clinical information in a way that can indicate real value.

For nursing, the following issues will be important work in relationship to its value determination:

1. A **practice-based workload management system** that represents the foundations and characteristics of clinical practice will need to emerge. Creating a tighter fit between skills and demands and reflecting the relationship between practice requisites and outcome expectations will be the foundation for good workload management. All workload systems will need to reflect measures of intensity and service requirements in a highly mobile and fast-paced clinical delivery infrastructure.

2. **Care protocols and standards** (packages) must be constructed around models of payment for clinical services in order to reflect real value determination and to ascertain which portion of service contribution, cost, and value is derived from nursing. These outcome and value delineations will form the foundation for indicators of high quality that will increasingly be used in the private and public payment process, where payment will be directly linked to quality and value.

3. As best practices emerge at local points of care and comparative models of quality are exemplified regionally, the **foundation of national best practices** is laid. A databank emerges to which all organizations have access and against which each organization can compare its individual, culturally specific, and organizationally unique practice processes. Currently the Center for Medicare and Medicaid Services hopes that by increasing the focus of payment on quality indicators, it is beginning to tie payment to quality and to reward those high-quality health systems with additional payment resources. This stimulus serves as an incentive for nurses and other clinical providers to refine their formulas for quality clinical practice and good patient outcomes.

As the relationship between quality and finance becomes more firmly established and the infrastructure of payment accommodates quality indicators, nursing will have to do a better job of tying practice processes to high levels of clinical expectations. Value-driven payment structures will increasingly force nursing to establish objective criteria for adequately and meaningfully measuring its value and financial contribution, forever altering nursing's role in health care delivery.

DETERMINANTS OF HEALTH, MOBILITY, AND THE CHANGING GROUND OF PRACTICE

In a social construct in which mass customization is driving society to more user-controlled opportunities and systems, the construct for health services is shifting. The emergence of the

Internet and the convenient, readily accessible service infrastructure built to support it has created a highly evolved system of service delivery. From Amazon.com© to eBay©, consumer and user utility, convenience, and cost-effectiveness are driving commercial social relationships. The locus of control for decision making is moving from the provider of service to the user of service. Such a move creates chaos in the delivery system, especially when the structures of delivery tend to favor the providers of service delivery. As technology increases the mobility and portability of service in health care, providers can exert less control over the variables influencing health care.

As a result of this emerging reality, it is increasingly apparent that addressing the underlying determinants of health and life management is critical to the health system's ability to thrive in the twenty-first century and, within the context of limited resources, to be able to make a sustainable impact on the health of the nation (Box 7-10). In addressing the future format of health care delivery and the context of nursing service provision over the next decade, the following factors are emerging concerns:

- Lifestyle and personal choice
- Employer-driven efforts to address health and illness
- Shifting role of the nurse

Lifestyle and Personal Choice

Over 80% of all illnesses treated to date in the American health care system relate to conditions of lifestyle and personal choice. If health is to be sufficiently addressed and positively affected over the next two decades, intervention at a national level must be related to lifestyle and personal choice. From media focus to information and knowledge systems, from basic education to health care counseling, from medical intervention to nursing care practices, all will be devoted to addressing the increasingly important and generally acknowledged requirement for changing social health practices. A greater number of nursing resources and services will be directed to this area of intervention as technology makes it possible to engage patients earlier and to address potential illnesses long before a late-stage intervention is required.

Employer-Driven Efforts to Address Health and Illness

Because employers provide a large portion of payment for health services, there is growing interest in employer-driven efforts to address health and illness within the context of worker engagement. Employers are seeking to become moderators of health care service to their employees. Employers' interest is not necessarily altruistic—they bear a significant burden

---

BOX 7-10   *The Emerging Influence of Health Practices*

- Lifestyle choices
- Nutrition
- Stress
- Social conditions
- Economic impact
- Creating healthy environments
- Lifelong health practices

in the cost of health care for their employees. The increasing cost of providing late-stage intervention due to inadequately addressed issues of health practices, lifestyle, information deficits, and other variables has driven employers to an increasing ownership of health care services.

Besides providing more directed and focused clinical services to their employees, employers are finding that they can have more control over the incidence of illness, the costs of those illnesses, and the growth in worker productivity. Over the next two decades the increasing focus on employer-driven control over health practices, education, and intervention will introduce a wider range of practice alternatives and site-based delivery of nursing and health care services. Because employees are also bearing an increased burden in the cost of their personal health care, their interest in addressing health care needs in employer-based settings will accelerate and engender a broader interest in health and lifestyle-based practices.

Shifting Role of the Nurse

Within the context of a complex multidimensional health delivery system, the role of the nurse is shifting dramatically. Fewer nurses will be used in hospital settings, and increasing numbers of nursing resources will be required in a wider variety of settings than have previously been available. From employer health and occupational services to community health services, from genetic services to health counseling services, from group medical practices to focused service settings and a whole array of emerging aging service configurations, nurses are expanding their practice horizons. This high mobility, widely variable, constantly changing environment for nursing care delivery creates the need for a nurse who is highly flexible, fluid, yet focused in the delivery of clinical services. This challenging transformation calls for a nurse who can provide a wide variety of clinical services. More important, this transformation calls for a change in the perception of what nursing is and a reconceptualization of nursing practice.

Managing the "journey" of health care delivery has been at the foundation of nursing practice since the time of Florence Nightingale. Health care context, role, and process are shifting the fundamental requisite to integrate, coordinate, and facilitate the health service journey. Nurses have always played this role and, although their circumstances may be changing, the demand and need for nurses to manage the health care journey is not changing. Nursing educators and service leaders must join forces to work through these considerable social, economic, and technologic shifts in health care, forcing the reconfiguration of nursing practice in the twenty-first century.

A stronger partnership between education and service will now be required to create a seamless intersection between formal academic preparation and continuing service learning. Indeed, nursing educators and nursing service leaders must now facilitate the provision of continual learning through the nurse's life span, ensuring that service-based opportunities for continuing education also relate to the advancement of academic preparation and enhancements in clinical practice. This new partnership must respect the unique character of nursing education and service yet, at the same time, reflect the intractable linkage between education and practice in the interest of advancing the nursing profession.

Summary

The future of nursing practice is fraught with multiple challenges and opportunities. The emerging twenty-first–century model of health care challenges the very foundations of twentieth-century nursing practice and calls the profession into a different discussion related to its future. Although the health care system is always evolving, now and then in the course of evolution, moments of revolution emerge, where time and intensity accelerate the demands and the pace of transformation. Nursing and health care are currently moving through just such a period. The challenge for the nursing profession is in ensuring that the response to its own transformation matches well the changes in the health system and, if possible, leads the engagement and embracing of such changes.

Moving from the twentieth-century fixed, institutional, manual, and mechanical model of health care intervention to a more fluid and mobile system of highly technologic, noninvasive, short-term, early-engagement health delivery processes is clearly the challenge of the time. The ability of the nursing profession to continue to thrive and significantly affect the health of the nation lies in the balance it creates while seeking to meet a largely different set of demands in the emerging health care system.

CRITICAL THINKING ACTIVITIES

1. Consider the following statement from the chapter: "No longer can nurses provide all of those activities of patient care that once were considered fundamental to nursing care." Based on your clinical experiences, what procedures considered "fundamental" to nursing care might be safely shifted to other types of care providers, including the family caregiver? Explain your choices.

2. Examine your most recent clinical experience and discuss how the work of nursing could be redesigned using recent technology (e.g., computer-based charting, PDA for determining drug interactions and lab values, a GPS locator system).

3. Imagine that you, as a nurse, consider developing a business to assist companies to implement employer-sponsored health initiatives. What type of programs could you develop that might be considered cost-effective for the employer and offer specific, improved health outcomes for employees? What financial savings for both the employer and the employee would result from such a program?

4. Consider the following statement from the chapter: "Indeed, many of the resource problems existing today can be tied directly to the inadequacy of the information management systems in most health care organizations." Based on your clinical experiences, how do problems and/or limitations in finding accurate patient information hinder your ability to provide patient care?

5. How can technology be used to develop a discharge teaching plan for an elderly client whose primary caregiver is unable to come to the hospital?

6. Consider the following statement from the chapter: "If health is to be sufficiently addressed and positively affected over the next two decades, intervention at a national level must be related to lifestyle and personal choice." What types of nationwide interventions might be appropriate to address lifestyle and personal choice that directly affect health?

Additional resources are available on-line at: http://evolve.elsevier.com/Cherry/

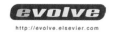

http://evolve.elsevier.com

REFERENCES

Alcott LM, Parsons EE: *Civil War nursing,* New York, 1984, Garland.

American Hospital Association, National League of Nursing Education (U.S.), Council of the Division on Nursing: *Manual of the essentials of good hospital nursing service,* Chicago, New York, 1942, American Hospital Association.

Andersen R, Rice TH, Kominski GF: *Changing the U.S. health care system: key issues in health services, policy, and management,* ed 2, San Francisco, 2001, Jossey-Bass.

Androwich I, American Medical Informatics Association, American Nurses Association: *Clinical information systems: a framework for reaching the vision,* Washington, DC, 2003, American Nurses Publishing.

Antony J, Preece D, NetLibrary Inc: *Understanding, managing, and implementing quality frameworks, techniques, and cases,* London, New York, 2002, Routledge.

Baer ED: *Enduring issues in American nursing,* New York, 2001, Springer.

Balkin K: *Health care: opposing viewpoints,* San Diego, Calif, 2003, Greenhaven Press.

Brown J, Duguid P: *The social life of information,* Boston, 2002, Harvard Business School Press.

Buerhaus P et al: Strengthening hospital nursing, *Health Affairs* 21(5):123-131, 2002.

Chaska NL: *The nursing profession: tomorrow and beyond,* Thousand Oaks, Calif, 2001, Sage Publications.

Committee on Health, Education, Labor, and Pensions: *Prescription drug costs: what drives increases?* Hearing of the Committee on Health, Education, Labor, and Pensions (#32), United States Senate, 106th Congress, 2nd session, July 18, 2000.

Davis JB: *The social economics of health care,* London, New York, 2001, Routledge.

Dorf RC: *Technology, humans, and society: toward a sustainable world,* San Diego, 2001, Academic Press.

Frampton SB, Gilpin L, Charmel PA: *Putting patients first: designing and practicing patient-centered care,* San Francisco, 2003, Jossey-Bass.

Frankel RM, Quill TE, McDaniel SH: *The biopsychosocial approach: past, present, and future,* Rochester, NY, 2003, University of Rochester Press.

Fukuyama F: *Our posthuman future,* New York, 2002, Farrar, Straus, and Giroux.

Geisler E, Krabbendam K, Schuring R: *Technology, health care, and management in the hospital of the future,* Westport, CT, 2003, Praeger.

Hein EC: *Nursing issues in the 21st century: perspectives from the literature,* Philadelphia, 2001, JB Lippincott.

IEEE Computer Society: *TC on distributed processing: proceedings of the Seventh IEEE International Workshop on Object-Oriented Real-Time Dependable Systems (WORDS 2002),* Los Alamitos, Calif, 2002, IEEE Computer Society Press.

Institute of Medicine (U.S.), Committee on Quality of Health Care in America: *Crossing the quality chasm: a new health system for the 21st century,* Washington, DC, 2001, National Academy Press.

Joel LA, Kelly LY: *The nursing experience: trends, challenges, and transitions,* ed 4, New York, 2002, McGraw-Hill.

Johnson BS: *Blueprint for action in hospital nursing; proceedings of the 1964 regional conferences sponsored by the Department of Hospital Nursing, National League for Nursing, and the Regional Councils of State Leagues for Nursing,* New York, 1964, National League for Nursing.

Kalow W, Meyer UA, Tyndale RF: *Pharmacogenomics,* New York, 2001, Marcel Dekker.

Lancaster L, Stillman D: *When generations collide,* New York, 2002, Harper Business Press.

Locsin RC: *Advancing technology, caring, and nursing,* Westport, Conn, 2001, Auburn House.

Maysys L: Effects of current and future information technologies on the healthcare workforce, *Health Affairs* 21(5):33-41, 2002.

McAlearney A: *Population health management,* Chicago, 2002, Health Administration Press.

Osborne H: *Partnering with patients to improve health outcomes,* Gaithersburg, Md, 2002, Aspen.

Porter-O'Grady T: Quantum mechanics and the future of healthcare leadership, *J Nurs Admin* 27(1):15-20, 1997.

Porter-O'Grady T: Profound change: 21st century nursing, *Nurs Outlook* 49(1):182-186, 2001.

Quaglini S, Barahona P, Andreassen S: *Artificial intelligence in medicine, Proceedings of the 8th Conference on Artificial Intelligence in Medicine in Europe, AIME 2001,* Cascais, Portugal, July 1-4, 2001, Berlin, New York, 2001, Springer.

Schappert SM, National Center for Health Statistics (U.S.): *Ambulatory care visits to physician offices, hospital outpatient departments, and emergency departments: United States, 1996,* Hyattsville, Md, 1998, U.S. Dept. of Health and Human Services, Centers for Disease Control and Prevention, National Center for Health Statistics.

Serruys PW: *Coronary lesions: a pragmatic approach,* London, 2002, Martin Dunitz.

Soukup SN, Beason CF: *Evidence-based nursing practice: enhancing health care through innovative nursing practice* (Sister Nayruta Soukup, Charlotte F Beason, guest editors), Philadelphia, 2000, WB Saunders.

Ulrich B: *Leadership and management according to Florence Nightingale,* Norwalk, Conn, 1992, Appleton & Lange Publishers.

U.S. House of Representatives, Committee on Government Reform, Subcommittee on Government Management Information and Technology: *H.R. 4401, the Health Care Infrastructure Investment Act of 2000,* Hearing before the Subcommittee on Government Management, Information, and Technology of the Committee on

Government Reform, House of Representatives, 106th Congress, second session, on H.R. 4401, to amend Title XVIII of the Social Security Act to provide for a moratorium on the mandatory delay of payment of claims submitted under part B of the Medicare program and to establish an advanced informational infrastructure for the administration of federal health benefits programs (July 11, 2000), Washington, DC, 2001, Government Printing Office.

Westwood JD: *Medicine meets virtual reality 02/10: digital upgrades, applying Moore's law to health*, Amsterdam, Washington, DC, 2002, IOS Press.

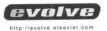

Legal Issues in Nursing and Health Care

Laura R. Mahlmeister, PhD, RN

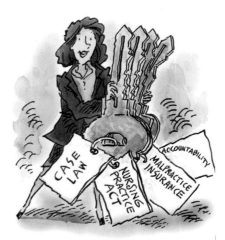

Knowledge of the law enhances the nurse's ability to provide safe and effective care.

VIGNETTE

Mary Clark is a registered nurse (RN) employed in the emergency department of a large for-profit hospital. The facility treats clients who are privately insured and individuals with Medicare coverage. Nurse Clark is the assigned triage nurse when Mr. Jones, a 48-year-old man, walks in for evaluation. He states that he has persistent, mild substernal pain that is now radiating laterally toward both shoulders. His skin is pink and dry, and he does not appear to be in obvious distress. He reports eating half of a garlic pizza and drinking three beers 1 hour ago. "I'm pretty sure it's just indigestion. This happened before when I ate garlic." He also tells the nurse, "I know I'm supposed to go to Community Hospital; I have 'Feel-Well' insurance, but I'm miserable and don't want to drive 10 miles across town in rush hour traffic with this much pain."

Mr. Jones is enrolled in a health maintenance organization (HMO). The HMO may not reimburse the for-profit hospital for Mr. Jones' visit if it is determined that his condition was not a true emergency after review by the HMO's utilization review department. In that case, Mr. Jones will have to pay out of pocket for the medical evaluation and care received in the emergency department. In this cost-conscious health care environment, the nurses in the emergency department are well aware of the financial losses the hospital has recently suffered as a result of unpaid emergency services. Nurses in this facility are expected to contribute to the facility's success in reducing operating costs.

Questions to consider while reading this chapter:

1. What is Nurse Clark's legal duty in this situation?
2. What legal principles underlie the nurse's obligations to the patient?

Additional resources are available on-line at: http://evolve.elsevier.com/Cherry/

3. What laws, if any, would govern the nurse's decision-making process in this case?
4. If Mr. Jones is not evaluated or treated and suffers a myocardial infarction while driving to Community Hospital, who would be legally accountable for his injuries? The nurse? The for-profit hospital? The HMO that may not have reimbursed for services?

KEY TERMS

Accountability Being responsible for one's actions; a sense of duty in performing nursing tasks and activities.

Advance directives Written or verbal instructions created by the patient describing specific wishes about medical care in the event he or she becomes incapacitated or incompetent. Examples include living wills and durable powers of attorney.

Adverse event An injury caused by medical management rather than the patient's underlying condition. An adverse event attributable to error is a preventable adverse event.

Case law Body of written opinions created by judges in federal and state appellate cases; also known as *judge-made law* and *common law.*

Civil law A category of law (tort law) that deals with conduct considered unacceptable. It is based on societal expectations regarding interpersonal conduct. Common causes of civil litigation include professional malpractice, negligence, and assault and battery.

Common law Law that is created through the decision of judges as opposed to laws enacted by legislative bodies (i.e., Congress).

Comparative negligence A type of liability in which damages may be apportioned among two or more defendants in a malpractice case. The extent of liability depends on the defendant's relative contribution to the patient's injury.

Criminal negligence Negligence that indicates "reckless and wanton" disregard for the safety, well-being, or life of an individual; behavior that demonstrates a complete disregard for another, such that death is likely.

Damages Monetary compensation the court orders paid to a person who has sustained a loss or injury to his or her person or property through the misconduct (intentional or unintentional) of another.

Defendant The individual who is named in a person's (plaintiff's) complaint as responsible for an injury; the person who the plaintiff claims committed a negligent act or malpractice.

Durable power of attorney for health care An instrument that authorizes another person to act as one's agent in decisions regarding health care if the person becomes incompetent to make his or her own decisions.

Error A failure of a planned action to be completed as intended, or the use of a wrong plan to achieve a specific aim.

Immunity Legal doctrine by which a person is protected from a lawsuit for negligent acts or an institution is protected from a suit for the negligent acts of its employees.

Liability Being legally responsible for harm caused to another person or property as a result of one's actions; compensation for harm normally is paid in monetary damages.

Licensing laws Laws that establish the qualifications for obtaining and maintaining a license to perform particular services. Persons and institutions may be required to obtain a license to provide particular health care services.

Malpractice Failure of a professional to meet the standard of conduct that a reasonable and prudent member of his or her profession would exercise in similar circumstances that results in harm. The professional's misconduct is unintentional.

Negligence Failure to act in a manner that an ordinary, prudent person (either lay person or professional) would act in similar circumstances, resulting in harm. The failure to act in a reasonable and prudent manner is unintentional.

Plaintiff The complaining person in a lawsuit; the person who claims he or she was injured by the acts of another.

Res ipsa loquitur Legal doctrine applicable to cases in which the provider (i.e., the physician) had exclusive control of events that resulted in the patient's injury; the injury would not have occurred ordinarily without a negligent act; derived from a Latin phrase meaning "the thing speaks for itself."

Respondent superior Legal doctrine that holds an employer indirectly responsible for the negligent acts of employees carried out within the scope of employment; derived from a Latin phrase meaning "let the master answer."

Risk management Process of identifying, analyzing, and controlling risks posed to patients; involves human factor and incident analysis, changes in systems operations, and loss control and prevention.

Standard of care In civil cases the legal criteria against which the nurse's (and physician's) conduct is compared to determine whether a negligent act or malpractice occurred; commonly defined as the knowledge and skill that an ordinary, reasonably prudent person would possess and exercise in the same or similar circumstances.

Statute or statutory law Law enacted by a legislative body; separate from judge-made or common law.

Tort Civil wrong or injury committed by one person against another person or a property. There are two types of torts—intentional and unintentional.

Vicarious liability Legal doctrine in which a person or institution is liable for the negligent acts of another because of a special relationship between the two parties; a substituted liability.

LEARNING OUTCOMES

After studying this chapter, the reader will be able to:

1. Differentiate among the three major categories of law on which nursing practice is established and governed.
2. Analyze the relationship between accountability and liability for one's actions in professional nursing practice.
3. Outline the essential elements that must be proven to prove a claim of negligence or malpractice.
4. Distinguish between intentional and unintentional torts in relation to nursing practice.
5. Incorporate fundamental laws and statutory regulations that establish the patient's right to self-determination in the health care setting.
6. Complete the critical thinking exercises at the end of the chapter to consolidate understanding of the relationship between nursing practice and the law.

CHAPTER OVERVIEW

The preceding vignette highlighted a growing clinical dilemma that nurses face in the complex, ever-changing health care system. Financial considerations may conflict with clinical concerns for patient well-being. In an increasingly complex health care environment, the nurse's ability to make appropriate decisions about the provision of patient care services is assisted by a sound knowledge of the laws governing practice. In the case of Mr. Jones, triage, assessment, medical evaluation, and treatment are regulated by a federal law known as the Emergency Medical Treatment and Active Labor Act (EMTALA) (COBRA, 42 U.S.C. 1395dd).

There also may be a specific state law regarding essential care and transport of patients in emergency departments. Additionally, sections of the Nursing Practice Act describing the professional conduct of the registered nurse (RN) would assist Nurse Clark in managing this clinical problem. Financial concerns become a secondary consideration for the nurse with this baseline knowledge of the law.

Each nurse must be able to describe his or her professional duty to the patient or client under the law and to recognize legal risks in practice. Knowledge of the law enhances the nurse's ability to provide safe and effective care in all settings. This chapter examines legal aspects of nursing practice. The concepts of law, professional accountability, legal liability, negligence, malpractice, and criminal offense are defined. Specific laws or statutes governing nursing practice are also reviewed. The reader is introduced to current, relevant information about case law, also known as common law or judge-made law, as it applies to professional nursing practice. Patients' rights are explored within the context of law and court opinions. Finally, the ongoing reports published by the Institute of Medicine (IOM) about medical errors are discussed, and specific strategies to reduce errors and legal risk are detailed.

SOURCES OF LAW AND NURSING PRACTICE

The actions of all individuals are regulated through two systems of principles known as laws and ethics. Laws enforce a minimum level of conduct by imposing penalties for violations of acceptable behavior (Hall, 2002). Laws are expressed in terms of "must" and "shall" and are based on a society's interest in prohibiting or controlling certain behaviors. Ethics are described in terms of "should" and "may" and address beliefs about appropriate behaviors within a societal context (Lagana, 2000). Chapter 9 presents an in-depth discussion about nursing ethics. Along with ethics, professional nursing conduct also is regulated by a variety of laws. There are two major sources of law:

- Statutory law
- Common law

The standards for professional nursing practice are in great part derived from both statutory and common law. The following section of the chapter deals with statutory law and describes how it governs and indirectly influences nursing practice.

STATUTORY LAW

The terms *law* and *statute* will be used interchangeably in this chapter. Laws that are written by legislative bodies such as Congress or state legislatures are enacted as statutes. The previously mentioned law, EMTALA, is an example of a federal statute. Violation of law is a criminal offense against the general public and is prosecuted by government authorities. Crimes are punishable by fines or imprisonment. The list of federal and state statutes that govern nursing practice has multiplied over the past 25 years. Nurses at all levels of practice must develop a greater depth and breadth of knowledge about laws related to professional practice, their specific practice setting (i.e., the emergency department in the case of EMTALA), and health care systems in general. Ignorance of the law is never a defense when the nurse violates a health care statute. A nurse who violates the law is subject to penalties, including monetary fines, suspension or revocation of his or her license, and even imprisonment in some instances (Steiner, 2003).

Federal Statutes

Federal laws have a major impact on nursing practice, mandating a minimum standard of care in all settings that receive federal funds (i.e., reimbursement for treatment of Medicare patients). For instance, nursing homes are a highly regulated industry that must meet both federal and state requirements in order to operate. Federal laws have established rules and regulations to ensure the confidentiality of patients' personal health information (Health Insurance Portability and Accountability Act, or HIPPA). Several federal laws protect the rights of patients who participate as subjects in research, by mandating the creation of institutional review boards and an appropriate informed consent process. The Federal False Claims Act makes it an offense to submit a false claim to the government for payment of health care services. Furthermore, the person who reports the false or fraudulent claim (often a whistle blower) is entitled to 15% to 25% of any monetary amount recovered by the federal government if the government wins the case in court. Nurses have been the recipients of these "bounties" in several recent false claim cases in which the federal government recovered several million dollars.

Three federal statutes that nurses must be familiar with and clearly understand are discussed in this section. The list is not comprehensive, but it includes examples of federal laws that directly affect nursing practice. Many federal laws are relevant to specific health care settings (i.e., mental health, nursing homes, emergency departments, maternity settings). When nurses are knowledgeable about the federal laws applicable to their area of practice, they will be able to more effectively advocate for patients in that setting.

Unfortunately, most nurses are unfamiliar with health care law and rely on authorities in their employment setting to know what is legal and therefore permissible. Automatically deferring to administrators or nurse managers about the legality of a particular issue is no longer acceptable behavior for the professional nurse. Each RN must take accountability for knowing the law and understanding how it relates to patient care and nursing practice. When concerns about work-related issues arise (e.g., a change in scope of practice for unlicensed staff or a reduction in RN staffing), the first question the nurse asks and answers should be, "Is this legal?" (Yorker and Mahlmeister, 2002).

Emergency Medical Treatment and Active Labor Law (COBRA, 42 U.S.C. 1395dd). This federal statute, often referred to as the "antidumping" law, was enacted in 1986 to prohibit the refusal of care for indigent and uninsured patients seeking medical assistance in the emergency department (Moy, 2003). This law also prohibits the transfer of unstable patients, including women in labor, from one facility to another. The law states:

- All persons presenting for care must receive the same medical screening examination and be stabilized, regardless of their financial status or insurance coverage, before discharge or transfer.

The Emergency Medical Treatment and Active Labor Law (EMTALA) is applicable to people presenting to non-emergency department settings such as urgent care clinics. It even governs the transfer of patients from an inpatient setting to a lower level of care in some parts of the United States (Roberts v. Galen of Virginia, Inc., 1997). Significant penalties can be levied against a facility that violates the EMTALA, including a $50,000 fine (not covered by liability insurance). The federal government also can revoke the facility's Medicare contract, and this could result in a major loss of revenue for the institution or even insolvency. Many legitimate concerns that nurses have about the discharge or transfer of patients could be promptly addressed if the nurse had a solid understanding of the EMTALA. This is not a daunting task. Nursing journals have published many articles about the EMTALA and the nurse's role in upholding this statute (Casaubon and Sparks, 2000; Lee, 2000; Snyder, 2003a).

Americans with Disabilities Act of 1990 (Public Law No. 101-336, 42 U.S.C. Section 12101). The intent of this law is to end discrimination against qualified persons with disabilities by removing barriers that prevent them from enjoying the same opportunities available to persons without disabilities. Recent court cases have established that, as a place of public accommodation, a health care facility must provide reasonable accommodation to patients (and family members) with sensory disabilities such as vision and hearing impairment (Aikins v. St. Helena Hospital, 1994; Negron v. Snoqualmie Valley Hospital, 1997).

This statute has relevance for all nurses. As patient advocates, nurses have a legal and ethical duty to provide appropriate patient and family education and to support the process of informed consent. The health care facility must have a policy that defines how it will meet the client's needs for education and information when there are vision or hearing disabilities. The policy also must describe how the nurse can obtain translators and special types of equipment needed to facilitate communication.

Patient Self-Determination Act of 1990; Omnibus Budget Reconciliation Act of 1990 (Public Law No. 101-508, Sections 4206 and 4751). This federal statute is a Medicare/Medicaid amendment intended to support individuals in expressing their preferences about medical treatment and making decisions about end-of-life care. The law requires that all federally funded hospitals:

- Inform adult patients, in writing, about their right under state law to make treatment choices. These choices include collaborating with the physician in formulating "do not resuscitate" (DNR) orders.
- Ask patients whether they either have prepared a "living will" or have executed a "durable power of attorney" for health care.

The law provides guidance to nurses who often are in the best position to discuss these issues with the patient (e.g., while completing a comprehensive admission assessment). (Legal considerations related to living wills, durable power of attorney, and DNR orders are discussed in the last section of this chapter.)

Health Insurance Portability and Accountability Act of 1996 (Public Law No. 104-191). The intent of this law is to ensure confidentiality of the patient's health information. The introduction of electronic medical records has provided additional impetus for introduction of this legislation. The statute sets guidelines for maintaining the privacy of health data. Legitimate concerns regarding the uses of and release of medical information, particularly to private entities such as insurance companies, led to the passage of this law. It provides explicit guidelines for nurses who are in a position to release health information. To maintain confidentiality of the patient's health information, all nurses must have a basic understanding of this federal law.

Nurses should also take note that HIPAA has whistle-blower protection for individuals who report in good faith any illegal disclosure of patients' health information (Aspen Health Law and Compliance Center, 2001).

State Statutes

In addition to federal laws, nursing practice is governed by state laws that delineate the conduct of licensed nurses and define behaviors of all health care professionals in promoting public health and welfare.

State Nursing Practice Act and Board of Nursing Rules and Regulations. One of the most important state laws governing nursing practice is the Nursing Practice Act (NPA). This law was enacted to define the scope and limitations of professional nursing practice. The aim of regulating practice in this manner is to protect the public and make the individual nurse accountable for his or her actions. State legislatures authorize the nurses' licensing board to promulgate administrative rules and regulations necessary to implement the NPA. Once these administrative rules and regulations are formally adopted, they have the same force and effect as any other law (*Nurse's Legal Handbook*, 2000).

Although nursing practice acts vary from state to state, they usually contain the following information:

- Definition of the term *registered nurse*
- Description of professional nursing functions
- Standards of competent performance
- Behaviors that represent misconduct or prohibited practices
- Grounds for disciplinary action
- Fines and penalties the licensing board may levy when the Nursing Practice Act is violated

For further exploration, excerpts from three separate state nursing practice acts can be found on-line (http://evolve.elsevier.com/Cherry/) to illustrate how the Nursing Practice Act defines the scope of practice for nurses.

Surprisingly, many nurses are not even aware that the Nursing Practice Act is a law, and they unknowingly violate aspects of this statute. They are not familiar with the administrative rules and regulations enacted by the licensing board. This is an unfortunate lapse because these administrative rules and regulations answer crucial questions that nurses have about the day-to-day aspects of practice and unusual occurrences. For example, rules promulgated by the Ohio Board of Nursing include the following section:

> At all times when a licensed nurse is providing direct nursing care to a client within the scope of the licensed nurse's practice as set forth in [the law] Section 4723.02 of the Revised Code, the licensed nurse shall display and identify applicable licensure as a registered nurse or as a licensed practical nurse. (Ohio Administrative Code, Section 4723-4-03, (H). 1996)

Based on this, an RN in Ohio who does not wear an identification badge that clearly displays his or her status as an "RN" is in violation of the law. In this era of health care redesign, knowledge of this administrative rule would be essential because many health care systems are attempting to remove the licensure status of health care professionals from identification badges. In these latter settings, all workers (even nurses and physicians) are identified by a generic title such as "patient care team member." An increasing number of licensing boards are considering amending administrative rules to require that the licensure status

(RN, LPN, or LVN) of each nursing staff member be clearly displayed on the worker's identification badge.

Each nurse should own a current copy of the Nursing Practice Act and the licensing board's administrative rules and regulations. The dramatic changes occurring in health care often lead to uncertainty among nurses about which functions constitute the exclusive practice of registered nursing and which patient care tasks may be lawfully delegated to LPNs, LVNs, or unlicensed assistive personnel. The Nursing Practice Act and licensing board rules and regulations provide essential information that clarify these important questions.

The Nursing Practice Act broadly defines the practice of registered nursing in accordance with nursing's rapidly evolving functions. In recent years, with the expansion of basic nursing functions and the development of advanced nursing practice, many states have revised their nursing practice acts. Licensing boards also have been authorized in some states to provide guidelines for the development of "standardized procedures." Standardized procedures are a legal means by which RNs may expand their practice into areas traditionally considered to be within the realm of medicine. The standardized procedure actually is developed within the facility where the expanded nursing functions have been approved. It is developed in collaboration with nursing, medicine, and administration. An example of a standardized procedure would be a written protocol authorizing a nurse to implement a peripherally inserted venous catheter for patients in the neonatal intensive care unit.

Violations of the Nursing Practice Act. State legislatures have given licensing boards the authority to hear and decide administrative cases against nurses when there is an alleged violation of the Nursing Practice Act or the nursing board's rules and regulations. Nurses who violate the Nursing Practice Act or board's administrative rules and regulations are subject to disciplinary action by the board. Research indicates that there has been an increase in the number of consumer complaints to licensing boards related to nursing misconduct (Malugani, 2000). Table 8-1 provides a synopsis of the licensing board procedure when a complaint is made about a nurse. Box 8-1 presents the more common grounds for disciplinary action by state boards of nursing. Penalties that licensing boards may impose for violation of the Nursing Practice Act include:

- Issuing a formal reprimand
- Establishing a period of probation
- Levying fines
- Limiting, suspending, or revoking the nurse's license

An estimated 6% to 8% of RNs in the United States are chemically dependent (Danis, 2003). The majority of disciplinary actions by licensing boards are related to misconduct resulting from chemical impairment, including the misappropriation of drugs for personal use and the sale of drugs and drug paraphernalia to support the nurse's addiction. When the nurse's license is limited or suspended because of problems related to chemical impairment, the ability to practice in the future often is predicated on successful completion of a drug rehabilitation program and evidence of abstinence. An increasing number of state licensing boards have established programs to guide nurses through the process of rehabilitation to reestablish licensure.

Nurse-Patient Ratios and Mandatory Overtime Statutes

As I travel across the United States speaking with nurses about the rapid and often daunting changes in health care, a common question I hear is this: "Isn't there a law prohibiting this—reduction in RN staff? floating? the use of nurse aides in this patient care situation?

Table 8-1	**Licensing Board Procedure When a Complaint is Filed**
ACTION	**CONSEQUENCE**
Complaint is made (initial complaint may be lodged by a telephone call or a letter mailed to the licensing board) Consumer (patient or family member) Nurse's employer or nurse manager Professional nursing organization State authority (i.e., Centers for Medicare and Medicaid Services [CMS], formerly the Health Care Financing Administration [HCFA])	Sworn complaints must be filed
Licensing board reviews complaint Examines evidence	Determination made by board Insufficient evidence to proceed Administrative review is scheduled Nurse is notified Rules of proceeding explained Witnesses called to testify Evidence is examined
Licensing board makes decision Nurse exonerated Nurse guilty of violating Nursing Practice Act	Case closed Disciplinary action Board issues formal reprimand Nurse placed on probation Nurse's license is not renewed Fines levied against nurse Nurse's license is suspended or revoked
Nurse may challenge licensing board decision Court reviews case (court action dependent on jurisdiction) Reviews licensing board ruling and conduct of proceedings *or* Court reviews case Case scheduled for trial	Nurse must file appeal in court Licensing board ruling reversed Licensing board can appeal ruling *or* Licensing board ruling is upheld Licensing board ruling overturned Board may appeal case to higher court *or* Licensing board ruling is upheld Nurse may appeal to a higher court

mandatory overtime?" Nurse staffing is influenced to some degree by federal law, through the rules for participation in Medicare, and by state laws. For instance, in 1999 California became the first state to enact a law (California Assembly Bill 394) that mandates the establishment of minimum nurse-patient ratios in acute care facilities. The law took effect in January 2004 and sets minimum nurse-patient ratios in critical care units, step-down and medical-surgical units, and maternity departments. The projected nursing shortage may prompt other states to follow suit. Legislation has been introduced in more than fifteen states to address the nursing shortage and, in particular, to limit or prohibit the use of mandatory overtime for nurses (US General Accounting Office, 2001).

Reporting Statutes

In 1973 the United States Congress enacted the Child Abuse Prevention and Treatment Act. The law mandated all states to meet specific uniform guidelines to qualify for federal funding

BOX 8–1   *Grounds for Disciplinary Action by State Boards of Nursing*

- Practicing without a valid license
- Failure to use appropriate nursing judgment
- Guilty of a felony
- Falsification of records
- Failure to complete nursing documentation
- Incorrect nursing documentation

- Failure to practice in accordance with nursing standards
- Inappropriate behavior/occurrence at work
- Medicare fraud
- Misappropriation of personal items

Adapted from Booth D, Carruth A: Violations of the nursing practice act: implications for nurse managers, *Nurs Manage* 29(10): 35-40, 1998.

of child abuse programs. All 50 states and the District of Columbia now have created laws that mandate reporting of specific health problems and the suspected or confirmed abuse of vulnerable individuals in society such as elders. Nurses often are explicitly named within the context of these statutes as one of the groups of designated health professionals who must report the specified problems under penalty of fine or imprisonment. The following are reportable in all states:

- Infant and child abuse
- Dependent elder abuse
- Specified communicable diseases (for example, bubonic plague)

An increasing number of states also require a report of suspected or confirmed domestic violence. For example, a California law (Assembly Bill 890) enacted in 1995 requires nurses and other health care workers to recognize and report symptoms of domestic violence to local law enforcement authorities or face a misdemeanor charge.

It is crucial that nurses understand the requirements of abuse reporting statutes as they apply to their practice setting. For example, pediatric nurses must have in-depth knowledge regarding child abuse reporting laws. Agency policies and procedures in the work setting may provide guidance in regard to reporting duties. If in doubt, the nurse should immediately contact his or her supervisor, an administrator, or the agency's compliance officer (the individual responsible for understanding and ensuring adherence to federal and state statutes) for additional guidance in the matter. In rare situations, where information is not available within the institution, the nurse may consult with the State Department of Health or the state nurses' licensing board for guidance in obtaining these reporting statutes.

In a recent Missouri case, a nurse failed to report a suspected case of child abuse to that state's division of family services and to the physician in charge of her emergency department as required by law. She was charged with two misdemeanors, which could result in punishment of up to 2 years in prison and $2000 in fines, if she is convicted (Goldsmith, 2003).

Nurses need not fear legal reprisal from individuals or families who are reported to authorities in suspected cases of abuse. Most legislatures have granted immunity from suit within the context of the mandatory reporting statute. A recent court decision upheld this doctrine of immunity. In the case of Heinrich v. Conemaugh Valley Memorial Hospital (1994), the family of an injured child initiated a lawsuit against a hospital that reported suspected child abuse after a state investigation found them innocent of the charge. The court ruled that the hospital and the physician who made the report in "good faith" were immune from litigation under a Pennsylvania Child Protective Service Law that required reports of suspected child abuse.

Institutional Licensing Laws

All facilities (i.e., hospitals, nursing homes, rehabilitation centers) providing health care services must comply with licensing laws promulgated by state legislatures. These laws are created to protect the public and ensure the safe and effective provision of health care services. Specific language usually is contained within health facility licensing statutes regarding the following issues:

- Minimum standards for the maintenance of the physical plant
- Basic operational aspects of major departments (nursing, dietary, clinical laboratories, and pharmacy)
- Essential aspects of patient rights and the informed consent process

Many state licensing laws mandate minimum levels of education, experience, or credentialing for department administrators such as nurses, anesthesia personnel, pediatricians, and obstetricians. Several states also require minimum nurse-patient ratios in critical care units and other specialty departments such as the operating room, nursery, or emergency department.

Health care restructuring and redesign have led to many changes in the way health care services are provided and the settings in which care is rendered. Not all change has been positive, and some redesign schemes have resulted in adverse outcomes for patients. Investigations by state authorities on report of patient injuries or death have discovered that in some cases health facilities have operated in violation of existing licensing laws. In the past, direct-care RNs generally could rely on their nurse managers to have a comprehensive knowledge of health facility licensing law and to create policies and procedures that implement and enforce applicable aspects of the law. The trend toward flattened management and reduction in staff development personnel has altered this picture. In an increasing number of settings, nurse managers have been replaced with nonnurse administrators who may have minimal knowledge of the health facilities licensing laws.

In light of these changes, direct-care nurses should have a working knowledge of current licensing laws as they relate to nursing care and patient care services. I have found that nurses who have serious questions regarding quality of care in their employment setting have been able to resolve these concerns in many instances, once they have read applicable sections of the health facility licensing law relevant to their setting. Bringing the pertinent section of the law to the attention of managers, administrators, or the risk management department often is the most effective strategy to resolve problems. In settings in which nurses are represented by union contracts, potential violations of health facility licensing laws may be most effectively addressed through union representatives (Mahlmeister, 2000a).

Internet access has allowed nurses to obtain rapid information about current institutional licensing laws. Information can be downloaded and printed in rapid fashion. On-line consultants may be available to respond to nurses' questions and concerns. Nurses also can obtain a copy of the health facilities licensing law for their employment setting through the State Department of Health or Public Health, Division of Licensing and Certification. Other states provide the statute and address questions through the Department of Health,

Division of Facilities Regulations or Division of Health Facilities Inspection or Division of Health Quality Assurance. The telephone number for this agency can be found in the white pages of the local telephone directory under the heading "State of _____" (e.g., Michigan). Nurses may call their licensing board or the state nursing association for guidance in reaching the appropriate authority to obtain a copy of the licensing law and to speak to a consultant about concerns.

COMMON LAW

In addition to statutory law, nursing practice is guided by common law, also known as decisional or judge-made law. Common law is created through cases heard and decided in federal and state appellate courts. Throughout the years judge-made law regarding nursing practice has accumulated in the form of written opinions. These opinions eventually contribute to the expected standard of nursing conduct (Hall, 2002). The body of written opinions about nurses also is known as nursing case law. The importance of nursing case law in establishing the current standard of practice cannot be overstated.

One of the most important cases to establish the expected conduct of nurses was Utter v. United Hospital Center, Inc. (1977). This West Virginia case affirmed that nurses were required to exercise independent judgments to prevent harm when caring for patients. Before the 1970s the issue of whether nurses were licensed professionals who made independent judgments was not clearly established. In the Utter case a patient whose arm was casted had signs and symptoms of compartment syndrome. The affected limb became progressively more edematous and eventually turned black. The nurses failed to activate the chain of command when the primary providers did not respond to their reports and requests for medical reevaluation. The patient's arm eventually had to be amputated. The court wrote:

> Nurses are specialists in hospital care who, in the final analysis, hold the well-being, in fact in some instances, the very lives of patients in their hands. In the dim hours of the night, as well as in the light of day, nurses are frequently charged with the duty to observe the condition of the ill and infirm in their care. If the patient, helpless and wholly dependent, shows signs of worsening, the nurse is charged with the obligation of taking some positive action . . . there was evidence that certain nurses did not fulfill their obligation.

The duty to prevent harm, known as the nurse's "affirmative duty," has been supported in numerous court decisions. In a recent case, Rowe v. Sisters of Pallottine Missionary Society (2001), a hospital and its emergency department nurses were found negligent for failing to question a physician's discharge order. A 17-year-old motorcyclist was admitted to the emergency department for an injury to his left leg. He complained of severe pain in his left knee and numbness in his left foot. The nurses were unable to find a pulse in the left leg or foot. The physician issued a discharge order and gave instructions, which included the application of ice and elevation of the affected leg. The next day the man sought emergency care at another hospital for worsening pain and swelling of his leg. An examination revealed a lacerated popliteal artery and dislocated knee. He underwent extensive surgery and suffers permanent impairment of the affected limb. The physician settled the suit against him for $275,000. The jury returned a verdict for the patient in excess of $880,000, and found the nurses negligent for failing to question the discharge order and invoke the chain of command to obtain additional medical consultation and advice.

Every nurse should understand the impact that nursing case law has on his or her current practice. Case law made in appellate court decisions has addressed a range of vital issues related to professional nursing, including:

- Nursing malpractice cases
- Questions concerning labor law and collective bargaining
- Lawsuits alleging wrongful termination
- Legal challenges to state board of nursing disciplinary action against a nurse's license
- Legal actions against the nurse instituted by medical licensing boards
- "Practicing medicine without a license" claims
- Lawsuits claiming violation of the nurse's civil rights, including free-speech issues and reasonable accommodation for nurses with disabilities

Efforts should be made by professional nurses to review case law as it is published and discussed in nursing journals. There has been a trend to incorporate "legal advice" columns into many practice journals, and journals often include discussions about nursing case law. There also has been a proliferation of nursing journals dedicated solely to legal issues in nursing practice. Table 8-2 lists examples of these publications.

In addition to contributing to the expected standard of nursing care through court decisions, common law also provides the courts with guidelines in deciding future cases containing similar facts about nursing practice. These decisions are called "legal precedents." The reliance of judges on previous court decisions to guide current opinions is based on the legal doctrine of stare decisis ("let the decision stand"). The principle of applying previous decisions to current cases most often occurs within the same jurisdiction or state in which the legal precedent was established. However, legal precedent may influence an opinion in cases heard on appeal in other regions of the United States.

Nurse managers in particular should have knowledge regarding the disposition of cases in their jurisdiction. A risk manager or agency attorney may assist any nurse in understanding how judge-made law in his or her state relates to expectations for nursing practice in the local community. Many medical libraries also subscribe to publications that review federal or appellate court decisions in health care law that are relevant to the local community. Although local jury verdicts do not contribute to common law, it is useful for managers and interested nurses to periodically review published reports of malpractice cases in the state and their immediate community. Medical libraries also often subscribe to a local "jury verdicts" publication. More information on finding nursing case law is available on-line (http://evolve.elsevier.com/Cherry/).

| Table 8-2 | **Examples of Journals Dedicated to Legal Issues in Nursing Practice** |

JOURNAL	PUBLISHER
Nursing Law's Regan Report (formerly *Regan Report on Nursing Law*)	Medica Press Inc., Providence, RI
Journal of Nursing Law	KRM Information Services, Inc., Eau Claire, WI
Legal Eagle Eye Newsletter for the Nursing Professions	*Legal Eagle Eye Newsletter,* Seattle, WA
Journal of Legal Nurse Consulting	American Association of Legal Nurse Consultants, Glenview, IL

CIVIL LAW

Two major categories of law have been created to deal with conduct that is considered unacceptable—criminal law and civil law. Nurses generally are more familiar with civil law and, in particular, the branch of civil law that deals with torts. Tort law is discussed first, with a discussion of criminal law following.

A tort is a civil wrong or injury committed by one person against another person or a property. The wrong results from a breach in one's legal duty regarding interpersonal relationships between private persons. This duty is established through societal expectations regarding interpersonal conduct (Hall, 2002). Civil suits almost always are brought by one person against another and generally are based on the concept of "fault." The person who initiates the civil lawsuit, the plaintiff, seeks damages for the wrongful behavior from the offending person, known as the defendant. The determination of whether wrongful behavior has occurred usually is determined by a jury, although in certain cases the right to a trial by jury can be waived by the private parties in the suit. In that case the judge considers the facts and determines the outcome. If the plaintiff succeeds in the civil lawsuit (plaintiff verdict), damages generally are awarded in the form of monetary compensation. Damages may include "hard" damages—financial reimbursement for treatment of injuries, loss of wages, rehabilitation services, or special equipment—and "soft" damages—monetary compensation for pain and suffering, loss of companionship, or mental anguish, among other things (*Nurse's Legal Handbook*, 2000).

Negligence and Malpractice

There are two types of torts: an unintentional tort or wrong and an intentional tort. An unintentional tort is an unintended wrong against another person. The two most common unintentional torts are negligence and malpractice.

Negligence is defined as the failure to act in a reasonable and prudent manner. The claim of negligence is based on the accepted principle that everyone is expected to conduct themselves in a reasonable and prudent fashion. This is true of lay persons, student nurses, and licensed professionals. A more formal definition of negligence is the failure of a person to use the care that a reasonably prudent and careful person would use under similar circumstances (Croke, 2003).

Malpractice is a special type of negligence—that is, the failure of a professional, a person with specialized education and training, to act in a reasonable and prudent manner (Hall, 2002). As state nursing practice acts have evolved to reflect the increasing professionalism of RNs, courts have begun to recognize the negligent acts of nurses as malpractice. Evidence of this change in perceptions is apparent in the increasing use of RNs as expert witnesses in malpractice cases.

In general, expert testimony is not needed in cases of "simple negligence," when the actions of the defendant are so obviously careless that even a lay person would recognize the conduct as negligent. In contrast, if the jury does not possess the special knowledge and information that professionals ordinarily have, an expert witness is required to establish whether the person breached the expected standard of care. In that case the breach in duty is not simple negligence, but malpractice.

Elements Essential to Prove Negligence or Malpractice. Although any patient (or surviving family member, in the case of a patient death) may sue the nurse and his or her employer, the following elements must be proved for the plaintiff to succeed in the case.

A. The nurse owed the patient or client a special duty of care based on the establishment of a nurse-patient relationship.

1. When the nurse accepts a patient assignment, it establishes the relationship and requires the nurse to meet his or her duty to the patient.
    a. The duty of the nurse is to possess the knowledge and skill that a reasonable and prudent nurse would possess and exercise in the same or similar patient care situation.
    b. The duty of the nurse as described is the standard of care.
2. A nurse-patient relationship also may be established through telephone communication in the case of a nurse who performs telephone triage and advice or via computer or audio-video systems that are now being introduced in some health care settings (Mahlmeister, 2000b).

B. The nurse has breached his or her duty to the patient or client.
    1. Evidence is presented that proves the nurse breached the standard of care.
    2. The standard of care is essentially what the nurse expert witness states that it is.
    3. The standard of care is derived from a multiplicity of sources; these are described in Box 8-2.

C. Actual harm or damage is suffered by the patient.

D. There is proximate cause or a causal connection between the breach in the standard of care by the nurse and the patient's injury.
    1. No intervening event is responsible for the injury.
    2. A direct cause and effect can be demonstrated.
    3. In some jurisdictions the nurse's breach in duty must only be proven to be a "substantial cause" of the patient's injury.

This last element merits further discussion. The relationship between the nurse's breach in the standard of care and the patient's injury must be established by the plaintiff. To prove "proximate cause," there must be a direct causal link. For example, a patient reports that he has an allergy to penicillin and wears a MedicAlert bracelet to that effect. A physician orders penicillin to treat the patient's infection. The nurse fails to check or ask the patient about allergies. The nurse administers the penicillin, and the patient suffers an anaphylactic reaction and dies. There is a direct connection between the nurse's actions and the patient's death. Proximate cause has been established.

One may ask what the physician's liability is in this case. The physician also owes a duty to the patient and may be found negligent for ordering penicillin, if he or she had knowledge of, or should have had knowledge of the allergy. However, even in the case of a physician's negligence—"I knew about the penicillin allergy, but forgot!"—the nurse has a separate and independent duty to the patient to prevent harm. The nurse must review the patient's medical record for information about allergies, ask the patient about allergies, and check the patient's identification band before administering a drug.

In some jurisdictions it only is necessary to prove that the nurse's actions were a *substantial* cause of the injury or harm to prove negligence. For example, in a large teaching hospital a nurse notes a significant change in a patient's vital signs, suggesting deterioration in his condition. A first-year resident is called to the bedside and made aware of the patient's status. The resident orders the nurse to simply continue observing the patient. The first-year resident remains immediately available in the unit and receives repeated reports of a continued decline in the patient's condition. There is a clear chain of command policy established in

BOX 8–2 Sources That Contribute to the Standard of Nursing Care

Federal Laws
Emergency Medical Treatment and Active Labor Law
Americans with Disabilities Act
Patient Self-Determination Act
Occupational Health and Safety Law

Federal Administrative Rules and Regulations
Rules and Regulations for Participation in Medicare

Federal Guidelines
Agency for Health Care Policy and Research Clinical Guidelines
National Institutes of Health Publications
Centers for Disease Control and Prevention Publications (Morbidity and Mortality Weekly Reports)

Nursing Case Law
Appellate court decisions

Professional Organizations
Standards and guidelines for practice
Nursing journals
Position statements
Technical bulletins and practice resources
Code of ethics

Manufacturer Guidelines
Durable medical equipment
Drugs and solutions
Disposable equipment and supplies

Agency Policies and Procedures
Job descriptions
Agency-specific documents
Nursing care plans
Care maps or critical pathways
Unit- or department-based standards of practice
Medical bylaws

State Laws
Nursing Practice Act
State reporting statutes
Health facility licensing laws

State Administrative Rules and Regulations
Licensing board rules

Board of Nursing Licensure
Position statements and advisories

the hospital, which takes into account varying levels of skill and expertise of the residents in training. There is also a chain of command policy to deal with unresolved disagreements between health care professionals and nonresponsive providers. Despite the existence of these policies, the nurse does not activate the chain of command.

The patient suffers hypovolemic shock caused by internal bleeding, and this leads to permanent anoxic brain damage. In this case the nurse's failure to obtain additional medical advice and consultation (a senior resident was physically present and available in the hospital) was a substantial cause of the patient's injury. These two examples illustrate that negligence may constitute a commission (inappropriate penicillin administration) or an omission (failure to activate chain of command) in care.

Negligence and the Doctrine of Res Ipsa Loquitur. In the majority of cases a plaintiff must retain a nurse expert witness because the jury does not ordinarily possess the scientific and technologic knowledge necessary to determine the required standard of care. When the negligent act clearly lies within the range of a jury's common knowledge and experience, the doctrine of res ipsa loquitur ("the thing speaks for itself") may be applied. For example, leaving a surgical instrument in the patient's body after an operation is one case in which the doctrine may apply (Hall, 2002). It would be obvious to any lay person that it is below that standard of care not to remove a surgical instrument.

Dickerson v. Fatehi (1997) illustrates this point. A woman who underwent neck surgery experienced severe pain in her right arm, hand, and neck after the procedure. Approximately 20 months later a second surgery was performed to determine the cause of the patient's continued pain. An 18-gauge hypodermic needle with a plastic attachment for a syringe was discovered in her neck and removed. The woman sued the surgeon and nurses involved in the original surgical procedure. The claims against the nurses included a failure to maintain a proper needle count and a failure to ensure the removal of the needle after surgery.

The court hearing this case dismissed the suit. On appeal the Supreme Court of Virginia reversed the lower court's decision and directed the case for trial. The Supreme Court held that in this particular case expert testimony was not necessary to establish the applicable standard of care and that the doctrine of *res ipsa loquitur* applied. A jury would be able to determine whether a reasonably prudent circulating nurse and scrub nurse should have made and reported an accurate needle count.

Gross Negligence. In some cases the negligent act of the nurse is so reckless and reflects such a conscious disregard for the patient's welfare that it represents gross negligence. When the nurse acts with complete indifference to the consequences for his or her patient, the court may award special damages meant to punish the nurse for the outrageous conduct. These damages are referred to as punitive damages. Each state has established standards to determine when punitive damages may be awarded. In Mobile Infirmary Medical Center v. Hodgen (2003), the jury awarded $2.5 million dollars in punitive damages (later reduced to $1.5 million dollars) when a new graduate, not yet licensed, administered five times the ordered dose of digoxin. The jury found that the new graduate had been improperly supervised by the novice nurse assigned as her preceptor by the shift charge nurse. The charge nurse was also found liable for failing to properly direct the preceptor in her role responsibilities. The Supreme Court of Alabama found, among other things, that the nurses acted callously and wantonly, the legal threshold that must be crossed before punitive damages can be awarded (Snyder, 2003b).

Another case in point is Manning v. Twin Falls Clinic and Hospital (1992). Punitive damages in the amount of $300 were awarded against an Idaho nurse for willful disregard of a terminally ill patient's comfort and physiologic stability during transfer from one unit of the hospital to another. The patient, who suffered from severe respiratory distress, required continuous oxygen administration. Despite the family's insistent and repeated requests that the nurse administer oxygen during the transfer, the nurse transported the patient without oxygen. The patient suffered a respiratory arrest and died shortly thereafter.

Nurses should be aware that as a rule malpractice insurance policies do not provide coverage for punitive damages. The purpose of punitive damages is not only to deter such egregious behavior from occurring in the future, but also to punish the nurse by requiring an out-of-pocket payment. Although the amount awarded in the Manning case was relatively modest, courts in some cases have levied damages in the thousands of dollars against nurses.

Criminal Negligence. Criminal negligence represents a case in which the negligent acts of the nurse (normally an unintentional civil wrong) also constitute a crime. In most states a nurse can be prosecuted when the conduct is deemed so reckless that the action results in serious harm or death to the patient. In 1997 two registered nurses and an advanced practice nurse licensed in Colorado were charged with criminal negligent homicide in the death of a newborn resulting from a medication error (Kowalski and Horner, 1998). In this case an oil-based form of penicillin was erroneously administered to the infant. The drug was administered at 10 times the physician's prescribed dose. This case is detailed in a 1998 article by Kowalski and Horner entitled "A Legal Nightmare: Denver Nurses Indicted" (see References). This article should be read by every student and graduate nurse.

The Colorado case reflects the changing perspective of our justice system when negligent acts of health care professionals result in patient death. In the event of an unanticipated patient death, it is more likely that the conduct of both basic and advanced practice nurses will be scrutinized by the criminal justice system (Garza, 2002). This shift may in part be a result of the public's increasing awareness of the magnitude of error in health care. It also may stem from consumer demands for greater accountability by health care systems and workers when injury or death occurs. Conservative estimates suggest that as many as 98,000 patients die each year as a result of the negligence and malpractice of health care providers (Institute of Medicine, 2000).

Other negative consequences that the nurse faces when criminal charges are filed include the loss of his or her job and disciplinary action by the state licensing board. Even when the criminal charges are not supported, the nurse's license can be suspended or revoked and out-of-pocket fines levied by the board if there is evidence of violation of the Nursing Practice Act.

An attorney may have to be retained to represent the nurse at considerable personal expense when criminal charges are filed. The nurse's malpractice insurance generally does not cover the attorney's fees in this case. Neither is the nurse's employer obligated to pay the legal fees of a nurse charged with a felony. In the Colorado case the nurse practitioner was immediately terminated. The two direct care nurses were permitted to work in nonpatient care areas of the hospital. The costs of the criminal defense of all three nurses were paid by the hospital.

Defenses Against Claims of Negligence. In some cases the nurse can use certain legal doctrines as a defense against a claim of negligence. These standard defenses are discussed in the next section. In no case may a nurse provide a defense of "only following the provider's orders" against allegations of negligence (NSO Risk Advisor, 2003; Tammelleo, 2000). The Nursing

Practice Act, licensing board rules and regulations, and nursing case law have delineated the nurse's independent duty to evaluate all provider orders before implementing them. In doing so, the nurse must consider two points:

- Is the order lawful?
- Is the order in this particular patient's best interest?

Each nurse has an absolute duty to take some positive action to prevent harm when orders are inappropriate or incomplete or when the actions of another health care provider endanger the patient's well-being. This principle of "affirmative duty" is well recognized in law and in ethics. The American Nurses Association "Code of Ethics for Nurses" (2001) and the American Medical Association's "Code of Medical Ethics" (2000-2001) recognize the central role of nurses in preventing patient harm.

Emergency Situations. Nursing care rendered in a life-threatening emergency may breach the standard of care required under ordinary circumstances. For instance, a woman who is 8 months' pregnant arrives in the labor and delivery suite. She is hemorrhaging because of a premature separation of the placenta (abruptio placenta). An emergency cesarean delivery is ordered by the doctor. The woman is near death as a result of blood loss. There also are clear signs of fetal distress. To expedite the surgical delivery, the operating room team does not observe the strict aseptic technique normally required during insertion of a Foley catheter into the woman's bladder and foregoes the lengthy abdominal scrub normally performed with an iodine solution.

The mother and infant are brought through the crisis safely, although the woman develops a skin infection at the site of the abdominal incision, which causes noticeable scaring. She also must be treated for a bladder infection, which resolves by discharge on the fourth postpartum day. She sues the nurses and physician. In this case the defense could argue that, to save the life of the mother and baby, the methods used were reasonable and prudent. Even a delay of seconds could have resulted in the death of the woman or her infant. Expert witnesses are produced to support the defense assertion that it would breach the standard of care in this particular situation to follow customary procedures in preparing the woman for surgery.

Governmental Immunity. For nurses working in federal or state health care facilities, a defense of governmental immunity may be used. Laws have been enacted that shield individual health care workers employed in federal or (some) state facilities from personal responsibility for damages awarded in malpractice cases. Nurses employed by the Department of Veteran Affairs, the U.S. Public Health Service, the National Aeronautics and Space Administration, and the Department of Defense are shielded from civil suits in the performance of professional duties. This immunity was granted through enactment of specific federal statutes, including the Federal Tort Claims Act of 1946 and the Federal Employees Liability Reform and Tort Compensation Act of 1988.

The intent of these laws was to substitute the U.S. government as the defendant in a malpractice suit. The government has waived its "sovereign immunity" against suit and pays the damages for injuries caused by the negligent acts of health care professionals employed in the aforementioned federal agencies.

State immunity statutes vary. In some instances, individual states have not waived their "sovereign immunity" from lawsuits. In those cases the state is not substituted for the individual health care provider in malpractice cases. Nurses and physicians are liable for their negligent acts in these states and are personally responsible for damages awarded. It may be imperative in this circumstance for the health care professional to have individual malpractice insurance. The nurse should seek the advice of an attorney to determine whether it would be prudent to purchase malpractice insurance (Hall, 2002).

Good Samaritan Immunity. Good Samaritan laws may limit a nurse's liability or shield the nurse from a malpractice claim if the nurse renders assistance in an emergency that occurs outside of the employment setting. Although in most states the nurse owes no legal duty to an accident victim, once the nurse makes a decision to stop and render aid (an ethical decision), a nurse-patient relationship is established. (Some states, including Vermont, Minnesota, and Wisconsin, have enacted "duty to rescue" or "compulsory assistance" laws.)

When the nurse renders care at the scene of an accident, he or she is required to render the standard of care that any reasonable and prudent nurse would render in a similar situation. To prevail in a malpractice suit under the Good Samaritan Law, the plaintiff must prove that the nurse intentionally caused the injury or was grossly negligent (*Nurse's Legal Handbook*, 2000). Therefore each nurse should be familiar with his or her state-specific Good Samaritan statute. Nurses also should be reassured by the fact that the preponderance of malpractice cases that invoke the Good Samaritan defense are settled in favor of the nurse.

Statutes of Limitation in Malpractice Cases

Each state has established a time limit in which a person may initiate a lawsuit. Although many states have established a time limit of 2 or 3 years from the date of the patient's injury or death in which the plaintiff must sue, statutes of limitation vary widely from state to state. In some jurisdictions a "termination of treatment" rule exists. It is predicated on the assumption that some injuries result from a series of treatments over time. In this case the statute of limitation does not begin to run until the treatment ends.

Other rules and regulations govern the "tolling" or running of the statutes of limitation. The court recognizes that an injured party cannot initiate a malpractice case until he or she discovers that some harm was done (discovery rule). This can occur when health care providers actually conceal the facts in the case of an injury through fraud, deceit, or concealment, as in the following:

- Fraudulent or misleading entries in the medical record
- Destruction of evidence
- Destruction of the medical record
- Lying to the patient about the cause of the problems

The statute of limitation also is altered when a foreign object is left in the patient's body. Until the foreign object is discovered, the statute of limitation does not begin to run. States have rules that regulate the tolling of the statute of limitation in cases involving mentally incompetent adults and minors. In the case of an adult patient who is so severely injured that there is a loss of mental capacity, the statute of limitation may not begin to toll until mental competence is regained. The statute of limitation varies in the case of minors and may only expire when the child reaches the age of majority (age 18 or 21 years) (Brent, 2001).

Each nurse should be familiar with the statute of limitation for his or her state. If the nurse suspects that some form of fraud or deceit has occurred relative to a patient's injury, the agency's risk manager or attorney should be contacted immediately. Major penalties and fines are applicable in cases in which health care providers deliberately deceive the patient or destroy evidence. These acts rise to the level of criminal misconduct and can result in loss of one's professional license.

When errors occur in practice, studies confirm that telling the patient (and family) about the mistake (voluntary disclosure) promptly results in far less severe ramifications for the clinicians and health care facility (Federico and Augello, 2003; Woods and Rozovsky, 2003). In 2001, the Joint Commission on the Accreditation of Healthcare Organizations (JCAHO) established a new patient safety care standard requiring that institutions have a process in place to disclose unanticipated outcomes to patients. Disclosure of errors and unanticipated adverse outcomes is a key element of the national patient safety movement (Federico, 2003).

When an unanticipated outcome occurs, the provider is generally responsible for discussing the situation with the patient and or family members. Other agency representatives may be involved in the disclosure process, including administrators, risk managers, or attorneys. The nurse should not assume responsibility for disclosure. It should be determined in advance who will speak with the patient (or family) and how questions and concerns about the patient's condition, subsequent treatment, and the cost of any required care will be addressed. Fear that disclosure will lead to a malpractice claim is a significant barrier to voluntary disclosure, despite research findings to the contrary. In fact, patients sue for many reasons, including mishandling of information about unanticipated outcomes, delayed communication about adverse events, and anger when they believe they have not been told the truth about events (Federico, 2003). If a nurse believes that providers have not disclosed essential information to the patient, concerns should be taken to the managers or administrators through the agency's line of authority.

Nursing Malpractice Insurance

With more states recognizing nursing malpractice as a legitimate claim in a civil suit, the question of whether nurses should carry malpractice insurance has become increasingly important (Hall, 2002). Nursing journals have published a number of articles that either address this question or describe the types of malpractice coverage the nurse should consider (Morrison et al, 1998; Tammelleo, 1997). An increasing consensus appears to recommend that all nurses purchase malpractice insurance as a result of changes in the health care system, civil law, and insurance company policies. Legal authors also are quick to note the fallacy of the assumption that having malpractice insurance increases the risk that the nurse will be targeted in a malpractice case. Lack of coverage will not discourage a lawsuit when there is a legitimate claim. Reasons given for the purchase of malpractice insurance by RNs include:

- Expanding functions of RNs and advanced practice nurses
- Floating and cross-training mandates
- Increasing responsibility for supervising subordinate staff
- Failure of some employers to initiate an adequate defense for nurses
- Insurance coverage limits that are lower than the actual judgment made against the nurse in a lawsuit

Other considerations that the nurse must take into account when considering malpractice insurance include whether he or she is employed by the federal government. In that case the nurse may be shielded from personal liability by federal tort statutes, although some states still uphold the doctrine of "sovereign immunity," making it impossible to sue a state-run medical facility for negligence. In those states it is a virtual necessity for nurses to purchase malpractice insurance because health care workers become the only available targets in a malpractice case.

Liability

Closely tied to the concepts of negligence and malpractice is that of liability. Liability asserts that every person is responsible for the wrong or injury done to another resulting from carelessness.

Personal Liability

Within the context of nursing practice, the nurse is always accountable for the outcomes of his or her actions in carrying out nursing duties. The rule of personal liability requires the professional nurse to assume responsibility for patient harm or injury that is a result of his or her negligent acts. The nurse cannot be relieved of personal liability by another professional, such as a provider or nurse manager, who asserts, "Don't worry, I'll take responsibility for the consequences."

In 1989 the ANA summarized the most frequent allegations of negligence leveled against nurses in malpractice cases. They are listed in Box 8-3. These charges have not substantially changed in the ensuing decades (Croke, 2003). Nurses may be educated to implement effective risk control strategies that reduce these claims. These personal and system-wide strategies are discussed in the next section.

Many nurses practice under the misconception that they are protected from personal liability when employed by a health care entity such as a hospital. I have heard nurses say, "Why would a patient sue me personally? I don't have the financial resources of this (hospital, nursing home, home health care agency)!" Nurses can and have been individually named in lawsuits and found negligent. Damages can be levied against the nurse's current assets and future earnings for negligent acts (LaDuke, 1999). Furthermore, as Tammelleo (1996) reports, hospitals have sued nurses to recoup financial losses suffered when they were required to pay damages for the alleged negligence of the nurses named in the malpractice case. Personal liability is illustrated in the case of Shelton v. Penrose/St. Francis Healthcare (1999).

> Gretchen Shelton was hospitalized for hip replacement surgery. After surgery she was fitted with a special brace to prevent posterior dislocation of her hip. Six days after surgery she was transferred to the rehabilitation unit in the hospital for daily physical therapy. During therapy her brace was removed. After the treatment, she was returned to her room and placed in a chair, where she fell asleep. Two nurses entered her room and proceeded to move her from the chair back to her bed without waking her or ascertaining whether her brace was on.

BOX 8–3 *Most Frequent Allegations of Nursing Negligence*

- Failure to ensure patient safety
- Improper treatment or negligent performance of the treatment
- Failure to monitor the patient and report significant findings
- Medication errors
- Failure to follow the agency's policies and procedures

Adapted from American Nurses Association: *Liability prevention and you,* Washington, DC, 1989, American Nurses Publishing, American Nurses Foundation/American Nurses Association.

During the transfer, her hip was dislocated, causing extreme pain. Ms. Shelton sued, claiming the nurses were negligent for failing to waken her and determine whether her brace was in place. One of the defense arguments was that the nurses would have ordinarily expected that her brace would have been on when she was returned to her room and were therefore not required to check the affected leg. The jury found the two nurses negligent, agreeing with the expert witness nurse. She concluded that, within a reasonable degree of nursing probability, the patient sustained the dislocation and pain as a result of a failure to assess the patient and correctly transfer her to bed. The hospital appealed, but the jury verdict was affirmed by the Supreme Court of Colorado.

Personal Liability with Floating and Cross-Training

New models of patient care often mandate floating and cross-training of patient care staff to enhance efficiency and reduce staffing costs. These new models of care have increased the personal liability of nurses (Croke, 2003). Professional nurses must be cognizant of state statutes and case law when asked to perform services outside of their usual area of practice. In no case is a nurse ever permitted to perform tasks or render services when he or she lacks the requisite knowledge and skill to act competently.

The Nursing Practice Act and the administrative rules and regulations of the licensing board provide explicit statutory language regarding the nurse's duty to provide safe and competent care. For example, the Administrative Rules of the Tennessee Board of Nursing (Revised, 2003) state:

> Each individual is responsible for personal acts of negligence under the law. Registered nurses are liable if they perform delegated functions they are not prepared to handle by education and experience, and for which supervision is not provided. In any patient care situation, the registered nurse should perform only those acts for which each has been prepared and has demonstrated ability to perform, bearing in mind the individual person's responsibility under the law.
>
> Tennessee Rules and Regulations of Registered Nurses
> Rule 1000-1-04 (3): Responsibility.

In addition to the laws governing practice in floating and cross-training situations, an increasing body of nursing case law also defines the limitation of assignments. Appellate court decisions have addressed the issue of when a nurse may safely refuse an assignment to float without risk of job termination. In Winkelman v. Beloit Memorial Hospital (1992), the Supreme Court of Wisconsin ruled that under certain circumstances a nurse had a right to refuse floating assignments without fear of reprisal.

> Nurse Winkelman was a skilled maternity nurse who was employed for 16 years at Beloit Memorial Hospital, working exclusively in the nursery. In 1987 the hospital created a new policy that required nurses in the maternity setting to float when the patient census was low in their unit. Nurse Winkelman was asked to float to an adult floor dedicated to the care of postoperative and geriatric patients. She notified her immediate supervisor that she did not feel qualified to float to that unit and that attempting to provide care in that setting would place the patients at risk. In her testimony the nurse said that she was given three choices: float, find another nurse who would float in her place, or take an unexcused absence day. She subsequently went home, and her employer construed her actions as "voluntary resignation of her employment." Nurse Winkelman then filed a complaint for wrongful discharge and breach of contract. A jury verdict was rendered in favor of Nurse Winkelman on the charge of wrongful discharge. The case was appealed and affirmed by the Supreme Court of Wisconsin.

The court found that the nurse had identified a fundamental and well-defined public policy in the Wisconsin Administrative Code, which stated that a nurse should not offer or perform services for which he or she is not qualified by education, training, or experience.

The nurse's right to refuse a floating assignment has not been supported in all cases. Courts have affirmed the right of a health care facility to redirect staff to meet the needs of patients. The New Mexico Supreme Court in Francis v. Memorial General Hospital (1986) held that the hospital was not prohibited from discharging a nurse who refused to float when the employer had made a reasonable offer to train the nurse for new responsibilities.

Nurse Francis, a critical care nurse, refused to float to an orthopedic unit, stating he did not feel qualified to care for orthopedic patients. The hospital then offered to provide him with an orientation to the floors where he might float in the future. When he refused the opportunity for orientation, he was terminated. The court upheld his discharge.

Although it is clear that nurses have a legal duty to refuse specific tasks that they cannot perform safely and competently, the prudent nurse should carefully consider the consequence of not floating. Careful negotiation with the nursing supervisor and the team leader making the actual assignment often can result in a satisfactory compromise. The floated nurse should clarify what aspects of professional nursing care he or she can safely carry out and which tasks are beyond his or her current capabilities. A reasonable supervisor will not insist that a nurse attempt to perform a task that he or she has no education, training, or current expertise to implement.

Another important strategy that may reduce the nurse's personal liability is to request that the team leader appoint a resource nurse who is skilled in the care of the patients on the unit. The resource nurse can assist the floated nurse as needed. It also is prudent practice for the floated nurse to enter a note in the medical record naming the resource or support nurse who will be available and responsible to assist with planning and evaluating care. For instance:

> Assumed care of Mrs. Jones after report completed. L. Doe, RN, will co-manage patient and assist with procedures, planning, and evaluation of care as needed.
>
> J. Smith, RN (floatee)

The Nursing Practice Act affirms that an RN ultimately is responsible for the quality of care provided to each patient, regardless of who actually is delegated the responsibility of carrying out the task. A claim of negligence may be leveled against the team leader who does not assign a competent "back-up" or resource nurse to assist the floatee. Only a nurse who is competent in the care of the patients normally treated in the setting (hospital, clinic, or home) can properly supervise a lesser skilled worker and evaluate the outcomes of care. The point is so critical that professional nursing organizations in California recently joined together to affirm this concept in law.

A section of the California Health Facilities Licensing for Hospitals (California Code of Regulations, Title 22, 1996; Revised 2003) now mandates:

> A registered nurse who has demonstrated competency for the patient care unit shall be responsible for nursing care . . . and shall be assigned as a resource nurse for those registered nurses and licensed vocational nurses who have not completed competency validation for that unit. Registered nurses shall not be assigned total responsibility for patient care . . . until all the standards of competency for that unit have been validated.
>
> Section 70214, Nursing Staff Development: (B) and (C)

Chapter 12 provides additional information about floating and accepting assignments.

Personal Liability for Team Leaders and Managers

The concept of personal liability extends to nurses who function as team leaders, supervisors, and upper-level managers. Team leaders, charge nurses, and managers are held to the standard of care of the reasonably prudent nurse employed in that role (Mahlmeister, 1999). Claims of negligence leveled against managers generally surround: (1) triage of patients and allocation of staff and equipment; (2) delegation of patient care tasks; (3) supervision of orientees, float staff, and subordinates; (4) reporting performance deficits in team members; and (5) supporting or invoking the chain of command process when indicated.

Nurse managers and administrators at the upper end of the management ladder also may be held liable for the following:

- Inadequate training
- Failure to periodically reevaluate staff competencies
- Failure to discipline or terminate unsafe workers
- Negligence in developing appropriate policies and procedures

The implementation of new models of care that alter staffing patterns and mixes "may place managers at the same risk for liability as the health care providers delivering the actual bedside care . . ." (Kreplick, 1996). The ANA affirms this view in the Code of Ethics for Nurses (2001).

> Although nurses in administration, education, and research have relationships with patients that are less direct, in assuming the responsibilities of a particular role, they share responsibility for the care provided by those whom they supervise and instruct. (p. 17)

The appropriate standard of care is established in the case of team leaders, charge nurses, managers, and leaders by expert nurse witnesses who function in those positions. An increasing body of case law in malpractice suits also is contributing to expectations about team leader and manager conduct. Although nurse managers and administrators generally are well aware of their particular liability risks, direct-care nurses who are relatively unfamiliar with the expanding role of team leaders or charge nurses may be particularly vulnerable to claims of negligence. Health care redesign has resulted in considerable flattening of the chain of command for nursing departments.

In September of 2003, The American Organization of Nurse Executives, the American Hospital Association and other health related organizations submitted an *amicus curiae* (friend of the court) brief in support of the unique role of the charge nurse (Brief Amici Curiae, July 24, 2003). These associations responded to a National Labor Relations Board invitation to file briefs to provide guidance on the meaning of the term *independent judgment* and the scope of discretion required for independent judgment with respect to the charge nurse. The brief asserts that

> The charge nurse's background in the hospital's organization and in nursing practice enables him or her to step in when there is crisis or conflict, quickly to assess the situation and identify needed resources. Charge nurses also direct other employees, sometimes making split-second decisions that can literally be a matter of life or death." (pp. 6-7)

Team leaders, regardless of their title or designation, have assumed greater responsibility for unit- or department-based functions, such as those listed in Box 8-4.

Any RN functioning in the role of team leader or charge nurse should review the following documents from administration:

- Detailed job description for the role, including how responsibilities are limited when the nurse is asked to lead team or serve as a charge nurse on an unfamiliar floor or department

BOX 8–4 *Typical Functions and Role Responsibilities of the Team Leader or Charge Nurse*

With flattened management the norm in an increasing number of redesigned health care settings, the "team leader" or "charge nurse" may be accountable for the following functions.

1. Staff assignments
2. Delegation of patient care tasks to unlicensed team members
3. Supervision of:
   a. Licensed practical or vocational nurses
   b. Unlicensed assistive personnel
   c. Temporary staff (floats, agency, or registry nurses)
4. Evaluation of the outcomes of care for licensed practical or vocational nursing staff and unlicensed team members
5. Triage of staff and equipment during acute patient events
6. Consultant for clinical problems
   a. Personal assessment or interview of patients
   b. Personal interpretation of data
   c. Advice about care or management of problems
7. Arbitrator in clinical disputes between patient care staff and primary providers
8. Traffic manager during acute patient events
9. Expert in operation of biotechnical equipment
10. Expert in unit operations
    a. Location of supplies and equipment
    b. Chain of command process
    c. Disaster plans

- Job descriptions for the team members assigned delegated tasks
- Formal period of training and mentoring in the role
- Validated proof of competence before team leading independently
- Guidelines regarding personal patient care assignment when also serving as team leader
- Chain of command model for the facility, department, or unit

Administrators and nurse managers should be aware of recent case law regarding incompetent charge nurses and team leaders. A jury directed a verdict in excess of $7 million against a hospital in a 1995 Illinois case, Holston v. Sisters of the Third Order (1995).

A charge nurse repeatedly refused a direct-care nurse's requests to personally evaluate a patient whose vital signs were rapidly deteriorating after gastric bypass surgery. The charge nurse also refused to call the patient's physician until the patient experienced cardiopulmonary collapse. Emergency surgery revealed that a central venous pressure catheter had migrated and perforated the cardiac muscle. The patient experienced cardiac tamponade and died approximately 1 week after this critical incident.

In a second case, Justin and Michelle Malovic v. Santa Monica Hospital Medical Center (1995), a California jury found a nurse manager negligent for failing to implement the chain of command. The case is described as follows:

The nurse manager failed to summon the chief of obstetrics when the primary obstetrician was unresponsive to a nonreassuring fetal heart rate. The primary nurse asked the nurse manager to personally evaluate the electronic fetal heart rate pattern. The manager did so but decided there was no need to call the chief of the department. This case was complicated by the fact that the managing obstetrician's practice already was under investigation, and the nurse manager was aware of this fact. The primary obstetrician eventually attempted a forceps birth over an unacceptably long period of time (1 hour). A subsequent cesarean delivery resulted in the birth of an infant who is now mentally retarded. The plaintiff's attorney successfully argued that, had the nurse manager called the chief of obstetrics, he would have effectively intervened, and the infant would have been born without damage.

This case illustrates the necessity of validating the strong clinical skill of all RNs who are being considered for a leadership role that includes clinical supervision and consultation. Effective risk management of an unresolved clinical problem requires direct-care nurses to consult early and frequently with team leaders or managers. Each consultation with the team leader or manager should be carefully documented in the patient's medical record to demonstrate that appropriate chain of command process has occurred. The employer will likely be named in any lawsuit under the rule of vicarious liability if the team leader or manager offers negligent advice. Vicarious liability is discussed in the next section of this chapter.

Personal Liability in Delegation and Supervision of Team Members

Team leaders and charge nurses who are responsible for delegation and supervision of team members must be absolutely clear about the legality of patient care assignments. They must determine whether it is reasonable and prudent to delegate a particular task based on their knowledge of the worker, the patient's status, and the current conditions in the work setting. The determination of whether a team leader or charge nurse has been negligent in delegating any particular patient care task or supervising subordinates will be based on these aforementioned considerations.

Mobile Infirmary Medical Center v. Hodgen (2003) is a case in point. A patient with cardiac problems sued after suffering catastrophic physical and mental disabilities when a graduate nurse, not yet licensed, administered five times the ordered dose of digoxin. The shift charge nurse assigned another nurse with only 7 months' experience to act as the graduate nurse's preceptor. The preceptor did not supervise the new graduate when she administered the drug. The jury found all three nurses negligent. The court criticized the shift charge nurse for assigning a novice nurse as a preceptor and for failing to give her explicit directions regarding the level of supervision required in the circumstances. The court also faulted the preceptor, who had never worked with the new graduate, for inadequate supervision. The jury awarded $2.5 million dollars in punitive damages.

Criteria for lawful and safe delegation have been spelled out by state boards of nursing and professional organizations such as the ANA, the American Association of Critical Care Nurses, and the National Council of State Boards of Nursing (ANA, 1996; AACN, 1995; NCSBN, 1995). These guidelines and a growing body of case law assist the nurse in making decisions about safe delegation of patient care. Singleton v. AAA Home Health, Inc., (2000) illustrates the professional duties of the registered nurse and the legal risks inherent in delegating nursing care to unlicensed assistive personnel.

> Rhea Polk, a patient with cardiac and renal disease, was released from the hospital with a discharge plan for home health care to be provided by skilled nursing staff. Orders were issued to provide treatment for a right hip decubitus, including packing with Betadine gauze. The wound did not heal, and surgical debridement was required. The surgeon discovered gauze embedded in the ulcerated wound, and this was determined to be the cause of the problem.

On behalf of Ms. Polk, Ms. Singleton sued the home health agency. Evidence uncovered during the trial indicated that the RN responsible for Ms. Polk's care had instructed home health aides in packing the wound and inappropriately delegated the task to them. The expert witness in the case asserted that the failure of an RN to properly inspect, clean, and treat the wound was the cause of the ulceration and need for surgery. The trial court rendered a verdict in favor of Ms. Singleton. The Louisiana Court of Appeal affirmed the verdict of the lower court on appeal.

It is important to note that, in addition to acting negligently in delegating the wound packing to a home health aide, the nurse had violated the Nursing Practice Act. Although this issue was not addressed in the Singleton case, courts have ruled in previous malpractice cases that a failure to adhere to the Nursing Practice Act (a law) and the administrative rules and regulations of the licensing board constitutes negligence per se (negligence as a matter of law).

Employer Liability

Although the nurse is never relieved of personal liability, the doctrine of vicarious or substituted liability permits a person to also sue the employer for the negligent conduct of nurses within the scope of their employment. Vicarious liability is based on the legal principle of respondent superior, a Latin term that means "let the master answer" (for the actions of subordinates or servants). Because the employer has some control over the worker, the courts have affirmed that the employer may be held responsible for the employee's negligent acts when injury occurs.

In a Texas case—Convalescent Services, Inc. v. Schultz (1996)—a nursing home was found negligent for failure of its nursing staff to provide appropriate skin care to an elderly client with Alzheimer's dementia. The patient developed severe pressure sores. He required surgery to repair the decubitus ulcers, experienced significant pain and suffering, and had a prolonged hospitalization. The suit claimed that the care provided by the staff in the nursing home was so substandard that it represented gross negligence. The jury awarded a verdict for the plaintiff and punitive damages for the gross negligence of the nursing staff. The appeals court upheld the ruling, which the nursing home had contested.

Corporate Liability

Hospitals and other health care facilities have evolved into dynamic systems that coordinate the care provided by a range of health care professionals (Hall, 2002; Brent, 2001). As a consequence of these changes, the courts have expanded the concept of corporate negligence in verdicts rendered against health care giants. The "standard of care" required of a health care corporation has been established through these cases but varies from state to state. Some jurisdictions have permitted JCAHO standards or State Department of Health licensing laws to define the "corporate standard of care." An agency's own medical bylaws or policies and procedures have been admitted as evidence of the appropriate corporate standard of care. In Thompson v. Nason Hospital (1991), the court elaborated four duties of a health care corporation:

1. Maintain safe and adequate physical facilities and equipment.
2. Select and retain competent physicians.
3. Oversee the acts of all persons who practice medicine within the facility as they relate to patient care.
4. Formulate, adopt, and enforce rules and policies to ensure quality of care.

In another case, Rodebush v. Oklahoma Nursing Homes, Ltd. (1993), the court found a nursing home liable for negligent hiring and supervision of a staff member, a nurse aide, who had a previous conviction of a violent felony: assault and battery with the intent to kill.

The criminal record was discovered only after the family of a patient in the nursing home filed a lawsuit. The suit was initiated when the family's elderly parent was injured by the nurse aide, who was intoxicated at the time of the incident. The jury awarded $50,000 in actual damages and $1.2 million in punitive damages against the corporation for failing to follow its own policies in hiring, training, and supervising employees and in investigating employee misconduct.

Health care facilities also have been found corporately liable for failing to have adequate numbers of qualified nursing staff assigned on each shift to meet the needs of patients. In Merritt v. Karcloglu (1996), a Louisiana hospital was found negligent for failing to have sufficient nursing staff to provide essential care. The hospital had a written policy that directed a nurse in the cardiac care unit to respond to "Codes" called in other areas of the hospital. A nurse assigned exclusively to an elderly, confused patient in the critical care unit was required to respond to a code. While she was out of the unit, her patient attempted to get out of bed, fell, and fractured her hip. She subsequently died, in part because of complications of her fall (pneumonia, decubitus development, sepsis). Her family sued and was awarded $500,000. The verdict was upheld on appeal. The hospital had a policy that required a nurse to be in "two places at one time," an impossible standard to meet.

A similar finding of negligence was found in an Arkansas case when a hospital failed to have sufficient nursing staff in a nursery to monitor newborns, HCA Health Services v. National Bank (1988). An unattended infant experienced a respiratory arrest and suffered permanent anoxic brain damage. The jury awarded $2 million in compensatory damages (for the cost of ongoing care) and $2 million in punitive damages for failing to provide an adequate number of qualified staff. The current nursing shortage is anticipated to grow in the first decade of this century. Nurses must develop a clear understanding of principles of safe staffing and advocate for appropriate staffing levels. Guidelines published by the ANA (1999) can assist nurses to ensure the efficient use of human resources and the delivery of quality care.

More recently, the courts have been asked to determine whether a hospital or an agency providing temporary nursing staff to that hospital was liable for the acts of an agency nurse (Ruelas v. Staff Builders Personnel Services, Inc., 2001). An agency nurse was alleged to have abused a patient during administration of an enema. (The precise nature of the abuse was not delineated.) The court affirmed that as a general rule, the employer (in this case Staff Builders) is legally liable for an employee's wrongful conduct. However in this case, Staff Builders had no practical or even theoretical right to control how its nurses carried out their clinical responsibilities in a particular setting. Although the agency is responsible for ensuring that the nurse has the requisite license, education, experience and certifications, the hospital has direct control and supervision of the nurse's actions. Staff Builders was dismissed from the lawsuit.

REDUCING LEGAL LIABILITY
Risk Management Systems

One of the most powerful allies the nurse has in any health care setting to facilitate positive change and reduce personal and corporate liability is the risk manager. The risk manager is a professional who tracks accidents and injuries that occur in the facility. The job of the risk manager is to establish and strengthen systems within the agency to reduce preventable patient injuries or deaths and to eliminate the loss of revenues as fines or the payment of damages through the insurance carrier. The risk manager may assist nurse managers in the development of effective policies and procedures to improve practice. Finally, the risk manager also is knowledgeable about federal and state administrative rules and regulations affecting health care systems, health care licensing laws, and health care case law. This knowledge is essential to prevent inadvertent violation of health care laws and to reduce claims of negligence and malpractice within the institution.

The Institute of Medicine (IOM) report "To Err is Human" (2000) recommends a "proactive" approach to risk management. Nurses are encouraged to anticipate the potential for errors, report "near misses," and work closely with the risk manager to reduce preventable adverse events. All health care providers are urged to develop "high-reliability" operating systems. This concept is derived from the airline and nuclear energy industries. Both have established excellent safety records despite the highly complex and dangerous nature of their operations. The IOM recommends creation of a nationwide mandatory reporting system for collection of information about adverse events and the development of performance standards that focus on patient safety. Nurses will play a central role in this process.

Incident Reports

Nurses are legally bound to report critical incidents to their nurse managers, agency administration, and the risk manager through a formal, intra-agency document generally entitled the "Unusual Occurrence" or "Incident Report." This form often is directed to the risk management department through the nurse's immediate manager. The nurse manager has an opportunity to review the written report and begin the process of risk control in a timely fashion, depending on the nature of the incident. The report then is forwarded (usually within 24 hours) to the risk manager. If an ongoing problem does not appear to be any closer to resolution as the nurse works through the formal chain of command, the nurse may speak directly to the risk manager for guidance and advice. However, in the usual course of events, the nurse would first address concerns with his or her immediate nurse manager.

Critical incidents that result in patient injury or death eventually may lead to a malpractice claim. Because state laws vary as to whether the incident report may be "discovered" by the plaintiff's attorney in a lawsuit, it is essential that the nurse follow appropriate procedures when completing and filing this document.

1. The nurse should describe all events objectively; avoid subjective comments, personal opinions about why the incident occurred, or assumptions about events that were not witnessed. For example, if a patient was found lying on the floor at the foot of his bed, the nurse should avoid the statement, "Patient fell out of bed—found on floor." That the patient fell out of bed is an unfounded assumption. The nurse should instead state, "Entered room. Patient discovered lying prone at the foot of the bed. Both upper and lower side rails were raised."
2. The nurse should never note in the patient's medical record that an incident report has been completed and filed. This may alter the protection from discovery normally provided the document in some states. The jury also will be made aware that an incident report has been filed because they have access to nurses' notes submitted in evidence during the trial.
3. The nurse should never photocopy the incident report for his or her personal files. Photocopying an incident report generally is prohibited by agency policy and may be expressly prohibited in writing on the incident report itself. Photocopying the incident report and taking it out of the agency violates patient confidentiality. It may fall into the hands of persons who are not authorized to read any information about the patient. It may fall into the hands of the plaintiff's attorney, should a lawsuit be filed, with damaging effects on the agency's ability to defend against the claims of negligence.

4. Physicians and advanced practice nurses should not write an order for an incident report to be filed. This brings the existence of an incident report to the attention of the plaintiff's attorney.

5. Report every unusual occurrence or incident. Do not assume that "everyone knows about the problem or event."

Box 8-5 lists circumstances under which incident reports should be filed.

INTENTIONAL TORTS IN NURSING PRACTICE

Ordinarily, in the course of carrying out one's nursing duties, breaches in the applicable standard of care are assumed to be unintentional acts. In other words, the nurse did not intend to harm the patient. As noted, this civil wrong is referred to as an unintentional tort. An intentional tort is a second category of civil wrong. It involves the direct violation of a person's legal rights. In this case the nurse intends to perform the offensive act, although normally most nurses do not mean to harm the patient. The following acts are intentional torts:

■ Assault
■ Battery
■ Defamation of character
■ False imprisonment
■ Invasion of privacy
■ Intentional infliction of emotional distress

BOX 8–5 *Circumstances Under Which the Incident Report Should Be Filed**

■ Patient or client injury
■ Unanticipated patient death
■ Malfunction or failure of durable medical equipment
■ Significant or unanticipated adverse reactions to ordered therapy or care
■ Inability to meet a patient's need(s) (ordered therapy, medications, treatments) after consultation with appropriate nurse mangers or providers. This may be related to:

System problems (e.g., pharmacy closed, drug not available)
Unresolved problem with order (e.g., incomplete or illegible order)
Lack of qualified staff to implement order to provide needed care (e.g., RN not available to perform task, and law stipulates that only an RN may perform)
Patient or family refusal of care (e.g., request for DNR orders)

■ Unresolved problems with physical plant that jeopardize patient well-being (i.e., crack in floor, loose carpet section, delay in repair)
■ Unethical, illegal, or incompetent practice that is witnessed
■ Patient complaint about provider or health care worker
■ Toxic spills, fires, other environmental emergencies
■ Violent behavior on part of family or patient

---

*This list is not comprehensive but is a representative list of occurrences that should be reported.

In the case of intentional torts, the plaintiff does not have to prove that the nurse breached a special duty or was negligent. The duty is implied in law (e.g., the duty to respect a patient's right to privacy). Generally, legal remedies for intentional torts include fines and punitive damages, although some intentional torts rise to the level of a criminal act (such as battery) and may result in a jail sentence. Some states such as California also have enacted penalties that include a term of imprisonment for willful and malicious breach of confidentiality in releasing information about a patient's human immunodeficiency virus (HIV) status.

Assault and Battery

Patients who agree to treatment or nursing care do not surrender their rights to determine who touches them. Assault is causing the person to fear that he or she will be touched without consent. Battery is the unauthorized or the actual harmful or offensive touching of a person. It is important to note that a charge of battery does not require proof of harm or injury. Nurses engaged in therapeutic procedures may face charges of battery if they touch the patient without his or her consent. It is essential that the nurse ask the patient's permission to proceed before initiating any procedure, particularly those of an invasive nature. Nurses also should document that the patient has given his or her permission for the treatment or procedure. Consider the following situation:

> A woman in active labor cries out through each contraction. The nurse has a standing order from the obstetrician for administration of an intravenous narcotic should the woman request pain relief. However, the woman refuses, being determined to experience a medication-free birth. As labor progresses, the woman's cries become so loud that other laboring women and visitors in the unit express concern and anxiety. Repeated efforts to assist the woman with breathing and relaxation exercises to reduce her vocalization have failed. The nurse finally says to the patient, "Look, if you don't stop screaming and making those horrible noises, I'm going to give you the pain medication your doctor has ordered, whether you want it or not. You're frightening the other patients!" She repeats this threat several times and in the presence of the woman's family. Although the woman continues to cry out, the nurse does not give the medication. The delivery of the infant is uneventful and without problems. After discharge from the hospital, the patient retains a lawyer, claiming she was threatened with being sedated against her will. She further asserts that the nurse's repeated threats to inject her with a narcotic created an unbearable level of anxiety that interfered with her ability to cooperate with other necessary procedures during the birth. This assertion could result in a charge of negligence or intentional infliction of emotional distress.

In this case the nurse is charged with assault (i.e., threatening the patient with unauthorized touching). Had the nurse actually carried out her threat of giving the medication, the charge could be expanded to assault and battery. Consequences for the nurse charged with assault may include the following:

- Imposition of fines and punitive damages
- State board of nursing disciplinary action
- Termination by the employer

When battery occurs, the nature of the touching may raise the offense to the level of a crime. In the aforementioned scenario, assume that the nurse decides to give the narcotic against the woman's will. She engages the assistance of a scrub technician to physically restrain the woman so that she can access a vein for the injection. The technician, becoming frustrated with the woman's resistance to the procedure, says, "You're going to be sorry if you don't stop struggling." The technician purposefully hyperextends the woman's arm and says, "There, maybe if it hurts enough, you'll stop this nonsense." A loud snapping sound is heard, and tests indicate that the technician has fractured the woman's arm. The charge of battery in this case may result in more serious ramifications, including punitive damages and a term of imprisonment. Both of these cases are fact-based events known to this author. Unfortunately, similar cases are noted in the nursing and legal literature each month.

In Duncan v. Scottsdale Medical Imaging, Ltd., 2003, a court affirmed that a patient could sue a nurse for battery when she gave an injection of a narcotic, fentanyl, despite a direct, verbal refusal by the patient. The patient told the nurse that she would only accept Demerol or morphine for pain control during a diagnostic procedure. The nurse lied, telling her that the medication was indeed Demerol, but instead gave the fentanyl. The patient suffered serious complications including breathing difficulties, vocal cord dysfunction, and posttraumatic stress disorder. Such conduct by the nurse could also result in disciplinary action by the state licensing board; however, this was not addressed by the court.

Defamation of Character

A person has a right to be free from attacks on his or her reputation (defamation of character). Libel is a form of defamation caused by written work. Slander refers to an injury to one's reputation caused by the spoken word. Nurses may be subject to a charge of libel for subjective comments meant to denigrate the patient that are placed in the medical record or in other written materials read by others. For example, a patient suffering from extreme pain who requested narcotics frequently was labeled as a "whiner," a "liar," and a "drug seeker" with an "addictive" personality. These comments were noted on the medical record, on the nursing Kardex, and in nurse's notes attached to a clipboard, which was kept on a wall peg outside of the patient's room.

The patient subsequently was found to have a severe intraabdominal infection that accounted for the intense pain he experienced. The patient sued for failure of the medical staff to identify and treat the infection. In the process of discovery, the patient, his family, and the attorney he had retained read the defamatory comments about his character. It was a distinct possibility that other family members, co-workers, and the patient's employer who visited may have read these subjective comments on the clipboard. A charge of libel was leveled against the nursing staff.

Nurses also may face charges of slander when they repeat similar types of subjective comments about patients in public places such as elevators or hospital cafeterias. All patient care staff must be extremely cautious about discussing the patient or their opinions about the patient in public places. Even in report rooms or conference rooms, nurses should consider who in the immediate vicinity could inadvertently overhear the conversation. In all circumstances, only objective, professional language should be used in discussing patients.

False Imprisonment

False imprisonment is defined as the unlawful restraint or detention of another person against his or her wishes. Actual force is not necessary to support a charge of false imprisonment. An adult of sound mind (mentally competent) has a right to refuse any treatment that has previously been agreed to (Klepatsky and Mahlmeister, 1997). If he or she refuses, the person can leave the facility (i.e., hospital, rehabilitation center, long-term care facility) whenever he or she chooses. The nurse has no authority to detain the patient, even if there is a likelihood of harm or injury as a result of discontinuing therapy.

The nurse has a duty to immediately notify the provider and appropriate nursing supervisors when a competent patients intends to leave "against medical advice" but may not in any way prevent the individual from leaving the facility. Many agencies request that a patient sign an "Against Medical Advice" (AMA) form when they intend to leave in contradiction to the plan of care and despite the absence of a discharge order. The form may provide the facility with a reasonable defense against a malpractice claim if the patient's condition worsen or an injury is sustained and a malpractice claim is filed. A more detailed discussion follows later in this chapter.

Intentional Infliction of Emotional Distress

When the nurse's behavior is so outrageous that it leads to the emotional shock of a patient, the court can compensate the patient for emotional distress. A recent case in the area of maternity nursing illustrates the potential for a claim of intentional infliction of emotional distress. In Roddy v. Tanner Medical Center, 2003, a woman brought suit against the hospital after she was treated in the emergency department for a miscarriage at approximately 10 weeks gestation. While en route to the hospital Ms. Roddy felt something large extrude from her vagina and she bled heavily. She reported to the emergency department nurse that whatever she had passed was still in her underpants with a great deal of blood. Ms. Roddy indicated that the nurse told her she would take whatever she could out of her clothes, and then the nurse placed the soiled clothes in a plastic bag.

Ms. Roddy was subsequently discharged home in stable condition after a gynecologic examination confirmed that she had passed the products of conception. When she returned home and began to remove her clothes from the plastic bag in order to launder them, the intact fetus dropped to the floor. Ms. Roddy claimed intentional infliction of emotional distress. The court permitted the case to go forward, indicating that there was evidence of "reckless disregard" of the rights of the patient.

Invasion of Privacy

Another basic right is to be free from interference with one's personal life. An invasion of privacy occurs when a person's private affairs (including health history and status) is made public without consent. The nurse has a legal and ethical duty to maintain patient confidentiality, and there may be serious repercussions when the nurse breaches this duty and violates this fundamental patient right.

With the explosion in electronic information systems, issues related to patient confidentiality and invasion of privacy are now being addressed by the federal and state legislatures. Statutes, including the federal law HIPAA, have been enacted to control access to electronic health data. Nurses are given passwords to access the patient's electronic medical record. Nurses should never share passwords with colleagues because this increases the risk of unauthorized access to the patient record.

In certain circumstances the law permits divulging information contained in the patient's medical record. These situations include reporting certain communicable diseases, child abuse, and gunshot wounds to the proper authorities. If a nurse is asked to provide information to any sources, the matter should immediately be referred to the agency's administrator or risk manager. In no case should the nurse personally divulge the information or provide copies of the patient's record to another person or agency. Another fact-based case known to this author illustrates the intentional torts of invasion of privacy and intentional infliction of emotional distress. Consider the following situation:

> A nurse works in a physician's office in a small, semirural community. The majority of the town's residents know each other. A patient being treated for several opportunistic infections has an HIV test performed. The nurse also is aware that the patient has been questioned by the physician about his sexual activities and that he has divulged that he is gay and has had unprotected sex with several male partners. When the test results are reported as positive, the nurse calls several close friends (who also know the patient) and reports the finding and information about the patient's sexual conduct. Before the patient is informed about his diagnosis by the physician, the man encounters two of the people who have been told about the HIV test result. They tell him that they know he is gay and infected with the HIV virus. He then discovers that the nurse has informed them about his condition. Suffering from intense shock and emotional pain, the man unsuccessfully attempts suicide.

In this case, the nurse's actions rise to the level of willful, malicious, and intentional infliction of emotional distress. The nurse faces serious charges and, in some states with HIV confidentiality laws, could face a prison sentence for intentionally violating the patient's confidentiality in a manner meant to harm the patient. It is likely that the nurse's license also will be revoked for her actions, and the board may impose a significant fine.

The Nurse and Criminal Law

A crime is an offense against society, defined through written criminal statutes or codes. A criminal act is deemed to be conduct so offensive that the state is responsible for prosecuting the offending individual on behalf of society. Legal remedies for crimes include fines, imprisonment, and in some states, execution (death penalty). Criminal acts are classified as either minor (misdemeanors) or major (felonies) offenses. Misdemeanor offenses that nurses are commonly charged with include the following:

- Illegal practice of medicine
- Failing to report child or elder abuse
- Falsification of the patient's medical record
- Assault and battery and physical abuse of patients

Felony acts may be committed against the federal government and generally involve drug trafficking offenses and, increasingly, fraud in billing for services of Medicare patients. Other serious criminal acts include theft, rape, and murder. A nurse found guilty of a felony generally serves time in prison and usually suffers the permanent revocation of his or her nursing license. Five RNs were indicted on 21 counts, including falsification of records, alteration of forms filed with the state department of health, and tampering with physical evidence in the death of a 97-year-old nursing home patient (Kelley, 2000). The woman died after being fed through a stomach tube attached to an enema bag. The nurses used the enema bag in lieu of the appropriate feeding receptacle because the proper receptacle was not available.

THE LAW AND PATIENT RIGHTS
Advance Directives

Society now recognizes the individual's right to die with dignity rather than be kept alive indefinitely by artificial life support. As a consequence, the majority of states have enacted "right-to-die" laws. These statutes grant competent adults the right to refuse extraordinary medical treatment when there is no hope of recovery. The term *advance directive* refers to an individual's desires regarding end-of-life care. These wishes generally are made through the execution of a formal document known as the "living will." Right-to-die statutes vary from state to state; therefore nurses must become familiar with their state-specific statute. Agency policies and procedures in the nurse's employment setting also will guide the nurse in an understanding of the patient's rights in this matter.

Living Wills. A living will is a formal document, a type of advance directive, in which a competent adult makes known his or her wishes regarding care that will be provided in the final stages of a terminal illness. A living will generally contains the following:

1. Designation of the individual (proxy or surrogate) who is permitted to make decisions once the patient is incapacitated and no longer able to make decisions (often referred to as "decisionally incompetent" or "decisionally incapacitated")
2. Specific stipulations regarding what care is acceptable and which procedures or treatments are not to be implemented
3. Authorization of the patient's physician to withhold or discontinue certain life-sustaining procedures under specific conditions

Although living wills are legal in every state, they may not be legally binding. In some cases a proxy is not recognized or sanctioned by the state statute. Living wills have been overturned, particularly when disputes arise among family members or significant others when the terminally ill patient is no longer able to make decisions. A living will may be revoked under any of the following conditions:

- There is evidence that the patient was not competent when the living will was executed.
- The patient's condition is not terminal.
- A state-imposed time for enforcement of the will has expired, and a new living will must be executed.
- The patient's condition has changed substantially, and the stipulations of the will no longer apply.

A living will must be written (in some cases using a state-specific document), dated, signed, and witnessed. If asked to witness a patient's living will, the nurse should refer the matter to the agency's risk manager. It may not be lawful in a particular state for the nurse to witness this document.

Medical or Physician Directives and "Do Not Resuscitate" Orders. A more specific type of living will that the patient may execute is known as the medical or physician directive. This document lists the desire of the patient in a particular scenario, such as whether he or she would want to be resuscitated if cardiopulmonary arrest occurs. "Do Not Resuscitate" (DNR) orders would be written by the physician based on written medical directives dictated by the patient. The medical directive, if properly executed, provides the physician with immunity from claims of negligence or intentional wrong-doing in the patient's death. The physician must also follow any state-specific statute and the agency's policies and procedures before writing a DNR order.

The nurse has an absolute duty to respect the patient's wishes in the case of DNR orders. A lawfully executed DNR order must be followed. Nurses have been sued for failure to observe DNR orders (Tammelleo, 1997). Claims against the nurse include battery, negligent infliction of pain and suffering, and "wrongful life" (Anderson v. St. Francis–St. George Hospital, 1992). When questions arise regarding the appropriateness of the DNR order or if the patient or a family member wishes the DNR order rescinded, the nurse must act promptly. The nurse should document the patient's or family's comments and immediately inform the physician and nurse manager. A patient may revoke a living will, including a DNR order, at any time.

Durable Power of Attorney for Health Care. An increasing number of health care law experts recommend that persons interested in writing a living will also seek legal assistance with executing a durable power of attorney for health care. This document authorizes the patient to name the person who will make the day-to-day and final end-of-life decisions once he or she is decisionally incompetent. With the current limitations in living wills, several states have enacted a "Uniform Durable Power of Attorney Act," which sanctions a durable power of attorney for health care. Living wills always require some degree of interpretation. Naming a proxy who is intimately knowledgeable about the person's true wishes is important to ensure that the patient's wishes will be carried out when he or she is no longer able to make decisions.

Nurses may be asked questions about living wills and durable power of attorney for health care by patients and their families. An important aspect of speaking to the patient about these issues is to provide the written materials about advance directives that are required under the federal statute, the Patient Self-Determination Act.

Informed Consent

For any patient to make meaningful choices about a particular procedure or treatment, the provider must convey certain material information. Under the doctrine of informed consent, the physician or advanced practice nurse has a duty to disclose information so that the patient can make intelligent decisions. This duty is mandated by federal statute (in the case of Medicare and Medicaid patients) and state law and is grounded as well in common law. In the case of both routine and specialized care, the primary provider must disclose the following:

- Nature of the therapy or procedure
- Expected benefits and outcomes of the therapy or procedure
- Potential risks of the therapy or procedure
- Alternative therapies to the intended procedure and their risks and benefits
- Risks of not having the procedure

This duty to disclose rests with the provider and cannot be delegated to the RN. When the nurse has reason to believe that the patient has not given informed consent for a procedure, the provider should be immediately notified. In no case should the nurse proceed with initiating any part of the therapy that he or she is responsible for implementing. The patient's questions or concerns should be documented in the medical record to indicate why there has been a delay in carrying out the procedure (Klepatsky and Mahlmeister, 1997). If the nurse is responsible for witnessing the patient's signature on a consent form for the specified procedure, this process also should be deferred until the provider has had an opportunity to clarify the patient's questions.

A variety of negligence claims arise out of the informed consent process. The provider may be alleged negligent for failure to obtain informed consent. Court decisions generally have upheld the provider's duty to obtain informed consent and have dismissed cases that have claimed hospitals and its nurses were negligent for "failing to obtain informed consent." With adoption in some states of the corporate negligence doctrine, an increasing number of appellate courts have ruled that hospitals and nurses may be liable for failure to obtain informed consent (Keel v. St. Elizabeth Medical Center, 1992; Karibjanian v. Thomas Jefferson University Hospital, 1989). When language barriers present an obstacle to providing informed consent, the agency has duty to obtain appropriate translators, fluent in medical terminology, to assist in the process (Gravely, 2001).

A Texas case (City of Irving v. Pak, 1994) illustrates the duty to ensure the patient's ability to communicate in English. A registered nurse and emergency medical technician were both employed as paramedics by the City of Irving. They responded to a call from Mr. Pak who complained of stomach pain. The paramedics examined him and decided not to transport the man to the hospital. The emergency medical tech alleged that he asked Mr. Pak whether he wanted to go to the hospital, and that Mr. Pak said "No." Mr. Pak asserted that he did not understand English and could not respond to the question appropriately. Mr Pak filed a malpractice claim against the nurse and other paramedic, stating that they failed to determine his ability to communicate in English and whether or not he had a life-threatening emergency. The paramedics requested a dismissal of the lawsuit, which was denied by the courts. The paramedics appealed the lower court decision. The appellate court did not address the nature of Mr. Pak's illness or injury but affirmed that Mr. Pak did indeed have a legitimate claim against the City of Irving and the paramedics.

In all cases, the reasonable and prudent nurse would be expected to notify the provider promptly when questions arise about whether the patient has given informed consent. In no case should the nurse attempt to convey information required for informed consent. As noted, providing information about the therapy remains the responsibility of the provider. Physicians have sued nurses for attempting to give the patient information, alleging interference with the patient–physician relationship, or for giving false or misleading information to the patient.

The Right to Refuse Treatment

As noted previously, an adult of sound mind has a right to refuse any treatment that has previously been agreed to. A Connecticut Supreme Court decision affirmed the fundamental right of adults to refuse medical treatment. In the case of Stamford Hospital v. Vega (1996), a woman who hemorrhaged after the birth of her infant refused blood on the grounds that it violated her beliefs as a Jehovah's Witness. The hospital obtained an emergency court order authorizing the facility to administer blood. The woman survived and was discharged in good health. Although it was a moot point (the blood already had been given), the family appealed the initial court decision authorizing the blood transfusion. The Supreme Court decided to hear the case and reversed the lower court's decision, stating the hospital did not have a right to substitute its decision for that of the patient.

If a patient under the nurse's care refuses treatment, the nurse has a duty to notify the primary provider. The same principles pertaining to the informed consent process apply to situations when the patient refuses care. The physician or advanced practice nurse should provide the patient with information about the consequences, risks, and benefits of refusing therapy. The provider also must explore any alternative treatments that may be available to the patient. Hospitals have a right to seek a judicial review when patients refuse specific types of lifesaving treatments, but current case law falls squarely in favor of the patient's right to self-determination.

Leaving Against Medical Advice. If a patient intends to leave the facility without a written order, the nurse also must act promptly to notify the provider. When circumstances suggest that the person may suffer immediate physical harm, the nurse must clearly articulate the dangers inherent in leaving. In the case of a competent elder, prompt notification of the immediate family also would be a reasonable and prudent action. The nurse should document all these actions and any communication with the aforementioned parties.

Almost all health care facilities have a document commonly known as the "Against Medical Advice" (AMA) form. Patients are asked to sign the AMA form when they decide to refuse or discontinue ordered therapy or intend to leave the facility. The value of the document in countering a claim of negligence should the patient or family later sue will depend in great part on the quality of the nurse's charting. A common allegation made in this case is that the patient was not fully apprised of the risks inherent in leaving the facility. If the primary provider has not arrived before the patient leaves, the nurse's notes should reflect the specific advice given the patient, which should include the fact that leaving the facility could:

- Aggravate the current condition and complicate future care.
- Result in permanent physical or mental impairment or disability.
- Result in complications leading to death.

This precautionary statement is reserved for situations in which the life and limb of the patient are at risk and the appropriate providers (physicians or advanced practice nurses) are not available to address the direct and indirect consequences with the patient.

Nurses have been charged with a variety of offenses when unlawfully detaining patients, including assault, battery, and false imprisonment (Snyder, 2001). These charges generally arise when well-meaning nurses try to prevent the patient from carrying out his or her intent. Actions that lead to a claim of false imprisonment include applying restraints, refusing to give the patient his or her clothes or access to a telephone, intimidating the patient by assigning a security person to guard his or her room, and sedating the patient against his or her will. As can be expected, in addition to civil penalties, the nurse faces disciplinary action by the licensing board when charges of false imprisonment are reported to the board.

The Use of Physical Restraints

One last, but equally important, area of patient rights to be discussed is the right of a competent adult to be free of restraint. Even patients with mental illness cannot be incarcerated or restrained without due process, and the institution must have the treatment and rehabilitation services necessary to reintegrate the individual into society (*Nurse's Legal Handbook*, 2000). Restraint of any kind is a form of imprisonment; and the reasonable and prudent nurse will closely adhere to all laws, rules, and policies pertaining to the use of restraints. The goal when restraints are clinically indicated is to use the least restrictive restraint and only when all other strategies to ensure patient safety have been exhausted. Patients may never be restrained physically or chemically because there is not enough staff to properly monitor them. Nurses have a legal and ethical duty to report institutions or individuals who violate patient rights through unlawful restraint.

As noted previously, one of the most common allegations leveled against nurses is a failure to ensure patient safety. Nurses in many practice settings must balance the right of patients to unrestricted control of their bodies and movements against the need to keep vulnerable patients safe from harm. The use of seclusion, chemical restraints, and physical restraints, including vests, mittens, belts, and wrist restraints, are all governed by federal and state statutes and accrediting bodies such as the JCAHO. Many nurses do not realize that even use of bed rails and chair trays falls under the category of physical restraints; these articles may not be used indiscriminately.

Violation of restraint statutes and the administrative rules and regulations promulgated to enact these laws can result in stiff penalties. The institution can lose its Medicare contract (decertification) and its JCAHO accreditation, effectively putting it out of business. Patients and family members may initiate civil suits for unlawful restraints, resulting in monetary damages if the plaintiff succeeds in the suit. Charges of assault, battery, and/or false imprisonment may be leveled against nurses who use restraints improperly. Claims of negligence may arise from improper monitoring of the patient who has been appropriately placed in restraints in compliance with applicable laws and hospital policy.

Careful nursing documentation is essential when restraints are applied. The patient's mental and physical status must be assessed at regular and frequent intervals as prescribed by law and the agency's policies. The chart must reflect these assessments and the frequency with which restraints are removed. Neurovascular and skin assessments of limbs or other body parts covered by the restraints also must be entered in the medical record. Written physician orders for restraints must be timed and dated, and renewal of orders must be accompanied by evidence of medical evaluations and nursing reassessments.

Based on the aforementioned information, some nurses are under the misconception that current law prohibits restraining patients until a written order is obtained. Nurses may lawfully apply restraints in an emergency, when in their independent judgment, no other strategies are effective in protecting the patient from harm. The physician must be contacted promptly to discuss the patient's condition and the need to restrain and to obtain an order for temporary continuance of restraints. The nurse is guided in the decision to restrain by knowledge of the laws, the agency's policies and procedures, qualifications of the staff, and conditions on the unit or in the department. In the case Estate of Hendrickson v. Genesis Health Ventures, Inc. (2002), the jury awarded a family more than $1 million for when it decided that the nursing home staff had failed to appropriately restrain a family member who had suffered a stroke. The patient had been admitted to a nursing home following a severe stroke and was paralyzed on her right side. Despite the hemiplegia, the patient was able to slide from one side of the bed to the other and had been found trapped between the mattress and side rail on previous occasions. Subsequently, the patient was found with her head wedged between the side of the mattress and the bed side rail and was dead. The jury noted that the patient's death had been foreseeable in this case, based on the staff previously finding the patient precariously trapped between the mattress and side rail. However, the staff had taken no protective action to prevent harm.

SUMMARY

Professional nursing practice is governed by an ever-widening circle of federal and state statutes and is constantly evolving in great part because of an accumulating body of nursing case law. The law provides guidance for every aspect of practice and can assist the nurse in managing the complexities of practice in a rapidly changing health care system. Knowledge is power, and the nurse who possesses a sound understanding of the law as it pertains to professional practice is empowered. Box 8-6 provides a list of Internet resources that can be accessed to learn more about legal issues in nursing.

This chapter has reviewed the major sources and categories of law influencing nursing practice. The reader has been introduced to the doctrines of civil and criminal law that affect all nurses. The chapter has explored issues related to the legal "rights" of patients who are served by professional nurses. As patient advocates, all nurses should keep these fundamental rights uppermost in their minds as they attempt to provide safe, effective, quality care in all settings.

BOX 8–6 Helpful Websites

American Association of Legal Nurse Consultants
www.aalnc.org.

Provides information about legal nurse consultants: credentialing process, standards of practice, publications, networking opportunities, continuing education

American Society for Healthcare Risk Management
www.ashrm.org

Provides information to consumers and members about risk management and risk control in health care settings; publications; news regarding health care laws and regulations

Federal Food and Drug Administration
www.fda.gov

Provides information about adverse events related to medication administration and use of durable medical equipment

Joint Commission for Accreditation of Healthcare Organizations
www.jcaho.org

Provides information regarding health care standards, sentinel event alerts, related health care law

National Council of State Boards of Nursing
www.ncsbn.org

Provides general information regarding nursing practice, nursing practice act; position statements regarding nursing conduct, such as delegation of nursing tasks

The American Association of Nurse Attorneys
www.taana.org

Website of the association of nurse attorneys; provides information on select laws; provides guidance for nurses interested in becoming attorneys

Centers for Medicare and Medicaid Services (CMS) (formerly the Health Care Financing Administration [HCFA])
www.cms.hhs.gov

Provides information about a wide range of health care law, Medicare program; offers access to other websites in health care law

CRITICAL THINKING ACTIVITIES

1. The nurse is asked to implement a new, complex, and invasive procedure and is concerned that this may violate the state's Nursing Practice Act. What are the logical steps to take to clarify the legal scope of nursing practice in this case? In what order should the nurse proceed?

2. A new graduate nurse is working in the pediatric intensive care unit. She has been employed a total of 5 months, 3 of which were spent in orientation. Her patient, a child with a cardiac defect and pneumonia, is very unstable and has required increasing supplemental oxygen during the night. This is the most complex and unstable patient the new nurse has cared for. The physician has been called four times during the night with reports of the deterioration in the child's status. Telephone orders have been issued each time but have not resulted in the patient's improvement. The nurse has kept her charge nurse apprised of the child's changing condition and physician's orders. The charge nurse advises her, "Try to get the doctor in here a little earlier this morning and make sure he sees your patient first; she's not looking good." Twenty minutes later the child arrests and cannot be resuscitated. What are the four elements that must be proved to uphold a claim of negligence? Can the child's family assert a claim of negligence against a new graduate with very limited experience and seniority? What duty, if any, did the charge nurse have to the child? Would the physician's knowledge of the child's condition serve as a defense against a claim of nursing negligence, particularly since the new graduate had spoken to the physician four times?

3. A nurse who works the night shift in an emergency department is told to prepare a pregnant woman in labor for transport to a high-risk perinatal center. The nurse is aware that there is an "antidumping" law governing transfer of emergency department patients and is unsure whether this transport is lawful. How can the nurse quickly determine the lawfulness of this transport at 3 o'clock in the morning? What resources should the nurse access for information? How would the nurse prioritize the process of obtaining clarification?

4. A nurse in an ambulatory setting administers a prescribed antibiotic. The "five rights" of medication administration are observed. However, the patient, who has no known allergies, experiences an anaphylactic reaction. The patient is skillfully resuscitated and promptly transported to the nearest hospital. Unfortunately, he suffers permanent hypoxic brain damage and severe disability. The family sues the clinic, physician, and nurse. What evidence must the plaintiff's attorney provide to prove the nurse was negligent? Can it be done? Why or why not? Explore the concepts of negligence and malpractice in this case to validate your answer.

5. A home health care agency hires a pediatric nurse case manager for children with severe disabilities. These children require 24-hour skilled nursing care by licensed professionals. The agency bills the insurance company (or government) for skilled nursing care. One day the case manager makes an unscheduled visit to the home of a client. She finds an unlicensed home health care aide providing technologically complex care requiring nursing judgment. She is told by the aide, "They just couldn't find a nurse today, and I've had a crash course in how to manage this child just in case we didn't have a nurse." What further information would the case manager need in this situation? What must be done, and in what order of priority? What laws must the nurse defer to in this case? What is the RN's liability in the situation? The agency's? The aide's?

6. At change of shift, a nurse working days in a nursing home is told by the night nurse, "Mr. Jones is always tied in a vest restraint at night, just to make sure he doesn't get out of bed and fall, but he's really upset. He just doesn't understand it's for his own good." The nurse quickly reviews Mr. Jones' record. He is noted to be a competent, compliant adult, without a psychiatric history or evidence of mental disorientation. He takes no medications that would alter his mentation. When the nurse enters the room, Mr. Jones is weeping. He states, "I feel like a criminal being tied up. I've urinated in my bed because no one answered my call light. I'm so humiliated." What is the relationship between Mr. Jones' right to self-determination in this case versus the need to protect patients from harm? How does the law guide the nurse in this situation? Are there civil liability issues related to restraining this patient? What charges could be leveled against the nurse for applying the restraint? Could the nurse be sued for *not* restraining Mr. Jones in this case? Would staffing levels influence the legal right of nurses to restrain patients?

Additional resources are available on-line at: http://evolve.elsevier.com/Cherry/

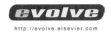

http://evolve.elsevier.com

REFERENCES

Aikins v. St. Helena Hospital, 843 F. Supp. 1329 (ND Cal, 1994).

American Association of Critical Care Nurses: *Delegation: a tool for success in the changing workplace,* Aliso Viejo, Calif, 1995, AACN.

American Medical Association: *Code of medical ethics,* Chicago, 2000-2001, AMA.

American Nurses Association: *Code of ethics for nurses,* Washington, DC, 2001, ANA.

American Nurses Association: *Protect your patient—protect your license,* Washington, DC, 1995, ANA.

American Nurses Association: *Registered professional nurses and unlicensed assistive personnel,* ed 2, Washington, DC, 1996, ANA.

American Nurses Association: *Principles for nurse staffing,* Washington, DC, 1999, ANA.

American Organization of Nurse Executives: *AONE signs onto amicus brief in support of charge nurse role* (09-26-2003)

Oakwood Health Care Inc. Petitioner: *Brief amici curieae in response to the National Labor Relations Board's July 24, 2003 notice and invitation to file briefs.* Case 7-RC-22141, September 22, 2003.

Anderson v. St. Francis–St. George Hospital, 614 N.E. 2d 841 (OH, 1992).

Aspen Health Law and Compliance Center: *HIPAA compliance handbook,* Gaithersburg, 2001, Aspen Publishers, Inc.

Booth D, Carruth A: Violations of the nursing practice act, *Nurs Manage* 29(10):35-40, 1998.

Brent N: *Nurses and the law,* ed 2, Philadelphia, 2001, WB Saunders.

Brief amici curiae American Hospital Association, American Organization of Nurse Executives, American Society for Healthcare Human Resources Administration, Michigan Health and Hospital Association in response to the National Labor Relations Board's July 24, 2003 Notice and invitation to file briefs. Filed September 22, 2003 United States of American Before the National Labor Relations Board.

Casaubon D, Sparks R: Patient dumping and EMTALA: How does it apply to you? *J Nurs Law* 7(2):35-41, 2000.

Chin v. St. Barnabas Medical Center, No. L11457-92 (NJ Super Ct Nov. 21, 1996).

City of Irving v. Pak, 885 S.W. 2d 189 (TX, 1994).

Convalescent Services, Inc. v. Schultz, 921 S.W. 2d 731 (Tex App, 1996).

Croke E: Nurses, negligence, and malpractice, *Am J Nurs* 103(9):54-64, 2003.

Danis S: The impaired nurse, Self-study module #153-C, *Nurs Spectr* 2003.

Dickerson v. Fatehi, 84 S.E. 2d 880 (VA, 1997).

Duncan v. Scottsdale Medical Imaging, Ltd, 70 P 3d 435 WL 21382470 (AZ, 2003).

Estate of Hendrickson v. Genesis Health Ventures, Inc., S.E. 2d WL1462267 (N.C. App., 2002).

Federico F: Disclosure: challenges and opportunities, *Forum* 23(2):2-3, 2003.

Federico F, Augello T: Disclosure from a risk manager's perspective: a conversation with Jeff Driver, *Forum* 23(2):10-12, 2003.

Fiesta J: Failing to act like a professional, *Nurs Manage* 25(7):15-17, 1994.

Francis v. Memorial General Hospital, 726 P 2d 852 (NM, 1986).

Garza M: The doctor as target: malpractice suit risks and how to avoid them, *OB-GYN Malpractice Prevention* 9(5):33-37, 2002

Goldsmith J: Negligent nurse or scapegoat? *Am J Nurs* 103(6):23, 2003.

Gravely S: When your patient speaks Spanish—and you don't, *RN* 65(5):65-67, 2001

Hall J: *Law and ethics for clinicians,* Amarillo, 2002, Jackhal Books.

HCA Health Services v. National Bank, 745 S.W. 2d 120 (AR, 1988).

Heinrich v. Conemaugh Valley Memorial Hospital, 648 A. 2d 53 (PA. 1994).

Holston v. Sisters of the Third Order, 650 N.E. 2d 985 (IL, 1995).

Hytha M: Nurses' strike tops long list of Kaiser woes, *San Francisco Chronicle,* July 17, 1997, pp A1 A11.

Institute of Medicine: *To err is human: building a safer health system,* Washington, DC, 2000, National Academy Press.

Institute of Medicine: *Keeping patients safe: transforming the work environment of nurses,* Washington, DC, 2004, National Academy Press.

Justin and Michelle Malovic v. Santa Monica Hospital Medical Center, Los Angeles County Superior Court, Case No SC019 167 (CA, 1995).

Karibjanian v. Thomas Jefferson University Hospital, 717 F. Supp. 1081, 1083-84 (ED Pa, 1989).

Keel v. St. Elizabeth Medical Center, 842 S.W. 2d 369 (KY, 1992).

Kelley T: Death at a nursing home leads to indictment of five, *New York Times,* November 7, 2000, p. B-1.

Kelley v. Kitahama, 675 So. 2d 1181 (La App, 1996).

Klepatsky A, Mahlmeister L: Consent and informed consent in perinatal and neonatal settings, *J Perinat Neonat Nurs* 11(1):34-51, 1997.

Kreplick J: Unlicensed hospital assistive personnel: efficiency or liability? Part II, *J Nurs Law* 3(2):7-21, 1996.

Kowalski K, Horner M: A legal nightmare: Denver nurses indicted, *MCN* 23(3):125-129, 1998.

LaDuke S: When the blaming stops: lessons in risk management, *J Nurs Law* 6(2):23-32, 1999.

Lagana K: The "right" to a caring relationship: the law and ethic of care, *J Perinat Neonat Nurs* 14(2):12-24, 2000.

Lee N: Update on EMTALA, *Am J Nurs* 9(100):57-58, 2000.

Mahlmeister L: A positive approach to managing short staffing, *Excellence Nurs Admin* 1(3):1-2, 2000a.

Mahlmeister L: The process of triage in perinatal settings: clinical and legal issues, *J Perinat Neonat Nurs* 13(4):13-30, 2000b.

Mahlmeister L: Professional accountability and legal liability for the team leader and charge nurse, *JOGNN* 28(3):300-309, 1999.

Malugani M: Nurse, interrupted, *Nurseweek* 13(18):1, 26-27: 2000.

Manning v. Twin Falls Clinic and Hospital, 830 P. 2d 1185 (ID, 1992).

Merritt v. Karcloglu, 668 So. 2d 469 (LA, 1996).

Mobile Infirmary Medical Center v. Hodgen, So. 2d, WL 2246334C (Ala, 2003).

Morrison D et al: Should nurses purchase their own professional liability insurance? *MCN* 23(3):122-123, 1998.

Moy M: *The EMTALA answer book,* 2004 edition, Gaithersburg, Md, 2003, Aspen Publishers.

National Council of State Boards of Nursing: *Delegation: concepts and decision-making process,* Chicago, 1995, NCSBN.

Negron v. Snoqualmie Valley Hospital, 936 P. 2d 55 (Wash App, 1997).

Nurse's legal handbook, ed 2, Springhouse, Pa, 2000, Springhouse Corporation.

Nursing Service Organization: Risk going toe-to-toe with a physician, *NSO Risk Advisor* 12(1):1-2, 2003

Roberts v. Galen of Virginia, Inc., 111 F. 3d 405 (6th Cir, 1997).

Rodebush v. Oklahoma Nursing Homes, Ltd., 867 P. 2d 1241 (OK, 1993).

Roddy v. Tanner Medical Center, 585 S.E. 2d 175 (GA, 2003).

Rostant D, Cady R: *Liability issues in perinatal nursing,* Philadelphia, 1999, JB Lippincott.

Rowe v. Sisters of Pallottine Missionary Society, WL 1585453 S.E. 2d (WV, 2001).

Ruelas v. Staff Builders Personnel Services, Inc., 18 P. 3d 138 (AZ App. 2001).

Shelton v. Penrose/St. Francis Healthcare, 984 P. 2d 623 (CO, 1999).

Siegel v. Long Island Jewish Medical Center, N.Y.S. 2d N.Y. Slip Op. 17790 WL 22439814 (NY, 2003).

Singleton v. AAA Home Health, Inc., WL 1693814, So. 2d (LA, 2000).

Snyder E: EMTALA: ER nurses failed to get EKG for patient with chest pains, court sees basis for lawsuit against hospital, *Legal Eagle Eye Newsletter for the Nursing Profession* 11(5):3, 2003a.

Snyder E: Digoxin overdose: $1.5 million punitive damages, *Legal Eagle Eye Newsletter for the Nursing Profession* 11(12):1, 4-5, 2003b.

Snyder E: Automatic blood pressure cuff: nurses ignored the patient, committed battery, *Legal Eagle Eye Newsletter for the Nursing Profession* 9(4):1, 2001.

Snyder E: Chain of command: court rules nurses should have gone over doctor's head, *Legal Eagle Eye Newsletter for the Nursing Profession* 8(2):1, 2000.

Stamford Hospital v. Vega, 674 A. 2d 821 (CT, 1996).

Stein T: On the defensive: more patients are naming nurses in malpractice suits, *Nurseweek* 13(11):1, 7, 2000.

Steiner, J: *2003 health law and compliance update,* New York, 2003, Aspen Publishers.

Tammelleo A: Are nurses often used as individual defendants? *Regan Report Nurs Law* 37(7):4, 1996.

Tammelleo A: Malpractice insurance: for your protection, *RN* 60(10):73, 75-77, 1997.

Tammelleo A: Nurse's failure to call for physician or supervisor, *Regan Report Nurs Law* 40(10):1, 2000.

Thompson v. Nason Hospital, 591 A. 2d 703, 707 (PA, 1991).

When and how do you tell patients about mistakes? *Healthcare Risk Manage* 19(5):54-55, 1997.

Winkelman v. Beloit Memorial Hospital, 483 N.W. 2d 211 (WI, 1992).

Utter v. United Hospital Center, Inc., 236 S.E. 2d 213 (WV, 1977).

United States General Accounting Office: *Nursing workforce: emerging nurse shortages due to multiple factors* (GAO-01-944), Washington DC, 2001.

Yorker B, Mahlmeister L: *Professional accountability and legal liability for nurses,* National Council's Learning Extension, Chicago, 2002, National Council of State Boards of Nursing, Inc. Retrieved on-line 8/22/04 (http://www.learningext.com/products/generalce/profacct/profacct.asp).

Woods J, Rozovsky F: *What do I say? Communicating intended or unanticipated outcomes in obstetrics,* San Francisco, 2003, Jossey-Bass.

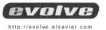
9

Ethical and Bioethical Issues in Nursing and Health Care

Carla D. Sanderson, PhD, RN

Ethical dilemmas
are the puzzles of life.

VIGNETTE

Jane Smith has accepted a position as the nurse manager in a very busy emergency department. Among Jane's many responsibilities is assigning nurses to work each shift, 24 hours a day, 7 days a week. Another responsibility is implementing the hospital's policy of offering all patients the right to an advance directive for end-of-life care. Jane must also ensure that each patient who enters the emergency department receives appropriate, high-quality care from competent, professional care providers who respect and respond to patients' individual needs and desires. With these responsibilities come challenges, sometimes so significant that the nurse manager is faced with ethical dilemmas.

Questions to consider while reading this chapter:

1. How will ethical and bioethical issues in nursing and health care affect my professional nursing practice?
2. What ethical theories and principles serve as a basis for nursing practice?
3. How can I assist patients and families who face difficult ethical decisions?

KEY TERMS

Accountability An ethical duty stating that one should be answerable legally, morally, ethically, or socially for one's activities.

Autonomy Personal freedom and right to make choices.

Additional resources are available on-line at: http://evolve.elsevier.com/Cherry/

Beneficence An ethical principle stating that one should do good and prevent or avoid doing harm.

Bioethics The study of ethical problems resulting from scientific advances.

Code of ethics Set of statements encompassing rules that apply to people in professional roles.

Deontology An ethical theory stating that moral rule is binding.

Ethics Science or study of moral values.

Nonmaleficence An ethical principle stating the duty not to inflict harm.

Utilitarianism An ethical theory stating that the best decision is one that brings about the greatest good for the most people.

Values Ideas of life, customs, and ways of behaving that society regards as desirable.

Veracity An ethical duty to tell the truth.

L E A R N I N G   O U T C O M E S

After studying this chapter, the reader will be able to:

1. Integrate basic concepts of human valuing that are essential for ethical decision making.
2. Analyze selected ethical theories and principles as a basis for ethical decision making.
3. Analyze the relationship between ethics and morality in relation to nursing practice.
4. Use an ethical decision-making framework for resolving ethical problems in health care.
5. Apply the ethical decision-making process to specific ethical issues encountered in clinical practice.

CHAPTER   O V E R V I E W

In a nursing education program, educators can only begin to introduce the nursing student to the complex and dynamic profession of nursing. Prelicensure nursing education is only an introduction to a discipline in which there are no knowledge boundaries. The abundance of nursing practice information is evident from a quick glance across the nursing textbook shelves in the college bookstore.

Most of that information addresses the "how to" aspects of nursing care. The scientific aspects of nursing care are evolving more rapidly than ever as a host of nurse researchers delve into questions about the safe, competent, and therapeutic aspects of professional nursing care. As quickly as nursing science produces new nursing knowledge, "how to" information is shared through professional journals, textbooks, and electronically through on-line Internet resources. The scientific aspects of care are evolving constantly through "how to" research.

A myriad of potential questions that surpass the "how to" body of knowledge is inherent in the profession of nursing. Everywhere in today's health care delivery system are potential questions of another nature—the "how should" questions. "How should" questions are challenging and sometimes evolve into ethical dilemmas. The "how should" questions that the emergency department nurse manager faces may sound something like this:

■ How should I determine the competency of an acutely ill 80-year-old patient who presents in the emergency department without an advance directive? Is her competency intact? How should I determine whether she is capable of giving an informed advance directive?

■ How should I act if her decision for her own end-of-life care is not consistent with what her family wants for her?

- How should I view her care? Is an emergency resuscitation effort for an 80-year-old considered ordinary and routine, or is it considered extraordinary and heroic?
- How should I respond to her if, in the course of efforts to stabilize her, she calls me in to ask me whether she is dying?
- How much of the truth is warranted?
- How should I decide when the availability of one-on-one trauma care beds becomes threatened and the decision must be made to move someone out of one bed to make room for this 80-year-old woman whose condition is rapidly deteriorating?
- Is the life of this 80-year-old woman any less significant than that of the 40-year-old father of four who has just been admitted after a tragic car accident?
- How should I make staffing assignments when the number of nurses on a given shift is insufficient to provide effective and adequate emergency department care to all?
- How should I feel when this 80-year-old patient is entered into a research study designed to test a new drug for flash pulmonary edema from congestive heart failure that has previously only been tested on a younger population?

This chapter introduces the nursing student to a different aspect of nursing care—the "how should" aspect, or as it is more appropriately called, the ethical aspect. Ethics is a system for deciding, based on principles, or what should be done. Socrates once said, "The unexamined life is not worth living." Ethics is about examining life in a way that will add a dimension to the understanding that goes beyond the scientific and moves toward a more complete and whole understanding of human existence.

NURSING ETHICS

Nursing ethics is a system of principles concerning the actions of the nurse in his or her relationships with patients, patients' family members, other health care providers, policy makers, and society as a whole. A profession is characterized by its relationship to society. Gallup polls in 2000, 2002, and 2003 indicated that the public ranks nursing as the most ethical of all professions. In 2001 the Gallup poll ranked nurses second only to firemen. Codes of ethics provide implicit standards and values for the professions. A nursing code of ethics was first introduced in the late nineteenth century and has evolved through the years as the profession itself has evolved and as changes in society and health have come about. Current dynamics such as the emerging genetic interventions associated with cloning and new threats to the effective delivery of health care as a result of significant nursing shortages bring nursing's code of ethics into the forefront. Box 9-1 illustrates the American Nurses Association (ANA) nursing code of ethics. Another nursing code of ethics is illustrated in Box 9-2.

BIOETHICS

Nursing ethics is part of a broader system known as bioethics. Bioethics is an interdisciplinary field within the health care organization that has developed only in the past three decades. Whereas ethics has been discussed since there was written language, bioethics has developed with the age of modern medicine. New questions surface as new science and technology produce new ways of knowing. Bioethics is a response to contemporary advances in health care.

BOX 9–1 *American Nurses Association Code of Ethics*

- The nurse, in all professional relationships, practices with compassion and respect for the inherent dignity, worth, and uniqueness of every individual, unrestricted by considerations of social or economic status, personal attributes, or the nature of health problems.
- The nurse's primary commitment is to the patient, whether an individual, family, group, or community.
- The nurse promotes, advocates for, and strives to protect the health, safety, and rights of the patient.
- The nurse is responsible and accountable for individual nursing practice and determines the appropriate delegation of tasks consistent with the nurse's obligation to provide optimum patient care.
- The nurse owes the same duties to self as to others, including the responsibility to preserve integrity and safety, to maintain competence, and to continue personal and professional growth.
- The nurse participates in establishing, maintaining, and improving health care environments and conditions of employment conducive to the provision of quality health care and consistent with the values of the profession through individual and collective action.
- The nurse participates in the advancement of the profession through contributions to practice, education, administration, and knowledge development.
- The nurse collaborates with other professionals and the public in promoting community, national, and international efforts to meet health needs.
- The profession of nursing, as represented by associations and their members, is responsible for articulating nursing values, for maintaining the integrity of the profession and its practice, and for shaping social policy.

Reprinted with permission from *Code for Nurses With Interpretive Statements*, 2001, American Nurses Publishing, American Nurses Foundation, American Nurses Association, Washington, DC, Available on-line (www.nursingworld.org/about/01action.htm#code).

Dilemmas for Health Professionals

Physicians, nurses, social workers, psychiatrists, clergy, philosophers, theologians, and policy makers are joining to address ethical questions, difficult questions, and right-versus-wrong questions. As they seek to deliver quality health care, these professionals debate situations that pose dilemmas. They are confronting situations for which there are no clear right or wrong answers. Because of the diverse society in which health care is practiced, there are at least two sides to almost every issue faced.

Every specialization in health care has its own set of questions. Life and death, quality of life, design of life, right to decide, informed consent, and alternative treatment issues prevail in every field of health care from maternal-child to geriatric care; from acute episodic to intensive, highly specialized care; and from hospital-based to community-based care. In every aspect of the nursing profession lie the more subtle and intricate questions of "how should" this care be delivered and "how should" one decide when choices are in conflict.

Many nursing students do not consider health care and the practice of nursing in terms of the personal and subjective side; rather they look at it only in terms of the technical and objective side. Yet there most definitely are factors that influence the way patients actually are treated, or at least the way they perceive their treatment, that go beyond the technical aspect. In many ways technology has changed the face of health care and created the troubling questions that have become central in the delivery of care.

BOX 9–2   *International Council of Nurses Code for Nurses*

- The fundamental responsibility of the nurse is fourfold: to promote health, to prevent illness, to restore health, and to alleviate suffering.
- The need for nursing is universal. Inherent in nursing is respect for life, dignity, and rights of humans. It is unrestricted by considerations of nationality, race, creed, color, age, sex, politics, or social status.
- Nurses render health services to the individual, the family, and the community and coordinate their services with those of related groups.

Nurses and People
- The nurse's primary responsibility is to those people who require nursing care.
- The nurse, in providing care, promotes an environment in which the values, customs, and spiritual beliefs of the patient are respected.
- The nurse holds in confidence personal information and uses judgment in sharing this information.

Nurses and Practice
- The nurse carries personal responsibility for nursing practice and for maintaining competence by continual learning. The nurse maintains the highest standards of nursing care possible within the reality of a specific situation.
- The nurse uses judgment in relation to individual competence when accepting and delegating responsibilities.
- The nurse, when acting in a professional capacity, should at all times maintain standards of personal conduct that reflect credit on the profession.

Nurses and Society
- The nurse shares with other citizens the responsibility for initiating and supporting action to meet the health and social needs of the public.

Nurses and Co-Workers
- The nurse sustains a cooperative relationship with co-workers in nursing and other fields.
- The nurse takes appropriate action to safeguard the patient when his or her care is endangered by a co-worker or any other person.

Nurses and the Profession
- The nurse plays a major role in determining and implementing desirable standards of nursing practice and nursing education.
- The nurse is active in developing a core of professional knowledge.
- The nurse, acting through the professional organization, participates in establishing and maintaining equitable social and economic working conditions in nursing.

From International Council of Nurses: *ICN code for nurses: ethical concepts applied to nursing,* Geneva, 1973, Imprimiéres Populaires.

Dilemmas Created by Technology

Advances in health care through technology have created new situations for health care professionals and their patients. For the very young and old and for generations in between, illnesses once leading to mortality have now become manageable and are classified as high-risk or chronic illness. Although people can now be saved, they are not being saved readily or inexpensively. Care of the acutely or chronically ill person sometimes creates hard questions for which there are no easy or apparent answers. Mortality for most will be a long, drawn-out phenomenon, laced with a lifetime of potential conflicts about what ought to be done. Even the nature of life itself and the technical manipulation of DNA is under investigation. Health care professionals who adhere to an exclusively scientific or technologic approach to care will be seen as insensitive and will fail to meet the genuine needs of the patient, needs that include assistance with these more subjective concerns.

ETHICAL DECISION MAKING

A professional nurse in the twenty-first century will be deemed competent only if he or she can provide the scientific and technologic aspects of care and has the ability to deal effectively with the ethical problems encountered in patient care. A competent nurse must be able to deal with the human dimensions of that care. The previously listed "how should" questions should be just as important as the "how to" questions surrounding day-to-day decision making in the emergency department or the care of the 80-year-old patient introduced previously. As the nurse seeks to understand the "how to" aspects of nurse management and patient care, such as how to best staff a busy emergency department at a time of nursing shortage and how to provide comfort measures for dyspnea and pharmacologic care against the threat of organ dysfunction, he or she also must seek to understand more.

Answering Difficult Questions

Care combining human dimensions with scientific and technical dimensions forces some basic questions:

- What is safe care?
- When staffing is inadequate, what care should be accepted or refused?
- What does it mean to be ill or well?
- What is the proper balance between science and technology and the good of humans?
- Where do we find balance when science will allow us to experiment with the basic origins of life?
- What happens when the proper balance is in tension?

No tension in balance is created in the effort to save the life of a dying healthy adolescent or set the broken leg of a healthy elderly adult. Science and the human good are not in conflict here. No conflict exists when there is a competent nursing staff, sufficient in number to provide quality care. However, what is the answer when modern medicine can save or prolong the life of an 8-year-old child but the child's parents refuse treatment based on religious reasons? Or what is the answer when modern medicine has life to offer a 30-year-old mother in need of a transplanted organ but the woman is without the financial means to cover the cost of the treatment? What is the answer when new discoveries allow some would-be parents to choose biologic characteristics of children not yet conceived? What is the answer when the emergency department is full of acutely ill patients and there are too few nurses expected for the next shift? At one end of the spectrum lies the obvious; at the other there is often only uncertainty. Health care professionals in everyday practice often find themselves striving somewhere between the two.

Balancing Science and Morality

If nursing care is to be competent, the right balance between science and morality must be sought and understood. Nurses must first attempt to understand not just what they are to do for their patients but who their patients are. They must examine life and its origins, as well as its worth, usefulness, and importance. Nurses must determine their own values and seek to understand the values of others.

Health care decisions are seldom made independently of other people. Decisions are made with the patient, the family, other nurses, and other health care providers. Nurses must make a deliberate effort to recognize their own values and learn to consider and respect the values of others.

The nurse has an obligation to present himself or herself to the patient as competent. The dependent patient enters into a mutual relationship with the nurse. This exchange places a patient who is vulnerable and wounded with a nurse who is educated, licensed, and knowledgeable. The patient expects nursing actions to be thorough since total caring is the defining characteristic of the patient-nurse relationship. The nurse promises to deliver holistic care to the best of his or her ability. The patient's expectations and the nurse's promises require a commitment to develop a reasoned thought process and sound judgment in all situations that take place within this important relationship. The more personal, subjective, and value-laden situations are deemed to be among the most difficult situations for which the nurse must prepare.

VALUES FORMATION AND MORAL DEVELOPMENT

A value is a personal belief about worth that acts as a standard to guide behavior; a value system is an entire framework on which actions are based. Diane Uustal, a well-known nurse ethicist, describes values as being a basis for what a person thinks about, chooses, feels for, and acts on (1992). Perhaps many nursing students come to the educational setting with an intact value system. No doubt anyone living in these times has faced many situations in which important choices had to be made. The options available to this generation are too numerous to avoid difficult choices. Values have been applied to those decisions. Yet often people do not take time to seriously contemplate their value system, the forces that shaped those values, and the life and world-view decisions that have been made based on them.

Examining Value Systems

To become a competent professional in every dimension of nursing care, nurses must examine their own system of values and commit themselves to a virtuous value system. A clear understanding of what is right and wrong is a necessary first step to a process sometimes referred to as values clarification, a process by which people attempt to examine the values they hold and how each of those values functions as part of a whole. Nurses must acknowledge their own values by considering how they would act in a particular situation.

A values clarification process (Uustal, 1992) is an important learning tool as nursing students prepare themselves to become competent professionals. The deliberate refinement of one's own personal value system leads to a clearer lens through which nurses can view ethical questions in the practice of their profession. A refined value system and world view can serve professionals as they deal with the meaning of life and its many choices. A world view provides a cohesive model for life; it encourages personal responsibility for the living of that life, and it prepares one for making ethical choices encountered throughout life. Tools to assist the reader in values clarification can be found on-line (http://evolve.elsevier.com/Cherry/).

Forming a world view and a value system is an evolving, continuous, dynamic process that moves along a continuum of development often referred to as moral development.

Just as there is an orderly sequence of physical and psychologic development, there is an orderly sequence of right and wrong conduct development. Consider an adult of strong physical prowess and strong moral character. With each biologic developmental milestone, there is a more mature, more expanded physical being; likewise, with each life experience that has right and wrong choices, there is a more mature, more virtuous person.

Learning Right and Wrong

The process of learning to distinguish right and wrong often is described in pediatric textbooks. Donna Wong describes such development in children (2003). Infants have no concept of right or wrong. Infants hold no beliefs and no convictions, although it is known that moral development begins in infancy. If the need for basic trust is met in infancy, children can begin to develop the foundation for secure moral thought. Toddlers begin to display behavior in response to the world around them. They will imitate behavior seen in others, even though they do not comprehend the meaning of the behavior that they are imitating. Furthermore, even though toddlers may not know what they are doing or why they are doing it, they incorporate the values and beliefs of those around them into their own behavioral code.

By the time children reach school age, they have learned that behavior has consequences and that good behavior is associated with rewards and bad behavior with punishment. Through their experiences and social interactions with people outside their home or immediate surroundings, school-age children begin to make choices about how they will act based on an understanding of good and bad. Their conscience is developing, and it begins to govern those choices they make (Hockenberry et al, 2003).

The adolescent questions existing moral values and his or her relevance to society. Adolescents understand duty and obligation, but they sometimes seriously question the moral codes on which society operates as they become more aware of the contradictions they see in the value systems of adults.

Adults strive to make sense of the contradictions and learn to develop their own set of morals and values as autonomous people. They begin to make choices based on an internalized set of principles that provides them with the resources they need to evaluate situations in which they find themselves (Hockenberry et al, 2003).

Understanding Moral Development Theory

Perhaps the most widely accepted theory on moral development is Lawrence Kohlberg's theory (1971). Kohlberg theorizes a cognitive developmental process that is sequential in nature with progression through levels and stages, which vary dramatically within society. At first morality is all about rules imposed by some source of authority. Moral decisions made at this level (preconventional) are simply in response to some threat of punishment. The good-bad, right-wrong labels have meaning but are defined only in reference to a self-centered reward-and-punishment system. A person who is in the preconventional level has no concept of the underlying moral code informing the decision of good-bad or right-wrong.

At some point people begin to internalize their view of themselves in response to something more meaningful and interpersonal (conventional level). A desire to be viewed as a good boy or nice girl develops when the person wants to find approval from others. He or she may want to please, help others, be dutiful, and show respect for authority. Conformity to expected social and religious mores and a sense of loyalty may emerge.

Not all people develop beyond the conventional level of moral development. A morally mature individual (postconventional level), one of the few to reach moral completeness, is an autonomous thinker who strives for a moral code beyond issues of authority and reverence. The morally mature individual's actions are based on principles of justice and respect for the dignity of all humankind and not just on principles of responsibility, duty, or self-edification (Kohlberg, 1971).

Moving Toward Moral Maturity

The rightness or wrongness of the complex and confounding health care decisions that are being made today depends on the level of moral development of those professionals entrusted with the tough decisions. Moving toward the level of moral maturity required for such decision making is, for most, a learning endeavor that requires a strong commitment to the task. Nurses must commit themselves to such learning.

The American Association of Colleges of Nursing (AACN) provides the profession with the results of a study in which the essential knowledge, skilled practice, and values necessary for nursing were delineated. From a consensus-building effort across the nation, the AACN has recommended seven values that are essential for the professional nurse. These values are described in Table 9-1.

The study and examination of these nursing values is a worthwhile endeavor for the nursing student. Students who seek to become morally mature health care providers will appraise the

Table 9-1	*Essential Nursing Values and Behaviors*	
ESSENTIAL VALUES	**ATTITUDES AND PERSONAL QUALITIES**	**PROFESSIONAL BEHAVIORS**
Altruism—concern for the welfare of others	Caring, commitment, compassion, generosity, perseverance	Gives full attention to the client when giving care; assists other personnel in providing care when they are unable to do so Expresses concern about social trends and issues that have implications for health care
Equality—having the same rights, privileges, or status	Acceptance, assertiveness, fairness, self-esteem, tolerance	Provides nursing care based on the individual's needs irrespective of personal characteristics Interacts with other providers in a nondiscriminatory manner
Esthetics—qualities of objects, events, and persons that provide satisfaction	Appreciation, creativity, imagination, sensitivity	Expresses ideas about the improvement of access to nursing and health care Adapts the environment so that it is pleasing to the client Creates a pleasant work environment for self and others Presents self in a manner that promotes a positive image of nursing
Freedom—capacity to exercise choice	Confidence, hope, independence, openness, self-direction, self-discipline	Honors individual's right to refuse treatment Supports the rights of other providers to suggest alternatives to the plan of care Encourages open discussion of controversial issues in the profession

Continued

Table 9-1	Essential Nursing Values and Behaviors—cont'd		
Human dignity—inherent worth and uniqueness of a person	Consideration, empathy, humaneness, kindness, respectfulness, trust	Safeguards the individual's right to privacy Addresses individuals as they prefer to be addressed Maintains confidentiality of clients and staff Treats others with respect, regardless of background
Justice—upholding moral and legal principles	Courage, integrity, morality, objectivity	Acts as a health care advocate Allocates resources fairly Reports incompetent, unethical, and illegal practices objectively and factually
Truth—faithfulness to fact or reality	Accountability, authenticity, honesty, inquisitiveness, rationality, reflectiveness	Documents nursing care accurately and honestly Obtains sufficient data to make sound judgments before reporting infractions of organizational policies Participates in professional efforts to protect the public from misinformation about nursing

From American Association of Colleges of Nursing: *Essentials of college and university education for professional nursing,* Washington, DC, 1986, American Association of Colleges of Nursing.

values of the nursing profession and strive to find a comfortable union of those values with their own. Furthermore, the study of ethical theory and ethical principles can provide a basis for moving forward as a morally mature professional nurse.

ETHICAL THEORY

Ethical theory is a system of principles by which a person can determine what should and should not be done. Although there are others, utilitarianism and deontology are theories that encompass modern moral thought and provide approaches for answering the question regarding what is right to do in a given ethical dilemma (Davis et al, 1997).

Utilitarianism

Utilitarianism is an approach that is rooted in the assumption that an action or practice is right if it leads to the greatest possible balance of good consequences or to the least possible balance of bad consequences. Utilitarian ethics are noted to be the strongest approach used in bioethical decision making. An attempt is made to determine which actions will lead to the greatest ratio of benefit to harm for all persons involved in the dilemma.

Deontology

Deontology is an approach that is rooted in the assumption that humans are rational and act out of principles that are consistent and objective and that compel them to do what is right. Ethics are based on a sense of a universal principle to consistently act one way. In bioethical decision making, moral rightness is the act that is determined not by the consequences it produces, but by the moral qualities intrinsic to the act itself. Deontologic theory claims that a decision is right only if it conforms to an overriding moral duty and wrong only if it violates that moral duty. All decisions must be made in such a way that the decision could become universal law. Persons are to be treated as ends in themselves and never as means to the ends of others.

ETHICAL PRINCIPLES

Perhaps the most useful tool for the morally mature professional nurse is a set of principles, standards, or truths on which to base ethical actions. Common ground must be established between the nurse and the patient and the family, between fellow nurses, between the nurse and other health care providers, and between the nurse and other members of society. A set of mutually agreed on principles makes it possible for people to come together to discuss ethical questions and move toward a sense of understanding and agreement (Husted and Husted, 1995).

The practice of ethics involves applying principles to the two ethical theories described, utilitarianism and deontology, or to other theories that are described elsewhere. Principles can permit people to take a consistent position on specific or related issues. If the principles, when applied to a particular act, make the act right or wrong in one situation, it seems reasonable to assume that the same principle, when applied to a new situation, can share similar features.

Three principles have proven to be highly relevant in bioethics: (1) autonomy, (2) beneficence, nonmaleficence, and (3) veracity. These principles are not related in such a way that they jointly form a complete moral framework. One may be relevant to a situation, whereas the others are not. Yet these principles are sufficiently comprehensive to provide an analytic framework by which moral problems can be evaluated.

Autonomy

Autonomy, the principle of respect for the person, or the principle of autonomy, is sometimes labeled as the primary moral principle. The umbrella concept says that humans have incalculable worth or moral dignity not possessed by other objects or creatures. There is unconditional intrinsic value for all persons. People are free to form their own judgments and whatever actions they choose. They are self-determining agents, entitled to determine their own destiny.

If an autonomous person's actions do not infringe on the autonomous actions of others, that person should be free to decide whatever he or she wishes. This freedom should be applied even if the decision creates risk to his or her health and even if the decision seems unwise to others. Concepts of freedom and informed consent are grounded in the principle of autonomy.

Beneficence, Nonmaleficence

In general terms, to be beneficent is to promote goodness, kindness, and charity. A different, yet related principle is nonmaleficence, a principle that implies a duty not to inflict harm. In ethical terms nonmaleficence is to abstain from injuring others and to help others further their own well-being by removing harm and eliminating threats, whereas beneficence is to provide benefits to others by promoting their good. The beneficence-nonmaleficence principle is largely a balance of risk and benefit. At times the risk for harm must be weighed against possible benefits. The risk should never be greater than the importance of the problem to be solved.

Although it may seem natural to promote good at all times, the most common bioethical conflicts result from an imbalance between the demands of beneficence and those acts and decisions within the health care delivery system that might pose threats. For instance, it is not always clearly evident what is good and what is harmful. Is the resuscitation effort of the 80-year-old woman good or harmful to her overall sense of well-being? How much beneficence is there in supporting someone toward a peaceful death? What is the balance between beneficence and nonmaleficence in an understaffed emergency department? Is it better to do as much good as you can with the limited resources you have or to refuse to assume care in an effort to avoid harm that can come from being understaffed?

Veracity

Most contemporary professionals believe that telling the truth in personal communication is a moral and ethical requirement. If there is the belief in health care that truth-telling is always right, then the principle of veracity can itself pose some interesting challenges.

In the past, truth-telling was sometimes viewed as inconvenient, distressing, or even harmful to patients and families. In fact, the first American Medical Association Code of Ethics in 1847 contained such a message:

The life of a sick person can be shortened not only by the acts, but also by the words or the manner of a physician. It is, therefore, a sacred duty to guard himself carefully in this respect, and to avoid all things that have a tendency to discourage the patient and to depress his spirits.

The belief that the truth could at times be harmful was held for many years. Only recently with the shift from a provider-driven system to a consumer-driven system has the history of silence begun to break. With this shift have come interesting questions. Is the provider-patient relationship generally understood by both parties to include the right of the provider to control the truth by withholding some or all of the relevant information until an appropriate time for disclosure? How much deception with patients is morally acceptable in the communication of a poor or terminal prognosis?

Difficult questions surface, but at the heart of the principle of veracity is trust. Health care consumers today expect accurate and precise information that is revealed in an honest and respectful manner. A few generations ago the trust factor may have been such that it was acceptable for providers to share parts of truth or to distort the truth in the name of beneficence. Today, however, for trust to develop between providers and patients there must be truthful interaction and meaningful communication. The moral conflict that results from being less than truthful to patients is too troublesome for today's practitioner. The deontologic theory of the health care provider having a duty to tell the patient the truth has taken precedence over the fear of harm that might result if the truth is revealed. The challenge today is to mesh together the need for truthful communication with the need to protect. Health care providers must lay aside fears that the truth will be harmful to patients and come to the realization that more often than not, the truth can alleviate anxiety, increase pain tolerance, facilitate recovery, and enhance cooperation with treatment. With a pledge toward human decency, health care providers must commit themselves to truth-telling in all interactions and relationships.

ETHICAL DECISION-MAKING MODEL

Theories provide a cognitive plan for considering ethical issues; principles offer guiding truths on which to base ethical decisions. Using these theories and principles, it seems appropriate to consider a system for moving beyond a specific ethical dilemma toward a morally mature and reasoned ethical action.

BOX 9-3 *Situation Assessment Procedure*

1. Identify the ethical issues and problems.
2. Identify and analyze available alternatives for action.
3. Select one alternative.
4. Justify the selection.

From Wright RA: *The practice of ethics: human values in health care,* New York, 1987, McGraw-Hill.

Many ethical decision-making models exist for the purpose of defining a process by which a nurse or another health care provider actually can move through an ethical dilemma toward an informed decision. Box 9-3 depicts one ethical decision-making model.

Situation Assessment Procedure

Identify the Ethical Issues and Problems. In the first step of assessment there is an attempt to find out the technical and scientific facts and the human dimension of the situation—the feelings, emotions, attitudes, and opinions. A nurse must make an attempt to understand what values are inherent in the situation. Finally, the nurse must deliberately state the nature of the ethical dilemma. This first step is important because the issues and problems to be addressed are often complex. Trying to understand the full picture of a situation is time consuming and requires examination from many different perspectives, but it is worth the time and effort to understand an issue fully before moving forward in the assessment procedure. Wright (1987) poses some important questions that must be addressed in this first step.

1. What is the issue here?
2. What are the hidden issues?
3. What exactly are the complexities of this situation?
4. Is anything being overlooked?

Identify and Analyze Available Alternatives for Action. In the second step a set of alternatives for action is established. The second step is an important step to follow. Because actions are based most commonly on a nurse's own personal value system, it is important to list all possible actions for a given situation, even actions that seem highly unlikely. Without deliberately listing possible alternatives, it is doubtful that the full consideration of all possible actions will take place. Wright's (1987) questions for the second step are these:

1. What are the reasonable possibilities for action, and how do the different affected parties (patient, family, physician, nurse) want to resolve the problem?
2. What ethical principles are required for each alternative?
3. What assumptions are required for each alternative, and what are their implications for future action?
4. What, if any, are the additional ethical problems that the alternatives raise?

Select One Alternative. Multiple factors come together in the third step. After identifying the issues and analyzing all possible alternatives, the skillful decision maker steps back to consider the situation again. There is an attempt to reflect on ethical theory and to mesh that thinking with the identified ethical principles for each alternative. The decision maker's own value system is applied, along with an appraisal of the profession's values for the care of others. A reasoned and purposeful decision results from the blending of each of these factors.

Justify the Selection. The rational discourse on which the decision is based must be shared in an effort to justify the decision. The decision maker must be prepared to communicate his or her thoughts through an explanation of the reasoning process used. According to Wright (1987), the justification for a resolution to an ethical issue is an argument wherein relevant and sufficient reasons for the correctness of that resolution are presented. Defending an argument is not an easy task, but it is a necessary step to communicate the reasons or premises on which the decision is based. A systematic and logical argument will show why the particular resolution chosen is the correct one. This final step is important to advance ethical thought and to express sound judgment. Wright's formula for the justification process is as follows:

1. Specify reasons for the action.
2. Clearly present the ethical basis for these reasons.
3. Understand the shortcomings of the justification.
4. Anticipate objections to the justification.

Usefulness and Application of the Situation Assessment Procedure

A procedure or model for ethical decision making is useful for individuals and groups alike. The more subtle and tenuous issues that arise in health care often are resolved within the context of the patient-provider relationship that exists between two people. Dilemmas resulting from questions about truth-telling, acknowledging uncertainty, paternalism, privacy, and fidelity are examples of issues that may be resolved between as few as two people.

Questions that are more encompassing often are addressed in group settings. Institutional ethics committees now are common within health care agencies. The purpose of the committee is to provide ethics education, aid in ethical policy development, and serve as a consultative body when resolution of an ethical dilemma cannot be reached otherwise. Although institutional ethics committees do not make legal decisions that are the province of the patient, the family, or the health care provider, a model such as the Situation Assessment Procedure can be a useful procedure to guide the thinking of a group that has been asked to provide counsel.

More and more nurses are finding themselves facing ethical dilemmas as members of hospital administration teams or policy-making bodies within professional organizations or governmental bodies. Nurses contribute a highly relevant perspective to discussions and decisions about safe and effective care in these times of change. The Situation Assessment Procedure can be applied to the decision-making process when procedures and policies are being developed to address conflicting variables.

Thus application of the Situation Assessment Procedure can occur on two levels. The procedure is applicable to the daily practice level of ethical decision making as patients and providers make choices between right and wrong actions. The procedure is equally applicable to the policy-making level where professionals come together to consider right and wrong choices that affect society as a whole. Professional organizations including the ANA have established committees such as the Ethics and Human Rights Committee, which allow nurses to meet to set policy for the practice of nursing. Inherent in the policy formation are questions that affect patient care. The Situation Assessment Procedure can be applied to difficult questions that arise in any setting in which the nurse is responsible for or contributes to ethical decision making.

BIOETHICAL DILEMMAS: LIFE, DEATH, AND DILEMMAS IN BETWEEN

Bioethical dilemmas are situations that pose a choice between perplexing alternatives in the delivery of health care because of the lack of a clear sense of right or wrong. It is imperative that every nursing student consider the potential dilemmas that might arise in a given practice setting. Concepts of life and death are central to nursing's body of knowledge, but a discussion of these concepts is incomplete unless the threats of conflict also are explored. A nursing student must not assume that conflict is rare or that it is to be dealt with primarily by other professionals on the health care team. Conflict must be addressed as the concepts of life and its origins, birth, death, and dying are addressed. However, conflict must also be addressed in the many varied situations that come up day after day in the practice of professional nursing.

Life

Entire textbooks are written to address the potential conflict that surrounds questions about the beginning of life. The most significant conflict that will be recorded in the historical accounts of the twentieth century will be the debate about when life begins. The abortion conflict became central in 1973 when the Roe v. Wade decision was made. Although the legal aspects of abortion have been resolved in courtrooms in the United States, the bioethical concerns continue to be debated 30 years later. The bioethical abortion conflict has been debated using ethical theories, ethical principles, value systems, rights issues, choice questions, and so on. Answers acceptable to society as a whole have not materialized; thus the right or wrong of abortion continues to rest with each person. Despite clear, generalizable answers to the abortion question, nurses serving in health settings for women and children must be prepared to face this morally laden issue.

Closely akin to the abortion question are newer questions about reproduction. Genetic screening, genetic engineering, stem cell therapy, and cloning are newer, highly advanced, and sophisticated techniques that bring with them the most ethically entangled questions ever encountered. Moving beyond the question about when life begins, health care providers in the twenty-first century must now address their patients' questions about the right or wrong of designing life itself through the manipulation and engineering of DNA. The entire human genome project with its rapidly developing advances has created a whole new dimension of bioethics.

Death

The second most debated conflict in health care involves the issue of death and dying. Since the development of lifesaving procedures and mechanical ventilation, questions about quality of life and the definition of death have escalated. With the advances in health care, it has become unclear what is usual care and what is heroic care. The purpose and quality of life of a person in a vegetative state continues to be debated and even legislated, as seen recently in court action in the State of Florida in 2003. Health care providers regularly contend with questions of cerebral versus biologic death in their dealings with patients and families.

The "dying with dignity" and "toward a peaceful death" concepts are examined in light of ever-evolving advances in life-prolonging care. Euthanasia and assisted suicide present the newest ethical questions surrounding the dying process. Because death is universal and part of human existence, every health care provider serving in every delivery setting must address the difficult end-of-life questions.

Dilemmas in Between

Life and death dilemmas receive the most attention in the written word through the media and in real-life drama played out in the news and on television and theater screens. However, a host of other questions comprise most ethical decision-making activities for the professional nurse in the practice of today's health care. Between questions of life and death are questions of existence, reality, individual rights, responsibility, equality, justice, and fairness. Added to these are an unlimited number of other questions that arise from the human dimension of caring.

It is in these ordinary, day-to-day situations of caring that many professionals find the most important and troublesome questions. Basic notions of individual and social justice are viewed in terms of fairness and what is deserved. A person has been treated justly when he or she has been given what is due or owed. Any denial of something to which a person has a right or entitlement is an act of injustice.

The Right to Health Care. Handling injustice has been a part of nursing since the days of Florence Nightingale, but as health care delivery has recently shifted to a managed care system, new questions of injustices have surfaced. The system has become more selective in the amount and type of treatment offered. A full range of diagnostic testing may not be available to every person seeking answers for perplexing illnesses. The particular benefit package offered through one insurance company may be more limited in scope of services than the benefit package offered through another company. Two families living side by side in a typical suburban neighborhood may be entitled to different health care services based on where they are employed. Perhaps one family has access to health care, and the other does not.

What right to health care do people have? Is each person entitled to the same health care package? Should ability to pay affect the specific level of entitlement? How ethical is the reality of gatekeeping in the managed care system? Are employers and insurance groups removing patient autonomy by choosing the least costly insurance plans (Lee and Estes, 2001)? Resolutions to such questions have been based largely on the doctrine of justice, which states that like cases should be treated alike and equals ought to be treated equally. Some have suggested that issues such as right to health care and distribution of health care are political, not bioethical, issues (Husted and Husted, 1995), but such issues grip at the core of nursing practice wherein access to health care and a respect for human dignity are paramount. Justice becomes a bioethical issue at the point that it affects whether, when, where, and how a patient will receive health care.

Allocation of Scarce Resources. The issues of organ transplantation and the allocation of scarce resources flow from the doctrine of justice. The problem of scarce medical resources is becoming more common. Which people in need of transplantation should receive organs when available organs are in shorter supply than the number of people who could benefit from them? The justice question is applicable to this situation. The utilitarians argue that the allocation decision should be framed so as to serve the greatest good for the greatest number of people affected. Should the selected recipient be the man with the largest, most loving family who does the greatest work for society? Or should a more universal law be applied? Should the people in need of organ transplantation be placed on a first-come, first-served list? Or should they be entered into a lottery? Distributive justice, or taking into consideration the needs, interests, and wishes of each patient, cannot alone answer allocation dilemmas. Who has the more meaningful life? Who has the best prognosis? Who can pay? As unjust as it may seem to some, these are the kinds of questions responsible parties must answer regarding the allocation of scarce resources. And what about the fact that nurses themselves are scarce resources? What about the challenge of the nurse's autonomous right to refuse to work in understaffed settings? Whose rights come first?

ETHICAL CHALLENGES

What about the doctrines of justice and freedom and the need for human experimentation and biomedical research? It is accepted that human experimentation is necessary for the progression of health care knowledge, but what about the risk for harm and the moral imperative that providers should, above all, do no harm? What about specifically problematic aspects of research such as the use of institutionalized or imprisoned research subjects or the practice of research on a viable fetus? Memories of harmful medical research and human experimentation such as the Nazi atrocities and the Tuskegee incident have resulted in governmental regulations involving the use of human subjects in medical research (Pence, 1998). The Nuremberg Code is a set of provisions for research that must be followed for the federal government to approve research. Institutional Review Boards are established within research institutions for the purpose of overseeing that the degree of risk to the subject is minimized, if not eliminated. Human experimentation tests the principles of autonomy and respect for personhood.

The Challenge of Veracity

Everyday issues that test the principle of veracity are the concepts of alternative treatment and acknowledging uncertainty. It is the nature of health science that new knowledge must come forth to abolish less effective dogma. However, new ignorance comes along with these new discoveries. Which treatment among two or more is best for a patient in a specific situation? Which of the new drugs should be used? Should every patient be subjected to every possible form of diagnostic evaluation? Should this patient be treated with surgery, medication, or both? And most important, should the patient be made aware of all these questions and various options for his or her care? Can patients comprehend medicine's esoteric knowledge, in general, and its accompanying certainties and uncertainties, in particular? Is disclosure of uncertainty ultimately beneficial or detrimental?

Acknowledging uncertainty is difficult for today's health care provider. As never before it seems that providers need to present themselves as confident, knowledgeable, and sensitive to their patients, who may see them as arrogant, dogmatic, and insensitive. Acknowledging uncertainty may be worth the effort. For the diagnostician, it may lighten the burden by absolving him or her of the responsibility for implicitly making decisions for which there may be conflicting answers. For the patient, knowing about the uncertainty may give him or her a greater voice in decision making and, in the event of treatment failure, may leave him or her better informed and more trustful of the caregiver. It seems that disclosure of uncertainty is ultimately beneficial to both parties. In fact, it seems that full disclosure and open communication through a commitment to veracity could prevent many everyday ethical situations. Optimum health care results from an exchange between patient and provider with open communication about the patient's wants and needs and the provider's judgment and advice. All too often time is not taken for open communication, and the exchange becomes one in which the patient listens to what the all-knowing and wise provider says about his or her needs. In this scenario, it is easy for the provider to assume a paternalistic attitude in the delivery of health care.

The Challenge of Paternalism

Paternalism is an action and an attitude wherein the provider tries to act on behalf of the patient and believes that his or her actions are justified because of a commitment to act in the best interest of the patient. Paternalism is a reflection of the "father knows best" way of thinking. The phenomenon of paternalism presumes, in the name of beneficence, to overlook the patient's right to autonomy. Thus in the process of attempting to act in the best interest of the patient, paternalism involves actions not based on the patient's choices, wishes, and desires. Paternalism interferes with a patient's right to self-determination and occurs when the provider believes that he or she can make a better decision than the patient.

Paternalism erodes the patient-provider relationship. Every provider must guard against actions and attitudes that are paternalistic. Perhaps in the past paternalism was associated with the white coat image of the physician as a sovereign god. Today paternalistic actions and attitudes can be found among nurses, pharmacists, physical therapists, occupational therapists, social workers, or anyone who assumes the image of the all-knowing in the delivery of care. The healthy patient-provider relationship is based on the open communication described previously, wherein patient choice and respect for personhood are deemed just as important as scientific knowledge and sound health care advice. The provider-patient relationship is built on trust when the right to confidentiality and privacy become ethical and legal obligations.

The Challenge of Autonomy

The provider-patient relationship makes way for the crucial legal concept of informed consent, which stipulates that the patient has the right to know and make decisions about his or her health. These decisions take the form of consent or refusal of treatment. Based on the principle of autonomy, the consent process must be voluntary and without coercion; the fully informed patient must clearly understand the choices being offered.

Informed consent dilemmas evolve from questions about whether patients are competent to make informed decisions and whether there are family members or surrogates to make those decisions by proxy. Difficult questions are posed for health care providers by the need for informed consent from minors, confused older adults, persons in emergency situations, and persons who are mentally compromised, imprisoned, inebriated, or unconscious. The burden of informed consent lies with the physician in most circumstances, although the nurse frequently is responsible for aspects of informing and obtaining consent.

In the latter part of the twentieth century another crucial concept of consent was introduced. Advances in technology and the potential to keep people alive for extended periods have brought about legislation aimed at giving people choices about end-of-life decisions while they are still healthy and well enough to make informed decisions. The opportunity for people to make advance directives is now common and is even a requirement for admission to hospitals and other health care agencies that receive federal dollars. People are not required to decide but must be given an opportunity to do so. Ideally the health care community will provide such an opportunity while the patient is well, perhaps in a community setting such as a public library or community center. Health care professionals such as nurses and other health care educators have an ethical obligation to educate the public about the use of advance directives. These opportunities can serve as excellent means of educating patients not only about advance directives but also about their rights in general, changes in health care delivery and managed care, and the role of the various health care providers. These are excellent opportunities to educate the public about the scope of practice of today's professional nurse.

The Challenge of Accountability

A host of specific ethical issues exists within the practice of nursing itself. Professional nursing is a complex profession that is unlike most others. The accountability factor in the practice of nursing is such that a keen sense of responsibility and personal integrity are necessary qualities for every practicing nurse. It is the nurse's ethical obligation to uphold the highest standards of practice and care, assume full personal and professional responsibility for every action, and commit to maintaining quality in the skill and knowledge base of the profession.

Failure to meet such obligations places the patient-nurse relationship at risk. Failure to be accountable for one's own actions places a tremendous burden on the relationship with the patient and poses ethical dilemmas for fellow nurse professionals. In health professions in which the safety and health of society is at stake, the obligation of professionals to police the practice of their colleagues is important.

There are public and legal official policing bodies such as the State Board of Nursing for matters of public record and formal conviction. However, there are countless situations in which the official policing body will never be involved, and the obligation to denounce a harmful action or potentially threatening situation falls to a fellow member of the profession. Sometimes known as "whistle blowing," the obligation to denounce is based on the fact that to remain silent is to consent to the action or threatening situation. Whether denouncing a chemical impairment, negligence, abusiveness, incompetence, or cruelty, the obligation is a moral one based at least in part on the principle of beneficence. Unless professionals of integrity blow the whistle on those whose actions are irresponsible and harmful, the wrong will continue, and the harm to others will escalate. In the end, the profession as a whole will suffer, and the well-being of society will be diminished.

S U M M A R Y

Professional nurses must be prepared to face any number of potential ethical conflicts in the day-to-day practice of their profession. They must realize that each situation is different and that recognizing this uniqueness demands that responsible parties seek a loving and humane solution to every situation that poses an ethical dilemma. When the answer remains clouded, the decision maker must choose the most appropriate action, given the situation, based on a variety of potentially applicable principles.

To think that dilemmas such as the ones described here are unlikely or far removed is to think that the surgery patient will not be troubled by pain or the trauma patient by anxiety or the cancer patient by fear. Ethical conflict is inherent in the practice of nursing and is played out in every practice setting every day. The challenge is not to escape the conflict but to meet it with expectancy and preparedness.

The profession of nursing often is described as a discipline of human caring. Those seeking a career in nursing must realize the multifaceted aspects of the profession. They also should appreciate the rich and diverse opportunities that will be afforded them. Braced with scientific knowledge and the resources for critical examination of health and illness, the professional nurse is provided access to life's most intimate and precious encounters. Perhaps more than any other health care provider, a sensitive and caring nurse is invited to join patients who are experiencing the most intense moments of their lives. Nurses are given the opportunity to embrace patients in their joy over the birth of a child or the good news of a successful surgery or chemotherapy treatment for cancer. They also are privileged to support patients and their families during the trials of waiting for the outcome of a tragic head injury or the last breath in a life devastated by terminal illness. To all of this, nurses are invited.

With such privilege comes responsibility. The purpose of this chapter has been to introduce nursing students to the idea that ethical conflict in health care abounds and to increase students' awareness of their role in resolving conflict. It is important for professional nurses to have a basic knowledge of the ethical thinking enterprise that is described in this chapter and realize that there are other resources for committed professionals to draw on in an effort to stay abreast of the issues they are likely to face in their practice. There are journals such as *The Hastings Center Report* and *Ethics in Medicine* that come from centers and institutes such as the Center for Health and Human Dignity; the Institute of Society, Ethics, and the Life Sciences; the Kennedy Institute Center for Bioethics; and the ANA Committee on Ethics and Human Rights. These groups prepare position statements and white papers on specific ethical dilemmas arising from today's health care practice. Learning centers, libraries, and websites generally provide access to these resources, although individual membership and subscriptions are available. Box 9-4 presents on-line resources available to learn more about ethics, bioethics, and the issues nurses are likely to face in their practice.

Bioethics and ethical decision making is a philosophic enterprise, a thinking activity. Many activities in nursing practice require an actual skill that involves training, practice, and technique development. For example, nursing students are introduced to the principles of intravenous line insertion while in a campus laboratory setting. They may have an opportunity to practice starting an intravenous line in a simulated setting before actually assuming the responsibility for starting one on a "real" patient. The first few times that students insert an intravenous line, their effort is based on a deliberate thinking through of each step and each principle of asepsis, circulation and blood flow, and positioning. In time, the principles of starting an intravenous line become a well-developed technique and skill activity.

BOX 9–4   *Helpful Websites*

ANA Center for Ethics and Human Rights
www.nursingworld.org/ethics/

Veterans Health Administration National Center for Ethics
www.va.gov/VHAETHICS/index.cfm

Center for Bioethics and Human Dignity
www.cbhd.org

Nursing Ethics Network
www.bc.edu/bc_org/avp/son/ethics/nen.html

The Nurse Friendly (nursing ethics and ethical issues; direct patient care)
From www.nursefriendly.com/nursing/directpatientcare/ethics.htm

The same process can be used when developing one's capacity for a critical thinking activity. This chapter has presented a vignette describing a nursing management situation laden with potential for ethical conflict within patient care. As nursing students move through their educational experience, they will be assigned to care for many patients. Every nursing management and patient care situation has the potential of presenting an ethical dilemma. As students are faced with ethical decisions, they refine their decision-making skills. Each time they reflect on ethical theories or consider ethical principles, students develop critical thinking skills. In time the professional nurse is able to refine what he or she has learned into a morally mature personal code of ethics. At that point, there is a liberating joy that comes from knowing that competence in professional nursing practice goes beyond technique and skill to include the ability to reason life's most difficult and challenging questions, and all for the benefit of another human being! Although it is not as easy as it may sound, it is well worth the effort.

Girded with truth, nurses must commit themselves to take a bold stance for what is right and against what is wrong. Nurses should feel empowered through their roles as primary patient advocates to voice their morality in the face of a new century that promises sweeping changes in health care delivery. Nurses must speak in support of patient choice and self-determination in the era of managed care. They must speak against the moral wrong of understaffed practice trends wherein patient safety is jeopardized. Nurses must monitor legislation that affects health care and study current issues such as assisted suicide and cloning. Professional nursing embodies a commitment, not just to think and act wisely in the administration of therapeutic nursing interventions, but also to think and act in accordance with specified values and basic principles of right and wrong. Nursing is making a commitment to all of the above.

CRITICAL THINKING ACTIVITIES

1. The 80-year-old patient had not issued a legal advance directive for her care before her hospitalization. Once admitted to the emergency department, she was in no condition to be counseled about the advance directive concept. Plan and implement a strategy that could have prevented this ethical dilemma.

2. During a brief stable period, the patient calls her nurse to her bedside late in the night. She asks the nurse whether the medication for her pneumonia is working. The nurse is fully aware that the aggressive antibiotic treatment not only is ineffective for the pneumonia but also is causing significant adverse effects. Discuss the nurse's ethical obligation to truth-telling versus the obligation to encourage, instill hope, and inspire a will to live.

3. Later that night, the patient expresses to her family and health care providers her desire to forego further resuscitation efforts. Her family does not agree with her decision. The health care providers believe that the patient is sufficiently competent to make her own choices. However, a second cardiac arrest occurs before legal action is taken. Discuss the issues involved when patients, their families, and health care providers disagree.

4. Late in the course of treatment, the physician is faced with a decision about whether to institute parenteral nutrition. The family asks the nurse manager about the choices involved in the decision. Describe how a nurse might respond to the family.

5. Given the entire scenario of this patient's care needs, describe the kind of professional nurse the patient deserves.

Additional resources are available on-line at: http://evolve.elsevier.com/Cherry/

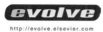

http://evolve.elsevier.com

REFERENCES

Davis AJ et al: *Ethical dilemmas and nursing practice*, ed 4, Stamford, Conn, 1997, Appleton & Lange.

The Gallup Organization: *Healthcare,* Sept 11-13, 2000a, Retrieved on-line January 26, 2001 (www.gallup.com/poll/indicators/ indhealth2.asp).

The Gallup Organization: *Honesty/ethics in the professions*, Nov 2000b. Retrieved on-line January 26, 2000 (www.gallup.com/poll/indicators/indhnsty_ethcs2. asp).

The Gallup Organization: *Dec 1, 2003.* Retrieved on-line Dec 2, 2003 (www.gallup.com/poll/releases/pr031201.asp).

Hockenberry MJ et al: *Wong's nursing care of infants and children*, ed 7, St Louis, 2003, Mosby.

Husted GL, Husted JH: *Ethical decision making in nursing*, ed 2, St Louis, 1995, Mosby.

Kohlberg L: Stages of moral development as a basis for moral development. In Beck CM, Crittenden BS,

Sullivan EV: *Moral interdisciplinary approaches,* Paramus, NJ, 1971, Newman.

Lee PA, Estes CL: *The nation's health,* ed 6, Boston, 2001, Jones and Bartlett Publishers.

Pence GE: *Classic works in medical ethics,* New York, 1998, McGraw-Hill.

Uustal D: *Values and ethics in nursing: from theory to practice,* ed 4, Greenwich, RI, 1992, Educational Resources in Nursing and Wholistic Health.

Viens DC: A history of nursing's code of ethics, *Nurs Outlook* 37:45-49, 1989.

Wright RA: *The practice of ethics: human values in health care,* New York, 1987, McGraw-Hill.

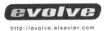

10

Health Policy and Politics: Get Involved!

Barbara Cherry, MSN, MBA, RN, and
Virginia Trotter Betts, MSN, JD, RN, FAAN

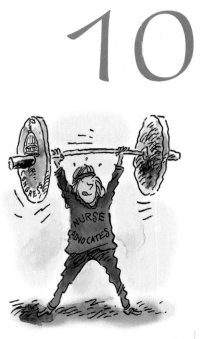

Nurses are powerful
advocates for health care.

VIGNETTE

Juan Hernandez is one of only four registered nurses (RNs) now staffing the 7 a.m. to 7 p.m. shift in a 12-bed medical intensive care unit after unlicensed assistive personnel (UAP) have replaced two RNs on this unit. Recently, a new unit policy was circulated stating, "all RNs will work overtime as necessary and determined by hospital administration." Juan was already concerned about the compromised safe delivery of patient care because of the decreased RN staff, the increase in UAP, and the increase in patient load and acuity. Although Juan feels a professional and moral obligation to ensure that adequate RN coverage is available for patient care, he also knows that the increased physical and mental strain of working over-time hours will be an additional detriment to quality care and patient safety. Juan understands that by mandating overtime, hospital administrators are failing to address the underlying issue of inadequate numbers of RNs to provide high-quality, safe patient care. Juan works with other RNs who have voiced these same concerns.

Juan realizes that, based on the Nursing Practice Act in his state, he has a professional responsibility to "implement measures to promote a safe environment for clients." He further understands that he is professionally accountable for his daily practice with each patient. Juan calls the State Nurses Association to discuss his concerns. He then discovers that other nurses around the state and across the United States are facing some of the same dilemmas. Although he has a professional responsibility to advocate for safe care for patients, issues of working hours are not currently protected under the Nursing Practice Act (NPA) or through any other state policy or regulation. Therefore Juan makes a commitment to participate

Additional resources are available on-line at: http://evolve.elsevier.com/Cherry/

211

in discussing political strategies for amending the NPA to protect himself and other RNs in refusing mandatory overtime assignments without being accused of unprofessional conduct.

Questions to consider while reading this chapter:

1. What types of local, state, and federal health policies affect Juan's nursing practice?
2. What are the major steps in health policy development that Juan must understand?
3. How can Juan apply the nursing process to develop an effective plan for policy development related to mandatory overtime assignments?
4. What types of grassroots political strategies can Juan use to ensure that policy makers hear his interests and concerns about safe patient care?

K E Y   T E R M S

Constituent A citizen who has the opportunity to vote for candidates in elections for representation at the local, state, and federal government level.

Constituent member association (CMA) The state professional organizational member of the American Nurses Association that represents all nurses at the state level (formerly known as the State Nurses Association).

Grassroots lobbying Advocacy by individual constituents in support of an organization's official position related to a policy issue.

Health policy A set course of action undertaken by governments or health care organizations to obtain a desired health outcome. Private health policy is made by health care organizations such as hospitals and managed care organizations, whereas public health policy refers to local, state, and federal legislation, regulation, and court rulings that govern the provision of health care services. Health policy as used in this chapter most often refers to public policies directly related to health care service delivery and reimbursement.

Lobbying An act of persuading or otherwise attempting to educate and convince policy makers to comply with a request, support a particular position on an issue, or follow a particular course of action.

Platform The statement of principles and policies of a political party, candidate, or elected official.

Policy maker A local, state, or congressional elected official who can propose legislation to be considered for public law.

Regulation Rules used to implement legislation and translate concepts into legal action.

Stakeholders Individuals, groups, or organizations who have a vested interest in and may be affected by policy decisions and actions being taken and who may attempt to influence those decisions and actions.

L E A R N I N G   O U T C O M E S

After studying this chapter, the reader will be able to:

1. Differentiate between policy and politics.
2. Discuss the roles of the legislative, administrative, and judicial levels of government.
3. Differentiate among federal, state, and local governments and their roles in governing and influencing health care and nursing practice.
4. Identify four policy issues of significant consequences to nurses and nursing.
5. Demonstrate knowledge needed to be a responsible and informed politically active nurse.
6. Use diverse technologic resources to obtain information about current health policy developments and political issues.

> CHAPTER > OVERVIEW

Perhaps at no other time in the history of the nursing profession has there been such an imperative for strong nursing leadership. The problems currently faced by the U.S. health care system—serious patient safety issues, a severe nursing shortage, unsatisfactory work environments, a fragmented delivery system, an aging population, the rising number of uninsured, and threats of major terrorists attacks—threaten the health and well-being of patients, families, and communities across the country. Nurses can no longer accept responsibility for the delivery of patient care without also addressing these very serious issues that jeopardize our health care system. Frequently, these critical issues can be resolved only through the policy process. Without a doubt, legislation and health policy will directly affect how health care is delivered and how the health care system responds to the very real threats it currently faces. Nurses must get involved now in the policy process and provide strong leadership to ensure the evolution to an efficient, effective health care system that promotes and protects the health and well-being of each person in our society.

This chapter explores the impact of governmental roles, structure, and action on health care policy and demonstrates how participation in the policy process can shape the U.S. health care system. Local, state, and federal legislative concerns, along with the involvement of professional nursing organizations in policy and politics, are discussed. The nurse's very important role in the policy process and involvement in political advocacy and campaigns are described. This chapter provides the reader with a basic understanding of policy development and political processes, ways to gain political savvy, and methods for getting politically involved.

NURSES' INVOLVEMENT IN HEALTH POLICY AND POLITICAL ACTION

Nurses' involvement in policy and politics has become more intense—and considerably more important—in recent years for the following reasons:

- National attention on the nursing shortage has intensified over the last few years.
- Evidence of serious patient safety issues has received national media attention and has become a major focus for policy makers.
- State and federal governments play a major role in health care and shape the evolution of the health care delivery system, the health care work force, and nursing practice.
- Nursing practice is directly affected by nurses' involvement in policy development and political action.

Decisions affecting the health care system, patient care, and the nursing profession will be made with or without the input of nurses. According to Mason, Leavitt, and Chaffee, "Patient care is indeed a political endeavor—one that is influenced by policies developed at all levels of government and by the private sector" (2002, p. 1). Thus it is absolutely essential that nurses become actively engaged in the legislative process and political action to ensure the development of health policies that are reflective of the nursing perspective.

WHAT IS HEALTH POLICY?

Health policy can be defined as a set course of action undertaken by governments or health care organizations to obtain a desired outcome. Private health policy is made by health care organizations such as hospitals and includes those policies instituted to govern employee practices and health care services provided by the organization. A hospital policy related to reporting medication errors is an example of private health policy. Public health policy refers to local, state, and federal legislation and regulations related to health care service delivery and reimbursement. The mandatory requirement for licensure to practice professional nursing is an example of public health policy. There is a close link between private and public policy in that the policies of health care organizations must conform to and are frequently implemented to comply with a public policy. Although it is vital that the RN be a leader in policy development at the health care organization in which he or she is employed, this chapter focuses on the development of public health policy and will be referred to simply as "health policy."

Health Policy at the Local, State, and Federal Level

Health policies may be developed and implemented at the local, state, or federal level and are characterized by the fact that they apply to all residents under the jurisdiction of the respective government. Local health policy applies only to those people who are residents of that local community, whereas health policy enacted at the federal level applies to all residents in the United States.

Local Health Policy. At the local level many cities or counties offer a variety of health care services to meet the needs of their residents. For example, as part of a city's health policy, free or reduced-rate immunizations may be offered to all children in the community. Allocating public funds to employee RNs in public schools is another example of local health policy. A more controversial policy is a community's requirement for tobacco-free public areas, such as restaurants and public buildings. Local health policy varies considerably across the United States, with some communities funding an extensive variety of health programs and others offering no or very limited health services. However, even the smallest communities are involved to some extent in health policy through partnerships with their state government to provide public health programs, such as safe drinking water, seat belt and child restraint laws, and emergency medical systems.

State Health Policy. Health policy at the state level has a powerful influence on the health and safety of each state's residents. In addition to its lead role in governing nursing practice through the Nurse Practice Act (NPA), each state also has health policies that may be even less visible. These policies include maintaining a safe meat supply through livestock inspections, ensuring safe food storage and preparation in restaurants, and ensuring that health care facilities provide safe, quality care through regulatory activities. Only when these activities fall short of preventing problems—as in recent cases of mad cow disease—do most states' residents realize the importance of these health policies.

State health policy also involves paying for some health care services. The Medicaid program, which pays for health care services for people at or below a specific income level and other qualified groups (as defined by federal/state agreement), is funded through a combination of state and federal funds. Many states also have a State Children's Health Insurance Program (SCHIP) that provides health insurance coverage to uninsured children who do not qualify for the Medicaid program. The SCHIP is funded though a partnership between federal and state governments. State governments are also the prime source of funding for mental health services, long-term care services for the elderly and disabled, and health care services for prisoners.

Federal Health Policy. Just as state health policies have an enormous impact on people's health and safety, the federal government plays a vitally important role in the health of Americans. The federal government's role in health care includes significant funding for health-related research; supplemental funding for education for health professionals, including nurses and physicians; and paying for individual health care services through Medicare, Medicaid, SCHIP, and the Veteran's Administration health care system.

Federal health policies have played and continue to play a monumental role in shaping nursing practice. The first federal policy to provide funding for nursing services was the Sheppard-Towner Act of 1921. This Act, which was passed by Congress despite objections from the American Medical Association (AMA), provided states with matching funds to establish prenatal and child health centers staffed by public health nurses with the goal of reducing maternal and infant mortality rates by teaching women about personal hygiene and infant care. Eventually, this highly successful program was discontinued when the AMA successfully persuaded Congress that physicians should perform these health activities (Starr, 1982).

Another example of legislation that significantly influenced nursing practice was the Hill-Burton Act, also known as the Hospital Survey and Construction Act, enacted in 1950. This Act provided federal funding for hospital construction and created a boom in the construction of hospitals across the country. As the number of hospitals increased rapidly, so did the need for nurses to staff the hospitals. Thus the nurse's role shifted from the community and public health to the acute care setting. Today federal legislation is affecting nursing practice through expanding reimbursement for advanced practice nurses and implementing policies to address the nursing shortage. Table 10-1 provides historic examples of how health policy enacted at the federal level affected nursing practice and health care. Current policy issues affecting nursing practice and health care are addressed later in this chapter.

Table 10-1	*Examples of Health Policies That Have Influenced Professional Nursing Practice*
LEGISLATION	**INFLUENCE ON PROFESSIONAL NURSING PRACTICE**
Nursing Practice Acts and registration of nurses was implemented by most states (1910).	Established scope of practice and minimal educational requirements for nurses
Sheppard-Towner Act (1921) funded prenatal and child health centers staffed by public health nurses.	First federal policy to provide funding for nursing services
Hill-Burton Act (1950), also known as the Hospital Survey and Construction Act, provided federal funding for hospital construction.	Caused a boom in hospital construction, which shifted nurses' primary employment setting from public health to hospitals
Medicare Program (1965) provided funding for health care services for the elderly and disabled.	Led to an increased number of hospitalized elderly and increased need for nurses in acute care settings
Renal Disease Program (1972) provided funding for dialysis treatments and renal transplants for patients with kidney failure.	Led to the development of a new area of nursing practice that is now a recognized specialty—nephrology nursing
Diagnostic Related Groups (DRGs) (1983) changed Medicare reimbursement to hospitals from fee-for-service to a fixed-fee method.	Forced hospitals to reduce patients' lengths-of-stay, cut costs, and reduce staff, including nurses; led to the development of new nursing roles—nursing case management and utilization review

HOW IS HEALTH POLICY DEVELOPED?

The development of health policy at the state or federal level is a complex, dynamic process that occurs in the following three ways (Mason and Leavitt, 2002):

- Enactment of legislation and the accompanying rules and regulations that carry the weight of law
- Administrative decisions made by various governmental agencies
- Judicial decisions that interpret the law

Numerous individuals and groups are involved in developing health policy, including elected officials, officials from governmental agencies, experts in the related area, citizens who may be affected by the policy, stakeholders such as corporate representatives who may be affected by the policy, and representatives from special interest groups who have a particular interest in the policy. As a special interest group, the American Nurses Association (ANA) represents nurses throughout the United States and carries a very strong voice in influencing health policy that may affect nursing practice. At the state level, the constituent member associations (CMAs) of the ANA are the policy voice of the profession.

The development of health policy involves all three branches of government: executive, legislative, and judicial. A basic knowledge of the function of the three branches of government is necessary to understand health policy development. Table 10-2 presents a very brief review of the three branches of the federal government and their roles in health policy. Although most state governments parallel the structure and functions of the federal government, there are differences among states. The nurse is encouraged to learn about the government structure of his or her state. In addition to understanding the branches of government, it is also important to understand the role of legislation and regulation in the development of health policy.

Legislation and Health Policy Development

The development of health policy refers to the steps through which an issue moves from a societal problem to an actual social program that can be evaluated. The legislative process is fundamental to the movement from a public problem to a viable program. Although there are many problems related to health care and nursing practice, most problems that will qualify for potential policy solutions are those that are brought to the attention of a policy maker who is willing to take definitive action through the legislative process.

Generally, individuals or groups approach policy makers with prepared legislative solutions to health problems, but policy makers may also learn of problems through their personal experiences and take action independently. At the federal level, only members of Congress can introduce legislation. The congressional member who introduces a specific piece of legislation becomes the sponsor of that legislation. Legislation is introduced by a member of Congress only after careful analysis of the problem, including the following:

- Public perception of the problem
- Definition of the problem
- Societal consequences and the number of people affected by the problem
- Degree of support and opposition from other members of Congress, special interest groups, corporate supporters, and the general public

Table 10-2	The Three Branches of the Federal Government		
	EXECUTIVE	**LEGISLATIVE**	**JUDICIAL**
Composition	Office of the President and 14 executive departments (State, Treasury, Defense, Agriculture, Energy, Housing and Urban Development, Justice, Commerce, Education, Health and Human Services, Interior, Labor, Transportation, and Veteran's Affairs)	Senate and Congress	U.S. Supreme Court, federal district courts, and U.S. circuit courts of appeals
Role in health policy	Recommends legislation and promotes major policy initiatives Implements laws and manages programs after they have been passed by Congress Writes regulations that interpret statutes (laws) Has the power to veto legislation passed by Congress	Possesses the sole federal power to enact legislation Able to originate and promote major policy initiatives Power to override a presidential veto	Judicial interpretations of the constitution or various laws may have a policy effect Resolve questions regarding agency regulations that may affect policy
Restrictions to power	Unable to enact a law without the approval of Congress (legislative branch)	U.S. Supreme Court may invalidate legislation as unconstitutional	Unable to recommend or promote legislative initiatives

After the problem is thoroughly analyzed and the decision is made to draft a piece of legislation, the staff members who work for the congressmen sponsoring the issue translate the idea into legal, technical, and constitutional language. Only then does the problem become a *bill* as a proposed legislative solution.

Steps in the Legislative Process

The official legislative process at the federal level begins when a bill or resolution is introduced by the sponsoring member(s) of Congress and is numbered, referred to a committee, and printed by the U.S. Government Printing Office. Following are the basic steps a bill follows in the legislative process (ANA, 2003).

Step 1: Referral to Committee. The bill is referred to a standing committee in the House or Senate according to carefully defined procedures.

Step 2: Committee Action. The bill may be referred to a subcommittee or be considered by the committee as a whole; it is examined carefully, and its chances for passage are determined. If the committee does not act on the bill, it is essentially dead.

Step 3: Subcommittee Review. Bills may be referred to a subcommittee for study and hearings; hearings provide committee members with the opportunity to obtain written or oral testimony about the bill from the executive branch, experts in the related area, and supporters and proponents of the bill.

Step 4: Mark Up. After hearings, the subcommittee may choose to "mark up" the bill, which means to make changes or amendments before recommending the bill to the full committee. The bill dies if the subcommittee votes not to refer the bill to the full committee.

Step 5: Committee Action to Report a Bill. After the full committee receives the bill from the subcommittee, the committee can conduct further hearings and study or vote on the subcommittee's recommendations. The full committee then votes on its recommendations to the House or Senate, a procedure known as "ordering a bill reported."

Step 6: Publication of a Written Report. The committee staff members prepare a written report about the bill that includes its intent, impact on existing laws and programs, position of the executive branch, and views of dissenting members of the committee.

Step 7: Scheduling Floor Action. The bill is scheduled on the calendar in either the House or the Senate, from where it originated for floor action. In the House, there are several different legislative calendars, and the Speaker and majority leader determine whether, when, and in what order bills are to be considered. There is only one legislative calendar in the Senate.

Step 8: Debate. Debate begins when the bill reaches the floor of the House or Senate; various rules govern the conditions and amount of time allowed for debate.

Step 9: Voting. After debate, the bill is passed or defeated by the members voting.

Step 10: Referral to Other Chamber. After a bill is passed by either the House or Senate, it is referred to the other chamber, where it normally follows the same process through committee and floor action; at this point the bill may be approved as received, rejected, ignored, or changed.

Step 11: Conference Committee Action. If only minor changes are made in Step 10, the bill will go back to the first chamber for concurrence. However, if the second chamber significantly alters the bill, a Conference Committee is formed to reconcile the differences between the House and Senate. The legislation will die if the conferees are unable to reach agreement. If members of the Conference Committee reach agreement, a conference report will be prepared with recommendations for changes to the bill. Both the House and Senate must approve the conference report.

Step 12: Final Actions. After the bill is approved by both the House and Senate in identical form, it is sent to the President, who may (a) approve and sign the bill into law, (b) take no action for 10 days while Congress is in session, after which time the bill automatically becomes a law, (c) veto the bill, or (d) take no action after Congress has adjourned, allowing the legislation to die.

Step 13: Overriding a Veto. If the President vetoes the bill, Congress may override the veto, which requires a two-thirds roll call vote of the members who are present in sufficient numbers for a quorum.

Although this legislative process appears to be a simple, straightforward method for creating public law, it is actually very complex and convoluted, with only a fraction of the legislation introduced actually making it through the final process to become law. In the first session of the 108th U.S. Congress (January 7, 2003, through October 31, 2003) 6413 measurers were introduced; only 103 of those actually became public law (Congressional Record, 2003). In other words, fewer than 2% of bills introduced in the first session of the 108th Congress actually became public law!

Once a bill finally becomes a law, implementation falls under the jurisdiction of one of the departments under the executive branch of government (see Table 10-2). At the federal level most health-related policies fall under the jurisdiction of the Department of Health and Human Services (DHHS) and its related agencies. The agency that will administer the law develops the regulations to implement the law. Implementation of new legislation can often be very different from what was intended when Congress passed the bill. It is important at this point that supporters of the new law take steps to ensure that the new law is implemented as intended by the policy makers, which leads us to the discussion about regulation and health policy.

HOW ARE HEALTH POLICY AND REGULATIONS CONNECTED?

The regulatory arena is an important but often overlooked area of political action that significantly affects nursing practice. An understanding of regulatory processes provides nurses with the knowledge necessary to become involved and affect the future of nursing. Regulation refers to the written set of rules issued by the government agency that has responsibility for administering the law. Because **regulations carry the force of the law**, they directly shape the implementation of health policy. Thus it is very important that the regulations reflect the intent of the law as enacted by Congress. As stated previously, supporters of any new law must be vigilant and involved in the development of regulations long after the legislation is adopted.

As regulations are being developed by the government agency, public hearings are held to allow individuals to comment on the content of the regulations. At this stage nurses can play an influential role in the final regulations by writing to the regulatory agency or speaking at public hearings. Once the proposed regulations are developed, they must be published and open to public comment for a specified length of time before being adopted. Comment is critical for the development of administrative law. Each comment received must be considered and responded to before final regulations are issued. The time interval between the interim and final rules is critical for assessing the impact of the proposed rules and requires concerted nursing action to react to the proposed rules either positively or negatively. Final published regulations carry the force of the law and will dictate how the law is actually implemented.

At the federal level the proposed, or interim, regulations are published in the *Federal Register*. The *Federal Register* (located on-line at http://fr.cos.com/) is the best source of information about proposed new rules and changes to existing rules for federal programs. It is printed every day and contains complete directions about where to send comments, as well as the deadlines for the public comment period. Most states have a parallel publication (e.g., *Texas Register*) with information about proposed rules and regulations at the state level.

A great deal of effort goes into the development of health policy, from the time a public problem is identified and a legislative solution is conceived until the health policy is actually implemented. By understanding and becoming involved in these processes, nurses can protect and influence nursing practice and create and direct change throughout the health care system.

HOW ARE HEALTH POLICY AND POLITICS CONNECTED?

Many people view politics as rather "shady" activities that occur in federal, state, and local governments to influence the outcomes of candidate elections and/or the passage of legislation. Mason and Leavitt (2002) have defined politics as "the process of influencing the allocation of scarce resources" (p. 9). Politics can also been defined as the process used to influence decisions and exert control over circumstances and events. As the reader will see, "influence" is the common denominator in any definition of politics. Political influence can come in many forms, including:

- Money
- Knowledge
- Relationships
- Information
- Talent
- Control over large groups of votes

Florence Nightingale was the consummate political nurse and understood how to use data (knowledge) to influence the British Parliament to allocate funds to reform British military hospitals and substantially improve the health and sanitary conditions for the troops.

Politics is a necessary part of the policy process when multiple interest groups such as elected officials, special interest groups, and corporate leaders are all competing to achieve their individual goals. The process becomes more interesting when you add the two-party political system and the varied agendas of the Democratic and Republican parties to the mix. Groups and individuals who have a stake in the fate of a piece of legislation (or the election of a candidate) use political strategies to obtain their desired outcome. Thus it is through effective political action that nurses can positively influence legislative and regulatory decisions and health policies that will affect nursing practice and the health of Americans. Following is a discussion of how nurses can get involved in the political process and use effective political strategies to influence health policy.

Getting Involved Through the Nursing Process

The first step for nurses to get involved in health policy development and politics is to learn to recognize nursing and health care issues that require policy action. During nursing school, students learn that the nursing process is the foundation of professional nursing practice. Once nursing students graduate, they appreciate the nursing process as the basis for making sound clinical judgments. Therefore use of the nursing process to identify broader professional and health care issues is no surprise to politically astute nurses.

As politically active nurses soon discover, effective involvement in policy development and political activities requires efforts similar to those used in the nursing process. Comparatively, the policy process and the nursing process are systematic approaches that involve the following:

1. Assessment: collection of information
2. Diagnosis: identification of the issue
3. Plan: development of an action plan
4. Implementation: implementation of the plan
5. Evaluation: evaluation of the intervention

Assessment. Collecting information and understanding the information collected are important initial steps in determining policy issues and how to handle them. As a nurse, one would not care for a patient without first knowing the patient's health problems and other factors that may affect his or her health. Once the nurse understands the health problems and other possible influencing factors, he or she has enough information to move to the next step in the process: identifying the patient's diagnosis. This same principle applies to health policy and political action. Information and material must be gathered from as many sources as possible before the health care issues amenable to policy intervention can be identified.

An excellent example of health policy assessment is provided by the Institute of Medicine's (IOM) 2001 report on the quality of long-term care. This report presents a comprehensive review of the quality of life and long-term care provided by nursing homes, home health agencies, residential care facilities, family members, and others. This report describes the current state of long-term care, identifies problem areas, and offers recommendations to federal and state policy makers, including recommendations for setting and enforcing standards of care, strengthening the caregiving workforce, addressing reimbursement issues, and expanding the knowledge base to guide caregivers in improving the quality of care (Wunderlich and Kohler, 2001).

Diagnosis. Once the information is gathered (system symptoms), it must be analyzed to identify the real issue or underlying problem that needs to be addressed. For a patient, the nursing diagnosis is determined after analysis of all objective and subjective data is completed. For an issue that may lend itself to a policy intervention, the collected information is analyzed and the parameters of the issue are determined.

A good example of diagnosing a health policy issue is related to the nursing shortage. Extensive data about the nursing shortage have been, and continue to be, collected and analyzed, thus providing policy makers and nursing advocates with the information needed to identify the underlying problem of the shortage, which is essential before policy interventions are developed.

Plan. After collecting the information and identifying the issue, the nurse is ready to develop a plan. Generally, an effective policy plan involves input from many people. The plan includes options and a determination of potential consequences for each option.

The U.S. health care system's quality and safety issues provide an excellent example of large-scale planning for a policy issue. Based on assessment and diagnosis of patient safety and the quality of care in America's hospitals, national organizations and federal agencies are working together to plan policy interventions to improve the safety and quality of health care. Key among these planning groups are the Leapfrog Group (LG), the Agency for Healthcare Research and Quality (AHRQ), and the IOM. The LG is a large, voluntary consortium of public and private health care purchasers whose goal is to recognize and reward big leaps in patient safety and consumer value. The AHRQ and the IOM have worked together to develop the congressionally mandated National Healthcare Quality Report, which will monitor the nation's progress toward improved health care safety and quality. LG, AHRQ, and IOM are making quality issues visible to policy makers and providing them with key recommendations and calls to action for policy interventions (Lang and Jennings, 2003).

Implementation. Once a policy option is selected, it must be implemented. Implementing a policy plan requires political action and a set of strategies. For example, through active membership in a state nurses' association and previous close working relationships with the state nurses' association lobbyist, a member of the Association of Operating Room Nurses learned about a regulatory issue of great importance to perioperative nurses. The issue involved the state administrative code dealing with licensure of hospitals and the use of RN circulators in the operating room. As part of a regulation review, the state department of health and social services proposed a change that would have allowed non-RNs to circulate in selected cases. Because of development and implementation of a policy plan by the nurses in that state, the state regulation continues to require assignment of an RN to circulating duties, with other personnel allowed only to assist with circulating duties (Oxhorn and Rosen, 1992).

This example raises at least two critical issues. First is the special relationship between the nursing profession and society. Nurses have a legal obligation to provide at least a "safe" standard of care to the persons they serve. Passively allowing use of non-RNs to circulate in even selected operative cases would jeopardize nurses' commitment and obligation to safeguard patients. Second is the connection between standards of practice and standards of education. RN circulators possess advanced skills, knowledge, and judgment that surpass the technical skills of non-RNs (Oxhorn and Rosen, 1992). This case is an excellent example to illustrate a nearly universal concept: what is good for nursing is good for patients and vice versa.

Evaluation. After implementing the plan, evaluation of the action must occur. The Needlestick Safety and Prevention Act, designed to protect health care workers from the approximately 800,000 needlestick injuries that occur in the U.S. annually, was signed into law in 2000. This law provides a good example of the importance of evaluation in demonstrating that (1) the law is appropriately implemented and enforced and (2) reductions in needlestick injuries and the associated savings are realized. To ensure that the law is enforced, nurses must proactively address compliance in the health care facilities in which they are employed. Following are some selected questions to use to evaluate whether your facility is in compliance with the law (Wilburn, 2001):

- Does a written exposure control program (ECP) exist?
- Does the annual review of the ECP include a review of the most recent technologic advances?
- Are frontline health care workers (nonmanagerial employees responsible for direct patient care) involved in the selection and evaluation of safety devices as required?
- Are needleless or shielded-needle IV line access products provided?
- Are purchasing decisions based on the safest and most effective options as opposed to simply the least expensive ones?
- Have health care workers received interactive training on the use of safer devices from a knowledgeable person, and have they been informed of the location of the ECP and the procedures to follow in case an exposure occurs?
- Is there a sharps injury log that is updated regularly with the details of all needlestick injuries, including device brand and type?

It is up to nurses to ensure ongoing compliance with the needlestick prevention law so that its intended outcome—preventing needlestick injuries to health care workers—is realized.

GRASSROOTS POLITICAL STRATEGIES

Grassroots political strategies are actions taken at the local level to influence policy makers. Nurses have a right to petition, lobby, or persuade policy makers to ensure that their interests and concerns are heard. Such actions (usually referred to as *lobbying*) provide those individuals and groups who are stakeholders in a particular issue an opportunity to be heard.

Lobbying also provides policy makers with information on which to base their decisions. Following are various methods through which nurses can be effective grassroots players:

- Registering to vote and voting in ALL elections
- Joining professional nursing organizations
- Working in political candidates' campaigns
- Attending "meet the candidates" town hall meetings
- Visiting with policy makers or their staff members
- Writing letters
- Sending e-mail or fax messages
- Telephoning
- Testifying at hearings

Registering to Vote and Voting in All Elections

Voting is a must for every nurse! However, voting is not enough. Informed voting is necessary to enhance nurses' political power to ultimately improve the health of patients and the nursing care that they receive. Nurses should become informed about the issues. Becoming informed involves reading legislative newsletters and finding out about policy makers' backgrounds, voting records, and current platforms. Discussing these issues with nurse colleagues and others in the community serves to enhance everyone's understanding of candidates and their positions.

Joining a Professional Nursing Organization

Another must for the professional nurse is to join a professional nursing organization. The value of the ANA, state nurses associations, and specialty nursing organizations is that together the nursing profession is much more powerful than each individual RN. As professionals in a collective, nurses know more, have more resources, and are able to pool their strengths and direct resources toward winning the health policy "game."

The ANA is the foremost recognized professional nursing organization in Washington, D.C., for federal health and public policy. This organization speaks for professional nurses, regardless of specialty. All nurses should consider ANA membership as one of their basic professional responsibilities. Nurses who choose to maintain membership in the specialty organization that represents their area of nursing practice have the additional advantage of receiving both clinical and health policy information related to that specialty.

Because professional nursing organizations monitor public policy and offer avenues for their members to learn about health policy, they serve as an invaluable resource for reliable information related to policy issues and policy makers. Generally, the information needed to make informed voting decisions does not come neatly packaged with the issues clearly identified. Obtaining this information and deciphering it requires skills that many nurses do not readily possess. Joining a professional nursing organization that has a political action committee (PAC) can help develop the necessary skills to understand political issues. A PAC is an arm of a corporation, association, or labor union formed to provide support either to persuade a policy maker to support a certain policy or program or, more often, to ensure that a policy maker who supports the organization's goals attains office or remains in office.

Professional nursing organizations may choose to endorse a specific candidate for office. Endorsement simply means that, in a particular political race, the nursing organization selects one candidate to support because of that candidate's platform or record supporting specific issues or goals. Although endorsement does not mean that everyone in the organization must vote for the selected person, it does mean that the organization has carefully screened the candidate and the nurse can be reasonably sure that the candidate will support nursing's interests.

Working in Political Candidates' Campaigns

Most political candidates are not health professionals and do not fully understand health-related issues. By becoming involved in political campaigns, nurses can (and should) educate and inform the candidates about health care issues. Other activities that the nurse may undertake on behalf of the candidates include assisting in writing health care position statements, working in campaign offices, attending local debates, displaying the candidates' political buttons and signs, and participating in fundraising events. Nurse supporters may also write letters to and/or call other nurses in the region to tell them about their support of the candidate and to ask for their vote. Having "nurse friendly" candidates win and become "nurse friendly" elected officials is critical to achieving nursing's policy agenda.

Participating in "Meet the Candidates" Town Hall Meetings

A strategy that nursing associations can use to determine which candidate(s) to endorse is to invite all candidates running for a particular office to a town hall meeting to discuss their platforms with nurses. Town hall gatherings with nurses allow the candidates to talk about their platform to a group of interested voters in a time-saving and cost-efficient manner. A town hall meeting affords nurses an opportunity to understand the candidate's platform and to voice their own opinions and concerns about health care issues.

Hosting a "Meet the Candidates" town hall meeting can be an exciting activity for student nurses and faculty. Nursing students at a hosting school should prepare for the town hall meeting as follows (TNA, 1995):

1. Before the town hall meeting, become familiar with each candidate's background, including his or her voting record on health policy issues, major contributors, personal occupations, family information, and hobbies. This information can provide insight into the candidate's positions on issues.
2. Identify current issues that would be relevant for discussion with the candidates. Collect and review information related to the issues and then prioritize the issues. Time may not be sufficient to discuss all of the issues of interest.
3. Prepare to give concise examples of how the issue affects the individual, community, health care consumers in the district, and other members of the nursing profession. Be prepared to debate arguments that unfavorably reflect one's position.
4. Plan the agenda for the meeting to allow ample time for discussion.
5. After introductions are made, listen carefully as each candidate presents his or her campaign platform; then be prepared to clearly and concisely discuss the issues with relevant examples as detailed in preceding paragraphs. Box 10-1 provides the correct titles to use when addressing state elected officials.
6. At the conclusion of the meeting, provide the candidate with contact information (names, addresses, telephone numbers, and e-mail addresses) for key members of your group.

Visiting With Policy Makers and Their Staff Members

Personal visits to policy makers and/or their staff members can be one of the most effective methods of lobbying for or against a health care policy. Nothing is more effective in communicating nursing's position than face-to-face contact between a policy maker and

BOX 10–1	*Speaking with the Governor, Lieutenant Governor, Legislators, or Staff*

Governor: Governor (last name)
Lieutenant Governor: Governor (last name)
Speaker of the House: Mr. Speaker or Madam Speaker
Senator: Senator (last name)
Representative: Representative (last name) or Mr. or Ms. (last name)
Staff: Mr. or Ms. (last name)

his or her staff and a group of well-informed nurses. Face-to-face meetings provide a great opportunity for nurses to educate policy makers about health care issues. Policy makers are very interested in information that will increase their knowledge about health care and help them plan for future health care policy.

Just as in the planning for a town hall meeting with candidates, similar preparation is necessary for personal visits with policy makers (TNA, 2004):

1. *Plan your visit.* Be clear about what you want to achieve and determine in advance which policy maker or staff member you want to meet. Remember, most elected officials have legislative staff members who are assigned to specific issues and can be very influential in supporting your cause and promoting it to the policy maker.

2. *Make an appointment.* Contact the policy maker's appointment secretary or scheduler to make an appointment. Be prepared to explain your purpose for the meeting and who you represent.

3. *Prepare for the meeting (perhaps the most important step!).* Become familiar with the policy maker's background, district represented, voting record on nursing issues, and personal occupation. Identify, collect, and review information about issues of critical importance. Policy makers are required to take positions on many different issues, but in some cases, they may lack important details about the pros and cons of a particular issue. Be ready to share examples and specific situations that clearly demonstrate the impact or benefits of an issue or piece of legislation.

4. *Be prompt and patient.* Policy makers' schedules often are unpredictable; if interruptions occur, be flexible. If the opportunity presents itself, meet with the legislative staff member.

5. *Be political.* Whenever possible, discuss the connection between your request or position on an issue and the constituency the policy maker represents. Tell the policy maker how you or your group can be of assistance to him or her within that constituency. When appropriate, ask for a commitment from the policy maker.

6. *Be responsive.* Be prepared to answer questions and provide additional information if requested by the policy maker. At the conclusion of the meeting, leave your name with an address and telephone number. Follow up the meeting with a "thank you" letter that outlines the points covered in the meeting and send along any additional information requested.

Writing Letters

Writing letters to policy makers can be effective if properly planned and implemented. The timing of a letter is important. It should be written early, before policy makers commit to vote a certain way. It is easier to convince an undecided policy maker than it is to get him or her to switch positions. A second very effective step is to send a follow-up letter immediately before the vote on the bill is scheduled. Information about voting schedules can be obtained online in most states. Guidelines for writing to policy makers include the following:

1. Type an individualized letter. Mass-produced form letters are easy to detect, may weaken your position, and should be avoided.
2. The purpose of the letter should be stated in the first paragraph. If the letter relates to a specific piece of legislation, identify it according to the assigned bill number.
3. Be courteous and concise, including key information and examples to support your position.
4. Use a proper salutation and closing (see Box 10-2).
5. The letter should be one page or less and should address only one issue.
6. Include a direct question to the policy maker. Request a written answer.
7. Thank the policy maker for his or her consideration of the issue.

BOX 10–2   *Writing a Letter to the Governor, Lieutenant Governor, Members of Congress, State Legislators, or Staff*

Governor: The Honorable (full name)
Governor of Alabama
State Capitol
Montgomery, AL 36106

Lieutenant Governor: The Honorable (full name)
Lt. Governor of Tennessee
State Capitol
Nashville, TN 37243

State Senator: The Honorable (full name) or Dear Senator (last name)
State Senate
P.O. Box _____
Capital City, State, Zip Code

State Representative: The Honorable (full name) or Dear Representative (last name)
State House of Representatives
P.O. Box _____
Capital City, State, Zip Code

U.S. Senator: The Honorable (full name) or Dear Senator (last name)
United States Senate
Washington, DC 20510

U.S. Representative: The Honorable (full name) or Dear Representative (last name)
U.S. House of Representatives
Washington, DC 20510

Staff: Mr. (full name) or Ms. (full name)
_____'s Office

Appropriate closing for letters to all of the above is "Sincerely yours," followed by your full name.

Sample letters to policy makers are available on this textbook's website (http://evolve.else-vier.com/Cherry/). Rosters of state legislators can be found on-line in most states. The roster contains contact information for each policy maker and usually includes information about his or her committee memberships. Contact information for members of the U.S. House of Representatives is available on-line (http://www.house.gov/). This site includes committee memberships, as well as links to individual Representatives' websites. Similar information for U.S. Senators is also available on-line (http://www.senate.gov/).

Sending E-Mail or Fax Messages

E-mail messages are quick and easy and may be helpful when speed is crucial. It is important to remember that conciseness is preferable when writing e-mail messages. The subject of the message should contain the number of the bill to which you are referring in the message. For example, "In opposition to Senate Bill 123" immediately focuses the reader. The message itself should be just a few short lines to relay a clear and strong message related to the issue. Brief examples of how the issue affects the policy maker's constituents are often very effective. Sending a facsimile (fax) may also be effective when time is of the essence. The message should be typed and should include the same information as a letter to the policy maker.

Telephoning

Telephoning is most useful when time is limited. It is an easy way to give the policy maker a sense of what his or her constituents believe about a certain bill. However, it is not an effective method for educating a policy maker or the legislative staff about an issue. The following list provides guidelines to use when telephoning a policy maker (TNA, 2004).

1. Telephone calls are usually taken by a staff member; ask to speak to the staff person assigned to the bill or issue for which the call is being made.
2. If the person is not available, leave a message.
3. After introducing yourself, give a brief and simple message such as "please tell Senator/ Representative (name) that I support (bill number).
4. You may briefly state your reasons for supporting or opposing the bill and ask for the policy maker's position on the bill.
5. Leave your name, telephone number, and address; if appropriate, ask for a written response to your telephone call (Box 10-3 is a sample telephone call).
6. If time permits, follow up the telephone conversation with a letter.

Testifying at Hearings

There is some debate concerning the effectiveness of testifying at hearings. Some believe (TNA, 1995), at least at the state level, that committee members frequently, but not always, decide how they will vote before a hearing begins. Others believe that testifying at a public congressional hearing is an effective method of lobbying. However, both sides of the debate agree that if someone plans to testify, preparation is extremely important. Usually persons submit a request to testify before the hearing occurs. The following guidelines are for testifying at state-level hearings (TNA, 1995):

1. Prepare a written statement and have enough copies for all committee members, along with one copy for the committee clerk.
2. Clearly document the facts in a brief, concise manner.
3. Organize testimony around key points.

BOX 10–3 *Sample Telephone Call to a Policy Maker*

"Hello, Senator (name's) office. How may I help you?"

"Hello, my name is (your name), and I am a registered nurse in (city, state). May I please speak with the person who handles health care issues? (Identify yourself again if you are transferred to the health specialist.)

I am calling because I want to let Senator (name) know that I am very concerned about (describe the issue, such as 'the vote on Senate Bill 123' or 'how the Violence in the Workplace Bill will affect my role in health care'). It is critical that the Senator (support or oppose issue, name, or bill description) because (give one to three brief reasons). More than 1 of every 100 adults in this country is a nurse, and 1 of every 44 registered female voters is a nurse. We, as nurses and voters, believe this issue to be very important."

"I appreciate your call today. I will make sure that the Senator gets your message. May I have your mailing address so that the Senator can contact you personally?"

"Yes, this is (name and address). Please make sure that the Senator knows that I (support or oppose issue, name, or bill description). Thank you for your time."

Substitute "Representative" for "Senator" when calling a member of the House of Representatives (Texas Nurses Association, 1995).

4. If testifying before a committee that includes the policy maker who represents your district, notify that policy maker.
5. Become familiar with the members of the committee and their home districts or constituencies.
6. Anticipate questions that may be asked. Prepare knowledgeable responses.

THE AMERICAN NURSES ASSOCIATION

The ANA is the professional nursing organization representing the nation's entire registered nurse population—approximately 2.7 million RNs. The ANA is composed of 54 CMAs, which represent state and U.S territory nursing associations, and 13 organizational affiliates (ANA, 2004a). ANA's organizational affiliates include the American Nurses Credentialing Center, the American Nurses Foundation, the American Academy of Nursing, and specialty organizations such as the American Association of Critical Care Nursing. A full list of ANA affiliated organizations and links to their websites can be found on the ANA website (www.nursingworld.org).

The two most recently established ANA organizational affiliates are the United American Nurses (UAN) and the Center for American Nurses *(CAN)*. Beginning in 2000, ANA began an organizational restructuring to better represent the needs of nurses in both right-to-work states and collective bargaining states, resulting in the creation of the UAN and *CAN*. The UAN is the labor union for nurses representing 100,000 RNs nationwide and is a full-fledged affiliate of both the ANA and the AFL-CIO (American Federation of Labor–Congress of Industrial Organizations) (ANA, 2004a). The *CAN*, established by the ANA House of Delegates to address the needs of individual nurses who are *not* represented by unions, offers noncollective bargaining workplace advocacy strategies, programs, and services to nurses *(CAN*, 2004).

Through its CMAs and organizational affiliates, ANA is the strongest voice in the nation advocating for the nursing profession and the health care consumer. The ANA "advances the nursing profession by fostering high standards of nursing practice, promoting the economic and general welfare of nurses in the workplace, projecting a positive and realistic view of nursing, and lobbying the Congress and the federal regulatory agencies on health care issues affecting nurses and the public" (ANA, 2004a). The ANA is at the forefront of policy initiatives pertaining to health care reform. Its priority issues are as follows (ANA, 2004a):

■ A restructured health care system that delivers primary health care in community-based settings

■ An expanded role for RNs and advanced practice nurses in the delivery of basic and primary health care

■ Obtaining federal funding for nurse education and training

■ Helping to change and improve the health care workplace to enhance the health and safety of the patient and the nurse

Through political and legislative activities, ANA has taken firm positions on various issues, including Medicare reform, patients' rights, the importance of safer needle devices, whistle-blower protection for health care workers, adequate reimbursement for health care services, and access to health care.

Nurses Strategic Action Team (N-STAT)

Nurses are impressive in their collective abilities to mobilize and take effective action in shaping national health care policy through the Nurses Strategic Action Team (N-STAT). N-STAT is an ANA program that unifies nurses' political voices across the country to enact measures to benefit health care for everyone and to defeat measures that would have serious negative impacts on the health care delivery system. N-STAT is composed of thousands of nurses around the country who stay informed on issues and contact their legislators about pending issues. Through Legislative Updates, N-STAT keeps members up to date on key bills as they move through the legislative process. Through Action Alerts, members are informed about when e-mails, phone calls, and letters will make the most impact (ANA, 2004b).

N-STAT empowers nurses by encouraging them to take action and make their opinions heard and understood by Congress and the public. N-STAT provides the structure and coordination for nurses across the country to be involved in grassroots lobbying. For example, N-STAT sends notices to nurses regarding impending legislation that affects health care. Enclosed with the notices are senators' names, addresses, and phone numbers to facilitate nurses' actions in making their opinions known to the policy makers. Therefore N-STAT makes the political process less intimidating by keeping nurses informed of political issues and providing strategies for making their opinions known.

CURRENT HEALTH POLICY ISSUES

Policy issues come and go as society, health care, and public needs and wants ebb and flow. However, a few topics will bear watching over the next decade, since it is unlikely that any of these will achieve a "perfect" solution. The importance of these topics will keep them on the policy agenda for many years to come.

Access to Care

In 2002, 43.6 million Americans—just over 15% of the population—were without health insurance coverage for a full year (U.S. Census Bureau, 2003). Lack of health insurance is the greatest barrier to accessing health care and has a tremendous impact on an individual's health.

Studies have consistently found that the uninsured receive inadequate health care. Consider these findings (Kaiser Commission on Medicaid and the Uninsured, 2001):

- 25% of uninsured children and 40% of uninsured adults have no regular source of health care.
- Uninsured individuals are more likely to delay or ignore needed treatment, resulting in conditions being diagnosed at a later stage.
- Uninsured individuals are more likely to be hospitalized for avoidable conditions.

The lack of health insurance has serious financial consequences as well. Approximately 50% of bankruptcies in the U.S. are related to medical causes or medical debt (Himmelstein and Weissman, 2001).

A variety of measures have been either proposed or enacted to deal incrementally with health care access since the failure of Congress to pass the Health Security Act of 1993, which would have provided universal coverage for health services. A successful access policy has been the State Children's Health Insurance Program (SCHIP), which has insured more than 5.3 million children since its passage in 1997 (Centers for Medicare and Medicaid Services, 2003). Other access proposals currently under debate include:

- Tax credits for private insurance coverage
- Expansion of Medicare to individuals between 55 and 65 years of age who lose group coverage
- Offering family coverage for parents and siblings of SCHIP enrollees

In another approach to improve health care access, the AMA (2004) is calling for transition from an employer-based health insurance system to an individually owned health insurance system. AMA advocates that this transition be accomplished though a change in the federal tax code. At the same time, in a recent statement, the Institute of Medicine has called for reexamining a national health insurance plan to achieve universal access for all Americans. Nurses must keep up to date on legislative actions related to health insurance and health care access—the upcoming policy debates will certainly be interesting!

Prescription Drug Coverage for Medicare Beneficiaries

Medicare became the health insurance mechanism for America's seniors and the disabled in the 1960s. Although Medicare provided coverage for hospitalizations and physician fees, there was no benefit for prescription drugs. The absence of a prescription drug benefit in the package of Medicare services has become a significant problem for the elderly. Over these past decades science has developed a vast array of pharmacologic interventions for most illnesses; the problem is that many older adults—the very patients many of these drugs would help most—are unable to afford them. In an effort to receive these treatments of choice, many seniors report being forced to choose between buying food or buying expensive prescription medications. Thus, advocates for the elderly and the disabled have pressed hard for many years to include a prescription drug benefit in Medicare. In December 2003, President George Bush signed into law a landmark bill passed by the 108th Congress adding a prescription drug benefit for Medicare enrollees. The prescription drug benefit is scheduled to be implemented in 2006 and will be available through private insurers and health plans under contract to Medicare.

This new plan is detailed in a 680-page legislative bill, which experts continue to analyze concerning its likely consequences. Such findings remain quite controversial. Opponents of the legislation are declaring that the new policy fails to provide sufficient coverage; supporters declare that it was the best compromise possible in 2003. Despite the continuing debate over this policy, it does represent the first major change to the Medicare benefit plan since its inception in the 1960s. The most important thing for nursing students to recognize, though, is the fact that the issue is not yet settled. Policy makers began developing legislative initiatives to amend the new law less than 3 months after it passed! In order to help support and improve the health and well-being of our nation's seniors, nurses must stay involved in legislation affecting Medicare.

Health Care Workforce and the Nursing Shortage

The American population is aging at a very rapid rate, and this demographic shift will demand greatly increased needs for health services over the next three decades. At the same time, the U.S. economy has exploded with new fields for study, work, and careers. Thus the numbers of individuals selecting health careers has decreased just as the need for these health services is increasing. No health profession has been hit as hard as professional nursing—a group that is aging faster than the population in general and whose retirees are outpacing new recruits. Both federal and state governments are currently evaluating proposals for health care professional recruitment and retention, and the nursing workforce is being given the highest priority among the health professions for policy intervention.

In January 2004, the Senate voted to approve Congress's long overdue $820 billion omnibus spending bill. Of special interest to the nursing profession and the health care community is the inclusion of $518 million in funding for hospital bioterrorism preparedness and $142 million in funding for nursing programs such as the Nurse Reinvestment Act. This funding reflects a $30 million increase in funding for nursing education, recruitment, and retention programs, which is the largest single-year funding increase for nursing workforce development since 1974. To further put the significance of this legislation into perspective, the same bill *reduced* funding for physician training by $14 million (ANA, 2004c). The Health Resources and Services Administration (HRSA) will administer the programs funded by this legislation. This funding increase is a testament to the influential voice of the ANA, the CMAs (state nurses associations), and individual nurses who actively supported the legislation. Nurses must continue to use their collective and individual strength to ensure further policy interventions to address the nursing shortage.

Patient Safety and Health Care Quality

In 1999, the IOM report *To Err Is Human: Building a Safer Health System* (IOM, 2000) placed the issue of medical mistakes and patient safety on the pages of many national newspapers, on the agendas of health care governing boards, and at the forefront of federal government legislation. The report concluded that up to 98,000 patients die each year as a result of medical errors. The IOM's most recent follow-up report, *Keeping Patients Safe: Transforming the Work Environment of Nurses* (Page, 2004) has focused national attention on the very important role nurses play daily in patient safety. Because the IOM is viewed as the nation's foremost authority on health care issues, policy makers pay close attention to their reports and recommendations. Thus, it is not surprising that patient safety, health care quality and nurses' work environments are currently receiving a great deal of attention and consideration for policy interventions at the state and federal levels.

Most recently, legislation has been introduced that would require hospitals that participate in the Medicare program to have safe nurse-to-patient ratios. The *Registered Nurse Safe*

Staffing Act of 2003 (HR3656) would require all hospitals to have an appropriate number of RNs with the appropriate level of experience and preparation to maximize the quality of care. The bill as currently written does not require specific nurse-to-patient ratios but rather requires the establishment of staffing systems that ensure appropriate staffing levels for quality patient care. A key provision of the bill is that it requires public posting of staffing information.

Another important piece of legislation to address patient safety and quality of care is the *Patient Safety and Quality Improvement Act* (HR663 or 720). The bill would create a confidential, voluntary reporting system in which health care providers could report information about errors to entities that would be known as Patient Safety Organizations (PSO). The PSOs would collect and analyze unique "patient safety data" and provide feedback on patient safety improvement strategies (AMA, 2003).

Nurses can review and track the progress of each of these proposed bills on the Library of Congress's "Thomas" website (www.thomas.loc.gov), which is designed to track the progress of all federal legislation. Simply enter the bill number, such as HR3536, and/or name of the bill and use the Search button to find information about a particular piece of legislation.

It is absolutely essential that nurses stay actively engaged in tracking these important pieces of legislation and advocating for passage of legislation that will improve patient safety, quality of care, and the work environment of nurses. Never before have nurses had such outstanding opportunities to improve the nursing profession and the quality of health care!

SUMMARY

Nurses are powerful advocates for health care. By understanding the policy and political processes presented in this chapter, nurses can make effective contributions to the development of health policies that promote a healthier society (Box 10-4 lists websites that will help nurses be more knowledgeable and active advocates for health care reform). Because nurses are the critical one-to-one link between organized nursing and policy makers, their basic professional responsibility is to be involved in professional nursing organizations and to be politically active in supporting meaningful health policies. Just as we learned from the first politically active nurse, Florence Nightingale, we can, as nurses, use health policy to make a difference in the lives of people we care for, as well as in our own lives and for the future of our profession.

BOX 10–4   *Helpful Websites for Health Policy and Political Activities*

Agency for Healthcare Quality and Research: Federal agency that sponsors and conducts research on health care outcomes; quality; and cost, use, and access; the information helps patients, clinicians, health system leaders, purchasers, and policy makers make more informed decisions and improve the quality of health care services—www.ahrq.gov

American Nurses Association: Professional nursing organization representing the nation's entire registered nurse population—www.nursingworld.org

Center for American Nurses: ANA affiliate organization for nurses who are not represented by unions; offers noncollective bargaining workplace advocacy strategies, programs, and services to nurses—www.nursingworld.org/can/

Centers for Medicare and Medicaid Services (CMS): Federal agency responsible for administering the Medicare program and parts of the Medicaid program—www.cms.hhs.gov

BOX 10–4 —cont'd

Department of Health and Human Services: Federal agency responsible for protecting the health of Americans and providing essential human services through more than 300 programs administered by 11 operating divisions—www.os.dhhs.gov

Federal Register: Best source of information about proposed rules and regulations for newly enacted legislation and changes to existing rules for federal programs—http://fr.cos.com/

Institute of Medicine: Part of the National Academy of Sciences, with a mission to advance and disseminate scientific knowledge to improve human health; provides objective, timely, authoritative information and advice concerning health and science policy to government, the corporate sector, the professions, and the public—www.iom.edu

Leapfrog Group: Large, voluntary consortium of public and private health care purchasers whose goal is to recognize and reward substantial gains in patient safety and consumer value—www.leapfrog.org

Library of Congress's "Thomas" website: Established to make federal legislative information freely available; tracks status of current legislation with historic information available as far back as the 104th Congress (1995)—www.thomas.loc.gov

United American Nurses: Labor union for nurses, representing 100,000 RNs nationwide; affiliate of both ANA and the AFL-CIO—www.nursingworld.org/uan/

United States House of Representatives—www.house.gov

United States Senate—www.senate.gov

CRITICAL THINKING ACTIVITIES

1. What statewide office is coming up for election in your state this year? Who are the candidates for the office? Do they have stated positions on health care issues? Do you agree or disagree with these positions? What questions would you ask concerning the candidates' positions on health care f given the opportunity to talk with them?

2. Identify and discuss health care issues that you perceive to be of great interest, not only to policy makers, but also to the public.

3. Identify a nursing issue that is of concern to you. What specific factors would help you determine whether this issue is feasible for policy action?

4. Identify the current health policy priorities for your state nurses association. Identify the benefits to you, your community, health care consumers in the district, and other members of the nursing profession that could come from supporting the proposed priorities. Develop a plan of action to educate your state senators and representatives about the priorities.

5. Determine how your state board of nurse examiners interprets the scope of nursing practice.

6. Review the methods by which grassroots lobbying can and does occur. Which methods would you choose if your plan is to maintain and improve the quality of patient care as it relates to the use of mandatory overtime as a routine staffing method? Explain your answer.

7. Use the Library of Congress's "Thomas" website (www.thomas.loc.gov) to track the status of the *Quality Nursing Care Act of 2004* (bill #HR3536) and the *Patient Safety and Quality Improvement Act* (bill #HR663 or Senate bill #720). Determine the positions of your state Senators and Representatives on these bills; if they are neutral or opposed to either bill, develop a plan of action for influencing their position.

Additional resources are available on-line at: http://evolve.elsevier.com/Cherry/

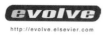

http://evolve.elsevier.com

REFERENCES

American Medical Association: *Patient safety, 2003*. Available on-line (http://www.ama-assn.org/ama/pub/category/6301.html).

American Medical Association: *Health insurance reform, 2004*. Available on-line (http://www.ama-assn.org/ama/pub/category/3373.html).

American Nurses Association: *Hill basics: the legislative processes, 2003*. Available on-line (http://vocusgr.vocus.com/grconvert1/webpub/ana/Profile.asp?Entity=PRAsset&EntityID=181&XSL=Asset&PublishType=GR+Asset).

American Nurses Association: *About us: statement of purpose, 2004a*. Available on-line (www.nursingworld.org).

American Nurses Association: *Join the nurses strategic action team, 2004b*. Available on-line (http://vocusgr.vocus.com/grconvert1/webpub/ana/Home.asp?XSL=GetInvolved&Entity=PRAsset&PublishType=Get+Involved).

American Nurses Association: *Update: House and Senate agree to $30 million increase for nursing workforce development: finalization pending, 2004c*. Available on-line (www.nursingworld.org).

Center for American Nurses: *About the Center for American Nurses, 2004*, Available on-line (http://nursingworld.org/can/).

Centers for Medicare and Medicaid Services: *SCHIP preliminary annual enrollment report* for *fiscal year 2002*. Available on-line, 2003 (http://cms.hhs.gov/schip/enrollment/).

Congressional Record: *2003 Résumé of congressional activity, 108th Congress*, Available on-line (http://thomas.loc.gov).

Himmelstein D, Woodhandler S: *Bleeding the patient: the consequences of corporate health care*, Monroe, Maine, 2001, Common Courage Press.

Institute of Medicine: *To err is human: building a safer health system* (Kohn L, Corrigan J, Donaldson M, editors), Washington, DC, 2000, National Academy Press.

Kaiser Commission on Medicaid and the Uninsured: *The uninsured and their access to health care*, Menlo Park, Calif, 2001, Kaiser Family Foundation.

Lang NM, Jennings BM: National health care quality initiatives: shaping or critiquing? *J Prof Nurs* 19(2): 59-60, 2003.

Mason DJ, Leavitt JK, Chaffee MW: Policy and politics: a framework for action. In Mason DJ, Leavitt JK, Chaffee MW, editors: *Policy and politics in nursing and health care*, ed 4, Philadelphia, 2002, WB Saunders.

Oxhorn V, Rosen S: Understanding the regulatory arena, *AORN J* 55(2):623-629, 1992.

Page A, editor: *Keeping patients safe: transforming the work environment of nurses*. Washington, DC, 2004, The National Academies Press.

Starr P: *The social transformation of American medicine: the rise of a sovereign profession and the making of a vast industry*, BasicBooks, 1982, HarperCollins Publishers.

Texas Nurses Association: *Capital Hill basics: communicating with elected officials, 2004*. Available on-line (http://capwiz.com/txnurses/issues/).

Texas Nurses Association: *Lobbying handbook for nurses*, Austin, 1995, Texas Nurses Association.

U.S. Census Bureau: *Health insurance coverage in the United States: 2002*. Report released in Sept, 2003, Available on-line (www.census.gov).

Wilburn S: Know your rights: ensuring your employer's compliance with federal needlestick law, *Am J Nurs* 101(3), 2001.

Wunderlich GS, Kohler PO: *Improving the quality of long-term care*, Committee on Improving Quality in Long-Term Care, Division of Health Care Services, Institute of Medicine. Washington, DC, 2001, National Academy Press.

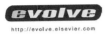
Cultural Competency and Social Issues in Nursing and Health Care

Susan R. Jacob, PhD, MSN, BSN, RN, and
M. Elizabeth Carnegie, DPA, RN, FAAN

PRIMARY
HEALTH
CLINIC

Clients deserve
culturally competent care.

VIGNETTE

When my instructor taught the session on cultural differences, she stressed the high alcoholism rates of Native Americans. I began to fear that my instructor and fellow classmates would stereotype me because of my Native American background, even though no one in my family drinks alcohol. We belong to the Mormon church, where drinking is not accepted. I wish the instructor had stressed the importance of not stereotyping.

Questions to consider while reading this chapter:

1. What preconceived ideas do you have about the following cultural groups: Hispanic, Appalachian, Moroccan, African-American, South African, Chinese?
2. What strategies can you implement to overcome prejudice?
3. How can nurses provide effective care to different cultural groups who each have a unique set of beliefs about illness?
4. How can nursing research affect the attitudes and beliefs of health professionals in regard to minority and marginalized populations?

KEY TERMS

Acculturation The process of becoming adapted to a new or different culture.
Assimilation The cultural absorption of a minority group into the main cultural body.

Additional resources are available on-line at: http://evolve.elsevier.com/Cherry/

Biculturalism Combining two distinct cultures in a single region.

Culture Shared values, beliefs, and practices of a particular group of people that are transmitted from one generation to the next and are identified as patterns that guide thinking and action.

Enculturation Adaptation to the prevailing cultural patterns in society.

Ethnicity Affiliation resulting from shared linguistic, racial, or cultural background.

Ethnocentrism Believing that one's own ethnic group, culture, or nation is best.

Marginalized population A subgroup of the population that tends to be hidden, overlooked, or on the outer edge.

Minority An ethnic group smaller than the majority group.

Prejudice Preconceived, deeply held, usually negative, judgment formed about other groups.

Stereotyping Assigning certain beliefs and behaviors to groups without recognizing individuality.

Transculturalism Being grounded in one's own culture, but having the skills to be able to work in a multicultural environment.

Worldview Perspective shared by a cultural group about general views of relationships within the universe. These broad views influence health and illness beliefs.

LEARNING OUTCOMES

After studying this chapter, the reader will be able to:

1. Integrate knowledge of demographic and sociocultural variations into culturally competent professional nursing care.
2. Provide culturally competent care to diverse client groups that incorporates variations in biologic characteristics, social organization, environmental control, communication, and other phenomena.
3. Critique education, practice, and research issues that influence culturally competent care.
4. Integrate respect for differences in beliefs and values of others as a critical component of nursing practice.

CHAPTER OVERVIEW

The United States has always been represented by a culturally diverse society. However, the volume of cultural groups entering our country is increasing rapidly. Professional nurses must provide care to persons of various cultures who have different values, beliefs, and perceptions of health and illness. This chapter explores cultural phenomena, including environmental control, biologic variations, social organization, communication, space, and time in relation to major cultural groups. It also examines different views toward health, illness, and cure. Federally defined minority groups, which include African-Americans, Asians, Hispanics, and American Indians, are emphasized, although the needs of marginalized populations such as the homeless, refugees, and the elderly also are addressed. The need for diversity in the health care force is explored, and strategies for recruiting and retaining minorities in health care are suggested. Also offered are strategies that nurses can use to increase their own cultural competence.

POPULATION TRENDS

The 2000 census shows a marked shift in the demographic and ethnic composition of the United States. Of the overall population, the percentage of whites is decreasing; this pattern is attributed to the rapidly growing Hispanic population, a large increase in Asian population, and a moderate increase in Americans of African descent (Stanhope and Lancaster, 2004). If migration trends continue, by the middle of the twenty-first century minority populations will outnumber Caucasians. Those who are currently minorities will become the majority. In many cities in the United States the number of persons from diverse cultural groups is increasing at such a rapid pace that minorities comprise more than half the population (Stanhope and Lancaster, 2004).

The aging population includes an increasing number of older adults whose ages exceed 85 years. By the year 2000 there were four million more Americans older than 65 years of age than there were in 1990. This demographic change introduces many interrelated social, economic, political, education, and health problems. The fact that people are living longer allows more opportunity for the development of chronic illness. Social isolation and depression that result from losses of friends and family will present a challenge for mental health care providers. Primary care providers are faced with identifying risks to independence and health for the aging population (U.S. Department of Health and Human Services, 2000).

Federally Defined Minority Groups

Federally defined minority groups are African-Americans, Hispanics, American Indians, and Asians/Pacific Islanders. Although tremendous strides have been made in improving health and longevity in the United States, statistical trends show a disparity in key health indicators among certain subgroups of the population (Nies and McEwen, 2001). There is a racial gap between African-Americans and Caucasians of 5.6 years, with average life expectancy being 75.2 years for Caucasians and 69.6 years for African-Americans. The infant death rate for African-Americans is twice that of Caucasians (Nies and McEwen, 2001). Although the ranking of health problems according to excess deaths differs among minority groups, six causes of death are considered priorities:

1. Cancer
2. Cardiovascular disease and stroke
3. Chemical dependency, as measured by deaths caused by cirrhosis of the liver
4. Diabetes
5. Homicides and accidents
6. Infant mortality (Nies and McEwen, 2001)

Marginalized Populations

Not only should the concern for culturally competent care focus on ethnic minorities and populations, who have a different heritage than Euro-Americans, but the needs of marginalized populations (Hall, Stevens, and Meleis, 1994), which are those populations that live on the periphery of society or in between, should be considered. Examples of such populations include gays and lesbians, older adults, recently arrived immigrants (e.g., from Russia, Afghanistan, and Rwanda), and groups that have been in this country for some time (e.g., from South America and the Middle East) who are less visible than the federally defined minorities (Lenburg et al, 1995). Their lives and health care needs often are kept secret and are understood only by them. Marginalized populations usually have considerable insights about their health care needs, although they often seem voiceless. This is in part a result of the different ways in which they both communicate and are silenced. It also may be because they feel even more peripheral or shut out from mainstream society when they are ill or experiencing a crisis.

ECONOMIC AND SOCIAL CHANGES

Changing world economics have had profound consequences, such as increased joblessness, homelessness, poverty, and limited access to health insurance and health care. Anxiety, hopelessness, depression, and despair commonly affect the individuals in our society who find themselves suddenly without a job and sometimes even without a home as a result of downsizing or other economic troubles. Dramatic changes in technology and specialization in the health care field have contributed to skyrocketing health care costs. Therefore not everyone can afford health care services. More minorities lack health insurance than the general population. Higher costs and lower wages for minority groups make it difficult to rise out of poverty (Stanhope and Lancaster, 2004).

Poverty

Most families with racially or ethnically diverse backgrounds have a lower socioeconomic status than that of the population at large. African-Americans, Hispanics, and American Indians have much higher rates of poverty than non-Hispanic Caucasians and Asians. The median family income of Asians is slightly higher than that of non-Hispanic Caucasians, which is consistent with Asians' high levels of education and the higher percentage of families with two wage earners (Council of Economic Advisers, 1999). However, opportunities for education, occupation, income earning, and property ownership that are available to upper- and middle-class Americans often are not available to members of minority groups (Stanhope and Lancaster, 2004).

The poor also suffer more than the population as a whole for nearly every measure of health. Substantial disparities remain in health insurance coverage for certain populations. Among the nonelderly population, approximately 33% of Hispanic persons lacked health insurance coverage in 1998, a rate that is more than double the national average. Mexican-Americans had one of the highest uninsured rates at 40%. For adults under age 65 years, 34% of those below the poverty level were uninsured. Lack of health care coverage has major implications for health (U.S. Department of Health and Human Services, 2000).

Minority members of society often live in poverty. This social stratification leads to social inequality. For instance, it is widely known that school systems and recreational facilities vary significantly between the inner city and the suburbs (Nies and McEwen, 2001). Residential segregation, substandard housing, unemployment, poor physical and mental health, and poor self-image are part of the cycle of poverty. This inequality is especially disturbing as it relates to health care. The United States has a history of providing the highest quality health care to those with the highest socioeconomic status and the worst health care to those with low socioeconomic status. Social, economic, and health problems have led to heated debates about the philosophy, scope and costs, and sources of funding for health care and insurance programs.

Violence

Changing economic and social conditions have contributed to the increasing level of violence in our society. Statistics indicate that homicide is the eleventh leading cause of death for all Americans and the leading cause of death among African-American males ages 15 to 34 years (Nies and McEwen, 2001). Businesses, schools, restaurants, playgrounds, and churches have become common settings for random acts of violence. Unemployment is associated with violence because it is an expectation in our society that people should be productive and gainfully employed. The inability to secure or hold a job may lead to feelings of inadequacy, guilt, and frustration, which in turn can precipitate acts of violence. Although the increasing incidence of violence affects all segments of society, those especially at risk are women, children, the elderly population, and culturally vulnerable groups. As Stanhope and Lancaster (2004) note, "Young minority males have the highest rates of unemployment in the United States, ranging close to 50%." This group also has the highest rate of violence, with homicide being a major problem for young African-American males. The differing rates of violence among races are more likely a result of poverty than race (Stanhope and Lancaster, 2004).

Societal changes have increased the tension between the empowered culturally dominant groups and the less visible vulnerable groups. This tension and behavioral response to tension has major implications for health care delivery and the education of nurses and other health care professionals (Lenburg et al, 1995).

ATTITUDES TOWARD CULTURALLY DIVERSE GROUPS

The range of attitudes toward culturally diverse groups can be viewed along a continuum of intensity, as illustrated in Fig. 11-1 (Lenburg et al, 1995).

The extreme negative manifestation of prejudice is hate in its many violent and nonviolent forms. Contempt is somewhat less intense but is highly problematic because it is so widespread and undermines many aspects of society. Tolerance reflects a more neutral attitude that accepts differences without attempting to convert them; it is the minimum-level attitude essential in democratic societies. Respect for diversity is manifested in behaviors that integrate differences into positive interactions and relationships. Respect is a demonstration of the inherent worth of the individual, regardless of differences. The most positive attitude is portrayed as a celebration (or affirmation) of the positive merits of cultural differences (i.e., of the value added to life experiences by multiple perspectives, traditions, rituals, foods, and art forms). The combination of ignorance of other cultures and arrogance about one's own culture fosters disrespect and hate. The deliberate attempt to discover and apply the positive benefits of cultural variation promotes respect and a celebration of the value of diversity, whereas perpetuating prejudice fosters narrow-mindedness and contempt. By integrating these perspectives as part of professional role behavior, educators can help students prepare for culturally competent practice in communities of diversity.

DIVERSITY IN THE HEALTH CARE WORKFORCE
Need for Diversity in the Health Care Workforce

Although the racial and ethnic makeup of the United States is moving rapidly toward greater diversity, recent workforce data document that less than 12% of all the RNs are minority

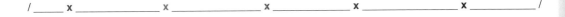

| Hate | Contempt | Tolerance | Respect | Celebration |

FIG. 11-1 A continuum of intensity of the range of attitudes toward culturally diverse groups.
(From American Academy of Nursing: *Promoting cultural competence in and through nursing education: a critical review and comprehensive plan for action,* Washington, DC, 1995, American Academy of Nursing.)

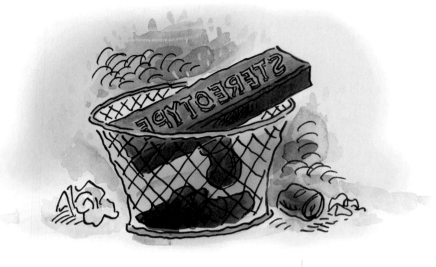

Stereotypes should be trashed.

nurses (Heller, 2002). "African Americans account for 4.2%, Asian or Pacific Islanders make up 3.4%, Hispanics 1.6%, and American Indians or Alaskan Natives 0.05% of the nursing workforce" (Stanhope and Lancaster, 2004). Members of some cultural groups are demanding culturally relevant health care that incorporates their beliefs and practices (Nies and McEwen, 2001). Consumers are becoming much more aware of what constitutes culturally sensitive and competent care and are less willing to accept incompetent care (Meleis et al, 1995). Since there is a lack of diversity and ethnic representation of health care professionals, there is limited knowledge about values, beliefs, experiences, and health care needs of certain populations such as immigrants, the elderly population, and gays and lesbians. Each of these groups has a unique set of responses to health and illness.

Nurses make up the largest segment of the workforce in health care delivery. Therefore, they have an opportunity to be proactive in changing health care inequities and access to health care (Heller, 2002). The changing health care system must reflect the community; and, as health care moves into the community, it is vital that partnerships be formed between health care providers and the community. For these partnerships to become a reality, minority representation in all health professions is vital. Factors inhibiting minority members from attaining a career in nursing include financial costs, inadequate career counseling, better recruitment efforts by other disciplines, and inadequate academic preparation, especially in the sciences (Sullivan, 1998).

Current Status of Diversity in the Health Care Workforce

Although most nurses are Caucasian women, the proportion of minority students graduating from nursing programs is increasing. In a survey conducted by the American Association of Colleges of Nursing (AACN) in 2003 (Table 11-1), minority representation in baccalaureate and higher-degree programs was highest among those identified as black or African-American (9.5%) and lowest among American Indian or Alaskan Native (0.6%). Graduates from Hispanic or Latino groups totaled 5.5%; and Asian, native Hawaiian, or other Pacific Islanders were

Table 11-1 Type of Degree by Race/Ethnicity and Nonresident Alien Status of Students Enrolled (Fall 2002) and Graduates (August 1, 2001, to July 31, 2002)

	Under Graduates				Doctoral			
	GENERIC	RN	TOTAL	MASTER'S	RESEARCH FOCUSED	CLINICAL-FOCUSED*	ND	POST-DOCTORAL
Students Enrolled (Fall 2002)								
RACE/ETHNICITY								
Asian, Native Hawaiian, or Other Pacific Islander	4,435	820	5,255	1,552	115	0	12	5
(%)	(5.2)	(2.7)	(4.6)	(4.6)	(3.7)		(4.4)	(7.6)
Black or African-American	9,340	3,638	12,978	2,903	210	5	21	5
(%)	(11.0)	(11.9)	(11.3)	(8.6)	(6.8)	(7.1)	(7.7)	(7.6)
American Indian or Alaskan Native (%)	484	218	702	197	16	0	0	0
	(0.6)	(0.7)	(0.6)	(0.6)	(0.5)			
Hispanic or Latino (%)	4,662	1,255	5,917	1,349	62	2	9	5
	(5.5)	(4.1)	(5.1)	(4.0)	(2.0)	(2.9)	(3.3)	(7.6)
White (%)	61,309	22,222	83,531	25,546	2,206	63	222	47
	(72.4)	(72.9)	(72.6)	(75.8)	(71.2)	(90.0)	(81.9)	(71.2)
Nonresident Alien (%)	881	274	1,155	514	397	0	6	4
	(1.0)	(0.9)	(1.0)	(1.5)	(12.8)		(2.2)	(6.1)
Unknown (%)	3,540	2,048	5,588	1,647	92	0	1	0
	(4.2)	(6.7)	(4.9)	(4.9)	(3.0)		(0.4)	
TOTAL	84,651	30,475	115,126	33,708	3,098	70	271	66
Schools reporting	474	497	553	335	81	2	4	21
Not reported	{764}	{209}	{973}	{473}	{0}	{0}	{0}	{0}
Graduates (August 1, 2001, to July 31, 2002)								
RACE/ETHNICITY								
Asian, Native Hawaiian, or Other Pacific Islander (%)	1,175	305	1,480	397	10	0	4	
	(5.0)	(3.1)	(4.5)	(4.3)	(2.2)		(7.5)	
Black or African-American	2.233	1,215	3,448	690	18	3	2	
American Indian or Alaskan Native (%)	161	66	227	61	0	0	0	
	(0.7)	(0.7)	(0.7)	(0.7)				
Hispanic or Latino (%)	1,318	378	1,696	349	6	0	4	
	(5.6)	(3.9)	(5.1)	(3.8)	(1.3)		(7.5)	
White (%)	17,751	7,280	25,031	7,306	362	12	38	
	(75.7)	(74.9)	(75.5)	(78.6)	(79.2)	(80.0)	(71.7)	
Non-Resident Alien (%)	168	107	275	197	57	0	5	
	(0.7)	(1.1)	(0.8)	(2.1)	(12.7)		(9.4)	
Unknown (%)	630	369	999	291	4	0	0	
	(2.7)	(3.8)	(3.0)	(3.1)	(0.9)			
TOTAL	23,436	9,720	33,156	9,291	457	15	53	
Schools reporting	469	477	541	316	81	2	4	
Not reported	{239}	{631}	{860}	{1,069}	{0}	{0}	{0}	

*There are two doctoral programs with a clinical focus: the Doctor of Nursing Practice program at the University of Kentucky and the DNSc program at the University of Tennessee Health Science Center.

NOTE: Percentages may not total exactly 100.0% because of rounding.

ND, Doctor of Nursing.

From American Association of Colleges of Nursing © 2003.

5.2% of the undergraduate students who responded to the survey. These totals lag behind the 72.4% reported Caucasian enrollment.

The number of men who graduate from basic registered nurse (RN) programs is increasing. In the AACN survey conducted in 2003, 8.4% of the undergraduate respondents were men (Table 11-2). Men continue to represent a minority in nursing, although recent recruitment efforts have focused more on men and minorities. Recent ad campaigns have highlighted men who were formerly firefighters, emergency responders, and law enforcement officers who have made the decision to pursue nursing as a career.

Recruitment and Retention of Minorities in Nursing

It is clear that we have been slow in preparing nurses to be reflective of our population, just as we have been unaware of the need for culturally sensitive patient care and sometimes less than welcoming to students different from the predominant population (Heller, 2002). Recruitment and retention of students from minority populations must not be separated. In other words, recruitment programs must have retention as their primary focus because

Table 11-2	Type of Degree by Gender of Students Enrolled (Fall 2002) and Graduates (August 1, 2001, to July 31, 2002)							
	Under Graduates				Doctoral			
	GENERIC	RN	TOTAL	MASTER'S	RESEARCH-FOCUSED	CLINICAL-FOCUSED*	ND	POST-DOCTORAL
Students Enrolled (Fall 2002)								
GENDER								
Female (%)	77,553	27,866	105,419	29,004	2,863	64	248	44
	(91.6)	(92.1)	(91.7)	(90.5)	(93.5)	(91.4)	(91.5)	(91.7)
Male (%)	7,113	2,398	9,511	3,035	200	6	23	4
	(8.4)	(7.9)	(8.3)	(9.5)	(6.5)	(8.6)	(8.5)	(8.3)
TOTAL	84,666	30,264	114,930	32,039	3,063	70	271	48
Schools reporting	481	494	558	334	78	2	4	21
Not reported	{749}	{420}	{1,169}	{2,142}	{35}	{0}	{0}	{148}
Graduates (August 1, 2001, to July 31, 2002)								
GENDER								
Female (%)	21,237	9,1025	30,342	8,924	369	12	45	
	(91.7)	(89.9)	(91.1)	(91.0)	(94.6)	(80.0)	(84.9)	
Male (%)	1,934	1,025	2,959	882	21	3	8	
	(8.3)	(10.1)	(8.9)	(9.0)	(5.4)	(20.0)	(15.1)	
TOTAL	23,171	10,130	33,301	9,806	390	15	53	
Schools reporting	466	487	545	306	68	2	4	
Not reported	{494}	{221}	{715}	{554}	{67}	{0}	{0}	

*There are two doctoral programs with a clinical focus: the Doctor of Nursing Practice program at the University of Kentucky and the DNSc program at the University of Tennessee Health Science Center.

NOTE: Percentages may not total exactly 100.0% because of rounding.

ND, Doctor of Nursing.

From American Association of Colleges of Nursing © 2003.

there is no point in recruiting minorities into nursing programs and then not helping them succeed.

Before World War II the only known effort to recruit minority students into nursing on a national scale was made by the National Association of Colored Graduate Nurses (NACGN), which had included recruitment of African-Americans into nursing as one of its objectives since its inception in 1908. During World War II a mechanism was set into motion by the federal government to produce additional nursing personnel by financing basic nursing education. This was done through the Cadet Nurse Corps. The Corps had a number of recruiters, two of whom were African-American. These two African-American nurses confined their recruiting to 82 African-American colleges and universities. By the end of the war, 21 African-American nursing schools had participated in the Corps, and well over 2000 African-American nurses had acquired their basic nursing education through this mechanism.

After the war, recruitment efforts for African-Americans at the national level reverted to NACGN, an organization that voted itself out of existence in 1949 and was dissolved in 1951. However, individual African-American schools in the North and South continued to recruit. In the South, law segregated the nursing schools, and in the North they were segregated by custom. In 1954 the unanimous Supreme Court decision in the case of Brown v. the Board of Education asserted "separate educational facilities were inherently unequal," making racial segregation in public schools unconstitutional. This decision was interpreted to mean that all kinds of educational discrimination would be considered, including nursing.

It was around the time of the Brown decision that schools of nursing were being accredited by national standards, and many schools, both African-American and Caucasian, did not measure up to the standards. As a result, numerous schools closed. With integration permitting African-American students to be admitted to formerly all-Caucasian schools, quality African-American schools had difficulty attracting enough students, and many more of those schools closed. However, the Caucasian schools that began admitting African-American students did not admit the same number that would have been admitted by the closed African-American schools. For example, many Caucasian schools admitted only one or two African-American students per class.

In the late 1960s many efforts were made to help the economically disadvantaged in this country. Although not all people of minority groups are economically disadvantaged, the vast majority of disadvantaged people are members of ethnic minority groups. Nursing, too, became concerned about the disadvantaged and began concerted efforts to recruit more members of minority groups into nursing schools. The Sealantic Fund, one of the Rockefeller Brothers' funds, was one of the first foundations that helped minorities enter nursing school. Sealantic funded projects in 10 universities in different parts of the country to recruit students from minority groups and help them achieve success. The best example of an ongoing project, funded by the Division of Nursing since 1971, is the National Student Nurses Association's "Breakthrough to Nursing" to accelerate the recruitment of minorities, including men.

In 1997 the American Nurses Foundation published a report of a project it had funded entitled Strategies for Recruitment, Retention, and Graduation of Minority Nurses in Colleges of Nursing. Through survey and interview analysis, Bessent and a cadre of knowledgeable leaders investigated the most effective approach to increase the nursing profession's representation of nurses of color (Bessent, 1997). Members of Chi Eta Phi, a national African-American nursing society with chapters throughout the country, serve as mentors to minority nursing students. As mentors, sorority members provide intellectual and inspirational stimulation along with counseling.

For the second time in the last 20 years, our country is experiencing a shortage of registered nurses. Estimates by the U.S. Department of Health and Human Services (2002) show a shortage of 140,000 nurses that will skyrocket to well over 800,000 by 2020.

The growing shortage presents unprecedented opportunities for the recruitment of minorities into nursing. Important strategies include making connections early at the middle school and high school levels, developing inclusive advertising campaigns, raising scholarship support, and providing mentoring and remedial support during educational programs (American Association of Colleges of Nursing, 2001).

In July 2002, the United States Congress adopted the Nurse Reinvestment Act to address the shortage by providing scholarships to nursing students, encouraging careers as nursing faculty, assisting in nurse education, and supporting career ladder partnerships between nursing scholars and practice settings. President George W. Bush signed the bill into law in August 2002. The U.S. Senate took a major step forward in supporting the Nurse Reinvestment Act when they accepted an amendment to the 2004 fiscal year.

The American Nurses Foundation (ANF), the only national philanthropic organization representing the nation's entire nursing profession, is collaborating with Congress in enacting the Nurse Recruitment Act to establish the National Nursing Service Corps and provide federal aid for nursing students and grants to improve nursing education, practice, and retention.

To develop strategies to deal with the current shortage of nurses, in October 2002 the American Nurses Foundation (ANF) launched an "Invest in Nursing Campaign," with a national steering committee to shape the direction and oversee the implementation of the campaign to raise $30 million. ANF, along with the American Nurses Association, is committed to promoting recruitment, retention, and diversity in nursing.

Just as contributions of diverse cultural groups are beginning to be valued, so must nursing programs value the need for diversity in their students and faculty and view this diversity as a strength. Diversity within nursing programs can increase the understanding and sensitivity of nurses and positively affect the way they provide care to their patients.

Strategies for Recruitment and Retention of Minorities in the Health Care Workforce

Recommendations of an American Academy of Nursing (AAN) expert panel on cultural competence (Meleis et al, 1995) include recruitment and retention of diversity in the workforce, raising consciousness, mentoring, and consultation. There also is a need to increase the number of nurse educators and researchers who are from diverse, marginalized, and vulnerable populations. Raising consciousness involves increasing the level of awareness of nurses and other health care professionals about the issues surrounding diversity. This can be accomplished by encouraging participation in forums related to different aspects of various cultural phenomena such as environmental control, communication, and health beliefs. Such forums might be offered by state and local professional nurses' organizations and health care facilities.

Another successful strategy for recruiting and retaining minorities in education and clinical practice is "matched mentoring," which would involve matching same-culture mentors and graduates either in the same institution or different institutions. A different mentoring strategy would involve teaching and modeling by nurses who have been trained in cross-cultural care. Cross-cultural nursing consultants in the care of specific groups are available to agencies, professional groups, licensing bodies, and individual nurses. Organizations should contact the Transcultural Nursing Society to obtain the names of consultants in the field of transcultural nursing.

Audiovisual media should be used to teach the importance of human health conditions cross-culturally. Video conferencing can provide international links for students and faculty members who cannot travel. Students from various cultures can share their clinical experiences. One of the greatest benefits is the discovery that thinking, values, and decision making differ in various cultures. Collaborative arrangements should be encouraged between colleges and universities so that exchange programs can be offered to students. Such exchanges can give students firsthand, in-depth experience with a culture different from their own. Interactive media can be used to gain a clearer perspective than can be obtained through printed material on particular cultures.

Strategies such as mentoring by same-culture professionals have been shown to be effective in recruiting and retaining minorities in nursing. In addition, the value of workshops, continuing education programs, and the use of consultants to promote culturally competent care should not be overlooked.

CULTURAL COMPETENCE

Health professionals, educators, and health care systems must all respond to the consequences of increasing cultural diversity for the future well-being of all populations. There is a shared responsibility to work collaboratively to achieve competence in nursing practice. It is evident that professional competence must incorporate cultural competence and the skillful use of knowledge and interpersonal and technical abilities (Lenburg et al, 1995). Evaluation of cultural competence in students, faculty, and staff is essential. It is essential that nurses take responsibility to:

- Be sensitive to and show respect for the differences in beliefs and values of others.
- Take responsibility to inquire, learn about, and integrate beliefs and values of others in professional encounters.
- Take responsibility to try to change negative and prejudicial behaviors in themselves and others.

In light of societal changes, responsible persons at all levels in education and health care delivery systems acknowledge the need to reassess the influence of culture on achieving expected health outcomes. There is an imperative need for nurse educators, administrators, students, and others to promote sensitivity to, acceptance of, and respect for the rights and mores of all individuals within the context of their cultural orientation and society as a whole. Nurses must be culturally competent because:

- The nurse's culture often is different from the client's culture.
- Care that is not culturally competent may be more costly.
- Care that is not culturally competent may be ineffective.

Specific objectives for persons in different cultures need to be met, as outlined in Healthy People 2000 (Stanhope and Lancaster, 2004). For this reason the expert panels of the American Academy of Nursing (AAN) were developed in 1992 and 1995 to draft proposals for promoting cultural competence in nursing.

Principles for Culturally Competent Care

The goal of culturally competent nursing care is to provide care that is consistent with the client's cultural needs. The AAN Expert Panel Report (1992) on culturally competent nursing care suggested the following four principles:

1. Care is designed for the specific client.
2. Care is based on the uniqueness of the person's culture and includes cultural norms and values.
3. Care includes empowerment strategies to facilitate client decision making in health behavior.
4. Care is provided with sensitivity to the cultural uniqueness of the client.

Nurses have a responsibility to become knowledgeable about the values, beliefs, and health care practices of the culturally diverse groups that are dominant in the nurse's particular practice area or region of the country. For example, nurses who work for the Indian Health Service must be culturally competent to care for American Indians and Alaskan Natives. Nurses who practice in California should strive to increase knowledge and understanding of Asian and Hispanic populations. In south Texas, where 70% of the population is Hispanic, cultural competence would ideally include the ability to speak Spanish.

Cultural Competence in Nursing Education

Since the 1960s there has been a united effort to include concepts sensitive to cultural diversity in nursing education. The National League for Nursing (NLN) has made this requirement mandatory for accreditation. The NLN specifies that the nursing curriculum should provide "learning experiences in health promotion and maintenance, illness care and rehabilitation for clients from diverse and multicultural populations throughout the life span" (NLN, 1996). Transcultural nursing was first introduced in the 1960s (Nies and McEwen, 2001). Since then some progress has been made, but only recently have nursing programs been systematically incorporating culturally diverse nursing care concepts into the curricula. Content about the health beliefs and practices of individuals from various cultural groups is essential. Information about the prevalence of health problems and disease incidence mortality rates, cultural factors related to situations such as birth and death, and specific culture-bound syndromes such as anorexia and bulimia should be essential content in nursing curricula and in continuing education programs for practicing nurses. The cross-cultural similarities and differences of roles and responsibilities of family members should be addressed, particularly in terms of support and health care functions of family members.

The AAN expert panel (1992) also recommended the following principles to be used in preparing nursing graduates who are sensitive to cultural diversity and global health care needs and able to provide culturally competent care:

- Nurses must learn to appreciate intergroup and intragroup cultural diversity and commonalities in racial/ethnic minority populations.
- Nurses must understand how social structural factors shape health behaviors and practices in racial/ethnic minorities (e.g., nurses must avoid a "blaming" and "victim" pattern).
- Nurses must understand the dynamics and challenges of biculturalism and bilingualism.
- Nurses must confront their own ethnocentrism and racism.
- Nurses must begin implementing and evaluating service provided to cross-cultural populations.

BOX 11-1   Anglo-American and Other Cultural Values

Anglo-American	Other Cultural Values
Personal control over the environment	Fate
Change	Tradition
Time dominates	Human interaction dominates
Human equality	Hierarchy, rank, status
Individualism, privacy	Group welfare
Self-help	Birthright inheritance
Competition	Cooperation
Future orientation	Past orientation
"Action-goal" work orientation	"Being" orientation
Informality	Formality
Directness, openness, honesty	Indirectness, ritual, "face"
Practicality, efficiency	Idealism, theory
Materialism	Spiritualism, detachment

CULTURAL BELIEF SYSTEMS

A value is a standard that people use to assess themselves and others. It is a belief about what is worthwhile or important for well-being. There is a tendency for people to be "culture-bound" (i.e., to assume that their values are superior, sensible, or right). Cross-cultural health promotion requires the nurse to work with clients without making judgments as to the superiority of one set of values over another. Box 11-1 provides a comparison of Anglo-American values and those of more tradition-bound countries.

Each culture has a value system that dictates behavior directly or indirectly by setting norms and teaching that those norms are right. Health beliefs and practices tend to reflect a culture's value system. Nurses must understand the patient's value system to foster health promotion.

CULTURAL PHENOMENA

Giger and Davidhizar (1999) have identified six cultural phenomena that vary among cultural groups and affect health care. These phenomena are environmental control, biologic variations, social organization, communication, space, and time orientation.

Environmental Control

Environmental control is the ability of members of a particular culture to control nature or environmental factors. Some groups perceive humans as having mastery over nature, others perceive humans to be dominated by nature, and still other groups see humans as having a harmonious relationship with nature (Spector, 2000a). People who perceive that they have mastery over nature believe that they can overcome the natural forces of nature. Such individuals would expect positive results from medications, surgery, and other treatment modalities. Persons who believe that they are subject to the forces of nature or that they have little control over what happens to them may not be compliant with treatments because they believe that whatever happens to them is part of their destiny. African-Americans and Mexican-Americans are most likely to subscribe to this view. Persons who hold the view of harmony with nature, such as Asians and American Indians, believe that illness represents a disharmony with nature. These clients may see medication as relieving only the symptoms and not curing the disease. Therefore they are more likely to rely on naturalistic remedies such as herbs or hot and cold treatments to effect a cure (Stanhope and Lancaster, 2004). Included in this concept are the traditional health and illness beliefs, the practice of folk medicine, and the use of traditional and nontraditional healers. Environmental control plays an important role in the way clients respond to health-related experiences and use health resources (Spector, 2000a).

Biologic Variations

Biologic variations such as body build and structure, genetic variations, skin characteristics, susceptibility to disease, and nutritional variations exist among different cultures. For example, babies who are born in Western culture tend to weigh more than babies born in other cultures. Other common variations include skin color, eye shape, hair texture, adipose tissue deposits, shape of ear lobes, and body configuration (Stanhope and Lancaster, 2004). For example, African-Americans have denser bones than Caucasians, which may account for the low incidence of osteoporosis in the African-American population. The size of teeth varies among cultures, with Caucasians having the smallest, followed by African-Americans, Asians, and Native Americans. Larger teeth can cause protruding jaws, a condition common in African-Americans, which does not represent an orthodontic problem (Nies and McEwen, 2001).

Laboratory values for some tests also vary among cultural groups. For example, serum cholesterol levels essentially are the same for African-Americans and Caucasians at birth. During childhood the levels are higher in African-Americans, but they are lower than in Caucasians in adulthood. This finding is interesting because of the high morbidity and mortality from cardiovascular disease in African-Americans (Nies and McEwen, 2001). The maternal mortality rate of African-Americans is three times that of Caucasians; occurrence of stomach cancer is twice as high among African-American men as Caucasian men; and occurrence of esophageal cancer is three times more common among African-Americans than the general population. Japanese-Americans have a lower incidence of cardiovascular and renal disease than the general population but a higher incidence of stress-related diseases such as ulcers, colitis, psoriasis, and depression. Native Americans have a higher incidence of streptococcal sore throat and gastroenteritis than the general population (Medcom, 1997). Native American women have the highest incidence of diabetes (Nies and McEwen, 2001).

Mexican-Americans have higher rates of obesity and diabetes than the general population, although they have lower rates of cardiovascular disease. The Mexican-American population has a pattern of less use of preventive services, including prenatal care, childhood immunizations, and vision, hearing, and dental care (Nies and McEwen, 2001).

Social Organization

Social organization refers to the family unit (nuclear, single-parent, or extended family) and the religious or ethnic groups with which families identify. Family is defined differently across cultures. For instance, in the African-American culture, family often includes people who are unrelated or distantly related. Families depend on the extended family for emotional and financial support in times of crisis. Mothers and grandmothers play important roles in African-American families and are involved in decision making, especially as it relates to health (Stanhope and Lancaster, 2004).

Communication

Communication differences include language differences, verbal and nonverbal behaviors, and silence. Language can be the greatest obstacle to providing multicultural care. If the client does not speak the same language as the nurse, a skilled interpreter is mandatory (Giger and Davidhizar, 1999). Comfort with direct eye contact during communication is an area that varies among cultures. Although some cultures such as Euro-Americans value direct eye contact as a sign of attention, other cultures such as African-Americans or American Indians, may view direct eye contact as rude behavior.

In the Asian culture it is considered important behavior to agree with those in authority. This aspect of the Asian culture has important implications for the nurse who is involved in patient education. The patient may seem compliant and nod his or her head as in agreement with the nurse's instruction even when the instruction is not clear or when the patient has no intention of carrying out the instruction (Stanhope and Lancaster, 2004).

Anglo-Americans tend to be informal in their style of communication, whereas other cultures may prefer a more formal style. Health professionals should not assume that a first-name basis is appropriate for client relationships. With any client, terms of endearment such as "honey" or "dear" are unacceptable and can be interpreted as disrespectful, derogatory, or condescending. The best solution to the challenge of different communication styles and preferences is always to ask the client how he or she prefers to be addressed.

If the nurse and the client do not speak the same language, an interpreter should be consulted. An interpreter can help the nurse establish rapport with the client and explain concepts to the patient in terms of cultural relevance that may be foreign to the nurse. When interpreters are needed, they should be selected carefully. Adult family members or friends are possible choices, as are bilingual staff and community volunteers. Nurses should be aware that some ethnic groups consider it a breach of confidentiality to have a stranger interpret, whereas certain individuals may not want other family members or friends to know the specifics of their medical condition.

The nurse also should be careful to consider the different dialects spoken in the same country and the particular culture's view of women and children. Children should not be used as interpreters because of the subject matter and because of certain cultural views of authority. Many cultures view adults as having more authority than children. In many cultures women would not be considered acceptable interpreters because of those cultures' view of women.

Nurses should be aware that AT&T has an interpreter service. A two-way calling system is arranged in which the nurse, the interpreter, and the client are on the telephone at the same time. This service is available in many hospitals, although many nurses and other health care professionals are unaware of this resource.

Space

People have different attitudes and comfort levels regarding the area immediately around them known as "personal space" or "intimate zone." There are vast cultural differences in the comfort level associated with the distance maintained between persons. Anglo-American nurses tend to feel comfortable with an intimate zone of 0 to 18 inches. This usually is the distance between the nurse and the patient when the nurse performs certain parts of a physical assessment such as an eye or ear examination. Entering this space could be uncomfortable for clients and nurses who have not had time to establish a trusting relationship. This discomfort would be increased for persons whose culture is not at all comfortable with such a limited personal space. For instance, Asians frequently believe that touching strangers is inappropriate;

therefore they have a tendency to prefer more distance between themselves and others, particularly health professionals whom they have not previously known. On the other hand, Mexican-Americans tend to be comfortable with less space because they like to touch persons with whom they are talking (Stanhope and Lancaster, 2004).

Time

Time orientation refers to the emphasis various cultures place on the present, past, or future. Present-oriented persons enjoy what they are experiencing at the moment and only move on to the next event or activity "when the time is right." Punctuality and "watching the clock" are definitely part of Western culture, but many cultural groups, such as American Indians, do not view time in the same way. This difference in time orientation can have implications for the present-oriented professional in the work setting, who may always be late for work without thinking it is an important issue. In addition, there are implications for health teaching. For example, when teaching medication schedules to a patient, it would be important to consider how that individual views time.

Clients who view the past as more important than the present or the future may focus on memories. For instance, the Vietnamese may take actions that they believe are consistent with the views of their ancestors and even look to those ancestors for guidance (Giger and Davidhizar, 1999). In the Asian culture time is viewed as being more flexible than in the Western culture and being on time for appointments is not a priority (Stanhope and Lancaster, 2004).

People who are future-oriented are concerned with long-range goals and health care measures that can be taken in the present to prevent illness in the future. These persons plan ahead in scheduling appointments and organizing activities. They may be seen as having "distant" or "cold" personalities because they are not always engaged in communication at the moment because they may be thinking about their plans for the future. On the other hand, persons who are oriented more to the present may be late for appointments because they are less concerned with planning ahead (Table 11-3).

PRACTICE ISSUES RELATED TO CULTURAL COMPETENCE
Health Information and Education

According to the Task Force on Black and Minority Health, minority populations are less knowledgeable about specific health problems than are Caucasians. African-Americans and Hispanics receive less information about cancer and heart disease than do nonminority groups. African-Americans tend to underestimate the prevalence of cancer, give less credence to the warning signs, obtain fewer screening tests, and are diagnosed at later stages of cancer than are Caucasians. Hispanic women receive less information about breast cancer than do Caucasian women. Hispanic women are less aware that family history is a risk for breast cancer, and only 29% have heard of breast self-examination. Successful programs to increase public awareness about health problems are being offered to minority groups, but efforts must be continued to reach more of the population. Families, churches, employers, and community organizations need to be involved in facilitating behavior changes that will result in healthier lifestyles. Education programs have the greatest impact on diseases that are affected by lifestyle such as hypertension, obesity, and diabetes. For example, if patients with diabetes could improve their self-management skills, 70% of complications could be prevented, saving human suffering and health care dollars (Nies and McEwen, 2001).

Table 11-3	**Variations Among Selected Cultural Groups**			
	AFRICAN-AMERICANS	**ASIANS**	**HISPANICS**	**AMERICAN INDIANS**
Verbal communication	Asking personal questions of someone met for the first time is seen as improper and intrusive	High respect for others, especially those in positions of authority	Expression of negative feelings is considered impolite	Speaks in a low tone of voice and expects that the listener will be attentive
Nonverbal communication	Direct eye contact in conversation often is considered rude	Direct eye contact with superiors may be considered disrespectful	Avoidance of eye contact usually is a sign of attentiveness and respect	Direct eye contact often is considered disrespectful
Touch	Touching another's hair often is considered offensive	It is not customary to shake hands with persons of the opposite sex	Touching often is observed between two persons in conversation	A light touch of the person's hand instead of a firm handshake often is used when greeting a person
Family organization	Usually have close, extended family networks; women play key roles in health care decisions	Usually have close, extended family ties; emphasis may be on family needs rather than individual needs	Usually have close, extended family ties; all members of the family may be involved in health care decisions	Usually have close, extended family ties; emphasis tends to be family rather than on individual needs
Time	Often present-oriented	Often present-oriented	Often present-oriented	Often present-oriented
Alternative healers	"Granny," "root doctor," voodoo priest, spiritualist	Acupuncturist, acupressurist, herbalist	Curandero, espiritualista, yerbo	Medicine man, shaman
Self-care practices	Poultices, herbs, oils, roots	Hot and cold foods, herbs, teas, soups, cupping, burning, rubbing, pinching	Hot and cold foods, herbs	Herbs, corn meal, medicine bundle
Biologic variations	Sickle cell anemia, Mongolian spots, keloid formation, inverted T waves, lactose intolerance, skin color	Thalassemia, drug interactions, Mongolian spots, lactose intolerance, skin color	Mongolian spots, lactose intolerance, skin color	Cleft uvula, lactose intolerance, skin color

Data from Giger JN, Davidhizar, RE: *Transcultural nursing,* ed 3, St Louis, 1999, Mosby; Spector RE: *Cultural diversity in health and illness,* ed 5, Upper Saddle River, NJ, 2000, Prentice Hall; Payne KT. In Taylor OL, editor: *Nature of communication disorders in culturally and linguistically diverse populations,* San Diego, 1986, College Hill Press.

Education and Certification

Increasingly more universities and colleges offer graduate programs in transcultural, cross-cultural, and international nursing. Many nurses have not been exposed to transcultural nursing in their basic education program. Therefore the availability of graduate study in this area often is an unrecognized possibility.

Transcultural nursing is the study of differences and similarities of various cultural health values and beliefs among different ethnic and minority groups (Medcom, 1997). The Transcultural Nursing Society has been certifying nurses in transcultural nursing since 1988. Certification as a certified transcultural nurse is based on oral and written examinations and evaluation of the nurse's educational and experiential background. Certification has increased recognition of transcultural nursing as a legitimate nursing specialty. Transcultural nurses are interested in finding a universal care for clients that will improve, maintain, and restore health and improve client satisfaction.

International Marketplace

Nurses trained in the United States work, teach, and consult in hundreds of foreign countries on every continent. They often are recognized as international pacesetters and are viewed as "commodities for import" by both the more developed countries and the less developed third- or fourth-world nations. Nurses can make a difference in the health outcomes of people all over the world. Technology has enhanced global communication and facilitated travel. As nurses help solve emerging health problems in countries throughout the world, they are the most valuable assets of the health care system. They will be called on to design, implement, and evaluate international projects, educational endeavors, and research with an intercultural focus. Therefore it is important that nurses understand the intercultural issues related to our global society (Nies and McEwen, 2001).

Nursing Literature

The number of journal articles about culturally diverse clients, transcultural nursing research, international nursing, and the inclusion of transcultural concepts in nursing curricula has increased considerably since the 1950s. The *Journal of Transcultural Nursing* is a refereed journal that was first published in 1989. This journal was created to advance transcultural nursing knowledge and practices; it focuses on theory, research, and practice dimensions of transcultural nursing and provides a forum for researchers. Other journals that address cultural issues include the *Western Journal of Medicine: Cross Cultural Issues,* the *Journal of Cultural Diversity,* the *Journal of Multicultural Nursing,* the *International Journal of Nursing Studies,* the *International Nursing Review,* and the *Journal of Holistic Nursing.* Nurse authors also need to be encouraged to publish articles related to clients' cultural views and health care needs in nursing specialty and practice journals that are more widely read by nurses who provide care on a daily basis to clients from diverse cultures.

Although research articles on transcultural issues are becoming a common feature in health care journals, there is a need for additional research that examines individual behavioral responses to normal life processes such as pregnancy, birth, death, and human growth and development. There also is a need for well-designed studies that explore the biologic, psychologic, sociologic, and spiritual differences within, between, and among cultural groups (Purnell and Paulanka, 1998). Even though there have been numerous research studies conducted on cultural diversity issues, a significant time gap often exists between the identification of findings and publication of results. The limited dissemination of research findings inhibits widespread acceptance of new interventions that could potentially improve health care practices of culturally diverse populations. Computer information technology and on-line networks help to narrow this gap and distribute research findings in a timely manner (Purnell and Paulanka, 1998).

Responsibility of Health Care Facilities for Cultural Care

Nursing policies should reflect openness to including extended family members and folk healers in the nursing care plan, provided their presence is not harmful to the client's well-being. For example, Hispanic clients may want the support of a curandero, espiritualista (spiritualist), yerbo (herbalist), or sabador (similar to a chiropractor). African-Americans may turn to a hougan (voodoo priest or priestess) or "old lady." American Indians may seek assistance from a shaman or medicine man. Clients of Asian descent may want the services of an acupuncturist or bonesetter. In some religions spiritual healers may be found among the ranks of the ordained and may be called priest, bishop, elder, deacon, rabbi, brother, or sister (Nies and McEwen, 2001). Most hospital chaplaincy programs have access to religious representatives available for patients of various religions.

Clients may need to consult with their support persons and folk healers before making medical decisions. Nurses must respect the client's right to privacy and allow time for the client to interact with his or her spiritual or cultural healers. Nurses must respect unconventional beliefs and health practices and work with clients to develop a plan of care that builds on their beliefs and incorporates nontraditional health practices that are not harmful. These nontraditional healers should be received with respect and provided privacy to enable the healers to interact with their patients (Nies and McEwen, 2001).

Health care facilities should provide resources for nurses and other health care professionals to assist with culture-specific needs of clients. Health care facilities should have a list of interpreters fluent in the major languages spoken by persons typically using the organization. Translators who have knowledge of health-related terminology would be more effective than those who do not. Gender, birth origin, and socioeconomic class need to be considered when selecting a translator. Gender is an important consideration because many cultures prohibit discussion of intimate matters between women and men. Birth origin of the client and translator should be determined because often there are many dialects spoken within the same country, depending on the particular region (Stanhope and Lancaster, 2004). Differences in socioeconomic class between client and interpreter can lead to problems of interpretation.

Clinical nurse specialists (CNSs) in transcultural nursing should be added to the staff of institutions serving large numbers of culturally diverse persons. The transcultural CNS could be a role model to the staff in delivery of culturally sensitive and competent care, provide inservice education to staff related to cultural differences, and conduct research related to cultural and social issues. In addition, consultants should be used to deal with specific cultural issues.

Continuing education programs for nurses should be offered by health care institutions. Programs should focus on promoting awareness of the nurses' own culturally based values, beliefs, and attitudes, cultural assessment, biologic variations of cultural groups, cross-cultural communication, and culture-specific beliefs and practices related to childbearing and childrearing, death and dying, issues of mental health, and cultural aspects of aging.

Recommended Standards for Culturally and Linguistically Appropriate Health Care Services (CLAS)

Culture and language have considerable impact on how patients access and respond to health care services. To ensure equal access to quality health care by diverse populations the Health Resources Services Administration (HRSA) with input from a national advisory committee of policymakers, providers, and researchers in their report "Assessing Cultural Competence in Health Care: Recommendations for National Standards and an Outcomes Focused Research Agenda" recommends the following standards for health care organizations:

- Promote and support the attitudes, behaviors, knowledge, and skills necessary for staff to work respectfully and effectively with patients and each other in a culturally diverse work environment.

- Have a comprehensive management strategy to address culturally and linguistically appropriate services, including strategic goals, plans, policies, procedures, and designated staff responsible for implementation.
- Utilize formal mechanisms for community and consumer involvement in the design and execution of service delivery, including planning, policy making, operations, evaluation, training and, as appropriate, treatment planning.
- Develop and implement a strategy to recruit, retain, and promote qualified, diverse, and culturally competent administrative, clinical, and support staff members that are trained and qualified to address the needs of the racial and ethnic communities being served.
- Require and arrange for ongoing education and training for administrative, clinical, and support staff in culturally and linguistically competent service delivery.
- Provide all clients with limited English proficiency (LEP) access to bilingual staff or interpretation services.
- Provide oral and written notices, including translated signage at key points of contact, to clients in their primary language informing them of their right to receive interpreter services free of charge.
- Translate and make available signage and commonly-used written patient educational material and other materials for members of the predominant language groups in service areas.
- Ensure that interpreters and bilingual staff can demonstrate bilingual proficiency and receive training that includes the skills and ethics of interpreting, as well as knowledge in both languages of the terms and concepts relevant to clinical or non-clinical encounters. Family or friends are not considered adequate substitutes because they usually lack these abilities.
- Ensure that the clients' primary spoken language and self-identified race/ethnicity are included in the health care organization's management information system as well as any patient records used by provider staff.
- Use a variety of methods to collect and utilize accurate demographic, cultural, epidemiologic, and clinical outcome data for racial and ethnic groups in the service area. Become informed about the ethnic/cultural needs, resources, and assets of the surrounding community.
- Undertake ongoing organizational self-assessments of cultural and linguistic competence; integrate measures of access, satisfaction, quality, and outcomes for CLAS into other organizational internal audits and performance improvement programs.
- Develop structures and procedures to address cross-cultural ethical and legal conflicts in health care delivery and complaints or grievances by patients and staff about unfair, culturally insensitive, or discriminatory treatment; difficulty in accessing services; or denial of services.
- Prepare an annual progress report documenting the organizations' progress with implementing CLAS standards, including information on programs, staffing, and resources.

CULTURAL ASSESSMENT

Cultural Self-Assessment

The first step to becoming a culturally sensitive and competent health care provider is to conduct a cultural self-assessment. The nurse should engage in a cultural self-assessment to identify individual culturally based attitudes about clients who are from a different culture. Cultural self-assessment requires self-honesty and sincerity and reflection on attitudes of parents, grandparents, and close friends in terms of their attitudes toward different cultures. Through identification of health-related attitudes, values, beliefs, and practices, the nurse can better understand the cultural aspects of health care from the client's perspective. Everyone has ethnocentric tendencies that must be brought to a level of consciousness so that efforts can be made to temper the feeling that one's own culture is "best." Box 11-2 shows a cultural self-assessment guide adapted from Swanson and Nies (1997) for the nurse who is not African-American but is caring for an African-American client.

Cultural Client Assessment

After the nurse performs a cultural self-assessment, he or she should obtain a cultural assessment for the client. Nursing assessments in institutional and community settings should include the gathering of data pertinent to cultural beliefs and practices. Cultural assessments lead to culturally relevant nursing diagnoses and give direction to effective nursing intervention. Basic cultural data include ethnic affiliation, religious preference, family patterns, food patterns, and ethnic health care practices. Cultural assessments should be used as an adjunct to other patient assessments. These data will give the nurse sufficient information to determine whether a more in-depth assessment of cultural factors is needed. A major reason that cultural assessments are performed is to identify patterns that may assist or interfere with a nursing intervention or treatment regimen (Giger and Davidhizer, 1999).

The nurse needs to find out whether the client's beliefs, customs, values, and self-care practices are adaptive (beneficial), neutral, or maladaptive (harmful) in relation to nursing interventions. For example, if a Mexican-American client who is diagnosed with hypertension insists on taking garlic instead of an antihypertensive, this could be harmful. If the client agrees to take the garlic in addition to the antihypertensive, this would be a neutral practice. An adaptive or beneficial practice would include daily exercise in addition to the garlic and antihypertensive.

In the case of Southeast Asians, dermal practices such as cupping, pinching, rubbing, and burning are a common part of self-care. The dermal methods are perceived as ways to relieve

---

BOX 11-2 *Cultural Self-Assessment*

- How do your parents, grandparents, other family members, and close friends view people from racially diverse groups?
- What is the cultural stereotype of African-Americans?
- Does the cultural stereotype allow for socioeconomic differences?
- Have your interactions with African-Americans been positive? Negative? Neutral?
- How do you feel about going into a predominantly African-American neighborhood or into the home of an African-American family? Are you afraid, anxious, curious, or ambivalent?
- What stereotypes do you have about African-American men, women, and children?
- What culturally based health beliefs and practices do you think characterize African-Americans? How are these different from your own culturally based health beliefs and practices?

From Swanson J, Nies M: *Community health nursing: promoting the health of aggregates,* ed 2, Philadelphia, 1997, WB Saunders.

headaches, muscle pains, sinusitis, colds, sore throats, diarrhea, or fever. Cupping involves placing a heated cup on the skin; as it cools it contracts, drawing what is believed to be toxicity into the cup. A circular ecchymosis is left on the skin. Pinching may be at the base of the nose or between the eyes. Bruises or welts are left at the site of treatment. Rubbing or "coining" involves rubbing lubricated skin with a spoon or a coin to bring toxic "wind" to the body surface. A similar practice is burning, which involves touching a burning cigarette or piece of cotton to the skin, usually the abdomen, to compensate for "heat" lost through diarrhea (Nies and McEwen, 2001). These practices nurture the client's sense of well-being and security in being able to do something to correct disturbing symptoms. In most cases the practice would be considered adaptive (beneficial) or neutral. However, if the client had a clotting disorder, the practices would pose a threat to physical integrity and therefore be considered maladaptive (harmful) (Nies and McEwen, 2001).

Cultural Client Nutrition Assessment

A cultural nutrition assessment should be obtained for clients who are minorities. It is necessary to assess the client's cultural definition of food. For example, certain Latin American groups do not consider greens to be food. Therefore when asked to keep a food diary, these individuals would not list greens, which are an important source of vitamins and iron, as food eaten even though they eat them. Frequency and number of meals, amount and types of food eaten, and regularity of food consumption are other important factors that should be considered.

Among Asian-Americans, dietary intake of calcium may appear inadequate because this group usually consumes a relatively low amount of dairy products. However, they commonly consume pork bone and shells, thus taking in adequate quantities of calcium to meet minimum daily requirements. In cultures in which obesity is a problem, it is helpful for the nurse to have an idea of food preferences to help the client select low-calorie, low-fat foods. Asians tend to prefer spicy foods that may lead to the high incidence of stomach cancer, ulcers, and gastrointestinal bleeding (Purnell and Paulanka, 1998).

Nurses should avoid cultural stereotyping as it relates to food—all Italians do not necessarily like spaghetti, nor do all Chinese like rice. However, knowing the clients' general food preferences makes it possible to develop therapeutic interventions that do not conflict with their cultural food practices (Stanhope and Lancaster, 2004). General food preferences of aggregate groups are described in Table 11-4.

Cultural Beliefs About Sickness and Cures

It also is important for the nurse to consider nontraditional beliefs of sickness and cure in various cultures. For example, there are conditions that are not classified as diseases in Western culture; yet for different cultural groups these are real diseases for which the group has medicines and treatments. Examples of such diseases include mal ojo, susto, bilis, and empacho.

Mal ojo, also called "evil eye," is thought to be caused by persons giving admiration. "According to this belief, some people are born with 'vista fuerte' (strong vision) with which they unwittingly harm others with a mere glance" (Swanson and Albrecht, 1993, p. 414). For example, a stranger who lovingly admires a Mexican-American baby by looking into the baby's face can cause mal ojo. An infant who has mal ojo sleeps restlessly, has fever and diarrhea, and may ultimately die. Treatment consists of rubbing the body with an egg for three consecutive

Table 11-4	Selected Food Preferences and Associated Risk Factors Among Selected Cultural Groups		
CULTURAL GROUP	**FOOD PREFERENCES**	**NUTRITIONAL EXCESS**	**RISK FACTORS**
African-Americans	Fried foods, greens, bread, lard, pork, and rice	Cholesterol, fat, sodium, carbohydrates, and calories	Coronary heart disease and obesity
Asians	Soy sauce, rice, pickled dishes, and raw fish	Cholesterol, fat, sodium, carbohydrates, and calories	Coronary heart disease, liver disease, cancer of the stomach, and ulcers
Hispanics	Fried foods, beans, rice, chili, carbonated beverages	Cholesterol, fat, sodium, carbohydrates, and calories	Coronary heart disease and obesity
American Indians	Blue cornmeal, fruits, game, and fish	Carbohydrates and calories	Diabetes, malnutrition, tuberculosis, infant and maternal mortality

Data from Andrews M, Boyle J: *Transcultural concepts in nursing*, ed 3, Philadelphia, 1998, JB Lippincott; Giger JN, Davidhizar RE: *Transcultural nursing*, ed 3, St Louis, 1999, Mosby; Jackson, Broussard: Cultural challenges in nutrition education among American Indians, *Diabetic Educ* 13(11): 47-50, 1987.

nights. The egg is broken and left under the bed overnight. In the morning if the egg appears to be cooked, then mal ojo is believed to have definitely caused the illness. For protection, mothers often adorn their children with red yarn around their wrists or amulets that usually are a deer's eyes (Nies and McEwen, 2001).

Susto, or "fright sickness," is an emotion-based illness that is common among Mexicans. An unexpected fall, a barking dog, or a car accident could cause susto. Symptoms include colic, diarrhea, high temperature, and vomiting. Treatment involves brushing the body with "ruda" for nine consecutive nights. The brushing is performed to allow the spirit that has been removed by the disease to return to the body. The treatment often is accompanied by burning candles and prayers in home or church (Nies and McEwen, 2001).

Bilis is a disease brought on by anger. It primarily affects adults and commonly occurs a day or two after a fit of rage. If untreated, bilis can cause acute nervous tension and chronic fatigue, although herbal remedies usually are effective (Giger and Davidhizar, 1999).

Empacho is a disease that can affect children or adults and is caused by food particles becoming lodged in the intestinal tract, causing sharp pains. To manage this illness, the afflicted person lies face down on the bed with his or her back bared. The curer pinches a piece of skin at the waist, listening for a snap from the abdominal region. This is repeated several times in hope of dislodging the material. Empacho usually is not a serious disease (Nies and McEwen, 2001).

It is important to determine how culturally diverse clients define health and illness and whether their health beliefs and practices differ from the norm in the Western health care system (Spector, 2000a). For example, the Chinese often find many aspects of Western medicine distasteful. They cannot understand why so many diagnostic tests are necessary and tend to believe that a "good" physician has the ability to diagnose by thoroughly examining the client's body. Chinese clients dislike painful procedures such as the practice of drawing blood. In their culture blood is seen as the source of life for the entire body, and they believe that it is not regenerated. They have a deep respect for their bodies and prefer to die with their bodies

BOX 11–3 | Health Traditions Assessment Model

Maintaining Health

Physical	Are there special clothes one must wear; foods one must eat, not eat, or combinations to avoid; exercises one must do?
Mental	Are there special sources of entertainment; games or other ways of concentrating; traditional "rules of behavior?"
Spiritual	Are there special religious customs; prayers; meditations?

Protecting Health and Preventing Illness

Physical	Are there special foods that must be eaten after certain life events such as childbirth; dietary taboos that must be adhered to; symbolic clothes that must be worn?
Mental	Are there special people who must be avoided, rituals for self-protection, familial roles?
Spiritual	Are there special religious customs, superstitions, amulets, oils or waters?

Restoring Health

Physical	Are there special folk remedies; liniments; procedures such as cupping, acupuncture, or moxibustion?
Mental	Are there special healers such as curanderos; rituals; folk medicines?
Spiritual	Are there special rituals and prayers, meditations, healers?

From Spector RE: *Cultural diversity in health and illness,* ed 5, Upper Saddle River, NJ, 2000a, Prentice Hall.

intact. Therefore it is not uncommon for the Chinese to refuse surgery that would be mutilating to the body (Spector, 2000a).

Health represents a balance within the body, mind, and spirit. It is strongly affected by the family and community. Spector (2000b) suggests a model for assessing health traditions (Box 11-3) and has also developed a guide that can be used to assess clients' personal methods for maintaining health, protecting (preventing) illness, and restoring health (Table 11-5).

S U M M A R Y

In a society as diverse as the United States, health care cannot come in one form to fit the needs of everyone. Culture has a powerful influence on one's interpretation of health and illness and response to health care. All clients have the right to be understood and respected, despite their differences. They have the right to expect health care providers to acknowledge that their perspectives on and interpretations of health are legitimate. Health care professionals must make a commitment to increase their knowledge, sensitivity, and competence in cultural concepts and care. Perhaps no other group in the health profession has recognized the impact of cultural diversity on outcomes of health care more than nursing. Nurses always have supported the concept of holistic care. By understanding the client's perspective, the nurse can be a better advocate for the client. With increased knowledge, sensitivity, respect, and understanding, therapeutic interventions can be maximized to promote the highest quality of health for clients in our multicultural society. Additional information can be found in the websites listed in Box 11-4.

Table 11-5   Assessment Guide for Personal Methods to Maintain, Protect (Prevent Illness), and Restore Health

	PHYSICAL	MENTAL	SPIRITUAL
Maintain health	Are there special clothes you must wear at certain times of the day, week, year? Are there special foods you must eat at certain times? Do you have any dietary restrictions? Are there any foods that you cannot eat?	What do you do for activities, such as reading, sports, games? Do you have hobbies? Do you visit family often? Do you visit friends often?	Do you practice your religion and attend church or other communal activities? Do you pray or meditate? Do you observe religious customs? Do you belong to fraternal organizations?
Protect health or prevent illness	Are there foods that you cannot eat together? Are there special foods that you must eat? Are there any types of clothing that you are not allowed to wear?	Are there people or situations that you have been taught to avoid? Do you take extraordinary precautions under certain circumstances? Do you take time for yourself?	Do you observe religious customs? Do you wear any amulets or hang them in your house? Do you have any practices such as always opening the window when you sleep? Do you have any other practice to protect yourself from "harm?"
Restore health	What kinds of medicines do you take before you see a doctor or nurse? Are there herbs that you take? Are there special treatments that you use?	Do you know of any specific practices your mother or grandmother may use to relax? Do you know how big problems can be cared for in your community? Do you drink special teas to help you unwind or relax?	Do you know any healers? Do you know of any religious rituals that help to restore health? Do you meditate? Do you ever go to a healing service? Do you know about exorcism?

From Spector RE: *Cultural diversity in health and illness,* ed 5, Upper Saddle River, NJ, 2000a, Prentice Hall.

BOX 11–4   Helpful Websites

Healthy People 2010
www.health.gov/healthy people/
www.omhrc.gov/clas/cultural/a.htm#project%20overview

U.S. Census Bureau: Money Income in the United States 1999
www.census.gov/hhes/income/income99/99tablea.html

American Cancer Society: Cancer Facts and Figures—1997: Racial and Ethnic Patterns
www.cancer.org/statistics

US Census Bureau: Poverty 1998: Poverty by Selected Characteristics, 1999
www/census.gov/hhes/poverty/poverty98/pv98est1.html

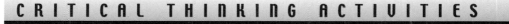

CRITICAL THINKING ACTIVITIES

1. What principles and actions must a staff nurse apply to provide culturally competent care?

2. What factors should a community nurse educator consider when planning a health promotion program for a minority group who does not speak English?
3. How can health care organizations promote the cultural competence of nursing staff?
4. What strategies can be used to recruit and retain minorities in nursing?

Additional resources are available on-line at: http://evolve.elsevier.com/Cherry/

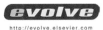

http://evolve.elsevier.com

REFERENCES

AAN Expert Panel on Culturally Competent Health Care: Culturally competent health care, *Nurs Outlook* 40(6):277-283, 1992.

American Association of Colleges of Nursing: *AACN issue bulletin: effective strategies for increasing diversity in nursing programs*, Washington, DC, 2001, AACN.

Assessing Cultural Competence in Health Care: *Recommendations for national standards and outcomes—focused research agenda.* Retrieved on-line February 14, 2004 (http://www.omhrc.gov/clas/cultural1a.htm#Project%20Overview).

Bessent H: *Strategies for recruitment, retention and graduation of minority nurses in colleges of nursing*, Washington, DC, 1997, American Nurses Foundation.

Council of Economic Advisers for the President's Initiative on Race: *Changing America: indicators of social and economic well-being by race and Hispanic origin, Washington*, DC, 1999, US Government Printing Office.

Giger JN, Davidhizer RE: *Transcultural nursing*, ed 3, St Louis, 1999, Mosby.

Hall J, Stevens P, Meleis A: Marginalization: a guiding concept for valuing diversity in nursing knowledge development, *Adv Nurs Sci* 16(4):23-24, 1994.

Heller B: Strategies for increasing student diversity in schools of nursing: lessons learned, *Hispanic Health Care International*, 1(2):68-70, 2002.

Lenburg C et al: *Promoting cultural competence in and through nursing education: a critical review and comprehensive plan for action*, Washington, DC, 1995, American Academy of Nursing.

Medcom: *Cultural assessment (film)*, Cypress, Calif, 1997, Medcom.

Meleis A et al: *Diversity, marginalization, and culturally competent healthcare issues in knowledge development*, Washington, DC, 1995, American Academy of Nursing.

National League for Nursing: *Criteria for the evaluation of baccalaureate and higher degree programs in nursing*, New York, 1996, National League for Nursing.

Nies M, McEwen M: *Community health nursing: promoting the health of populations*, ed 3, Philadelphia, 2001, WB Saunders.

Purnell L, Paulanka B: *Transcultural health care*, Philadelphia, 1998, FA Davis.

Spector R: *Cultural diversity in health and illness*, ed 5, Upper Saddle River, NJ, 2000a, Prentice Hall.

Spector R: *Guide to heritage assessment and health traditions*, Upper Saddle River, NJ, 2000b, Prentice Hall.

Stanhope M, Lancaster J: *Community health and public health nursing*, ed 6, St Louis, 2004, Mosby.

Sullivan EJ: *Differences: reflections, second quarter*, Indianapolis, 1998, Sigma Theta Tau.

Swanson J, Albrecht M: *Community health nursing: promoting the health of aggregates*, Philadelphia, 1993, WB Saunders.

Swanson J, Nies M: *Community health nursing: promoting the health of aggregates*, ed 2, Philadelphia, 1997, WB Saunders.

U.S. Department of Health and Human Services, Public Health Service: *Healthy people 2000*, Washington, DC, 1990, U.S. Government Printing Office.

U.S. Department of Health and Human Services, Public Health Service: *Healthy people 2010: national health promotion and disease prevention objectives*, Washington, DC, 2000, US Government Printing Office.

U.S. Department of Health and Human Services: *Projected supply, demand, and shortage of registered nurses*: 2000-2020, Washington, DC, 2002, US Government printing Office.

SUGGESTED READINGS

Andrews M, Boyle J: *Transcultural concepts in nursing care*, ed 3, Philadelphia, 1999, JB Lippincott.

Fadiman A: *The spirit catches you and you fall down*, New York, 1997, Farrar, Straus and Giroux.

Health Resources and Services Administration, Bureau of Health Professions: *A national agenda for nursing workforce racial/ethnic diversity*, Washington, DC, 2000, US Department of Health and Human Services, National Advisory Council on Nursing Education and Practice.

Huff RM: *Promoting health in multicultural populations: a handbook for practitioners*, Thousand Oaks, Calif, 1999, Sage.

Leininger M: Transcultural nursing education: a worldwide imperative, *Nurs Health Care* 15(5):254-257, 1994.

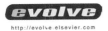
12

Workplace Advocacy and the Nursing Shortage

Alexia Green, PhD, RN, FAAN, and
K. Lynn Wieck, PhD, RN

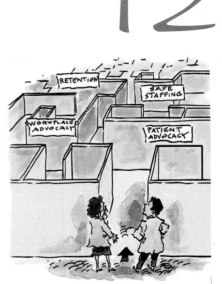

A changing workplace requires nurses to embrace workplace advocacy to ensure quality health care delivery.

VIGNETTE

As a new graduate, 26-year-old Elena Gonzalez is searching for her first position as a registered nurse (RN) in a large metropolitan city in the Southwest United States. As part of her education, she learns about the importance of the nurses' role in advocating for a workplace conducive to delivering safe and effective quality health care. She also understands that the workplace is filled with complex issues—nursing shortages, staffing issues, potential exposure to blood-borne diseases—affecting the nurse, the patient, the organization, and the profession. As a result of the nursing shortage, Elena receives many offers from various organizations with promises of sign-on bonuses and other incentives. However, she wisely chooses not to accept a job on its "face value" and decides to investigate her opportunities more thoroughly. Using the Internet, she searches the websites of hospitals in her target area. She is looking for the answers to questions like these: Have any organizations within my area received magnet hospital status? Which organizations have shared governance models? Are nurses encouraged to participate in shared governance? What is the content and length of orientation for new nurses? What is the organization's philosophy regarding staff mix designations? Does the organization have a conflict resolution process? What is the organization's turnover rate, and what is the average longevity of staff nurses? Answers to these questions are accessible on health workforce websites, from hospital nurse recruiters, or from the nurse educators in charge of the hospital orientation program. Armed with answers to these and other questions, Elena decides to accept a position with a large tertiary care center that she believes has created an environment most supportive of ensuring the delivery of quality patient care. However, she knows that with the acceptance of this position, her role as a workplace and patient advocate has not ended; rather, it has only just begun.

Questions to consider while reading this chapter:

1. What workplace advocacy strategies can Elena use to promote quality patient care and a safe work environment?
2. What is the value of shared governance to Elena's individual nursing practice?
3. If Elena becomes concerned about floating assignments, what questions can help guide her decision about accepting such assignments?
4. What on-line resources are available to help Elena learn more about important workplace issues and workplace advocacy?
5. How can Elena gain increased marketability of her nursing expertise?

K E Y   T E R M S

Patient advocacy The nurse and the nursing profession's powerful voice at the local, state, and national levels in supporting policies that protect consumers and enhance accountability for quality by promoting safer health care systems. Patient advocacy is a cornerstone of the nursing profession, and patients depend on nurses to ensure that they receive quality care. Workplace advocacy is a component of patient advocacy.

Professional practice advocacy Professional activities that encompass two primary mechanisms to promote and maintain a professional practice environment: workplace advocacy and collective bargaining.

Workplace advocacy An array of activities that promote power bases to afford nurses an optimal professional work environment. The objective is to equip nurses to skillfully use a range of external and internal workplace strategies that are complementary in nature, focus on strengthening nursing's voice, and ensure nurse involvement in workplace decisions affecting nursing care. Workplace advocacy uses universally empowering strategies while supporting effective and efficient patient care.

Workplace issues An array of complex issues that confront nurses in the workplace on a daily basis. These complex issues not only affect the nurse, but also the patient, the organization, and the profession. Examples include the nursing shortage, adequate staffing levels, errors in health care delivery, and violence in the workplace.

L E A R N I N G   O U T C O M E S

After studying this chapter, the reader will be able to:

1. Describe workplace advocacy as a means of improving the quality of health care delivery.
2. Identify issues that affect the practice of professional nursing in the health care workplace.
3. Identify available resources to assist in improving the workplace environment.
4. Define the role of nurses in advocating for safe and effective workplace environments.
5. Describe both internal and external workplace strategies that support efficient and effective quality patient care.
6. Identify unique opportunities within the organization to improve the work environment for nurses.

In today's modern health care system, nurses are faced with many workplace issues. These complex issues affect not only the nurse, but also the patient, the organization, and the profession. This chapter attempts to identify a few select critical issues currently facing nurses and the nursing profession, including the nursing shortage, appropriate staffing, patient safety and advocacy, and workplace rights and safety. Professional practice advocacy is defined, and specific strategies under the domain of workplace advocacy are highlighted. To be a successful and accountable professional, nurses must recognize current issues and know where to seek support for workplace advocacy.

PROMOTING A PROFESSIONAL PRACTICE ENVIRONMENT

Professional nurses are seeing the dawn of an era of involvement and control in the work environment that was unheard of a decade ago. Important research is validating the contribution and value of registered nurses in the following areas:

- Improved patient outcomes (Needleman et al, 2002)
- Prevention of premature mortality (Aiken et al, 2002)
- Increased hospital profitability (McCue, Mark, and Harless, 2003)

Within this context of the important contributions that nurses make to patients, hospitals, and health care in general, we find nurses challenged to deliver care against all kinds of barriers and with dwindling resources. Nurses' strong concern and commitment to patient care and their role as patient advocates often places them in direct conflict with those who have more control, such as physicians and administrators of health care organizations. How the nurse reacts to this conflict, how the nurse continues to advocate for patients in this environment, and what powers the nurse can call on to improve care for patients are issues of a new focus for the profession as we enter the twenty-first century—a focus called "professional practice advocacy." Professional practice advocacy has been described as an umbrella of professional activities encompassing two primary mechanisms to promote and maintain a professional practice environment: workplace advocacy and collective bargaining (a detailed discussion about collective bargaining can be found on-line at http://evolve.elsevier.com/cherry/).

Professional Practice Advocacy

Professional practice advocacy, as defined by the American Nurses Association (ANA) in 1999, encompasses the programs and services intended to promote and support professional practice standards in the workplace. Included are those activities supportive of nurses' advocacy for their patients, professional practice self-determination, and the exercise of their employment rights and responsibilities. As we visit Elena Gonzalez 6 months after she assumed her new position, we find that she has become involved in advocating for a safe work environment. Elena and the other nurses working on the medical unit are concerned because retractable needle devices are not available on their unit. The patients on the medical unit often have diagnoses of hepatitis B infection, and the nurses are worried about needlestick injuries. Where will they find information about needlestick safety and other workplace safety issues? Are there laws that require hospitals to implement safety measures to protect their staff against blood-borne pathogens? What legal rights do nurses have to demand safe needle devices? Is there an avenue to work with hospital administrators to decrease the costs associated with unsafe practices and to move toward a user-friendly work environment? All of these questions are related to professional practice advocacy, specifically workplace advocacy. Examples of professional practice advocacy are included in Box 12-1.

Workplace Advocacy

As a component of professional practice advocacy, workplace advocacy promotes power bases that afford nurses optimal work environments. The objective is to equip nurses to skillfully use a range of external and internal workplace strategies. These strategies are to be complementary in nature, focusing on strengthening nursing's voice and ensuring nurses' involvement in workplace decisions affecting nursing care. ANA defined workplace advocacy in 1993 as: "an array of activities which are initiated to address the many and varied employment and workplace challenges nurses face on a daily basis. As the definition of advocacy implies, these activities range from supporting and sustaining efforts to more innovative and assertive measures. Workplace advocacy is inherent in the role and responsibility of each professional nurse" (Young, Hayes, and Morin, 1993, p. 1). Workplace advocacy uses universally empowering strategies while supporting effective and efficient patient care. Elena and her colleagues will be empowered to improve the workplace when they find the answers to their questions. By knowing where to seek information and other resources to solve workplace problems, nurses promote safe and effective workplaces.

In 2000 the ANA committed to supporting the profession through workplace advocacy strategies with the formation of the Commission on Workplace Advocacy (CWPA). Commitment to workplace advocacy was further refined in 2003, with structural changes within ANA resulting in the creation of the Center for American Nurses *(CAN),* formally the CWPA. The *CAN* (located on-line at http://nursingworld.org/can) is an independent national professional association established by the ANA House of Delegates to address the needs of individual nurses who are *not* represented by collective bargaining in their employment setting. *CAN's* (2004) purposes are to:

1. Offer noncollective bargaining workplace advocacy strategies, programs, and services to nurses
2. Support nurses in personal and professional growth and development in the practice setting in order to promote positive work-related experiences

---

BOX 12–1   *Examples of Professional Practice Advocacy*

Promoting and protecting the occupational safety and health of nurses
Using nurse practice acts and other legislative and regulatory protections
Using the political process to influence legislative and regulatory agencies for the protection of nurses and patients
Providing education regarding employment rights and responsibilities
Developing skills related to public relations, media presentations, and conflict resolution
Building coalitions and support groups to enable nurses to speak and advocate for their professional practices
Negotiating and administering strong and effective employment contracts
Participating in committee structures of the hospital to ensure a nursing voice in safety and workplace issues

Adapted from American Nurses Association: *Definition of professional practice advocacy adopted by House of Delegates (internal document),* Washington, DC, 1999, ANA.

3. Collaborate with others to provide services and to develop policies that positively affect the work environment for all nurses
4. Provide education to nurses on workplace issues
5. Promote and provide leadership and mentoring in the workplace environment
6. Conduct, evaluate, and support workplace-related research

Currently there are 37 state nurses associations, along with the Federal Nurses Association, that are *CAN* members. Developing an effective workplace advocacy program is a complex multifaceted role for the individual nurse and professional organizations such as the national and state nurses associations. The Texas Nurses Association (TNA), a leader in workplace advocacy, identified five opportunities and challenges for workplace advocacy programs (Box 12-2). Other examples of workplace and patient advocacy will be discussed, along with specific workplace issues, in the following sections of the chapter.

BOX 12–2   *Five Opportunities/Challenges for Workplace Advocacy Programs*

1. Identify mechanisms within health care systems that provide opportunities for RNs to affect institutional policies.
   - Shared governance
   - Participatory management models
   - Magnet hospital identification
   - Statewide staffing regulations

2. Develop conflict resolution models for use within organizations that address RNs' concerns about patient care and delivery issues.
   - Identification of the reporting loop
   - Appointment of a final arbiter in disputes

3. Seek legislative solutions for workplace problems by reviewing issues of concern to nurses in employment settings and introducing appropriate legislation, such as:
   - Whistle-blower protection
   - "Safe Harbor" peer review
   - Support for rules outlining strong nursing practice standards

4. Develop legal centers for nurses, which could provide legal support and decision-making advice as a last recourse to resolve workplace issues.
   - Provide fast and efficient legal assistance to nurses
   - Earmark precedent setting cases that could impact case law and health care policy

5. Provide RNs in practice with self advocacy and patient advocacy information, such as:
   - Laws and regulations governing practice
   - Use of applicable nursing practice standards
   - Conflict resolution and negotiation techniques
   - Identifying state/national reporting mechanisms that allow RNs to report concerns about health care organizations and/or professionals

Adapted from Texas Nurses Association: *Workplace advocacy program*, Austin, Tex, 2001, Author, Available on-line (www.texanurses.org).

THE NURSING SHORTAGE

The nursing profession has a long history of cyclic shortages, which have been documented since World War II (Minnick, 2000). The acute cyclic shortage impacting the nation during the late 1990s and the early 2000s was a direct result of the struggle to implement managed care as a means of controlling the escalating cost of health care. As we move further into the twenty-first century, the profession faces another shortage, one that promises to be much more complex and long-lasting and threatens to dwarf all shortages to date (Nevidjon and Erickson, 2001).

At a time when the U.S. nursing population is aging and more nurses are moving into primary care settings, an increasing number of baby boomers are also aging, resulting in a higher demand for quality health care. As a result, there is a need for more nurses, especially those who deliver specialized care. Professional nursing is the largest U.S. health care occupation, and according to the Bureau of Labor Statistics (2003), employment opportunities for professional nurses will grow more rapidly than all other U.S. occupations through 2010. By 2010, the United States is projected to need almost 1 million more registered nurses than will be available. The demand for registered nurses is projected to increase by 40% in 2020, whereas the supply will have increased by only 6% (U.S. Department of Health and Human Services, 2002). Planning for an adequate workforce will be one of the most critical challenges of the new century. Although the current nursing shortage is related to both supply and demand issues, a closer look at several confounding variables provides an insight into the complexity of the shortage and the need for an array of actions.

Health Care is No Longer a Favored Employer

In examining the shortage of nurses, which is also accompanied by a shortage of other health care workers, the attractiveness of careers in health care, especially hospital care, has declined over the last two decades (American Hospital Association, 2001). In a single generation health care has moved from a favored to a less favored employment sector. The American Hospital Association (2001) framed this insight by five observations:

1. In an earlier manufacturing economy, health care was considered high-tech, but in our current information economy, young people view health care as low-tech.
2. In the 1960s, 1970s, and 1980s health care was considered safe, secure, and prestigious employment, but in today's labor market health care is seen as chaotic and unstable.
3. In a traditional society, health care was one of only a few employment options for women, but in contemporary society health care is one of many choices.
4. In a long-stay hospital system, such as that of the 1960s, 1970s, and 1980s, nurses had strong, supportive relationships with patients, but in today's short-stay hospital system nurses are focused on disease protocols, regulatory compliance, and documentation.
5. In a mass-production society in which production schedules controlled work hours, the 24-hour/7-days-a-week demands of hospitals were seen as an unattractive, but necessary, burden; however, in an information society in which more people are able to schedule work time at their own convenience, these demands are considered unacceptable.

The identification and recognition of these changes, along with the other changes identified in the following paragraphs, provide hospitals and health care systems with the unavoidable requirement to redesign work and workplace environments so that they are able to attract, retain, and develop the best RN workforce.

Insufficient Nursing School Enrollments and Recruitment

One factor contributing to the aging of the nursing workforce is that younger birth cohorts (i.e., those born after 1955) are smaller in population size, as well as significantly less likely to choose nursing as a career (Buerhaus, Staiger, and Auerbach, 2000). Evidence of this trend was seen in the decline in nursing school enrollments, which dropped by 20.9% between 1995 and 1998 (Carpenter, 2000). Since many young nurses are attracted to the excitement of a critical care setting, acute care settings in particular have been hit hard by this decline in younger nurses entering the workforce. The declining size of graduating classes of professional nurses resulted in a shrinking supply of RNs wanting to work in critical care settings (Buerhaus, Staiger, and Auerbach, 2000). A second factor contributing to the shrinking nursing workforce is the expanded career opportunities for women outside of nursing. Women currently make up 90% of the professional nursing workforce (Bednash, 2000). The first factor of an overall smaller number of individuals available to enter the workforce is beyond the control of the profession; however, we are challenged to make our profession attractive to young men and women as a viable career alternative.

Numerous efforts are presently underway to recruit more students into nursing. Twenty-one of the nation's leading nursing and health care organizations formed a coalition, called Nurses for a Healthier Tomorrow, in an attempt to provide long-term help (Sigma Theta Tau International, 2000). According to the coalition, highly visible patient and professional complaints about managed care in the early 1990s have discouraged young people from entering the nursing profession. The first phase of the coalition's work also reveals that students from second through tenth grades are confused about the training involved to become a nurse, are unsure of job security and career advancement possibilities, and voice a lack of compelling reasons to become a nurse. Another group working on recruitment into nursing is the National Student Nurses Association, which has produced a video titled *Nursing: The Ultimate Adventure*, which is targeted at junior and senior high school students.

Unfortunately, even when attempts to recruit more people into nursing have been successful, most schools and universities find themselves unable to expand their nursing programs to accept the qualified applicants because they are faced with a serious shortage of nursing faculty. National and statewide efforts have resulted in increases in nursing school enrollments for 3 consecutive years (2001-2003); yet these increases continue to fall below the projected need to reverse the nursing shortage (AACN, 2003). Enrollments in entry-level baccalaureate programs in nursing increased by 15.9% in fall 2003 over the previous year. Though this increase continues a 3-year upward trend, this growth is still not sufficient to address the current RN shortage, which is expected to intensify over the next 10 years. By 2020 the deficit of nurses will be near 1 million, almost three times that of many allied health workers (O'Neil, 2003).

Along with the need to recruit into the profession, nursing must continue to examine the ways in which new nurses are introduced into the nursing work culture. Adequate orientation, mentoring, and preceptor programs are absolutely essential to introducing and retaining new nurses. Several health care organizations eliminated these programs during the 1990s for reasons associated with cost reduction during reorganization efforts. Many health care organizations are now working to rebuild these programs (ANA, 2000a).

Educational Preparation

During past shortages, employers have hired RNs, regardless of their degree preparation (American Association of Colleges of Nursing [AACN], 2001). The current and projected demands for RNs requires not simply more RNs, but more RNs of the right type and right educational and skill mix to handle increasingly complex care demands. Demand has intensified for more baccalaureate-prepared nurses with critical thinking, leadership, case management, and health promotion skills who are capable of delivering care across a variety of structured and unstructured health care settings. Additionally, baccalaureate level education has been associated with lower patient mortality (Aiken et al, 2003). Demand has also increased for experienced RNs; for nurses in key clinical specialties such as critical care, emergency department, operating room, and neonatal intensive care; and for master's- and doctoral-prepared RNs in advanced clinical specialties, teaching, and research.

Historically nursing has sought to educate its way out of a nursing shortage, primarily by producing more associate degree graduates. According to Bednash (2000), one challenge is to overcome perceptions that nursing is not intellectually stimulating by rewarding advanced education such as a baccalaureate degree over an associate degree or diploma. Currently few health care organizations differentiate practice or provide significant financial differentials based on educational preparation of the professional nurse.

Faculty Shortage

Presently, one of the most critical problems facing nursing and nursing workforce planning is the aging of nursing faculty (AACN, 2003). According to the AACN in 2002, the mean age of nursing faculty has steadily increased to 53.3 for doctoral faculty and 48.8 for master's faculty. Unfortunately, the shortage of faculty is contributing to the current nursing shortage by limiting the number of students admitted to nursing programs. In 2002, an AACN survey determined that 5283 qualified applications to nursing schools were not accepted; and an insufficient number of faculty were cited by 41.7% of schools as a reason for not accepting all qualified applicants (Berlin, Stennett, and Bednash, 2003). Faculty salaries continue to be a major contributor to the faculty shortage. According to the AACN (2003), academic institutions, especially those faced with budget cuts, generally cannot compete with nonacademic employers. In fall 2001, the median academic-year salaries for instructional faculty with doctoral degrees in public institutions with the ranks of associate and assistant professors were $59,772 and $51,897, respectively. Most schools point to budget constraints when reporting too few faculty. However, 30% said faculty shortages were due to increasing job competition from higher-paying clinical sites (AACN, 2003).

Nurse Retention

Contributing to the disenchantment with nursing is the lingering cynicism caused by the downsizing of hospitals in the 1990s. Unsettled by restructuring, downsizing, and other management fads some organizations implemented during the 90s, many nurses believe that health care no longer offers the stability and job security it once did (Gelinas and Bohlen, 2002). Compounding health care's image problem is the knowledge that nursing is often physically and emotionally demanding, and exposes nurses to pathogens and work-related injuries. Additionally, in today's telecommuting, Internet-connected society, where people are accustomed to defining their own schedules and workspace, the demands of 24/7/365 staffing, on-call work, and mandatory overtime seem increasingly unattractive (AHA, 2001).

Past nursing shortages have proven that the retention of professional nurses is a key to any organization's success. As shortages occur, nurses are often enticed away from one organization to another with lucrative sign-on bonuses, shift differentials, and promises of a work environment that promotes professional autonomy. Once a shortage has abated, the monetary rewards of joining a particular organization tend to quickly fade. Further complicating the nurse retention issue is the likelihood that younger generation nurses, like their 20-something-aged counterparts in corporate America, find that frequent job change is a means to increased marketability and positive career sculpting (Tulgan, 2003). The ability of an organization to retain nurses primarily depends on the creation of an environment conducive to professional autonomy. The importance of autonomy in professional practice is a critical issue for nurses. Nurses want to work in an environment that supports decision making and effective nurse-physician relationships as interdependent and essential concepts of nursing practice (Gleason, Sochalski, and Aiken, 1999). Furthermore, younger nurses want opportunities to engage in entrepreneurial activities, practice free agency, and have balance in their lives (Wieck, Prydun, and Walsh, 2002).

Magnet Hospitals

One of the most successful retention models focuses on promoting standards for professional nursing practice and recognizing quality, excellence, and service. In 1980, recognizing a critical and widespread national shortage of nurses, the American Academy of Nurses undertook a study to identify a national sample of what are referred to as "magnet hospitals" (i.e., those that attract and retain professional nurses in their employment) and to identify the factors that seem to be associated with their success in doing so (McClure et al, 1983). This landmark study, entitled Magnet Hospitals: Attraction and Retention of Professional Nurses, identified workplace factors such as management style, nursing autonomy, quality of leadership, organizational structure, professional practice, career development, and quality of patient care as influencing nurse job satisfaction and low turnover rates in the acute care setting. As a result, the ANA began a program recognizing hospitals with excellent nursing recruitment and high retention rates. Out of 165 hospitals initially participating, only 41 were deemed magnet hospitals for their ability to support nurse autonomy and decision making in the workplace.

As the magnet hospital program evolved, it sought to combine the strengths of the original study with quality indicators identified by ANA and the standards of nursing practice as defined in ANA's Scope and Standards for Nurse Administrators so that both quantitative and qualitative factors of nursing services were measured. With its link between quality patient care and nursing excellence, the Magnet Recognition Program for Nursing Excellence has reached a coveted level of prestige within the nursing community and among acute care facilities. Magnet status is now seen as the single most effective mechanism for providing consumers and nurses with comparative information, a seal of approval for quality nursing care. Research has shown (Aiken, Havens, and Sloane, 2000) that magnet hospital nurses have higher levels of autonomy, more control over the practice setting, and better relationships with physicians. Nurses advocating for a strong workplace should advocate for their hospital to achieve magnet hospital status.

Aging Workforce and Retention

As the nation works to increase the supply of professional nurses through education, nursing and the health care system must develop strategies that will retain the older, expert professional nurse within the nursing workforce. The following statistics detail the extent of the aging workforce issue:

- In 2000, the national average age of professional nurses was 44.3 years.
- In 2000, RNs under 30 years of age represented only 10% of the total nurse population.

■ In 2005, large cohorts of baby boomer RNs will begin to reach the age (55 years) at which RNs have historically begun to reduce their labor participation (Minnick, 2000).

■ Professional nurses over the age of 40 now represent nearly 60% of the workforce (Buerhaus, Staiger, and Auerbach, 2000).

The shortage will worsen by 2010, when almost all of these RNs will have reached retirement years. A review of the literature shows that very little research has been done, particularly within nursing, about the impact of the aging workforce and potential accommodations that may need to be made to retain the experienced nurse (ANA, 2000b).

For hospitals and other health care organizations, the challenge in helping nurses achieve long-term careers and retaining an aging nursing population is to create an environment in which both baby boomer nurses and generation X nurses (and beyond) can thrive (Ulrich, 2001). Many organizations have added on-site day and sick care for children of younger nurses. Because of the aging workforce, organizations will need to consider adding adult day care to assist older nurses who are caring for aging parents. Creative staffing plans with shorter shifts and identified respite periods may help extend the work life of aging nurses. Technology has provided many workplace accessories that reduce the physical demands on nurses that can potentially result in injury or stress, especially to aging nurses. ANA's "Handle With Care" initiative aims at eliminating lifting in the hospital environment by using technology and assistive devices to do the heavy work (ANA, 2003). Ergonomic issues are important for staff of any age, but additional attention will be needed as the workforce ages. Organizations that strategically plan for an aging workforce will be best positioned to deliver quality health care to their customers.

Emerging Workforce Recruitment and Retention

In addition to planning for retention of an aging workforce, health care is challenged to become the employer of choice for the younger emerging workforce. The younger generation, born between 1969 and 1985, presents unique problems for the health care environment. Tulgan (2003) has written extensively about the work and management expectations of today's young worker who expects balance and perspective in the workplace. The overall goals of the 20-something generation are to start at the top, avoid long hours, and have fun on the job (Bradford and Raines, 1992). It is evident that this description does not fit very many jobs in health care, although it neatly typifies the young entrepreneurial "dot.com" industry executive. Many young workers desire to be entrepreneurs and seek to take advantage of free-agent type career options (Pink, 2001). Again, these options are limited in the current health care environment, where round-the-clock patient care is mandatory, including weekends and holidays.

Our young nurse described at the beginning of the chapter, Elena, will be searching for opportunities to gain advanced training, education, and certification as she seeks to make herself more marketable in her professional nursing role. She expects feedback on her performance to help refine her skills and build her confidence. She also expects her manager to take a personal interest in her, to know her name and to help her build a competitive portfolio. Many managers are unaware of these expectations in emerging workforce employees and contribute to their hastened exit from the workplace by not attending to their personal and career needs.

Today's typical hospital workplace may have members of four generations working together at the same time. The resulting clash of ideas, incentives, and goals make the work of today's manager extremely difficult. The younger generation has clear expectations of what they want in a manager, educator, and leader (Wieck, Prydun, and Walsh, 2002). They are seeking a manager who is approachable, supportive, receptive, and motivating. They want to be taught by and led by someone who serves as a coach, mentor, and guide who gets to know them personally (Bradford and Raines, 1992).

Today's fast-paced health care environment holds many attractions to young people who are comfortable with technology and who excel at multitasking. Hospitals are high-tech environments with lasers in surgery and technologically advanced machinery at all levels of care. However, young workers want to have fun and balance in their lives as well. The serious, overworked, and frustrated demeanor of many older colleagues is a turn-off to younger workers who do not plan to stay more than 2 or 3 years at any one institution anyway (Tulgan, 2003). They want to learn all they can, achieve certifications and training, and then move on to negotiate a better work situation at a different institution. Hospitals see this as lack of loyalty. Young workers see this as smart career sculpting. Hospitals are greatly challenged to make the work environment one that embraces the young worker by allowing for career investment and personal achievement. Managing multiple generations and various cultures within one setting is a great challenge for today's health care managers.

Foreign Nurse Recruitment

Long relied on as a remedy for nursing shortages has been the recruitment of foreign nurses. However, this method of resolving the U.S. nursing shortage is particularly problematic for two reasons. First, the current shortage is worldwide; therefore recruitment of foreign nurses results in an intensified shortage in the country from which the nurses were recruited. Second, the Employment and Training Administration has recognized the status of RNs as a permanent shortage profession, which, combined with the rules surrounding the granting of visas, makes foreign nurse recruitment open to abuse (Tabone, 2000).

Abuse of nurses from foreign countries is a possibility because of their vulnerable status, limited social support, and language challenges. Any indication that foreign nurses are being deprived of their rights or unfairly treated in compensation or work requirements should be reported to the state nurses association. Monitoring of foreign nurses' employment falls under the authority of the U.S. Department of Labor.

A primary example of foreign nurse abuse occurred in Texas during the 1990s, when many foreign nurses were employed in the state and the prevailing wage fell $3 per hour. In addition, many foreign nurses suffered abuses in living conditions, as well as through sexual harassment (Tabone, 2000). An investigation conducted by the U.S. Departments of Labor, Justice, and Immigration resulted in the conviction of the owner of multiple long-term care facilities (Tabone, 1998). The owner was convicted of operating an alien-smuggling ring that exploited foreign nurses and jeopardized fair labor standards in Texas. He was found guilty of obtaining fraudulent visas; recruiting nurses from the Philippines, Jamaica, and Korea; and paying them substandard wages in long-term care facilities in Texas and Oklahoma. The fraud was uncovered by an investigation instigated by the TNA, who advocated on behalf of the foreign nurses and nurses living in west Texas. Back wages totaling approximately $1.5 million were awarded to the foreign RNs (Tabone, 2000). State nurses' associations such as the TNA are committed to preventing foreign nurse abuse and related wage abuses of RNs, both foreign and domestic.

Recruitment of foreign nurses brings many other challenges and hurdles. Many of these challenges relate to the complicated and costly immigration and credentialing processes.

There is no consistent standard of nursing education worldwide. Therefore, the credentials of foreign nurses must be assessed before licensure is considered. Most scrutiny of credentials is done by the Commission on Graduates of Foreign Nursing Schools (CGFNS). Credentialing requirements and utilization of CGFNS information varies from state to state. In addition, the U.S. Department of Labor's visa program has become much more stringent since the terrorist attacks of September 11, 2001, making international recruitment much more cumbersome (Farrington and Martucci, 2003).

Ethical issues related to foreign nurse recruitment are also emerging as more and more industrialized countries are relying on the importation of foreign nurses to meet their health care needs, while at the same time depleting those resources in underdeveloped countries. An example of this has been reported in Bostwana, where the HIV epidemic is now being threatened not so much by unwillingness to acknowledge the problem, lack of access to drugs, or inadequate public health infrastructure, but by the fact that other nations are recruiting their nurses away in sufficient numbers to deteriorate the health of the nation (Dugger, 2003).

Compensation

Buerhaus (1998), a leading nursing workforce researcher, found that during the 1980s professional nursing hourly wages increased by approximately 3% each year. Unfortunately, during the 1990s nursing salaries remained flat as hospitals dealt with mounting financial pressures from Medicare cuts and managed care belt-tightening. Low compensation levels during the 1990s have definitely contributed to the current nursing shortage. In 1996 the national average annual salary of an RN in a staff nurse position was $38,567 (Moses, 1998). Salary compression has long plagued the nursing profession, with little opportunity for extended growth of salary as nurses gain more experience.

Again, as in past nursing shortages, health care agencies are moving to offer relocation bonuses and other financial and fringe benefits to attract nurses. To ease the shortage, hospitals and other health care employers are using sign-on bonuses of up to $10,000, increased recruitment of foreign nurses, new concessions in flexible scheduling, and a growing reliance on "traveling nurses" (Carpenter, 2000). All of these mechanisms result in considerable expenditures by health care organizations. Many believe that these recruitment-related costs could be better spent by increasing basic compensation levels of professional nurses. As past shortages have abated, so has the offering of financial bonuses and differential pay scales.

Fortunately, a sharp increase in RN wages occurred in 2002, with real earnings increasing nearly 5% (Buerhaus, Staiger, and Auerbach, 2003). The *Nursing 2003* annual salary survey reported the average salary for all respondents was $49,634, an 8.3% increase from the 2002 average (Robinson and Mee, 2003). This increase reflects the acceleration in the demand for RNs that occurred in 2001 and 2002, along with increasing collective bargaining activity and several labor strikes. According to Spetz and Given (2003), the economic principle that wage changes can bring supply and demand into balance, and thus rectify shortages, predicts that the increases in RN wages, if continued, will end the nursing shortage in the near future. However, the current nursing shortage is unique, and concerted additional efforts must be made to rectify the problem. Historically, nursing shortages have lasted 3 to 8 years and have been followed by periods of equilibrium or surpluses of similar length. Spetz and Given (2003) believe this is unlikely to happen unless substantial wage growth occurs and graduations increase significantly over the next 10 years. According to projections, cumulative real wage growth between 2002 and 2016 would need to exceed 55.4% to substantially affect the abatement of the shortage.

The emerging workforce, aged 18 to 35 years, has compensation expectations that differ from previous generations (Tulgan, 2003). This generation prefers to work in an outcomes-based environment, where pay is based on achievement or merit, not on longevity. They seek opportunities for entrepreneurial projects where they can compete for financial rewards. They prefer alternative work models, such as working on-line and extended breaks in employment, to ensure balance in their work and personal lives. The 24-hour-a-day work environment of the hospital precludes many of the alternatives to balance work and personal life that attract young people into a profession. This fact may be one of the reasons that young persons are opting out of health careers. Those choosing to remain in health care should see substantial growth in wages over the next 10 to 15 years.

Work Environment

According to the ANA (2000b), the work environment is a significant contributor to the difficulty in recruiting and retaining RNs. Although pay rates continue to be a problem, the work environment is a primary motivator for individual professional nurses making employment choices. Several studies have shown that one of the primary factors for the increasing nurse turnover rate is workload and staffing patterns. In a 1998 study by the Hay Group (Healthcare, 1998) examining the nursing shortage, nurse managers, RNs, and licensed practical nurses all cited "insufficient supply of qualified managers and experienced staff" as the most likely reason for the current and growing shortage. Other studies indicate that the primary reason for nurse turnover is increased market demand (Mercer, 1999). Thus the primary causes underlying turnover are alternative career prospects or dissatisfaction with the job or the supervisor. Tulgan (2003) has suggested that the immediate supervisor is the most important person in the workplace. He suggests that the midlevel supervisor is the lynchpin of corporate America. The challenge of managing a workplace with four generations present at the same time is a daunting task for most supervisors. The second most cited reason for turnover was workload and inappropriate staffing. These issues are fundamental problems that stand separate from the issues related to the supply of and demand for nursing services. Unless issues related to the work environment are addressed, strategies to increase the overall supply of nurses are unlikely to be successful (ANA, 2000b).

APPROPRIATE STAFFING AND MANDATORY OVERTIME

Appropriate staffing levels and the increased requirement for mandatory overtime are the two largest contributing factors to dissatisfaction within the workplace. An understanding of how managed care has affected our health care system provides a background as to why nurses have major concerns about adequacy of staffing levels. In response to declining reimbursement for services during the 1990s, health care systems eagerly sought and implemented the advice of consulting firms to reduce the cost of health care. These consultants brought with them accounting expertise and new models for care delivery that decentralized the majority of diagnostic and support services to patient care units and then cross-trained the unit staff to provide those services. A perceived outcome of decentralizing services and cross-training unit staff was that patients would have exposure to fewer personnel, personnel could spend less time off their units, and employers could reconfigure staff and eliminate unnecessary positions. Consequently, during the 1990s, many nursing positions—particularly experienced, higher paid nursing positions— were eliminated or downgraded, whereas lesser-skilled, lower-salaried unlicensed personnel were hired as replacements to function as part of the team under the direction of an RN.

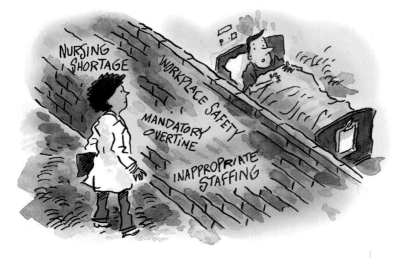

Professional nurses are struggling to deliver patient care against all kinds of barriers and with dwindling resources.

Appropriate Staffing

During this tumultuous time frame of downsizing, cross-training, and cost-cutting, nurses and other health professionals challenged the efficacy of using unlicensed personnel to deliver care to patient populations who were more acutely ill and required high-tech care and whose lengths of stay were being reduced to keep costs in check. The mix of staff continued to be diluted with increasing numbers of unlicensed personnel and elimination of nursing middle managers and executive level staff. These factors further decreased the support, advocacy, and resources necessary to ensure that nurses could provide optimum care. Although not currently required in today's health care system, standardized and mandatory reporting of data about staffing patterns could objectively quantify the effects of staffing on the safety and quality of care for patients, as well as the safety and quality of work life for nurses and other health care workers and lead to dramatic changes in staffing patterns. For example, standard reporting of patient complications and incidents (i.e., falls, postoperative pulmonary complications, medication errors) for a group of patients, along with the ratio of RNs present to provide care to that same group of patients, would provide objective data about the effect of RN staffing on patient outcomes.

Floating and Mandatory Overtime

By the late 1990s an emerging shortage of professional nurses began to further complicate staffing levels. The shortage resulted in (1) professional nurses being required to "float" to other patient care units for which they had little or no orientation, experience, or support; and (2) the implementation of mandatory overtime and/or mandatory on-call requirements by some employers. The practice of requiring nurses to work mandatory overtime spread across the United States in the year 2000. In studies of mandatory overtime in other industries, the U.S. Department of Labor found that increasing scheduled work time increased time lost to absenteeism and increased injuries, and it usually required 3 hours of work to produce an additional 2 hours of productivity (Thomas, 1990). In the health care sector mandatory overtime by medical residents is implied to be linked to significant numbers of patient deaths as a result of care delivery by exhausted residents (Worth, 1999).

Nurses believe that employers' ability to mandate last-minute overtime or to use peer pressure as a negative motivator relieves the employers' sense of urgency to find safer and more appropriate staffing. Although nurses are fully cognizant and concerned about inadequate staffing, they are also resentful that they bear the personal, professional, and legal burden for this problem that is in large part a direct result of earlier changes in skill mix and care delivery models made acceptable by national imperatives to work swiftly to reduce the cost of health care (ANA, 2000a). By the late 1990s many nurses began to unite to push mandatory overtime and inadequate staffing issues to the forefront through professional practice advocacy mechanisms.

Advocating for Safe Staffing

Many nurses across the country are concerned about the inadequacies of staffing and are struggling with excessive and unsafe overtime work to meet patient care needs. Health care delivery systems underwent significant changes during the 1990s as the nation moved toward managed care. Many believe that the vigorous downsizing and layoffs of professional nursing staff during the 1990s demonstrate that professional nurses were not valued for their contribution to safe, accessible, quality care (ANA, 2000b). Before accepting a position with an organization, professional nurses should ask the questions identified in Box 12-3 regarding safe staffing. Resources to help professional nurse decision making relative to adequate staffing and mandatory overtime are included in Box 12-4.

The immediate concern for most nurses in a staffing conflict is whether or not to accept an assignment. Many times this comes down to a disagreement between the nurse manager making the assignment and the staff nurse asked to accept the assignment. Box 12-5 identifies a set of questions to help the staff nurse in making a decision to accept or not accept an assignment. These questions are designed to help the staff nurse think critically about the assignment so that, if there is a problem, the nurse can be clear in telling the manager what makes her or him uncomfortable with the assignment.

Mandatory overtime and adequate staffing levels have become a legislative issue at both the national and state levels of government (Jordan and Tabone, 2000). The first state to pass legislation addressing nurse staffing levels was California in 1999. The California bill requires all acute care facilities to provide minimum nurse-to-patient ratios and to adopt written policies and procedures for training and orientation of nursing staff (ANA, 1998c). Although the California bill passed in 1999, implementation is still fraught with problems. According to the California Department of Health Services, hospitals statewide will have to hire a combined 5000 additional nurses at an annual cost of about $900 million to comply with the rules, scheduled to take effect January 1, 2004. Under the new California rules, the first such regulations in the nation, nurses will not have to care for more than eight patients at a time. The rules also call for one nurse per five patients in medical-surgical units by 2005, as well as one nurse per four patients in specialty care and telemetry units and one nurse per three patients in step-down units by 2008. In addition, the regulations state that licensed vocational nurses can comprise no more than 50% of the licensed nurses assigned to patient care and that only registered nurses can care for critical trauma patients (AACN, 2003).

Federal legislation was introduced in the fall of 2003 to provide patient protection by limiting the number of mandatory overtime hours a nurse may be required to work in certain health care facilities to which payments are made under the Medicare Program. Multiple bills

---

BOX 12–3 *Questions to Ask About Safe Staffing Before Accepting Employment*

1. Who is the chief nursing officer, to whom does she or he report, and does she or he have authority over staffing?
2. Who controls the staffing budget?
3. Is the level of staffing an active and ongoing discussion in the organization, and do staff nurses have input?
4. Does the organization have a shared governance model?
5. When, where, and how is staffing input obtained from staff nurses?
6. How do ratios in the organization compare with recommendations of national/regional organizations such as the American Organization of Nurse Executives and the Association of Critical Care Nurses?
7. What is the content and length of orientation for new nurses?
8. What is the philosophy regarding staff mix designations?
9. What is the frequency of floating to other nursing units?
10. What are the criteria used by the organization in determining competency of cross-trained staff?
11. What resources does the organization use to supplement staff during peak census?
12. If concerns arise about the adequacy of staffing, where and to whom is it appropriate to voice those concerns?
13. How are overtime, on-call time, and cancellation of regularly scheduled shifts handled?
14. Does the organization mandate overtime? If so, can the staff nurse refuse to participate without repercussions?
15. What is the turnover rate, and what is the average longevity of staff nurses?
16. What opportunities for advancement exist in the organization, such as clinical ladders or other systems of recognition?
17. Where does the organization expect discussions about staffing or practice issues to take place?
18. Is there a conflict resolution process in place?

Adapted from Texas Nurses Association: *Nurse staffing task force document (internal document)*, Austin, Tex, 1999, Author, Available on-line (www.texanurses.org).

---

would amend title XVIII of the Social Security Act to protect nurses and patients from mandatory overtime (AACN, 2003).

Realistic concerns about nurses' ability to provide safe care were amplified by the release of the three Institute of Medicine (IOM) documents: *The Adequacy of Nurse Staffing in Hospitals and Nursing Homes* (Wunderlich, Sloan, and Davis, 1996), *To Err Is Human: Building a Safer Health Care System* (Kohn, Corrigan, and Donaldson, 2000), and *Keeping Patients Safe: Transforming the Work Environment of Nurses* (Page, 2004). The number of nursing staff available to provide in-patient nursing care is linked to patient safety by a substantial and growing number of research studies. Recently Aiken et al (2002), have shown that an increased patient load is related to more patient deaths, as well as higher levels of stress and burnout in nurses. The hope is that nurses will use this information in ongoing efforts to advocate for appropriate staffing to improve patient and financial outcomes.

Shared Governance as a Method of Advocating for Excellence in Nursing Practice

Introduced in the 1970s, shared governance has been identified by RNs as a key indicator of excellence in nursing practice (McDonagh et al, 1989; Metcalf and Tate, 1995; Porter-O'Grady, 1984, 1991, and 2003). The concept of professional practice models such as shared governance

BOX 12–4	Resources for Decision Making Related to Adequacy of Staffing and Mandatory Overtime

Principles of Nurse Staffing
Outlines the critical considerations needed to determine appropriate staffing. Single copies are free to members of ANA's constituent member associations by calling 1-800-274-4ANA and asking for PNS-1. Multiple copies can be ordered from 1-800-637-0323 or these on-line sources:
www.nursesbooks.org
http://nursingworld.org/readroom/stffprnc.htm

ANA Consumer Alert
"ANA Calls Hospital Staffing Practices Unsafe":
www.nursingworld.org/pressrel/2000/pr0420b.htm

Nursing Quality Indicators: Definitions and Implications; Guide for Implementation
1-800-637-0323
www.nursesbooks.org
http://nursingworld.org/quality/

State Nurses Association
ANA's Constituent Member Associations
www.nursingworld.org

BOX 12–5	Questions to Ask in Making the Decision to Accept a Staffing Assignment

1. **What is the assignment?**
   Clarify the assignment. Do not assume. Be certain that what you believe is the assignment is indeed correct.

2. **What are the characteristics of the patients being assigned?**
   Don't just respond to the number of patients; make a critical assessment of the needs of each patient, his or her age, condition, other factors that contribute to special needs, and the resources available to meet those needs. Who else is on the unit or within the facility that might be a resource for the assignment? Do nurses on the unit have access to those resources? How stable are the patients, and for what period of time have they been stable? Do any patients have communication and/or physical limitations that will require accommodation and extra supervision during the shift? Will there be discharges to offset the load? If there are discharges, will there be admissions, which require extra time and energy?

3. **Do I have the expertise to care for the patients?**
   Am I familiar with caring for the types of patients assigned? If this is a "float assignment," am I crossed-trained to care for these patients? Is there a "buddy system" in place with staff familiar with the unit? If there is no cross-training or "buddy system," has the patient load been modified accordingly?

4. **Do I have the experience and knowledge to manage the patients for whom I am being assigned care?**
   If the answer to the question is no, you have an obligation to articulate limitations. Limitations in experience and knowledge may not require refusal of the assignment but rather an agreement regarding supervision or a modification of the assignment to ensure patient safety. If no accommodation for limitations is considered, the nurse has an obligation to refuse an assignment for which she or he lacks education or experience.

Continued

| BOX 12–5 | *Questions to Ask in Making the Decision to Accept a Staffing Assignment—cont'd* |

5. What is the geography of the assignment?

Am I being asked to care for patients who are in close proximity for efficient management, or are the patients at opposite ends of the hall or on different units? If there are geographic difficulties, what resources are available to manage the situation? If my patients are on more than one unit and I must go to another unit to provide care, who will monitor patients out of my immediate attention?

6. Is this a temporary assignment?

When other staff are located to assist, will I be relieved? If the assignment is temporary, it may be possible to accept a difficult assignment, knowing that there will soon be reinforcements. Is there a pattern of short staffing, or is this truly an emergency?

7. Is this a crisis or an ongoing staffing pattern?

If the assignment is being made because of an immediate need on the unit, a crisis, the decision to accept the assignment may be based on that immediate need. However, if the staffing pattern is an ongoing problem, the nurse has the obligation to identify unmet standards of care that are occurring as a result of ongoing staffing inadequacies. This may result in a request for "safe harbor" and/or peer review.

8. Can I take the assignment in good faith? If not, you will need to get the assignment modified or refuse the assignment.

Consult your individual state's nursing practice act regarding clarification of accepting an assignment in good faith. In understanding good faith, it is sometimes easier to identify what would constitute bad faith. For example, if you had not taken care of pediatric patients since nursing school and you were asked to take charge of a pediatric unit, unless this were an extreme emergency such as a disaster (in which case you would need to let people know your limitations, but you might still be the best person, given all factors for the assignment), it would be bad faith to take the assignment. It is always your responsibility to articulate your limitations and to get an adjustment to the assignment that acknowledges the limitations you have articulated. Good faith acceptance of the assignment means that you are concerned about the situation and believe that a different pattern of care or policy should be considered. However, you acknowledge the difference of opinion on the subject between you and your supervisor and are willing to take the assignment and await the judgment of other peers/supervisors.

Adapted from Texas Nurses Association: *Workplace advocacy program*, Austin, Tex, 2001, Author, Available on-line (www.texasnurses.org).

has attracted the attention of nursing over the last decade in response to maintaining nursing job satisfaction, quality care, and fiscal viability. During the past 15 years, there has been proliferation of such models to redesign care delivery roles and systems and restructure the governance of professional nursing.

The importance of shared governance is that such models provide an organizational framework for nurses in direct care to become committed to nursing practice within their organizations. The implementation of such models allows nurses to have an active role in decision making by providing maximum participation and accountability for the outcomes of those decisions. Shared governance models render both a structure and an environment that empowers staff to make care decisions. Attributes of shared governance include independence, accountability, and autonomy over nursing practice, which are important factors in nursing job satisfaction. Shared governance results in more than job satisfaction; it includes as equally important increased efficiency and better patient outcomes.

The delegation of decision making to the professional doing the work is often referred to as participatory management and may be the first level of nursing governance in a regular hierarchic organization. However, self-governance goes beyond participatory management through the creation of organizational structures that allow nursing staff to govern issues of nursing practice and nursing service delivery. An example is the Safety Committee that Elena (in our opening vignette) was elected to by her colleagues after she initiated inquiries as to why safe needle devices were not available on her nursing unit.

Shared governance of nursing services often develops in phases. These phases offer organizations the opportunity to adjust to the changing roles and decision-making authority of nurses. Each phase provides greater autonomy to practicing nurses in determining practice policy. However, the structure allows nursing delivery decisions to be integrated with other policy needs of the organization. Box 12-6 provides an overview of potential developmental phases for shared governance. As a shared governance model is developed in the health care organization, it is important that it does not become isolated from other organizational problem solving and policy-making bodies such as quality improvement, ethics, and risk management.

Not all health care organizations place quality patient care at the top of their agenda; rather they focus more on bottom-line profits. In these situations nurses may find themselves

---

BOX 12–6   *Three Developmental Phases of Shared Governance*

Phase 1

- Staff nurse representatives—members of clinical forums, have authority for designated practice issues and some authority for determining roles, functions, and processes.
- Managers—members of management forums, responsible for facilitation of practice through resource management and allocation.
- Executive committee—administrative and staff membership, often in disproportionate numbers, accept recommendations from staff nurses and managers.
- Chief nurse executive—retains final decision-making authority.

Phase 2

- Staff nurse representatives—members of nursing committees that are designated for specific management and/or clinical functions.
- Managers—serve on same committees with staff nurses.
- Committee chairs—appointed by chief nurse executive.
- Nursing cabinet—composed of multiple committee chairs that make final decisions on recommendations from the committees.

Phase 3

- Staff nurse representatives—belong to councils with authority for specific functions.
- Council chairs—make up management committee charged with making all final operational decisions.

Adapted from Texas Nurses Association: *Workplace advocacy program*, Austin, Tex, 2001, Author, Available on-line (www.texasnurses.org).

BOX 12–7 *Questions to Ask About Shared Governance Models*

Access to the Process
■ Are nurses encouraged to participate in shared governance?
■ How do nurses become involved in the shared governance process?
■ What is the ratio of staff nurses to managers involved in shared governance within the organization?
■ Is adequate work time allowed to participate in governance councils?

Implementation and Communication of Action
■ How does the organization communicate shared governance decisions with staff nurses?

Effectiveness of the Process
■ How did shared governance improve nursing care delivery in the organization?
■ Do nurses feel shared governance within their organization is beneficial to their practice?

Outcomes of the Process
■ Does the organization have outcomes data related to shared governance?
■ If so, how have that data impacted changes in nursing practice?

Adapted from Texas Nurses Association: *Workplace advocacy program*, Austin, Tex, 2001, Author, Available on-line (www.texas-nurses.org).

challenged to provide quality care. Therefore it is important that nurses have access and input to the various organizational structures in place, the decisions of which affect the nurse and patient. Nurses need to be integral members of such organizational structures as quality improvement and ethics committees. Staff nurses need to know who their representatives are and how to access such committees. Box 12-7 identifies questions that should be asked about shared governance or participatory management models when nurses are trying to identify the organization that would be most conducive to the delivery of quality nursing care.

Nurses working under shared governance models should have access to conflict resolution procedures that define the processes they should follow if they are in disagreement with the organization. However, organizations without shared governance models may also have systems in place that could be of assistance. Examples of these are open-door policies, ombudsman programs, or dispute-resolution processes. When seeking dispute resolution, the nurse may use a third party or resources internal to the organization to assist in the resolution. Some states have processes that can assist in resolving patient care or professional issues. These processes include peer review, safe harbor, and mandatory reporting.

PATIENT ADVOCACY AND SAFETY

Patient advocacy is a cornerstone of the nursing profession, and patients depend on nurses to ensure that they receive proper care. Although nurses have always advocated for their patients, it has only been during the last 25 years that the recognized role of the nurse as "patient advocate" has begun to clearly emerge. The evolution of the nurse's role in patient advocacy has changed from a vague assertion of ethical-legal responsibility in the mid-1970s to a "rights" framework in the 1980s (Mallik and Rafferty, 2000). This "rights" framework has only intensified in the 1990s and will continue to do so as we move through the new century.

Today's health care systems have created an environment in which errors and adverse events are attributed to complex systems and complicated uses of technology. This complex environment demands that the nursing profession assert its powerful voice in the role of patient advocate by supporting public policies that protect consumers and enhance accountability for quality by promoting safer health care systems.

Errors in Health Care

Errors in the health care system carry a high cost for all involved. Based on findings of two major studies, errors in health care delivery kill approximately 44,000 people in U.S. hospitals (Brennan et al, 1991; Cook, Woods, and Miller, 1998). Another study estimates the number higher, at 98,000 (American Medical Association, 1999). Even using the lower figures, more people supposedly die from health care errors each year than from highway accidents, breast cancer, or AIDS (Centers for Disease Control and Prevention, 1999). No health care setting is immune from errors, including hospitals, outpatient clinics, retail pharmacies, long-term care facilities, and homes. Over 7000 deaths that occur in multiple settings annually are attributed to medication errors alone (Occupational Safety and Health Administration, 1998; Phillips, Christenfeld, and Glynn, 1998).

During late 1999, the IOM's *To Err Is Human* report (Kohn, Corrigan, and Donaldson, 2000) quickly seized the attention of the entire health care delivery system, providers, policy makers, and the public on the seriousness of errors in health care. It described a fragmented health care system that is prone to errors and detrimental to the goal of safe patient care. The IOM report concentrated on those errors (acknowledged to be the vast majority) that result from mistakes rather than those caused by incompetence of the health care provider. The IOM report recommended a variety of legislative, regulatory, and voluntary corrective actions designed to improve the safety of health care delivery systems (Swankin and LeBuhn, 2000). Since the release of the reports, many nursing organizations have attempted to demonstrate the linkage between nurse staffing and the prevention of patient adverse events and errors. Health care errors and adverse patient incidents include:

- Transfusion and medication errors
- Equipment or device failure
- Wrong-site surgery
- Preventable suicides
- Falls
- Burns
- Mistaken identity

In another report, the IOM focused on the quality of care in the long-term care industry. This report cited a need for effective government oversight and ample nurse staffing to boost the quality of care provided in long-term care (Hallam and Lovern, 2000). The IOM made sweeping recommendations intended to improve the long-term care workforce, such as improving the work environment through competitive wages, career development, work design, and better supervision. The report also outlines a role for federal and state governments in establishing minimum staffing levels and competency standards.

Following their now famous report on medical errors, the IOM released *Crossing the Quality Chasm: A New Health System for the 21st Century* (2001) to define a vision for improving the quality of our nation's health care system. The most recent IOM report entitled *Keeping Patients Safe: Transforming the Work Environment of Nurses* (Page, 2004) builds on the previous IOM reports by examining patient safety from the perspective of the work environment in which nurses provide patient care. The report provides evidence of the critical role nurses have in the health care system. The report found evidence that the typical work environment of nurses is characterized by many serious threats to patient safety. These threats were found in all four of the basic components of all organizations, including:

- *Leadership and management:* Frequent failure to follow management practices necessary for safety, leading to a loss of trust in hospital administration by nurses, along with the reduction of clinical nursing leadership at multiple levels leading to a diminished voice for nurses in patient care
- *Workforce:* Unsafe workforce deployment as evidenced by a wide variation in nurse staffing levels across hospitals and nursing homes and a need for all health care professionals (nurses and physicians alike) to have better training and active involvement in interdisciplinary collaboration and teamwork
- *Work processes:* Unsafe work and workspace design including long work hours, insufficient technology to support tasks such as medication administration, and undue time commitment to document patient information and care processes resulting in insufficient time for patient care
- *Organizational culture:* Punitive cultures that hinder the reporting and prevention of errors

The 2004 IOM report goes on to recommend that no single action can, by itself, keep patients safe from health care errors. It recommends defenses be created in all four organizational components—leadership and management, the workforce, work processes, and organizational culture (Page, 2004). Specific recommendations focus on the following:

- Transformational leadership and evidence-based management
- Maximizing workforce capability
- Design of work and workspace to prevent and mitigate errors
- Creating and sustaining a culture of safety

Whistle-Blower Protection

Nurses want the assurance that, if they are acting within the scope of their practice, they will be able to speak up for their patients through appropriate channels without fear of retaliation. Whistle-blower legislation has been advocated for at the federal level and has actually passed in some states. Whistle-blower protection basically prohibits health care organizations from retaliating against nurses when the professional nurse in good faith discloses information or participates in agency investigations. Specifically, whistle-blower protection protects nurses who speak out about unsafe situations from being fired or subjected to other disciplinary actions by their employers.

An example of how whistle-blower protection promotes workplace advocacy is illustrated by a recent case in Texas. A Texas jury awarded a nurse formerly employed by a large health science center $810,000 in her lawsuit filed under the Texas Whistle-Blower Act (Tabone, 2000). She witnessed patients, who in her assessment were not in imminent danger of death, having their rights to informed consent disregarded. Patients refusing treatment were treated

BOX 12–8   Things to Know About Whistle-Blowing

If you identify an illegal or unethical practice, reserve judgment until you have adequate documentation to establish wrongdoing.

Do not expect those that are engaged in unethical or illegal conduct to welcome your questions or concerns about this practice.

Seek the counsel of someone you trust outside of the situation to provide you with an objective perspective.

Consult with your state nurses association or legal counsel if possible before taking action to determine how best to document your concerns.

Remember, you are not protected in a whistle-blower situation from retaliation by your employer until you blow the whistle.

Blowing the whistle means that you report your concern to the national and/or state agency responsible for regulation of the organization for which you work or, in the case of criminal activity, to law enforcement agencies as well.

Private groups such as the Joint Commission on Accreditation of Healthcare Organizations or the National Committee for Quality Assurance do not confer protection. You must report to a state or national regulator.

Although it is not required by every regulatory agency, it is a good rule of thumb to put your complaint in writing.

Document all interactions related to the whistle-blowing situation and keep copies for your personal file.

Keep documentation and interactions objective.

Remain calm and do not lose your temper, even if those who learn of your actions attempt to provoke you.

Remember that blowing the whistle is a very serious matter. Do not blow the whistle frivolously. Make sure you have the facts straight before taking action.

Adapted from Tabone S: 2000 update: foreign nurse recruitment, *Texas Nurs* 74(8):9, 15, 2000.

despite their protests to doctors. This nurse sought counsel from her state nurses association and, based on their recommendations, documented her concerns about these incidents according to the hospital's policies and tried to work within the system to stop what she believed to be serious patient rights violations. The nurse further protected herself by documenting her interactions with those who were retaliating against her for speaking out and reported the situation to the State Board of Nurse Examiners, the Texas Department of Health, and the local police department. She was eventually terminated by the employing hospital. However, the jury found that she acted in accordance with the state nursing practice act in reporting her concerns about patient care practices and upheld her suit for defamation and wrongful termination (Tabone, 2000). Box 12-8 provides an overview of "Things to Know About Whistle-Blowing." Nurses should check with their state nurses association to assess the status of whistle-blower protection in their state.

Nursing Quality Indicators

Major changes in systems of care and nurse staffing are occurring with little data to justify or demonstrate the potential effects on safety and quality of patient care. Many organizations, including the National Nursing Research Roundtable, the National Institute of Nursing Research, and the major federal supporter of health systems and health outcomes research, the Agency for Healthcare Quality and Research, are working collaboratively to promote collection and publication of data that link nurse staffing mix with patient outcomes. A critical and pioneering component of this work has been the initiation of research to examine linkages between

BOX 12–9	*Ten Nursing–Sensitive Quality Indicators for Acute Care Settings*

Mix of RNs, LPNs, and unlicensed staff caring for patients
Total nursing care hours provided per patient day
Pressure ulcers
Patient falls
Patient satisfaction with pain management
Patient satisfaction with educational information
Patient satisfaction with overall care
Patient satisfaction with nursing care
Nosocomial infection rate
Nurse staff satisfaction

Adapted from American Nurses Association: *Quality indicators for acute care settings*, Washington, DC, 2001, ANA, Available on-line (www.nursingworld.org).

professional nurse staffing, processes of care, and patient outcomes in acute care settings. Because of limited research in this area, the ANA took the lead in the design and implementation of ongoing, comprehensive, broad-based research efforts to establish and quantify the impact of professional nurse staffing on processes of care and patient outcomes. The initial step in the identification of nursing-sensitive indicators focused on the acute care setting. However, the work has now moved into testing of quality indicators appropriate for community-based nonacute health care settings. Box 12-9 lists the nursing-sensitive quality indicators for acute settings. The National Database of Nursing Quality Indicators, established in late 1997, continues to receive data and issue reports about the data analyses of participating facilities (ANA, 1998b).

Numerous states have introduced and passed legislation that calls for states to collectand disseminate nursing data to the public, including nurse staffing patterns and patient outcomes, such as nosocomial infections, patient fall rates, decubitus ulcers, and patient satisfaction (ANA, 1998c). This information provides an important guide to consumers, providers, and institutions when making purchasing decisions about health care services.

WORKPLACE SAFETY

Nurses are battling to provide safe, quality care for patients in an environment that is becoming increasingly dangerous. The occupational safety and health of nurses continues to be an ongoing concern for both individual nurses and professional nursing associations. Workplace injuries for all industries cost Americans $125.1 billion, the equivalent to nearly triple the combined profits reported by the top five Fortune 500 companies during the same year (Texas Tech University Health Sciences Center, 2001). There were 5100 workplace fatalities in 1999, and for women workers homicides were the leading cause of workplace deaths. Box 12-10 describes categories of health hazards in the health care workplace.

Needlesticks

Of particular concern are the growing phenomena of exposure to blood-borne diseases. Health care workers in the United States experience at least 800,000 needlestick

---

BOX 12–10   *Categories of Health Hazards in the Health Care Workplace*

Biologic Hazards
Bacteria, viruses, fungi, or parasites that may be transmitted by contact with infected patients or contaminated body secretions/fluids (e.g., human immunodeficiency virus, hepatitis B and C, tuberculosis, and varicella)

Ergonomic Hazards
Musculoskeletal injury to the back and extremities resulting from lifting, standing for long periods, and repeated hand motions

Chemical Hazards
Medications, solutions, gases (such as ethylene oxide, formaldehyde, glutaraldehyde, waste anesthetic and laser gases), cytotoxic agents, pentamidine, latex, PVC plastics, Di-ethylhexyl phthalate (DEHP)

Psychologic Hazards
Stress, shift work, mandatory overtime, verbal abuse by patients and other health care providers

Physical Hazards
Radiation, lasers, noise, electricity, violence

Adapted from American Nurses Association: *Occupational safety and health: 1998 ANA House of Delegates Status Reports,* Washington, DC, 1998a, ANA.

---

injuries annually. These injuries account for the majority of all exposures to blood-borne pathogens (ANA, 1998a). The Centers for Disease Control and Prevention (1997) reported results of research showing that the use of safer needlestick devices (including blunting intravenous catheters and retractable needles) reduced worker injuries by up to 76% without significant patient complications, and health care workers generally accepted the safer devices.

Legislative initiatives at the federal and state levels are being passed to ensure that nurses and other health care workers are protected from blood-borne diseases in the workplace. The most significant piece of legislation passed to date occurred at the federal level during fall 2000 when the Needlestick Safety and Prevention Act was signed into law (The American Nurse, 2000). The ANA was instrumental in advocating for passage of this legislation. The Needlestick Safety and Prevention Act amends the existing Blood-Borne Pathogen Standard administered by the Occupational Safety and Health Administration to require the use of safer devices to protect from sharps injuries. It also requires employers to solicit the input of non-managerial employees responsible for direct patient care who are potentially exposed to sharps injuries in the identification, evaluation, and selection of effective engineering and work-practice controls. This bill also requires employers to maintain a sharps injury log to contain, at a minimum, the brand of device involved in the incident, the department or work area where the exposure incident occurred, and an explanation of how the incident occurred. The log will become an important source of data for researchers to determine the relative effectiveness and safety of devices now on the market and those that may be developed in the future (The American Nurse, 2000).

Ergonomic Injuries

Although nurses have suffered from back and other musculoskeletal disorders for decades, it is only during the last decade that these injuries are being directly attributed to the workplace. There are strong data demonstrating the problem of overexertion injuries in hospitals, nursing homes, and home care settings over the last decade. Of the disabling injuries in nursing, 67% were caused by sprains and strains, mostly overexertion injuries to the back or trunk from lifting patients (The American Nurse, 2000). Back injuries are particularly troublesome for nurses. ANA's new lifting initiative, "Handle With Care," is aimed at reducing the number of nurses who suffer career-ending or career-altering back and limb injuries (ANA, 2003). New ergonomic standards were released in fall 2000 by the National Institute of Occupational Safety and Health and should help protect nurses from disabling back injuries and musculoskeletal disorders. The ANA was instrumental in advocating for the passage of this legislation. The standard includes work restriction protections, and the "action trigger" in the standard focuses on identification of hazards, which is crucial in preventing back injuries and musculoskeletal disorders.

Barriers to Reporting a Workplace Injury

Many nurses find themselves suffering from workplace injuries, which they are reluctant to report because of perceived potential negative consequences to their employment status (De Castro, 2003). Reporting a work-related injury or illness is not always easy. According to an ANA survey, 75% of nurses who responded to a survey stated they did not report injuries that occurred on the job. De Castro (2003) identified the following barriers to reporting work-related injuries or illness:

- Fear of repercussions such as disciplinary action
- Stigmatization as a complainer
- Harassment by supervisors and coworkers
- Denial of opportunities for promotion
- Termination of employment

In addition, nurses often blame themselves for work-related injuries or illnesses via their own perceptions of failing to be more careful. It is important for nurses to report injuries and illnesses in order to ensure a safe workplace. According to De Castro (2003) reporting helps pinpoint trends and areas of need in health and safety by providing insights into conditions that lead to injury or illness. Every organization should have specific policies concerning reporting of workplace injuries and illness. The ANA provides a *Workplace Health and Safety Guide for Nurses* and information concerning nurses health and safety rights. New guidelines issued by the U.S. Department of Labor—Occupational Safety and Health Administration (OSHA) Recordkeeping Standard—require employers to show employees how to report a workplace injury or illness by using the OSHA 300 Log. The OSHA standard also prevents discrimination against employees who report a work-related injury, illness, or fatality.

Workplace Violence

Workplace violence has become a major societal issue. The National Institute for Occupational Safety and Health estimates that, for all businesses across the United States, 2 million workers are attacked annually in the workplace and a more alarming 6 million are threatened (Antai-Otong, 1998). One-sixth of all violent crimes occur in the workplace, including 8% of all rapes, 7% of all robberies, and 16% of all assaults. Furthermore, 10% of all workplace violence involves handguns.

Causative factors of workplace violence are multivariate (Antai-Otong, 1998). The continuing pressures in health care delivery to contain costs have resulted in shortened hospital stays, with many patients being discharged with unstable medical and psychiatric conditions that pose even greater dangers for nurses in all practice settings (Antai-Otong, 1998) The frequency with which health care organizations reorganize is also increasing, resulting in job insecurity, disloyalty, apathy, stress, tension, and feelings of helplessness and devaluation. Settings where these factors seem to be the most amplified are high-stress practice areas, including emergency departments, acute care psychiatry and intensive care units, and long-term care units or facilities. These factors, along with increased workloads and dwindling resources, further heighten the incidence of violence in the health care workplace (Antai-Otong, 1998).

An example of workplace violence can be illustrated by an incident that occurred in early 2001 in a west Texas hospital. A prison inmate with complaints of gastrointestinal bleeding was accompanied to the emergency department of a large hospital by two prison guards (Queen, 2001). The inmate managed to confiscate the keys to his handcuffs, becoming free and brandishing a gun while threatening the guards, emergency staff, and other patients. He then barricaded himself and two nurses in a room, where he sexually assaulted the nurses and held a SWAT team at bay for nearly 2 hours. Apparently the guards responsible for the inmate did not follow many routine safety procedures; it was later discovered that the inmate's gun was fake.

Nurses must proactively advocate for safe workplaces. This should occur through a comprehensive organizational assessment to identify high-risk environments and psychologic conditions and populations that threaten workplace safety (Antai-Otong, 1998). Failure to recognize behavioral cues such as pacing, yelling, and verbal and physical threats further compromises the safety of nurses and patients. Staff education is essential to proactively address the identification and response to high-risk behaviors, which can lead to violence. Nursing safety is imperative and includes adequate staffing levels, adequate staff training, and environmental safeguards.

Advocating for a Safer Workplace

The ANA has emerged as a leader in health care worker health and safety, working in collaboration with other nursing organizations, including the *CAN*, American Association of Occupational Health Nurses, Association of Operating Room Nurses, the Emergency Nurses Association, and other labor unions representing health care workers (ANA, 1998a). The *CAN* advocates for administrative controls such as adequate staffing and health and safety committees, engineering controls such as ventilation and safer needlestick devices, and personal protective equipment such as respirators and synthetic gloves that will prevent exposure to hazardous substances and/or prevent illness or injury from unavoidable exposure. Although the health care industry is a dangerous place to work, many of the risks are avoidable and dangerous exposures preventable. Box 12-11 identifies resources available to improve the safety of the workplace for both nurses and patients.

S U M M A R Y

This chapter has covered a variety of significant workplace issues and identified professional practice strategies for the nurse to use to improve the workplace environment and quality of patient care. A rapidly changing health care environment, significantly affected by an

BOX 12–11 *Helpful Websites/Resources*

Workplace Health and Safety Guide for Nurses: OSHA and NIOSH Resources
Occupational Health and Safety Series: Your Health and Safety Rights
http://nursingworld.org/osh/

American Nurses Association—Safe Needles Save Lives Campaign
www.needlestick.org

American Nurses Association—Pollution Prevention Kit for Nurses
www.nurses-books.org
or 1-800-637-0323 to request publication 9811LA

Citizens Advocacy Center—unique support program for public members who serve on health care regulatory
boards and governing bodies as representatives of consumer interest
www.cacenter.org

FDA MedWatch Program—report reactions to latex products and other chemical exposures
1-800-FDA-1088 (fax 1-800-FDA-0178)

Health Care Without Harm—neonatal exposure to DEHP and opportunities for prevention
www.noharm.org (for educational brochure, click on Library)

Information on Mercury
www.epa.gov/seahome/mercury/src/mercmed.htm
or www.nwf.org/greatlakes/resources/mercury.html

National Academy of Sciences—IOM reports
www.nap.edu

National Institute of Occupational Safety and Health
www.cdc.gov/niosh/publistd.html

National Institute of Occupational Safety and Health—Ergonomics Standards
www.cdc.gov/niosh/publistd.html

National Institute of Occupational Safety and Health—Latex Allergy Alert
Education information on identifying latex allergy
1-800-45-NIOSH (to request publication No. 97-195)

National Institute of Occupational Safety and Health—What Every Worker Should Know: How to Protect Yourself
from Needlestick Injuries
Educational brochure on needlestick prevention
1-800-35-NIOSH (to request publication No. 000-135)

National Institute of Occupational Safety and Health—Health Hazard Evaluation
Demonstrates the problem of indoor air causing illness to hundreds of health care workers
1-800-35-NIOSH (to request report HETA 96-0012-2652)

Nightingale Institute for Health and the Environment
www.nihe.org

The Environmentally Preferable Purchasing (EPP) Work Group—resources for healthy hospitals
www.geocities.com/EPP_how_to_guide/

U.S. Department of Labor—Occupational Safety and Healthy Administration Recordkeeping Web Page: demonstrates how to report a workplace injury or illness using the OSHA 300 log and prohibits discrimination against
employees who report a work-related injury, illness, or fatality
www.osha.gov/recordkeeping/index.html

aging workforce and shortage of nurses, creates a challenge for all nurses. Nurses must be aware of the issues facing the profession and know where to seek assistance, information, and resources to address workplace issues. Working together with the resources of such organizations as the ANA, nurses can create a workplace that promotes career satisfaction and quality patient care.

CRITICAL THINKING ACTIVITIES

1. How will the nursing shortage affect you as an individual? How will the shortage affect the profession of nursing and health care delivery?
2. What activities can health care organizations undertake to promote retention of nurses? How can health care organizations retain the older, more experenced nurse?
3. Determine whether your clinical practice site has a conflict resolution process. Does your state provide whistle-blower protection? How would you proceed if you believed there was cause for concern about patient safety in your clinical practice site?
4. Is your clinical practice site in compliance with the Needlestick Safety and Prevention Act (2000)?
5. Does your clinical practice site have a plan for handling workplace violence? Have nurses and other health care providers been educated on the use of the plan?

Additional resources are available on-line at: http://evolve.elsevier.com/Cherry/

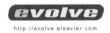

http://evolve.elsevier.com

REFERENCES

Aiken L et al: Hospital nurse staffing and patient mortality, nurse burnout, and job dissatisfaction, *J Am Med Assoc* 288(16):1987-1993, 2002.

Aiken L et al: Educational levels of hospital nurses and surgical patient mortality, *J Am Med Assoc* 290(12): 1617-1623, 2003.

Aiken L, Havens D, Sloane D: The Magnet Nursing Services Recognition Program: a comparison of two groups of magnet hospitals, *Am J Nurs* 100(3):26-34, 2000.

American Association of Colleges of Nursing: *Media talking points: the emerging nursing shortage, 2001.* Available on-line (www.aacn.nche.edu/MembersOnly).

American Association of Colleges of Nursing: *Increase in nursing school enrollments for the third consecutive year: increase falls below projected need to reverse the nursing shortage, 2003.* Available on-line (www.aacn. nche.edu/Media/News Release/ 2003Dec10.htm).

American Hospital Association: *Workforce supply for hospitals and health systems: issues and recommendations, American Hospital Association Policy Forum, 2001.* Available on-line (http://www. ahapolicyforum.org/policyresources/Workforce B0123.asp).

American Medical Association: *Hospital statistics,* Chicago, 1999, American Medical Association.

American Nurses Association: *Occupational safety and health, 1998 ANA House of Delegates Status Reports,* Washington, DC, 1998a, ANA.

American Nurses Association: *Nursing facts: nursing's quality indicators for acute care settings and ANA's safety and quality initiative,* Washington, DC, 1998b, ANA.

American Nurses Association: *Safety and quality initiatives: state legislative trends and analysis: special report to the 1998 House of Delegates,* Washington, DC, 1998c, ANA.

American Nurses Association: *Definition of professional practice advocacy adopted by House of Delegates (internal document),* Washington, DC, 1999, ANA.

American Nurses Association: *Opposing the use of mandatory overtime as a staffing solution: summary of proceedings: 2000 ANA House of Delegates,* Washington, DC, 2000a, ANA.

American Nurses Association: *Nursing workforce and the environment of care: status report 2000 ANA House of Delegates,* Washington, DC, 2000b, ANA.

American Nurses Association: *ANA launches "Handle With Care" ergonomic campaign, 2003.* Available on-line (http://www.nursingworld.org/pressrel/2003/pr0917.htm).

Antai-Otong D: Proactive responses to workplace violence: nurses' roles in health promotion, *Tex Nurs* 72(7): 4-7, 1998.

Bednash G: The decreasing supply of registered nurses: inevitable future or call to action, *JAMA* 283(22): 2985-2987, 2000.

Berlin LE, Stennett J, Bednash, GD: *2002-2003 enrollment and graduations in baccalaureate and graduate programs in nursing,* Washington, DC, 2003, American Association of Colleges of Nursing.

Bradford LJ, Raines C. *Twentysomethings: managing and motivating today's new workforce,* Denver, Colo, 1992, Merrill-Alexander Publishing.

Brennan T et al: Incidence of adverse events and negligence in hospitalized patients: results of the Harvard Medical Practice Study I, *N Engl J Med* 324: 370-376, 1991.

Buerhaus P: Is another RN shortage looming? *Nurs Outlook* 46:103-108, 1998.

Buerhaus P, Staiger D, Auerbach D: Implications of an aging registered nurse workforce, *JAMA* 283(22):2948-2954, 2000.

Buerhaus, P, Staiger, D, Auerbach, D: Is the current shortage of hospital nurses ending? *Health Affairs* 22(6):191-198, Nov-Dec, 2003.

Bureau of Labor Statistics, U.S. Department of Labor: *Occupational outlook handbook, 2002-2003 edition, Registered Nurses.* Retrieved October 3, 2003, on-line (http://www.bls.gov/oco/ocos083.htm).

Carpenter D: Going . . . going . . . gone? *Hosp Health Networks* 74(6):32-36, 38, 40-42, 2000.

Center for American Nurses: *About the Center for American Nurses.* Available on-line, 2004 (http://nursingworld.org/can/).

Centers for Disease Control and Prevention: Evaluation of safety devices for preventing percutaneous injuries among health-care workers during phlebotomy procedures—Minneapolis–St. Paul, New York City, and San Francisco, 1993-1995, *MMWR* 46(2):21-25, 1997.

Centers for Disease Control and Prevention, National Center for Health Statistics: Births and deaths: preliminary data for 1998, *National Vital Statistics Rep* 47(25):6, 1999.

Cook R, Woods D, Miller C: *A tale of two stories: contrasting views of patient safety,* Chicago, 1998, National Patient Safety Foundation.

De Castro B: Barriers to reporting a workplace injury, *AJN* 103(8):112, 2003.

Dugger C: Botswana says a brain drain is crippling its war against AIDS, *New York Times*, November 13, 2003, p 7.

Farrington C, Martucci, F: Public finance: nursing shortage update, *FitchRatings*. Retrieved on-line, May 13, 2003 (www.fitchratingscom).

Gelinas L, Bohlen, C: *Tomorrow's work force: a strategic approach,* Dallas, Tex, 2002, VHA.

Gleason S, Sochalski J, Aiken L: Review of Magnet hospital research: findings and implications for professional nursing practice, *J Nurs Admin* 29(1):9-19, 1999.

Green A, Jordan C: Common denominators: shared governance and workplace advocacy—models for nurses to gain control over their practice, *OJIN*, 9(1), 2004.

Hallam K, Lovern E: IOM sets sights on long-term care, *Mod Healthcare* 30(22):32-33, 2000.

Healthcare Information Resource Center: *1998 nursing shortage study,* Walnut Creek, Calif, 1998, Hay Group.

Institute of Medicine: *Report brief: Crossing the quality chasm: a new health system for the 21st century,* 2001. Available on-line (http://www.iom.edu/file.asp?id=4124).

Jordan C, Tabone S: Mandatory overtime and on call: growing concerns for nurses, *Tex Nurs* 74(8):4-6, 2000.

Kohn L, Corrigan J, Donaldson M: *To err is human: building a safer health system,* Washington, DC, 2000, Institute of Medicine, National Academy Press.

Mallik M, Rafferty A: Diffusion of the concept of patient advocacy, *J Nurs Scholarsh* 32(4):399-404, 2000.

McClure M et al: *Magnet hospitals: attraction and retention of professional nurses: American Academy of Nursing Task Force on Nursing Practice in Hospitals,* Kansas City, Mo, 1983, American Nurses Association.

McCue M, Mark B, Harless D: Nurse staffing, financial performance, and quality of care, *J Health Care Finance* 29(4):54-76, 2003.

McDonagh K et al: Shared governance at Saint Joseph's Hospital of Atlanta: a mature professional practice model, *Nurs Admin Q* 13(4):17-28, 1989.

Mercer W: *Attracting and retaining registered nurses—survey results,* Chicago, 1999, William M Mercer.

Metcalf R, Tate R: Shared governance in the endoscopy department, *Gastroenterol Nurs* 18(3):96-99, 1995.

Minnick A: Retirement, the nursing workforce, and the year 2005, *Nurs Outlook* 48:211-217, 2000.

Moses E: *The registered nurse population,* Rockville, Md, 1998, US Department of Health and Human Services.

Needleman J et al: Nurse-staffing levels and the quality of care in hospitals, *N Engl J Med* 346(22):1715-1722, 2002.

Nevidjon B, Erickson J: The nursing shortage: solutions for the short and long term, *Online J Issues Nurs* 6(1):Manuscript 4, 2001 (www.nursingworld.org/ojin/topic14/tpc14_4.htm).

O'Neil E: *Centering on where we need to focus now, The Center for the Health Professions, 2003* (http://futurehealth.ucsf.edu/from_the_director.html).

Occupational Safety and Health Administration: *The new OSHA: reinventing worker safety and health,* 1998 (www.OSHA.gov/oshinfo/reinvent.html).

Page A, editor: *Keeping patients safe: transforming the work environment of nurses,* Washington, DC, 2004, Institute of Medicine, National Academy Press.

Phillips D, Christenfeld N, Glynn L: Increase in U.S. medication-error deaths between 1983-1993, *Lancet* 351(43):644, 1998.

Pink D: *Free agent nation,* New York, 2001, Werner Books Inc.

Porter-O'Grady T, Finnigan S: *Shared governance for nursing: a creative approach to professional accountability,* Rockville, Md, 1984, Aspen Systems Corp.

Porter-O'Grady T: Shared governance and new organizational models, *Nursing Economics,* 5(6): 281-286, 1987.

Porter-O'Grady T: Shared governance for nursing part II: putting the organization into action, *AORN Journal,* 53(3):694-703, 1991.

Porter-O'Grady T: Researching shared governance: a futility of focus, *JONA* 33(4):251-252, 2003.

Queen S: Inmate charged in UMC sex assaults: fake gun used to hold two nurses hostage, *Lubbock Avalanche Journal,* January 5, 2001, p 1A.

Robinson ES, Mee CL: Nursing 2003 salary survey, *Nursing* 33(10):50-53, 2003.

Sigma Theta Tau International: *Nurses for a healthier tomorrow, 2000.* Available on-line (www.nursesource.org).

Spetz J, Given R: The future of the nurse shortage: will wage increases close the gap? *Health Affairs* 22(6): 199-206, 2003.

Swankin D, LeBuhn R: *Promoting patient safety: collaboration between regulators and health care organizations,* Washington, DC, 2000, Citizen Advocacy Center.

Tabone S: TNA advocates for fair labor: smuggler is sentenced, *Tex Nurs* 72(6):3, 1998.

Tabone S: 2000 update: foreign nurse recruitment, *Tex Nurs* 74(8):9, 15, 2000.

Thomas H: *Effects of scheduled overtime on labor productivity: a literature review and analysis,* Document 60, November 1990, Austin, Tex, 1990, Construction Industry Institute.

Texas Tech University Health Sciences Center: Workers' comp fast facts, *Safety Reporter* 47(3):4, Lubbock, Tex, 2001, Texas Tech University Health Sciences Center.

The American Nurse: New federal measure protects nurses from needlesticks, *Am Nurse* 32(6):1, 8, 2000.

Tulgan B: *Managing Generation X,* New York, 2003, WW Norton and Company.

Tulgan, B *Generational shift: what we saw at the workplace revolution, RainmakerThinking, Inc. Executive Summery: Key findings of 10-year work place study, 2003.* Available on-line (http://www.rainmakerthinking.com).

Ulrich B: Editors note: Generation RN: organizations, nurses of all ages work together to achieve professional longevity, *NurseWeek* 6(2):4:2001. Available on-line (www.nurseweek.com/ednote/01/012201b.asp).

U.S. Department of Health and Human Services, Health Resources and Services Administration: *Projected supply, demand, and shortages of registered nurses, 2000-2020,* Washington, DC, 2002, U.S. Government Printing Office.

Wieck K, Prydun M, Walsh T: What the emerging workforce wants in its leaders, *J Nurs Scholarsh* 34(3):283-288, 2002.

Worth R: Exhaustion that kills, *Washington Monthly* 31(1):25-20, 1999.

Wunderlich G, Sloan F, Davis C: *Nursing staff in hospitals and nursing homes: is it adequate? Committee on the Adequacy of Nurse Staffing in Hospitals and Nursing Homes,* Washington, DC, 1996, Institute of Medicine, National Academy Press.

Young S, Hayes E, Morin K: Developing workplace advocacy behaviors *J Nurs Staff Dev* 11(5):265-269, 1993.

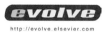

http://evolve.elsevier.com

13

Emergency Preparedness and Response for Today's World

Linda D. Norman, DNS, RN, and
Elizabeth E. Weiner, PhD, RN, BC, FAAN

Partnering to respond to disaster.

VIGNETTE

Jane Wolverton works as a staff nurse on a medical-surgical unit at the Culverton General Hospital. She is in a patient room giving an IV medication when the news program announces that there has been an explosion at a chemical plant that is thought to be the result of a terrorist bomb. The plant has 400 workers, including her husband.

Questions to consider while reading this chapter:

1. How do we prepare for threats against our nation's security?
2. How are response efforts coordinated so that the needs of the local area are met?
3. How do I protect myself in various situations designed to harm others?
4. How do hospitals organize themselves to manage disaster situations while continuing to communicate with other external agencies?
5. Where can I find current information about this ever-changing area?

KEY TERMS

All hazards approach A process approach for all sectors to prepare for any emergency or disaster situation that may occur.

Additional resources are available on-line at: http://evolve.elsevier.com/Cherry/

Biologic agents Microorganisms or toxins from living organisms with infectious or noninfectious properties that produce lethal or serious effects in plants and animals.

Chemical agents Solids, liquids, or gases with chemical properties that produce lethal or serious effects in plants and animals.

Comprehensive emergency management A broad style of emergency management, encompassing prevention, preparedness, response, and recovery (Landesman, 2001).

Consequence management Measures to protect public health and safety, restore essential government services, and provide emergency relief to governments, businesses, and individuals affected by the consequences of terrorism.

Containment Limitation of an emergency situation within a well-defined area.

Credible threat Situation in which the FBI determines that a terrorist threat is credible and confirms the involvement of a weapon of mass destruction (WMD) in the developing terrorist incident.

Crisis management Measures to identify, acquire, and plan the use of resources needed to anticipate, prevent, and/or resolve a threat or act of terrorism.

Decontamination The physical process of removing harmful substances from personnel, equipment, and supplies.

Disaster condition A significant natural disaster or man-made event that overwhelms the affected state, necessitating both federal public health and medical care assistance.

Disaster medical assistance teams (DMATs) Regionally organized teams consisting of physicians, nurses, and other health care providers that can be sent into areas outside their own regions to assist in providing care for ill or injured victims at the location of a disaster or emergency. DMATs provide triage, medical or surgical stabilization, and continued monitoring and care of patients until they can be evacuated to locations where they will receive definitive medical care. Specialty DMATs can Iso be deployed to address mass burn injuries, pediatric care requirements, chemical injury or contamination, etc.

Emergency As defined in the Stafford Act, any occasion or instance for which, in the determination of the President, federal assistance is needed to supplement state and local efforts and capabilities to save lives and protect property, public health, and safety; includes emergencies other than natural disasters.

Incident command system (ICS) A multiagency operational structure that uses a model adopted by the fire and rescue community. ICS can be used in any size or type of disaster to control response personnel, facilities, and equipment. ICS principles include use of common terminology, modular organization, integrated communications, unified command structure, action planning, manageable span-of-control, predesignated facilities, and comprehensive resource management. The basic functional modules of ICS (e.g., operations, logistics) can be expanded or contracted to meet requirements as an event progresses.

Lead agency As defined by the FBI, the federal department or organization assigned primary responsibility to manage and coordinate a specific function—either crisis management or consequence management. Lead agencies are designated on the basis of their having the most authority, resources, capabilities, or expertise relative to accomplishment of the specific function. Lead agencies support the overall lead federal agency during all phases of the terrorism response.

Major disaster As defined under the Stafford Act, any natural catastrophe (including any hurricane, tornado, storm, high water, wind-driven water, tidal wave, tsunami, earthquake, volcanic eruption, landslide, mudslide, snowstorm, or drought) or, regardless of cause, any fire, flood, or explosion in any part of the United States that, in the determination of the President, causes damage of sufficient severity and magnitude to warrant major disaster assistance under the Stafford Act to supplement the efforts and

294 UNIT TWO Current Issues in Health Care

available resources of states, local governments, and disaster relief organizations in alleviating the damage, loss, hardship, or suffering caused thereby.

Mass casualty incident (MCI) A disaster situation that results in a large number of victims who need the response of multiple organizations.

Mitigation Those activities designed to alleviate the effects of a major disaster or emergency or long-term activities to minimize the potentially adverse effects of future disasters in affected areas.

National disaster medical system (NDMS) A nationwide medical mutual aid network between the federal and nonfederal sectors that includes medical response, patient evacuation, and definitive medical care. At the federal level, it is a partnership among the Department of Health and Human Services (DHHS), the Department of Defense (DOD), the Department of Veterans Affairs (VA), and the Federal Emergency Management Agency (FEMA).

Nuclear weapons Weapons that release nuclear energy in an explosive manner as the result of nuclear chain reactions involving fission and/or fusion of atomic nuclei.

Personal protective equipment (PPE) Equipment designed to shield or isolate individuals from chemical, physical and biologic hazards (Barbera and Macintyre, 2003, p. 211).

Preparedness Activities that build capability and capacity to address potential needs identified by the threat and vulnerability study.

Recovery Activities designed to return responders and the facility to full normal operational status and to restore fully the hospital's capability to respond to future emergencies and disasters (Barbera and Macintyre, 2003, p. 52); activities traditionally associated with providing federal supplemental disaster relief assistance under a Presidential major disaster declaration. These activities usually begin within days after the event and continue after response activity ceases. Recovery includes individual and public assistance programs that provide temporary housing assistance, as well as grants and loans to eligible individuals and government entities to recover from the effects of a disaster.

Response Activities to address the immediate and short-term effects of an emergency or disaster. Response includes immediate actions to save lives, protect property, and meet basic human needs. Based on the requirements of the situation, response assistance will be provided to an affected state under the federal response plan.

Scene assessment The act of reviewing the location of an event to look for information that might help to determine treatment options.

Technical operations Actions to identify, assess, dismantle, transfer, dispose of, or decontaminate personnel and property exposed to explosive ordnance or WMD.

Terrorist incident As defined by the FBI, a violent act or an act that is dangerous to human life, in violation of the criminal laws of the United States or of any state, and intended to intimidate or coerce a government, the civilian population, or any segment thereof in furtherance of political or social objectives.

Triage Process of prioritizing which patients are to be treated first; first action in any disaster response (Veenema, 2003b, p. 153).

Weapon of mass destruction (WMD) As defined by Title 18, U.S.C. 2332a, (1) any destructive device as defined in section 921 of this title, [which reads] any explosive, incendiary, or poison gas, bomb, grenade, rocket having a propellant charge of more than four ounces, missile having an explosive or incendiary charge of more than one-quarter ounce, mine or device similar to the above; (2) poison gas; (3) any weapon involving a disease organism; or (4) any weapon designed to release radiation or radioactivity at a level dangerous to human life.

*Adapted from FEMA: *Appendix A: Terms and Definitions* (http://www.fema.gov/).

LEARNING OUTCOMES

After studying this chapter, the reader will be able to:

1. Describe educational competencies for professional nurses related to mass casualty events.
2. Describe the interaction between local, state, and federal emergency response systems.
3. Examine the roles of public and private agencies in preparing for and responding to a mass casualty event.
4. Compare and contrast chemical, biologic, radiologic, nuclear, and explosive agents and treatment protocols.
5. Access resources related to disaster preparedness on the Internet.
6. Communicate effectively (using correct emergency preparedness terminology) in regard to a mass casualty incident.

CHAPTER OVERVIEW

A NEW URGENCY FOR EMERGENCY PREPAREDNESS AND RESPONSE

The last decade has seen an accelerated pattern of terrorist attacks on U.S. property around the world, including some on domestic soil. Examples include the New York World Trade Center bombing in 1993; the bombing of the Murrah Federal Building in Oklahoma City in 1995; the attacks on the United States embassies in Kenya and Tanzania in 1998; the attack in 2000 on the U.S.S. Cole, an American warship refueling in Yemen; and the anthrax scare in 2002 (Johns Hopkins Evidence-Based Practice Center, 2002). None of these events, however, had the same impact as the events of September 11, 2001, when the United States experienced devastating well-coordinated attacks in New York City and Washington, D.C., that led to the deaths of over 3000 people.

The growing number of attacks has caused our country to realize that we can no longer adequately thwart all terrorist activity. A more reasonable approach has been the recent movement to plan and improve *responses* to a variety of hazards, called an *all hazards approach*. Nurses have traditionally received disaster education as a part of community health content within nursing education programs as it related to natural disasters. They have not, however, routinely received education related to biologic, chemical, nuclear, explosive, or radiologic hazards. It is imperative that all health care providers become knowledgeable about how to provide care for victims of all types of hazards.

It is recognized by all federal agencies that the most serious void for health care providers is in the area of *bioterrorism* attacks. Unlike the other hazards, these situations place the health care providers in a different position of being "first responders." Traditionally, first responders to emergencies have been the police, firefighters, and emergency medical technicians who respond with ambulances. In a covert biologic event, however, victims will first appear in emergency rooms, physician offices, nurse-managed clinics, or even in school health settings. Health care professionals need to be able to identify symptoms, data patterns, and other irregularities. If they fail to recognize or report significant events, an attack could go unrecognized until it is too late.

The purpose of this chapter is to describe the various components of our nation's local, state, and federal disaster response system and how these components interrelate in the event of a mass casualty incident. The kinds of agents that may be used in a terrorist attack are described along with the activities and response systems related to the preimpact and impact phase of a disaster. International efforts to develop a nurse workforce that can competently respond to mass casualty events are also discussed. As nursing students read the chapter, they will be particularly interested to note how standard triage and patient care priorities change when care is provided during a mass casualty incident. Additionally, readers will find an extensive list of resources about emergency preparedness and disaster management provided at the end of the chapter.

THE BASICS OF EMERGENCY PREPAREDNESS AND RESPONSE

Nurses have significant experience in dealing with natural disasters and are familiar with the work of the Red Cross in bringing disaster relief to affected areas. A *disaster condition* is defined as a significant natural disaster or man-made event that overwhelms the affected state and necessitates both federal public health and medical care assistance (FEMA, 2003). The disaster condition must be declared of significant impact to warrant federal resources.

In some situations, the number of victims is so large that multiple organizations will be called to respond. A mass gathering is usually defined as a group of 1000 persons or more (Veenema, 2003b). When casualties occur at this level, the event is termed a *mass casualty incident*. Although the situation may be unfamiliar for some nurses, it is important to remember that the nursing fundamentals practiced in other settings and during smaller crises will generally still be applicable (Veenema, 2003b).

Traditionally, triage that is practiced in most health care agencies categorizes patients into low risk, intermediate care, and critically ill (those who need immediate care to save their lives). With such large numbers, however, there is a paradigm shift to change priorities into doing the greatest good for the greatest number of people. Care is given to those patients who have the greatest chance of survival (Ihlenfeld, 2003). In addition, nurses will find themselves in positions where there is a lack of necessary resources, and they will then have to come up with creative solutions.

Terrorism has created the need for us to prepare against agents that we previously thought were no longer threats. The Department of Homeland Security (DHS) defines *terrorism* as an act of violence that is dangerous to human life, in violation of the criminal laws of the United States, and used to intimidate or coerce a government, the civilian population, or any segment thereof in furtherance of political or social objectives. Ultimately, terrorists plan their attacks with the intent to create fear in the public sector. With this in mind, strategies to offset terrorist activities must include calm and effective communication.

These new threats involve a variety of different agents, but a standardized nomenclature has been developed for five categories using the acronym *CBRNE,* which stands for *c*hemical, *b*iologic, *r*adiologic, *n*uclear, and *e*xplosive. Table 13-1 describes the similarities and differences related to the CBRNE agents.

STAGES OF DISASTER

Veenema (2003b) describes three phases of the disaster continuum: preimpact, impact, and postimpact. In the preimpact phase, activities are focused on planning, preparedness, prevention, and warning. In the impact stage, all efforts are directed to responding to the disaster, initiating the emergency management system, and mitigating the effects of the hazard. During the postimpact phase, which usually begins 72 hours after the disaster and may

Table 13-1	CBRNE Agents			
AGENTS	**ACTION**	**ADVANTAGES**	**DISADVANTAGES**	**TREATMENT**
Chemical	Agents injure or kill through variety of means: vesicant, nerve, blood, respiratory	Spread easily through air; cause immediate effects; require decontamination	Less toxic than biologic agents; need to be used in large quantities; subject to dispersion by wind; terrorists need to protect themselves; require trained HAZMAT teams	Dependent on agent used; in some cases have agent specific medications; decontamination; use of PPE by personnel
Biologic	Disease-causing organisms (bacteria, viruses, toxins)	Available; small quantities can have large effect; spread through large areas; can remain in air or on surfaces; difficult to prepare against	Delayed effects; production hazardous to terrorists; difficult to develop	Dependent on agent used; most cause flu-like symptoms plague and smallpox most contagious; timing of specific treatment critical; in some cases can have vaccinations
Radiologic	Ionizing radiation able to strip electrons from atoms, causing chemical changes in molecules; expression may be delayed; radiation depends on time, distance, shielding, and quantity of radioactive material	Available; psychologic impact likely to be substantial; often used in conjunction with explosive devices ("dirty bomb")	Delayed effects of radiation materials; difficult to shield against	Dirty bomb causes immediate effects (radiation burns/acute poisoning) and long-term effects (cancer/contamination of drinking water); decontamination must occur before patient care can be safely provided by the health care worker
Nuclear	Depends on yield of nuclear weapon, but consists of blast range effects, thermal radiation, nuclear radiation, and radioactive fallout	Requires decontamination; contamination can remain for many years; psychologic impact likely to be substantial	Large, heavy, and dangerous weapons; hazardous to terrorist; expensive and difficult to make weapons of this type	Symptomatic treatment of thermal burns, shrapnel injuries, and radioactive fallout; depends on distance from source and time of exposure
Explosive	Most common method for terrorists; capable of violent decomposition; pressure/temperature changes and propellants cause injury and/or death	Easy to find materials to construct explosive device; large devices can be placed in abandoned vehicles; smaller devices can be placed on bodies of persons willing to commit suicide by lignting the device	Volatile ingredients could cause premature explosion of device, thus creating danger for terrorists; government agencies have improved training and processes for identifying incendiary devices	Symptomatic; often requires treatment for burns

continue for 2 to 3 years, a network of activities is designed to enhance recovery, rehabilitation, and reconstruction. Evaluation of the disaster preparedness and response plan is a major activity that needs to be included in the postimpact phase. The following sections will describe components of the preimpact and impact phases of a disaster.

Preimpact Phase

Every disaster, regardless of the cause, begins as a local event. Each locale has the responsibility for responding to the emergencies within its community first. Thus, the heaviest burden falls on the local community when a mass casualty occurs. Assistance from state and federal levels is appropriated when the local system is unable to provide the necessary level of care. It is imperative, then, that communities plan for the services that will be needed in a time of disaster and train the providers within each agency about responding to all hazard types of mass casualty events. Efforts must be directed toward the interrelationship of roles and responsibilities of the agencies and services that will needed at the time of a disaster (Fig. 13-1).

The key elements of a community preparedness program should include the following: (1) assessing the community for risks and determining the types of events that may occur, (2) planning the emergency activities to ensure a coordinated response effort, and (3) building the capabilities that are necessary to respond to the consequences of the events (CDC, 2001). There must be agreements between agencies within the community and between neighboring communities for such entities as emergency response units, hospitals, long-term care facilities, clinics, and health departments to be able to provide mutual aid and transfer of people and materials during a time of disaster. Agreements should be in place that address issues related to credentialing health care providers who may be shared between institutions.

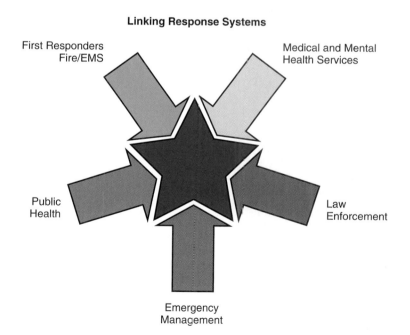

FIG. 13-1 Agencies and services involved at the time of a disaster. (From http://www.bt.cdc.gov/planning/CoopAgreementAward/presentations/mmrs-oep10minbriefing-jim11.pdf).

Plans and contracts need to be developed with school systems, YMCAs, or other large facilities to provide shelter for large numbers of victims. The interface with volunteer agencies such as the Red Cross also needs to be arranged. Each agency should have a well-developed emergency operating plan (EOP) that includes its responsibilities and capabilities for responding to a mass casualty event, an identified chain of command, and a plan for interaction with other community agencies. Agency personnel should be knowledgeable about their role in the EOP and receive education concerning the ways to respond to all types of hazards.

There are several federal level programs designed to assist communities in planning their emergency response to a mass casualty event and to provide assistance during a time of disaster. Agency and community EOPs should outline their relationship with the federal system. Fig. 13-2 illustrates the relationship among local, state, and federal response systems. Following is a description of the key components of the federal response system.

Metropolitan Medical Response System (MMRS). MMRS, currently funded through the DHS, was initiated in 1996 to enhance local planning and emergency response system capability to care for victims of a terrorist incident. Since its inception, 127 MMRS jurisdictions have been initiated. The MMRS builds a cadre of specialty trained responders and equipment. The system is coordinated with area statewide planning systems and integrates the efforts of all of the emergency response teams. The MMRS includes plans for expanding hospital-based care, enhancing emergency medical transport and emergency department capabilities, locating specialized pharmaceuticals to respond to a terrorist event, managing mass fatalities, and providing mental health care for the community, victims, and health care providers. Scenarios designed to test the effectiveness of the MMRS in the community in providing an integrated response to a terrorist incident are conducted on a regular basis.

National Disaster Medical System (NDMS). NDMS is a partnership among FEMA, the Veteran's Administration (VA), Department of Defense (DOD), and Department of Health and Human Services (DHHS) and is the lead federal agency for medical response under the National Response Plan. The purpose of NDMS is to supplement state and local resources during disasters and major emergencies, thus supporting the MMRS activities. The NDMS is activated when state and local resources are insufficient to provide care for the victims of the disaster incident. Major components of the NDMS include (1) teams of health care providers with supplies and equipment, (2) patient evacuation from the disaster area to an unaffected area, and (3) arrangements for hospitalizations in both federal hospitals and a voluntary network of nonfederal acute care hospitals in the case of a national emergency. There are more than 7000 participating health care professionals in the NDMS system, including four rapid response WMD trained teams. Included in the NDMS are disaster medical assistance teams (DMAT), disaster mortuary operational response teams (DMORT), veterinary medical assistance teams (VMAT), and urban search and rescue (USAR).

Commissioned Corps Readiness Force (CCRF). CCRF is an initiative led by the Surgeon General; it is an additional asset that is capable of responding in times of extraordinary need when the public health needs exceed the ability of the local or state agencies. CCRF is composed of more than 1400 health care professionals that can be deployed to respond to a disaster, either as a large group or in small numbers to support the DMAT effort.

Strategic National Stockpile (SNS). SNS is a program that is jointly managed by the DHS and the DHHS to assist the state and local public health capacity to respond to national emergencies.

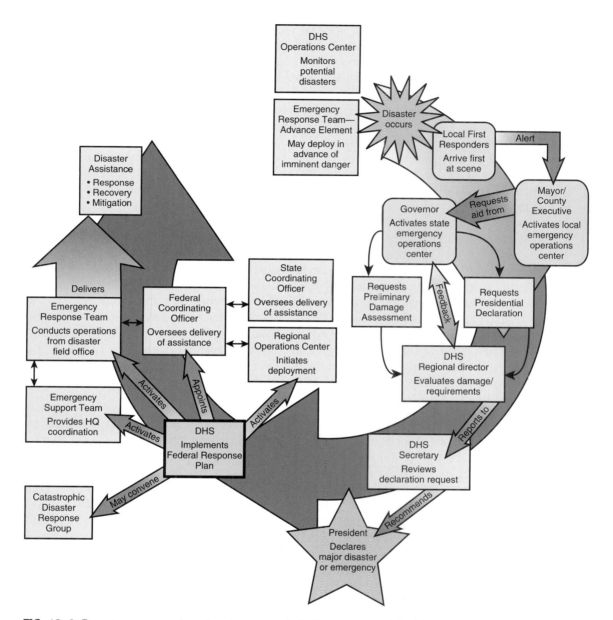

FIG. 13–2 Emergency response flows from the community to the state to the federal level. (From FEMA: *Federal Response Plan, 2003*, http:www.fema.gov/rrr/frp).

The SNS has a national repository of antibiotics, chemical antidotes, antitoxins, IV administrations, airway supplies, and other medical/surgical items. This stockpile is designed to replenish and enhance the supplies of local and state agencies during a time of emergency. A 12 hour "push-pack" of supplies can be deployed within 12 hours of the decision to activate the SNS. The community emergency plan should include procedures to receive the push package.

Follow-up pharmaceutical or medical supplies can be shipped within 24 to 36 hours if required. This supply can be tailored to the specific needs of the event if the needs are known at that time (CDC, 2003).

Community emergency operating plans must include strategies for the community's interaction with these various state and federal response teams and systems in order to efficiently utilize the services and materials provided for mass casualty response. Hospital EOPs should include descriptions of the federal responses and how they will be incorporated into the emergency operations.

Impact Phase

Response Activities. Response activities are first initiated during the impact phase of disasters. These activities begin at the time of the event and are focused on providing the first emergency response to victims of the disaster, stabilizing the situation, and providing adequate treatment for the victims. This phase requires the interaction of emergency responders from fire and police departments, emergency medical services, hazardous materials teams, health care agencies, health departments, and other agencies to be able to triage and provide assistance to the victims and stabilize the scene. Usually the first unit responding establishes an incident command post from which to coordinate the activities. However, as other units arrive and as the cause of the incident becomes known, one of the law enforcement agencies may assume control if there is suspicion of a crime prior to the establishment of a community-based emergency operations center (EOC).

Incident Management. Emergencies breed chaos, and it is essential to bring order to the situation for an effective response. The incident management system (IMS) has become a popular solution; it was first used by firefighters to control disaster scenes in a multijurisdictional and interdepartmental manner. IMS consists of four functions: planning, operations, logistics, and finance and administration. The system is designed to expand from one person or agency performing all roles to having hundreds of people involved in the process. An efficient IMS requires a hierarchical chain of command led by the incident manager or commander. Job assignments are consistently followed by assigned personnel who refer to a specific job action sheet. An IMS will be established at the scene of the disaster and will include representatives of all agencies needed to provide the emergency services.

At the time of a mass casualty, each hospital system will initiate their emergency response plans. The IMS was adapted for hospital use in 1992 and tested by six hospitals in California (HEICS III, 2003a). Structures may vary from hospital to hospital, but most are using the system called the Hospital Emergency Incident Command System (HEICS). The assumption is that in a time of crisis, communication will be improved if all disaster responders begin from a common structure. HEICS defines responsibilities, reporting channels, and common terminology for hospitals, fire departments, local governments, and other agencies. The HEICS can be customized for organizations of varying sizes. HEICS has been used by hospitals in the United States, Canada, Germany, New Zealand, Japan, South America, and Saudi Arabia (HEICS III, 2003b). The HEICS template can be downloaded on-line at no charge (http://www.emsa.cahwnet.gov/dms2/heics3.htm). Regardless of the structure of the IMS, the ultimate aim is to coordinate the safe and effective response of emergency resources to an incident.

In the HEICS system, there is only one incident commander, supported by clearly identified levels in the command structure. The hierarchy of command is important so that there

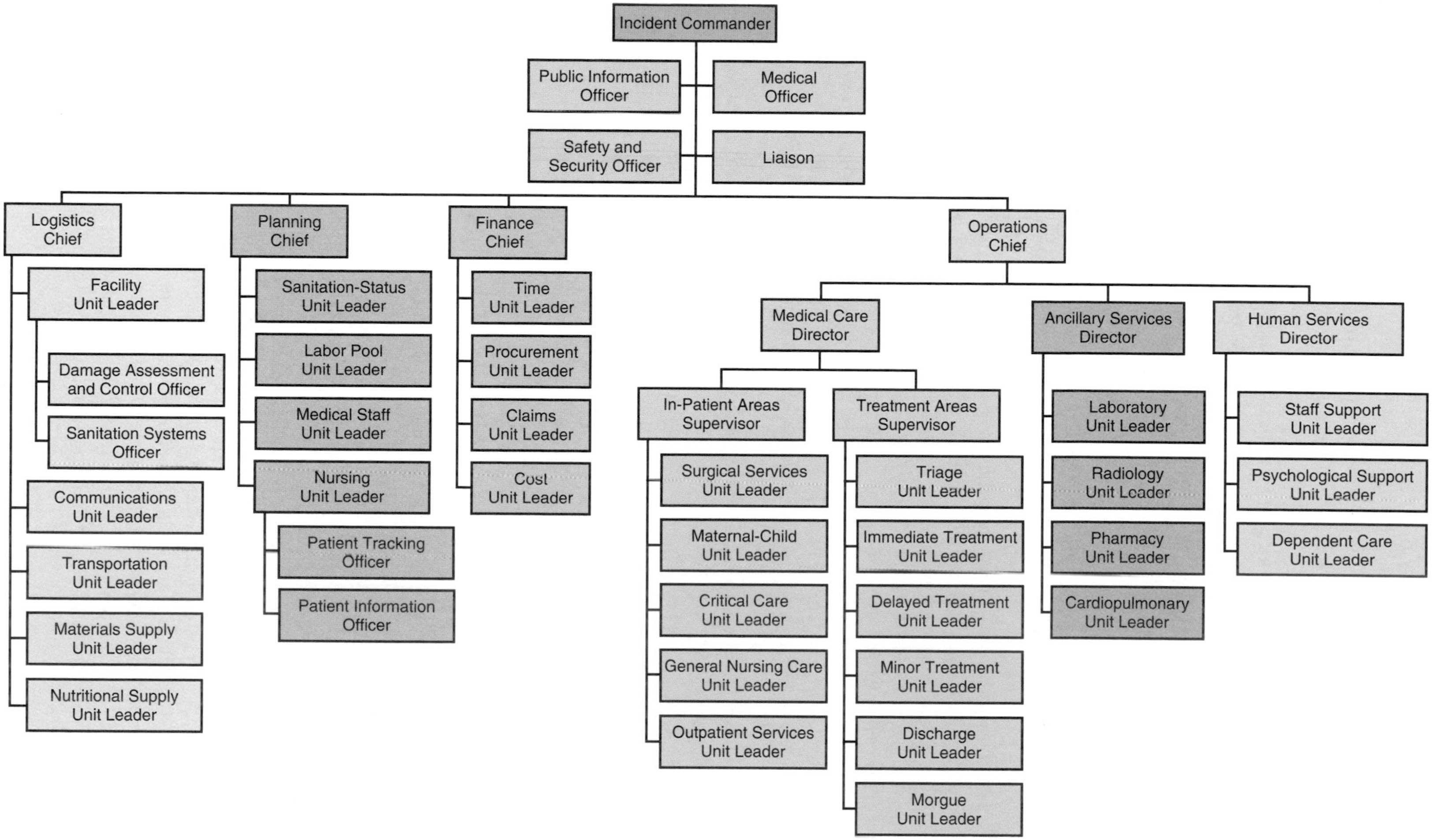

FIG. 13-3 HEICS organizational chart. (From California Emergency Medical Services Authority, www.emsa.ca.gov/dms2/heics.asp).

is no confusion as to who reports to whom or about who is managing the incident. The chain of command is established to allow for communication to flow from the top down or the bottom up.

It is important to understand that although a community event may trigger the establishment of an EOC using incident management, the local hospitals may establish their own centers in order to manage the incident within that hospital. Careful attention is paid, however, to designate a liaison officer to coordinate the response between the community EOC and the hospital EOC. Successful use of incident command principles depends on a unified command structure with a clearly established chain of command, along with incident objectives and strategies.

Fig. 13-3 illustrates the typical HEICS organization. The positions at the top of the organizational chart are typically seen across a wide variety of organizations. As the chart expands downward, positions are usually customized to meet the organizational needs of individual groups. For example, a large academic health sciences center is likely to have different position descriptions (below the top levels) than a local community hospital with fewer employees and functions.

Event Recognition. At the time of impact, it is rare that the extent of the incident or the causative agent is known. Emergency responders at the scene will assess the potential for contamination and set up appropriate triage and decontamination procedures, performing field decontamination before transporting victims to health care facilities. Responders must utilize personal protective equipment (PPE) before providing primary triage for victims to prevent themselves from being exposed to the agent and becoming victims as well.

Health care facilities should be notified of the event and the possibility of contamination as soon as possible. In the Sarin gas incident in Tokyo, many walking victims appeared at the hospital emergency rooms and clinics before the arrival of the first ambulance. Approximately 20% of the house staff and other transporting personnel suffered effects of the gas as a result of lack of information of the causative agent at the time the first victims began arriving (Ohbu et al, 1997). Security personnel must limit access to the hospital and should be equipped with the appropriate level of PPE. When receiving contaminated victims, the health care facility's first responsibility is to protect their patients, staff, and facility, then to provide medical care for the contaminated victims, and finally, to protect the environment from decontamination waste runoff (Macintyre et al, 2000).

Personal Protection and Safety. Personal protection and safety are important regardless of the situational factors causing a disaster. What is important to note, however, is that situational factors will dictate how to be personally protected and safe. Protecting the lives of emergency responders takes precedence over other incident issues because, if emergency responders are exposed or injured, they will not be able to provide care to others.

To understand how to provide protection, responders must be familiar with the routes of exposure (i.e., the routes or pathways into the body). Chemical, biologic, radiologic, and explosive devices can enter the body through one or more routes: inhalation, ingestion, absorption, and injection. Dispersed chemical and biologic agents usually enter the body through inhalation or ingestion. Nerve agents in liquid form can be absorbed by the skin. Radiologic agents can be inhaled, absorbed, or ingested. Explosive materials can inject shrapnel into bodies.

Because of the varied routes of exposure, protective equipment must be designed to impede the most vulnerable route(s), thereby blocking the agent from entering the body. Specially designed PPE is available in a variety of levels, each level designed to meet specific protection needs:

- **Level A** equipment provides a totally encapsulated chemical resistant suit, including supplied air. As a result, maximum respiratory and skin protection is provided. In addition, this level of equipment is used to provide protection against liquid splashes or in situations where agents are still unidentified.
- **Level B** provides a chemical splash–resistant suit with hood and self-contained breathing apparatus (SCBA). It provides maximum respiratory protection but less skin protection than level A.
- **Level C** equipment is chemical-resistant clothing with a hood and an air-purifying respirator. The respirator can remove all anticipated contaminants and concentrations of chemical materials, thus providing adequate protection against airborne biologic agents and radiologic materials.
- **Level D** protection may consist of a uniform or "scrubs" and is appropriate when it has been determined that no respiratory or skin hazard is present.

Although each level provides some protection, it is important to understand the limitations of all PPE. Typically, first responders to community emergencies are firefighters, police, and emergency medical technicians. These professionals have traditionally been trained in the effective use of PPE and can be a good community resource. In addition, hospital infection control personnel can be an excellent resource for the use of PPE. As health care providers assume the care of patients who may have been contaminated, it is important to note whether they have been decontaminated and require no further protective equipment or what additional level of protection is required.

If a situation arises that requires the use of PPE, one must keep in mind that some procedures will be difficult to complete while wearing this equipment. The gloves will limit range of motion, and hoods will limit peripheral vision. In addition, proper fluid and electrolyte levels are very important for those wearing PPE because perspiration is not allowed to evaporate and may result in overheating. A rotation schedule for caregivers needs to be implemented so that caregivers in PPE do not wear the equipment for more than 30 minutes without a break. If given the opportunity, every caregiver should have the experience of wearing PPE before an actual event. Unfortunately, the cost of maintaining this equipment is a prohibitive factor for most organizations. Fig. 13-4 illustrates the donning of level C PPE. Note the importance of helping one another put on and remove this equipment.

Decontamination. Initial decontamination will begin at the scene of the incident. However, secondary decontamination may be needed at the health care facility where the victim will be treated. Victims who may transport themselves to the facility will also need to have decontamination procedures performed before treatment. Hospitals should have decontamination facilities; however, free-standing clinics or health care provider offices will probably not have a space for decontamination. These issues should be addressed in the health care facility's emergency operating procedures.

Decontamination from chemical exposures usually includes removal of the victim's clothing and washing with soap and water. Outdoor facilities with shower heads and soap dispensing units are used for mass casualty incidents. Health care providers wearing PPE will be

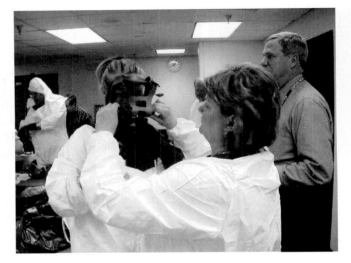

FIG. 13–4 Donning PPE. Elizabeth Weiner and Margaret Irwin help each other put on personal protective equipment (PPE) during an educational session at the Noble Training Center.

assigned to assist with the decontamination procedures and monitor victims for deterioration during the decontamination process.

Whenever possible, separate areas for sexes should be available to protect privacy during the decontamination process. Careful labeling of clothing and valuables is necessary because all items may be considered criminal evidence (Macintyre et al, 2000).

Communication Within the Health Care Facility. At the initial time of the event, when news stories are first breaking, staff, patients, and families may hear of the incident before the EOP and the HEIC system have been initiated. In this case, it is crucial for the facility information officer to take charge of communicating with the news media and for administrators to initiate a plan to communicate within the health care facility. Crisis intervention strategies to prevent group panic must be instituted immediately. Communication officers need to do the following:

- Determine the effects the crisis will have on the audience
- Speak clearly and simply about the facts
- Be direct, honest, and to the point
- Reassure and calm the audience (JCAHO, 2002)

Regular updates of information (every 30 minutes) need to be planned and distributed to all hospital units as quickly as possible (Veenema, 2003b).

Patients and families need to be informed of measures that will be taken with the initiation of the EOP, such as early discharge or relocation of less ill patients to other areas of the hospital or to other facilities. Family members may not be able to leave the hospital to return home; arrangements will need to be made to care for them, including providing medications that they take regularly (Staten, 2002).

Mechanisms for staff to contact their families or significant others should be initiated as soon as possible. Arrangements need to be made for the care of children, other dependents, and pets for those staff members who will be staying at the hospital for extended periods of time. Places to provide rest and measures to encourage staff to rest should be determined.

INTERNATIONAL NURSING COALITION FOR MASS CASUALTY EDUCATION (INCMCE)

The INCMCE is an international coalition consisting of organizational representatives of schools of nursing, nursing accrediting bodies, nursing specialty organizations, and governmental agencies interested in promoting mass casualty education for nurses. The vision of the organization is to be the point of influence for public policy that affects the welfare of the public through nursing practice, education, research, and regulation for mass casualty incidents. The mission of INCMCE is to ensure a competent nurse workforce to respond to mass casualty events. Their strategic plan has been developed in the priority areas of awareness, response, and research.

Dean Colleen Conway-Welch from Vanderbilt University, in conjunction with the Office of Emergency Preparedness, agreed to host the INCMCE and led the first meeting in March 2001. After the events of September 11, 2001, interest in the INCMCE grew. Organizational representatives constitute the full membership of the group, which meets annually. Associate members receive communication regarding the work of the INCMCE and are eligible to become subject matter experts.

Early important work of the INCMCE involved the development of competencies for nurses graduating from all programs. The document was developed by a task force (chaired by Joan Stanley from the American Association of Colleges of Nursing [AACN]) and has been reviewed and revised by INCMCE members. The revised document was then reviewed by another level of representatives for validation. This final version was accepted by the INCMCE during their July 2003 meeting. A copy of the current competencies can be found on-line (www.incmce.org).

The competencies provide the framework for the development of on-line learning modules under the direction of Elizabeth Weiner, Associate Director of the INCMCE. She has outlined the modules for development and placed them into a curriculum grid that can also be found on the INCMCE website. Funding for the development has been provided from HHS and DHS, by the Health Resources and Services Administration (for curriculum innovation), and by the Agency for Healthcare Research and Quality (to determine the effectiveness and efficiency of the on-line modules). A unique aspect of the modules is that they are being developed using the "How People Learn" framework (derived from a comprehensive review of the educational literature for the National Research Council). The INCMCE website will provide the capability to present the modules as they are completed and to announce current INCMCE activities.

S U M M A R Y

Preparing for a mass casualty event requires a complex set of activities. Nurses need to be aware of the emergency response system at the local, state, and federal levels and how they should interface with the systems. They should be involved in developing and evaluating the emergency response plans for their health care agencies and communities. Nurses are well positioned to serve in leadership roles within health care agencies during the time of a disaster because of their excellent skills in communication and collaboration. Content on disaster management needs to be included in nursing education programs and provided in continuing education courses for practicing nurses. Determining the competencies for nurses related to disaster management will be key to the development of the educational programs. Following is an extensive list of resources the reader can use for further information about emergency preparedness.

INTERNET RESOURCES RELATED TO EMERGENCY PREPAREDNESS AND RESPONSE

KEY GOVERNMENT WEBSITES

Centers for Disease Control and Prevention
http://www.bt.cdc.gov/emcontact/index.asp

Agency for Healthcare Research and Quality (AHRQ)
http://www.ahcpr.gov/

Federal Emergency Management Agency
http://www.fema.gov

Department of Defense
http://www.defenselink.mil/

Department of Health and Human Services
http://www.ndms.dhhs.gov/

U.S. Department of Health and Human Services—Bioterrorism
http://www.hrsa.gov/terrorism/bioterror.htm

U.S. Department of Homeland Security
http://www.dhs.gov/dhspublic/

U.S. Department of Homeland Security—Kit and plan information
http://www.ready.gov/

U.S. Army Medical Research Institute of Infectious Diseases
http://www.usamriid.army.mil

USAMRIID Virtual Naval Hospital
http://www.vnh.org/BIOCASU/toc.html

U.S. National Response Center
www.nrc.uscg.mil

Federal Legislation

Legislative information on the Thomas website of the Library of Congress
http://thomas.loc.gov/

NONGOVERNMENT WEBSITES

World Health Organization
http://www.who.int/csr/delibepidemics/en/

American Red Cross
http://www.redcross.org/

Medical NBC Online
http://www.nbc-med.org/others/

Pan American Health Organization
http://165.158.1.110/english/ped/pedhome.htm

Bioterrorism and Disaster Response
http://www.nursingworld.org/news/disaster/

Kansas University Medical Center
http://www2.kumc.edu/safety/grant/resource.htm

How Biologic and Chemical Warfare Works
http://science.howstuffworks.com/biochem-war3.htm

Mental Health Resources

National Mental Health Information Center
http://www.mentalhealth.org/cmhs/EmergencyServices/default.asp

David Baldwin's Trauma Information
http://www.trauma-pages.com/

GENERAL PREPAREDNESS—ALL HAZARDS
Key Websites

Disaster Preparedness and Response for Nurses
http://www.nursingsociety.org/education/case_studies/cases/SP0004.html

Journals

Disaster Management and Response
http://www2.us.elsevierhealth.com/scripts/om.dll/serve?action=searchDB&search
    DBfor=home&id=mmd

Australasian Journal of Disaster and Trauma Studies
http://www.massey.ac.nz/~trauma/

Books/Handbooks/Manuals

Barbera JA, Macintyre A: *Jane's Mass Casualty Handbook: Hospital Emergency
    Preparedness and Response,* Coulsdon, Surrey, United Kingdom, 2003,
    Jane's Information Group, WX 215 B2341.
To order: http://catalog.janes.com/catalog/public/index.cfm?fuseaction=home.
    Product InfoBrief&product_id=9242

Veenema TG, editor: *Disaster Nursing and Emergency Preparedness for Chemical,
    Biological, and Radiological Terrorism and Other Hazards*, New York, 2003,
    Springer Publishing Co.
To order: http://www.springerpub.com/books/nursing/pub_2143_8.html

Videos

Disaster Preparedness for Healthcare
To order: http://www.medfilms.com/videos/disaster-prep.shtml

GENERAL PREPAREDNESS—CHEMICAL
Key Websites

CDC Chemical Agent List
http://www.bt.cdc.gov/agent/agentlistchem.aspWebsites

Handbooks/Manuals

Veterans Administration: *Chemical Terrorism: General Guidance Pocket Guide*
http://www.oqp.med.va.gov/cpg/BCR/G/chemcard_5_16_02dgs.doc

Videos

Chemical Terrorism for Healthcare
To order: http://www.medfilms.com/videos/chemical-terror.shtml

GENERAL PREPAREDNESS—BIOLOGIC
Key Websites

CDC Bioterrorism Agents List
http://www.bt.cdc.gov/Agent/Agentlist.asp

WHO Preparedness for Deliberate Epidemics
http://www.who.int/csr/delibepidemics/en/

Infectious Diseases Society of America (IDSA)
Bioterrorism Information and Resources
http://www.idsociety.org/Template.cfm?Section=Bioterrorism&Template=/
TaggedPage/TaggedPageDisplay.cfm&TPLID=27&ContentID=5022

Handbooks/Manuals

U.S. Army Medical Research Institute of Infectious Diseases:
USAMRIID Medical Management of Biological Casualties Handbook, ed 4, Fort
Detrick, Md, 2001, International Medical Publishing Inc.

Veterans Administration: *Biological Terror Consideration General Guidance Pocket Guide*
http://www.oqp.med.va.gov/cpg/BCR/G/Biocard_5_16_02dgs.doc

Webcasts/Videos

AHRQ—Free Web-Assisted Audioconference Calls on Bioterrorism and Health System Preparedness
http://www.ahcpr.gov/news/ulp/biotconf.htm

Bioterrorism for Healthcare (video)
To order: http://www.medfilms.com/videos/bioter-for-healthcare.shtml

GENERAL PREPAREDNESS—RADIOLOGIC/NUCLEAR
Key Websites

Centers for Disease Control and Prevention
http://www.bt.cdc.gov/radiation/dirtybombs.asp

Handbooks/Manuals

Veterans Administration: *Terrorism with Ionizing Radiation: General Guidance Pocket Guide*
http://www.oqp.med.va.gov/cpg/BCR/G/radcard_5_16_02dgs.doc

Other Radiologic/Nuclear Resources

Time Online Edition
http://www.time.com/time/nation/article/0,8599,182637,00.html

American Society for Therapeutic Radiology and Oncology (radiation disaster management information)
http://www.astro.org/government_relations/government_relations_topics/disastermanagement.htm

U.S. Nuclear Regulatory Commission
http://www.nrc.gov/reading-rm/doc-collections/fact-sheets/dirty-bombs.html

Dirty-Bomb Fact Sheets
http://www1.va.gov/emshg/docs/Radiologic_Medical_Countermeasures_062003.pdf

Videos

Radiological Terrorism for Healthcare and Radiological Incidents
http://www.medfilms.com/videos/radiological-terror.shtml

EDUCATIONAL AND TRAINING PROGRAMS
Educational Programs

University of California–Los Angeles
http://www.cphd.ucla.edu/

University of Rochester
Masters Program Leadership in Healthcare Systems
Disaster Response and Emergency Preparedness Track
http://www.urmc.rochester.edu/son/AcademicPrograms/lhcs.cfm

The Disaster Mental Health Institute (DMHI), a State of South Dakota Board of Regents Center of Excellence
http://www.usd.edu/dmhi/

University of Alabama at Birmingham
http://www.bioterrorism.uab.edu

Center for the Study of Bioterrorism, Saint Louis University School of Public Health
http://www.bioterrorism.slu.edu/

Saint Louis University—Disaster Preparedness for Nurses Certificate
http://www.ed-x.com/courselistings/courseinfo.asp?NewsID=24323

Columbia University Mailman School of Public Health—Basic Emergency Preparedness
http://cds.osr.columbia.edu/bepcourse/index.htm

University of Minnesota Center for Infectious Disease Research and Policy
http://www.cidrap.umn.edu/cidrap/

Vanderbilt University School of Nursing—Emergency Response Management Certificate
http://www.mc.vanderbilt.edu/nursing

Training Programs

American Red Cross
http://www.redcross.org/

Biological and Chemical Warfare and Terrorism: Medical Issues and Response
http://www.swankhealth.com/USAMRIID.html

Compendium of Federal Terrorism Training (FEMA)
http://www.fema.gov/compendium/index.jsp

Emergency Management Institute (FEMA)
http://training.fema.gov/emiweb/

U.S. Army Medical Research Institute of Infectious Diseases
http://www.usamriid.army.mil/education/index.html

CDC Public Health Training Network
http://www.phppo.cdc.gov/phtn/default.asp

North Carolina Center for Public Health Preparedness
http://www.sph.unc.edu/nccphp/training/all_trainings/at_biot_ph.htm

CDC Emergency Preparedness and Response
http://www.bt.cdc.gov/Training/index.asp

Bioterrorism CE Credit
http://www.abqaurp.org/module.asp?CourseID=11

INCIDENT COMMAND SYSTEM RESOURCES
Hospital Emergency Incident Command System

Hospital Emergency Incident Command System Update Project
http://www.emsa.cahwnet.gov/Dms2/download.htm

Incident Management Systems

International Federation of Red Cross and Red Crescent Societies: History and Development of Incident Management System
http://www.ifrc.org/docs/pubs/health/chapter10.pdf

The Public Health Role in Incident Management Systems
National Association of County and City Health Officials (NACCHO)
http://www.naccho.org/general910.cfm

Incident Command System

U.S. Response Team Committee Document on ICS
http://nrt.org/production/nrt/home.nsf/resources/Publications1/$File/ICS_UC_Technical_Assistance_Document.pdf

CRITICAL THINKING ACTIVITIES

1. Choose one of your primary acute care clinical training sites and locate and review its emergency response plan. What is the facility's role in community, state, and regional plans? How does the facility's plan compare with information presented in this chapter?

2. After reviewing a health care facility's emergency response plan, interview staff nurses and nurse managers in the facility. Ask them to describe their responsibilities in the facility's emergency response plan. Determine who makes the decision about when to don personal protective equipment and what level is required.

3. How could security and confidentiality be maintained during a mass casualty incident?

4. If you were asked develop a program to present to a community lay audience about emergency preparedness, what information would be most important to relay?

Additional resources are available on-line at: http://evolve.elsevier.com/Cherry/

evolve

http://evolve.elsevier.com

REFERENCES

Barbera J, Macintyre AG, editors: *Jane's mass casualty handbook: hospital emergency preparedness and response*, Surrey, United Kingdom, 2003, Jane's Information Group, Ltd.

Centers for Disease Control: *Strategic national stockpile: emergency preparedness and response, 2003*. Available on-line (http://www.bt.cdc.gov/stockpile/index.asp).

Centers for Disease Control and Prevention: *The public health response to biological and chemical terrorism: interim planning guidance for state public health officials*, Atlanta, Ga, 2001, U.S. Department of Health and Human Services.

Federal Emergency Management Agency: *Federal response plan, 2003*. Available on-line (http:www.fema.gov/rrr/frp).

HEICS III: *Hospital emergency incident command system update project: about the HEICS III project, 2003a*. Available on-line (http://www.emsa.cahwnet.gov/Dms2/HISTORY.HTM).

HEICS III: *Hospital emergency incident command system update project: frequently asked questions about the hospital emergency incident command system, 2003b*. Available on-line (http://www.emsa.cahwnet.gov/dms2/faqs.htm).

Ihlenfeld JT: A primer on triage and mass casualty events, *Dimens Crit Care Nurs* 22(5):204-207, 2003.

Johns Hopkins Evidence-Based Practice Center: *Training of clinicians for public health events relevant to bioterrorism preparedness* (AHRQ Publication No. 02-E011), Rockville, Md, 2002, Agency for Healthcare Research and Quality.

Joint Commission Resources: *Guide to emergency management planning in health care*, Oakbrook Terrace, Ill, 2002, Joint Commission Resources, Inc..

Landesman LY: *Public health management of disasters: the practice guide*, Washington, DC, 2002, American Public Health Association.

Macintyre AG et al: Weapons of mass destruction events with contaminated casualties: effective planning for health care facilities, *JAMA* 283(2):242-249, 2000.

Ohbu S et al: Sarin poisoning on Tokyo subway, *South Med J* 90(6):587-93, 1997.

Staten PA: Heighten your emergency preparedness, *Nurs Manage* 33(5):20, 2002.

Veenema TG: Chemical and biological terrorism preparedness for staff development specialists, *J Nurses Staff Develop* 19(5):215-222, 2003a.

Veenema TG, editor: *Disaster nursing and emergency preparedness for chemical, biological, and radiological terrorism and other hazards*, New York, 2003b, Springer Publishing Co.

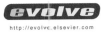

14

Nursing Informatics and Clinical Information Systems

Leslie H. Nicoll, PhD, MBA, RN

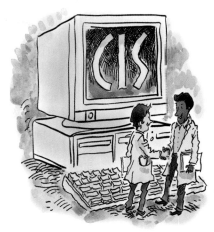

Clinical information systems
offer nurses and other
team members information
when, where, and how they need it.

VIGNETTE

The certified informatics nurse welcomed everyone to the committee meeting. She was chairing the group that would have responsibility for selecting, implementing, and evaluating the nursing service module of the new clinical information system (CIS) for the institution. "We have a big job ahead of us," she told the group, "but I know we are up to it."

Two years later the system was on-line. The group looked back on 24 months of hard work: developing specifications for the system, putting out a request for proposals to meet the specifications, reviewing bids and selecting a vendor, installing the equipment, training the staff, and finally going 'live." They felt enormously rewarded for all their hard work. They all knew that the new system would decrease nursing costs, help save nurses time, and ultimately benefit their patients. It was a proud moment.

Questions to consider while reading this chapter:

1. What strategies could the certified informatics nurse use to help the nursing staff adjust to the new CIS system?
2. How will the new CIS decrease nursing costs? Save nursing time? Benefit patients?

Additional resources are available on-line at: http://evolve.elsevier.com/Cherry/

KEY TERMS

Clinical information system (CIS) The software and associated hardware that supports the entry, retrieval, update, and analysis of patient care information and associated clinical information related to patient care.

Computer literacy The knowledge and understanding of computers combined with the ability to use them effectively.

Data capture The collection and entry of data into a computer system.

Decision support systems Software programs that process data to produce or recommend decisions by linking with an electronic knowledge base controlled by established rules for combining data elements; the knowledge base and rules mimic the knowledge and reasoning an expert nurse would apply to data and information to solve a problem.

Electronic health record (EHR) All information about an individual's lifetime health status maintained electronically.

Hardware The physical computer and its components, such as the central processing unit (CPU), the monitor, and the screen.

Internet 1. With a lower case "i," any collection of distinct networks working together as one. 2. With an upper case "I," the worldwide "network of networks" that are connected to one another, using specific protocols.

Knowledge delivery systems An automated system that updates the knowledge base with new evidence, research, reports, and other pertinent information that is critical for accurate decision making. An ideal knowledge delivery system filters the information based on relevance and quality and alerts and directs the user to the new information as it is imported.

Lexicon Entire stock of words belonging to a branch of knowledge, such as nursing (Encarta, 2003).

Software Programs that run the computer (programs that perform different tasks, such as statistics or word processing, are known as applications).

Taxonomies Classification systems used to organize electronic data and information.

Three waves of computing The three eras in the development of modern computing: phase I, the mainframe era; phase II, the personal computer (PC) era; and phase III, ubiquitous computing.

Ubiquitous Present everywhere.

URL Universal resource locator; the system of addresses used on the Internet.

Vendor An individual or company that sells products.

Virtual reality An artificial environment created with computer hardware and software and presented to the user in such a way that it appears and feels like a real environment.

World Wide Web (www) The graphic part of the Internet. The www is based on hypertext and allows the creation and transfer of multimedia objects.

LEARNING OUTCOMES

After studying this chapter, the reader will be able to:

1. List the components that are integral to a nursing specialty and discuss how nursing informatics meets these requirements.
2. Describe educational pathways that exist for nurses interested in pursuing nursing informatics as a specialty.
3. Summarize the major points in the evolution of computer technology.
4. Predict future trends in computing as they relate to health care and nursing practice.
5. Use established criteria to evaluate the content of health-related sites found on the Internet.

NURSING INFORMATICS

The prevalence of computers in society has made it imperative for nurses to integrate the use of computers into their professional practice. Because it is no longer an option, nurses must make good use of computer technology to work toward the goal of improved patient care and positive patient outcomes. Students, clinical nurses, educators, researchers, and administrators are all benefiting from computer technology. Students are using word processing programs to prepare course assignments and accessing course assignments via the Internet; they also learn nursing skills using computer-assisted instruction (CAI) programs. Educators use computers to post course assignments for access via the Internet and to prepare audiovisual materials for class presentations, papers for publication, and posters for display at professional conferences. Administrators plan their budgets with spreadsheet programs to manage costs for sound financial management. Researchers are collecting data via the Internet and then analyzing the data with statistics programs. Nurses in clinical settings retrieve patient data, document their interventions, and view laboratory and other results through electronic patient records. These are just a few examples of how computers and their associated technology are influencing nursing practice.

Although all nurses are involved with computers to some degree, there are nurses who have chosen to specialize in the area of nursing practice that relates to computers. This field is known as *nursing informatics (NI)*. This is a relatively new specialty within the profession of nursing. It is only within the past 15 years that it has been named, recognized as a specialty, and defined by the nursing profession. Academic programs to prepare nurses with expertise in informatics have been established; the American Nurses Credentialing Center (ANCC) has developed a certification examination to allow nurses who demonstrate beginning levels of competency to be certified in nursing informatics and use the credential NI (Gassert, 2000; Newbold, 1996). There is tremendous potential for nurses within this specialty to have a major impact on the way care is planned and delivered in the current complex health care environment.

What Is Nursing Informatics?

"Informatics" was coined from the French word *informatique*. It was first defined by Gorn (1983) as computer science plus information science. Informatics is more than just computers—it includes all aspects of technology and science, from the theoretic to the applied. Learning how to use new tools and building on capabilities provided by computers and related information technologies also are important parts of the field of informatics (Ball, Hannah, and Douglas, 2000).

Nursing informatics refers to that component of informatics designed for and relevant to nurses. Several definitions of nursing informatics have been developed since 1984, but the one that generally is accepted has been set forth by the American Nurses Association (ANA), which states:

> Nursing informatics is the specialty that integrates nursing science, computer science, and information science in identifying, collecting, processing, and managing data and information to support nursing practice, administration, education, research, and the expansion of nursing knowledge (ANA, 1994).

Embedded in this definition are the many components of nursing informatics: information processing, language development, applications of the system's life cycle, and human-computer interface issues. In addition, the definition provides guidance for content that is relevant to curricula for nurses studying to become informatics specialists (Gassert, 2000).

The Specialty of Nursing Informatics

There are many specialties in nursing that cover a range of interests and clinical domains, such as perioperative nursing, community health nursing, and administration. What makes a practice area a specialty? According to Styles (1989) the following attributes are necessary:

- Differentiated practice
- A research program
- Representation of the specialty by at least one organized body
- A mechanism for credentialing nurses in the specialty
- Educational programs for preparing nurses to practice in the specialty

In 1992 the ANA acknowledged that nursing informatics possessed these attributes and designated nursing informatics as an area of specialty practice.

Differentiated Practice. For more than two decades nurses have been working in hospitals and other settings to help with the selection, development, installation, and evaluation of information systems. This early role function of the NI continues to be important, but, with the constant changes in health care, the scope of practice has expanded, and job opportunities are increasing rapidly. Hersher (2000) describes several current and future roles for nurses in informatics, both traditional and nontraditional. Some of these include:

- *User liaison:* A nurse in this role is involved in the installation of a CIS and interfaces with the system vendors, the users, and management of the health care institution. Generally, the nurse working in this role is employed by the health care institution.
- *Clinical systems installation:* In this role the nurse works for the vendor who has developed and sold the CIS to a health care institution. The nurse-installer helps train the users of the system and troubleshoots problems during the conversion to the new system. The nurse-installer often serves as the liaison between the health care institution and the vendor and in most cases works closely with the system coordinator for the health care institution, who may very well be a nurse.
- *Product manager:* A nurse in this role is responsible for constantly updating a current product and keeping abreast of new developments in the field. Product managers interface with marketing staff, clients, technical staff, and management. Applications that nurse product managers have developed include decision-support systems, nurse staffing systems, scheduling systems, acuity systems, and bedside and handheld terminals. Although product managers typically have been employed by vendors, many health care institutions are starting to develop this role.
- *Systems analyst/programmer:* In this role the nurse works in the information systems department, helping analyze and maintain the system or programming. To be effective in this role, the nurse needs a strong working knowledge of the CIS. In many cases the nurse will work on all aspects of the CIS, not just the nursing applications.

These are just a few examples of the types of roles nurses in informatics are filling. Other examples that Hersher (2000) describes include chief information officer, consultant, network administrator, data repository specialist, and clinical information liaison. Settings also vary, as nurses move from the hospital-based acute care sites to community-based sites, which include insurance companies, utilization review organizations, integrated health networks, and health care associations. Clearly, nurses working in informatics have met the criterion of differentiated practice.

Research Program. In 1986 Schwirian proposed a framework for research in nursing informatics. At that time research in the field was practically nonexistent. Since then, however, there has been rapid development; researchers have reported their studies at national and international conferences and published in a variety of peer-reviewed journals. In nursing the peer-reviewed journal *CIN: Computers, Informatics, Nursing* serves as the premier source of published research in nursing informatics as it has since its inception in 1984.

The National Institute of Nursing Research (NINR) has provided direction for much of the research that is ongoing in nursing; informatics is no exception. In 1988 a panel of experts was convened to establish broad priorities for the NINR; this ultimately led to the development of the National Nursing Research Agenda (NNRA). Seven specific broad priorities were identified within the NNRA; the sixth identified priority was "Information Systems." Subsequent Priority Expert Panels were called together to further develop each priority area and make recommendations for future research. The Priority Expert Panel on Nursing Informatics published the results of its deliberations in *Nursing Informatics: Enhancing Patient Care* in 1993 (NINR, 1993). These were the six goals identified by the panel:

1. Establish nursing languages, including lexicons, classification systems, and taxonomies, and standards for nursing data.
2. Develop methods to build databases of clinical information (including clinical data, diagnoses, objectives, interventions, and outcomes) and management information (including staffing, charge capture, turnover, and vacancy rates) and analyze relationships among them.
3. Determine how nurses use data, information, and knowledge to give patient care and how care is affected by differing levels of expertise and by organizational factors and working conditions. Determine how to design information systems accordingly.
4. Develop and test patient care decision support systems and knowledge delivery systems that are appropriate for nurses' needs, with consideration for expertise, organizational factors, and working conditions.
5. Develop prototypes and eventually working models of nurse workstations linked to an integrated information system and equipped with tools to provide nurses with all the information needed for patient care, research, and education at the point of use.
6. Develop and implement appropriate methods to evaluate nursing information systems and applications, particularly as to their effects on patient care (NINR, 1993).

Research is ongoing in each of these priority areas. In particular, great strides have been made in the area of developing and testing standardized languages. Both the ANA and the National League for Nursing (NLN) have provided leadership and support for these efforts. In addition, the ANA has established criteria for recognizing nursing classifications and standardized nursing languages. These criteria are promulgated through the ANA Committee for Nursing Practice Information Infrastructure, which recognizes languages that have met the criteria. Currently there are 13 standardized languages that have been recognized by the ANA:

- North American Nursing Diagnosis Association (NANDA) Taxonomy
- Omaha System
- Home Health Care Classifications (HHCC)
- Nursing Interventions Classification (NIC)
- Nursing Outcomes Classification (NOC)

- Patient Care Data Set (PCDS)
- PeriOperative Nursing Data Set (PNDS)
- Nursing Management Minimum Data Set (NMMDS)
- SNOMED CT
- Nursing Minimum Data Set (NMDS)
- International Classification for Nursing Practice (ICNP®)
- ABCodes
- Logical Observation Identifiers Names and Codes (LOINC®)

These 13 languages were uniquely developed to document nursing care. They were designed to record and track the clinical care process for an entire episode of care for patients in the acute, home, and/or ambulatory care settings (ANA, 2003). Research is underway to continue to test and refine the languages so that they fulfill their stated goal of capturing nursing practice to promote positive patient outcomes.

Representation of the Specialty by an Organized Body. There are many organizations devoted to nursing informatics at the local, regional, national, international, and even virtual level. These range from small, grassroots efforts in local communities to large, formal organizations with thousands of members. No matter what the size or geographic location, these groups provide education, networking, and support for nurses interested in informatics. Annual conferences provide the opportunity for members to share their research and innovations and to meet with informatics colleagues from around the world (Newbold, 2003; Nicoll, 2003).

The American Nurses Informatics Association (ANIA) was established in 1992 to serve the needs of informatics nurses in southern California. It has since grown and expanded and become a national organization with members throughout the United States. You can learn more about the ANIA on-line (www.ania.org). Another organization that started with a regional focus, Capital Area Roundtable on Informatics in Nursing (CARING), has also grown to more than 850 members in 47 states/territories and 12 countries. CARING can also be accessed on-line (www.caringonline.org).

Nonnursing associations such as the American Medical Informatics Association (AMIA) and the Health Information and Management Systems Society (HIMSS) have nursing informatics work groups. In these organizations, NIs have taken leadership roles and are well represented on the organizational committees.

Credentialing Nurses in the Specialty. When nursing informatics was recognized as a specialty by the ANA in 1992, work began to establish a process by which nurses could be credentialed in informatics. The ANCC, which offers certification examinations for a variety of specialties in nursing, describes certification as a formal, systematic mechanism whereby nurses can voluntarily seek a credential that recognizes their quality and excellence in professional practice and continuing education (ANCC, 1993). For many nurses becoming certified is a professional milestone and validation of their qualifications, knowledge, and skills in a defined area of nursing practice.

To be eligible for the nursing informatics examination, which was first offered in 1995, a nurse must meet the following requirements:

- Possess an active registered nursing license in the United States or its territories
- Have earned a baccalaureate or higher nursing degree or a baccalaureate degree in a relevant field, including science (biology, anatomy, physiology, etc.), professional

disciplines (engineering, computer science, psychology, physical therapy, etc.), or academic liberal arts, (mathematics, English, philosophy, history, etc.)

- Practiced actively as a registered nurse for at least 2 years
- Practiced at least 2000 hours in the field of nursing informatics within the past 5 years or completed at least 12 semester hours of academic credits in informatics in a graduate program in nursing and a minimum of 1000 hours in informatics within the past 5 years
- Earned 30 contact hours of continuing education credit applicable to the specialty area within the past 3 years (ANCC, 2003b)

The requirements for eligibility to take the Informatics Nurse certification exam were expanded to include either a baccalaureate or higher degree in nursing or a baccalaureate degree in a relevant field. Allowing a degree in another field recognizes informatics nurses who were prepared as nurses at the diploma or associate degree level and completed their baccalaureate degrees in another field. This was the route taken by many of the first nurses who entered the field of informatics. Nurses who certify with a baccalaureate or higher degree in nursing will receive an RN, BC as their credential, whereas those who certify with a degree in a related field will receive an RN, C.

The nurse who successfully passes the examination is certified as a generalist in informatics nursing. The ANCC is planning to offer an examination for a specialist in informatics nursing in the future. Once certified, the nurse must be recertified every 5 years. In the first year the examination was offered, 83 nurses became certified in informatics (Newbold, 1996). Since then, more than 500 nurses have become certified in the specialty (ANCC, 2003a).

Education in Informatics. There are both formal and informal opportunities for education in informatics. The first formal educational programs that offered specific degrees in nursing informatics were established within the past decade, and the number of programs has been increasing steadily. However, because educational options were limited, many nurses are currently practicing in informatics who have been prepared for their role through on-the-job training or by receiving education for the role outside of nursing. For example, a nurse may have a bachelor of science degree in nursing (BSN) plus a second degree in computer science or information technology. Nurses have been successful in educating themselves using formal and informal resources. Nurses considering a career in informatics need to carefully consider options that are available and plan their educational programs accordingly.

At the graduate level, students can pursue either a master's or doctoral degree with a major in informatics (Moore-Cox, 2003). Programs that offer such an option are available at Case Western Reserve University, Central Missouri State University, Duke University, University of Colorado Health Science Center, and the Universities of Arizona, Maryland, and Utah (Moore-Cox, 2003; Snyder-Halpern, 2004). Although each program is unique, there are similarities. For example, students pursuing master's level education will take approximately 42 semester credit hours of course work, which are divided among core courses (such as theory, research, policy, and advanced nursing), courses in nursing informatics (such as programming, database design, systems analysis and design, clinical decision-making, informatics models, and practice activities), and support courses. Similarly, students at the University of Arizona, University of Utah, and the University of Maryland may pursue doctoral study with substantive course work in nursing informatics. Again courses are taken in nursing theory, research, statistics, and nursing informatics. As with any doctoral degree, a dissertation is required.

Another option are graduate programs that allow a student to pursue an emphasis or minor in nursing informatics. In these programs students take 6 to 12 credit hours of course work in informatics. Students can pursue this type of study at Excelsior College, Loyola of Chicago, Northeastern University, Slippery Rock State College, and the Universities of California, Iowa, and Pennsylvania.

Many schools offer individual courses in nursing informatics at both the graduate and undergraduate level. The Nursing Informatics Working Group of AMIA (NIWG) has identified a number of such programs (Georgia College and State University, Lewis University, Lewis-Clark State College, Oregon Health Sciences University, Western Michigan University, and the University of North Carolina), although it is likely that this list is incomplete (see http://www.amia.org/working/ni/education/cat3.html). If you are interested in formal study in informatics, check with schools and colleges of nursing in your locale to see what is available.

These are the formal programs in nursing informatics, but many universities have courses in computer science and information technology. Interested students are able to self-design programs that meet their individual learning needs. Programs at the University of Texas at Austin, University of California San Francisco, and the University of Wisconsin at Madison have been identified as having particularly strong concentrations of courses available in informatics (Gassert, 2000).

Informal Education. For many nurses graduate education is not an option or personal choice, but they still desire to become more knowledgeable about informatics. In this case many informal opportunities exist, including networking through professional organizations, keeping abreast of the literature by reading journals, and attending professional conferences.

Organizations vary in their scope, services offered to members, and the types of educational programs offered. Anyone interested in learning more about informatics should become active in at least one related organization. As a member a nurse has access to the meetings, publications, and educational offerings that the organization provides. Getting on mailing lists or visiting organizational sites on-line also allows a nurse to keep abreast of different opportunities available through each organization. Box 14-1 provides a listing of Internet addresses for some of the larger organizations.

Reading journals and newsletters is another way to become more knowledgeable about informatics. Offerings range from trade magazines that are not related to health but are important sources of information, such as *PC Magazine* or *Byte*, to specialized journals in nursing such as *CIN: Computers, Informatics, Nursing.* Since 1995 *CIN: Computers, Informatics, Nursing* has offered continuing education credit for articles published in the journal. The AMIA publishes the *Journal of the American Medical Informatics Association,* a publication source for much of the research that has been conducted related to informatics. A nurse interested in informatics should become familiar with the journals that are available, subscribe to those that are most interesting, and read others in the library. Keep in mind, though, that more information is published every month than anyone could possibly hope to keep abreast of—thus the need for networking! Colleagues can alert one another to articles of interest that are in journals they might not regularly read.

Finally, conferences provide an excellent source of education. At a conference the nurse is able to hear the latest information directly from experts in the field. Larger conferences usually have vendor exhibits that provide the opportunity for hands-on demonstrations of

BOX 14–1 *Helpful Websites*

American Medical Informatics Association (AMIA)
www.amia.org

Nursing Informatics Working Group of AMIA
http://www.amia.org/working/ni/main.html

American Nursing Informatics Association
www.ania.org

Healthcare Information and Management Systems Society (HIMSS)
www.himss.org

International Medical Informatics Association (IMIA)
www.imia.org

Special Interest Group on Nursing Informatics of IMIA (IMIA-NI)
http://www.imia.org/ni/index.html

a variety of commercial products. Conferences vary in size, focus, location, and cost. For those interested in nursing informatics, nursing conferences especially are helpful. Local organizations, such as CARING, sponsor a variety of half-day or 1-day conferences. Rutgers, the State University of New Jersey, has an annual informatics conference; in 2004 they celebrated their twenty-second year of successful implementation. The University of Maryland hosts a week-long institute on informatics every summer at the Baltimore campus. ANIA has an annual conference, usually held in the spring, with a call for abstracts, posters, and vendor exhibits. In addition, nonnursing organizations such as the HIMSS and AMIA have nursing sessions at their annual meetings. Nonnursing sessions also are often of great interest to nurse attendees (Nicoll, 2003).

CLINICAL INFORMATION
Clinical Information Systems

Clinical information systems (CIS) are changing the way that health care is delivered, whether in the hospital, the clinic, the provider's office, or the patient's home. With capabilities ranging from advanced instrumentation to high-level decision support, the CIS offers nurses and other clinicians information when, where, and how they need it. Increasingly, CIS applications function as the mechanisms for delivering patient-centered care and for supporting the move toward the computer-based patient record (CPR) and the lifetime electronic health record (EHR).

What exactly is a CIS? Definitions vary, often from organization to organization. Semancik (1997) describes a CIS as a collection of software programs and associated hardware that supports the entry, retrieval, update, and analysis of patient care information and associated clinical information related to patient care. The CIS is primarily a computer system used to provide clinical information for the care of a patient.

A CIS can be patient-focused or departmental. In patient-focused systems, automation supports patient care processes. Typical applications found in a patient-focused system include order entry, results reporting, clinical documentation, care planning, and clinical pathways.

As data are entered into the system, data repositories are established that can be accessed to look for trends in patient care. Departmental systems evolved to meet the operational needs of a particular department, such as the laboratory, radiology, pharmacy, medical records, or billing. Early systems often were stand-alone systems designed for an individual department. A major challenge facing CIS developers is to integrate these stand-alone systems to work with one another and with the newer patient-focused systems.

Computerized Patient Records

A CIS is not the same as a CPR (computerized patient record) or an EHR (electronic health record). Ideally, the CPR/EHR will include all information about an individual's lifetime health status and health care maintained electronically. The CPR/EHR is a replacement for the paper medical record as the primary source of information for health care, meeting all clinical, legal, and administrative requirements. However, the CPR/EHR is more than today's medical record. Information technology permits much more data to be captured, processed, and integrated, which results in information that is broader than that found in a linear paper record.

The CPR/EHR is not a record in the traditional sense of the term. "Record" connotes a repository with limitations of size, content, and location. The term traditionally has suggested that the sole purpose for maintaining health data is to document events. Although this is an important purpose, the CPR/EHR permits health information to be used to support the generation and communication of knowledge. Figs. 14-1 and 14-2 illustrate selected screens from a patient's CPR.

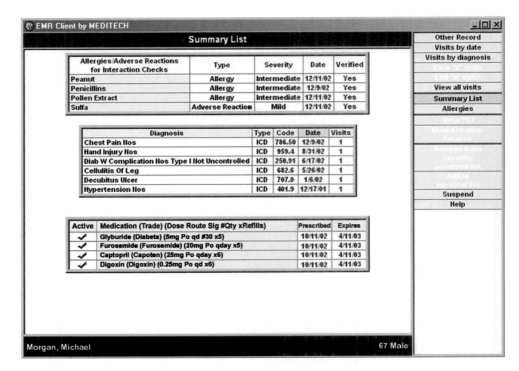

FIG. 14–1 Computerized patient record—summary screen. (Image provided courtesy Meditech—Medical Information Technology, Inc., Westwood, Mass).

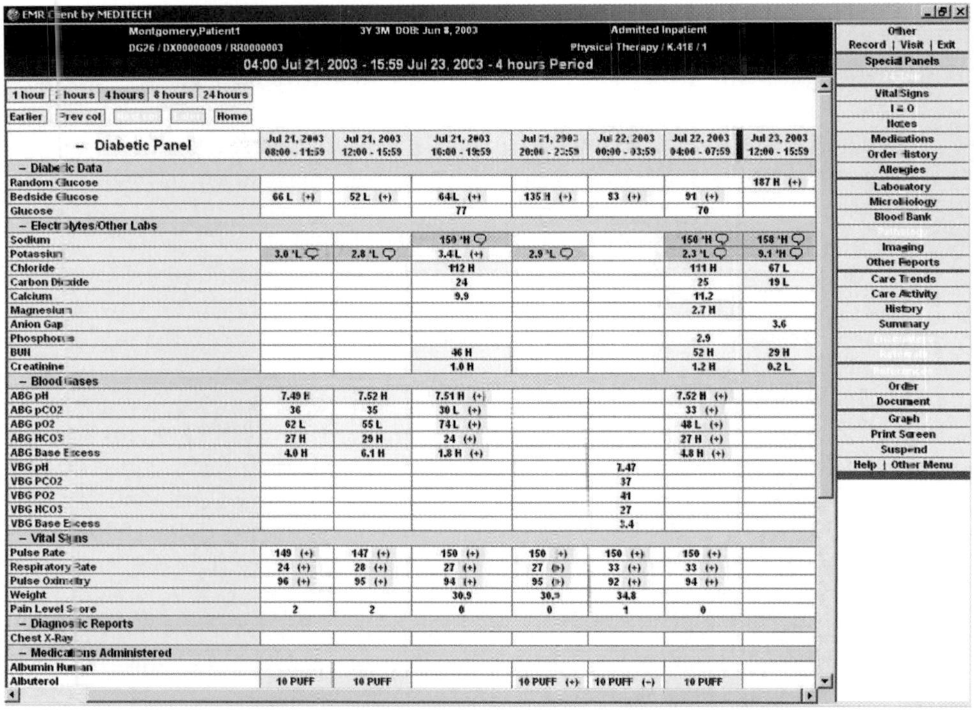

– Diabetic Panel	Jul 21, 2003 08:00 - 11:59	Jul 21, 2003 12:00 - 15:59	Jul 21, 2003 16:00 - 19:59	Jul 21, 2003 20:00 - 23:59	Jul 22, 2003 00:00 - 03:59	Jul 22, 2003 04:00 - 07:59	Jul 23, 2003 12:00 - 15:59
– Diabetic Data							
Random Glucose							187 H (+)
Bedside Glucose	66 L (+)	52 L (+)	64 L (+)	135 H (+)	83 (+)	91 (+)	
Glucose			77			70	
– Electrolytes/Other Labs							
Sodium			159 H			156 H	158 H
Potassium	3.0 L	2.8 L	3.4 L (+)	2.9 L		2.3 L	9.1 H
Chloride			112 H			111 H	67 L
Carbon Dioxide			24			25	19 L
Calcium			9.9			11.2	
Magnesium						2.7 H	
Anion Gap							3.6
Phosphorus						2.9	
BUN			46 H			52 H	29 H
Creatinine			1.0 H			1.2 H	0.2 L
– Blood Gases							
ABG pH	7.49 H	7.52 H	7.51 H (+)			7.52 H (+)	
ABG pCO2	36	35	30 L (+)			33 (+)	
ABG pO2	62 L	55 L	74 L (+)			48 L (+)	
ABG HCO3	27 H	29 H	24 (+)			27 H (+)	
ABG Base Excess	4.0 H	6.1 H	1.8 H (+)			4.8 H (+)	
VBG pH					7.47		
VBG PCO2					37		
VBG PO2					41		
VBG HCO3					27		
VBG Base Excess					5.4		
– Vital Signs							
Pulse Rate	149 (+)	147 (+)	150 (+)	150 (+)	150 (+)	150 (+)	
Respiratory Rate	24 (+)	28 (+)	27 (+)	27 (+)	33 (+)	33 (+)	
Pulse Oximetry	96 (+)	95 (+)	94 (+)	95 (+)	92 (+)	94 (+)	
Weight			30.9	30.9		34.8	
Pain Level Score	2	2	0	0	1	0	
– Diagnostic Reports							
Chest X-Ray							
– Medications Administered							
Albumin Human							
Albuterol	10 PUFF	10 PUFF		10 PUFF (+)	10 PUFF (–)	10 PUFF	

FIG. 14–2 Computerized patient record—diabetic screen. (Image provided courtesy Meditech—Medical Information Technology, Inc., Westwood, Mass).

The health care delivery system is dramatically changing, with a strong emphasis on improving outcomes of care and maintaining health. The CPR/EHR needs to be considered in a broader context and is not applicable only to patients (i.e., individuals with the presence of an illness or disease). Rather in the CPR/EHR the focus is on the individual's health, encompassing both wellness and illness.

As a result of this focus on the individual, the CPR/EHR is a virtual compilation of nonredundant health data about the person across his or her lifetime, including facts, observations, interpretations, plans, actions, and outcomes. Health data include information on allergies, history of illness and injury, functional status, diagnostic studies, assessments, orders, consultation reports, and treatment records. Health data also include wellness information such as immunization history, behavioral data, environmental information, demographics, health insurance, administrative data for care delivery processes, and legal data such as informed consents. The who, what, when, and where of data capture are also identified. The structure of the data includes text, numbers, sounds, images, and full-motion video. These are thoroughly integrated so that any given view of health data may incorporate one or more structural elements.

Within a CPR/EHR, an individual's health data are maintained and distributed over different systems in different locations, such as a hospital, clinic, physician's office, and pharmacy. Intelligent software agents with appropriate security measures are necessary to access data across these distributed systems. The nurse or other user who is retrieving these data must be able to assemble it in such a way as to provide a chronology of health information about the individual.

The CPR/EHR is maintained in a system that captures, processes, communicates, secures, and presents the data about the patient. This system may include the CIS. Other components of the CPR/EHR system include clinical rules, literature for patient education, expert opinions, and payer rules related to reimbursement. When these elements work together in an integrated fashion, the CPR/EHR becomes much more than a patient record—it becomes a knowledge tool. The system is able to integrate information from multiple sources and provide decision support; thus the CPR/EHR serves as the primary source of information for patient care.

A fully functional CPR/EHR is a complex system. Consider a single data element (datum), such as a person's weight. The system must be able to capture, or record, the weight, then store it, process it, communicate it to others, and present it in a different format such as a bar graph or chart. All of this must be done in a secure environment that protects the patient's confidentiality and privacy. The complexity of these issues and the development of the necessary systems helps to explain why few fully functional CPR/EHR systems are in place today.

Data Capture. Data capture refers to the collection and entry of data into a computer system. The origin of the data may be local or remote from patient-monitoring devices, from telemedicine applications, directly from the individual recipient of health care, and even from others who have information about the recipient's health or environment, such as relatives and friends and public health agencies. Data may be captured by multiple means, including key entry, pattern recognition (voice, handwriting, or biologic characteristics), and medical device transmission.

All data entered into a computer are not necessarily structured for subsequent processing. For example, document imaging systems provide for creation of electronically stored text but have limitations on the ability to process that text. Data capture includes the use of controlled vocabularies and code systems to ensure common meaning for terminology and the ability to process units of information. As noted earlier, great strides have been made in the development of standardized nursing languages. These languages provide structured data entry and text processing, which result in common meaning and processing.

Data capture also encompasses authentication to identify the author of an entry and to ensure that the author has been granted permission to access the system and change the CPR/EHR.

Storage. Storage refers to the physical location of data. In CPR/EHR systems health data are distributed across multiple systems at different sites. For this reason, common access protocols, retention schedules, and universal identification are necessary.

Access protocols permit only authorized users to obtain data for legitimate uses. The systems must have backup and recovery mechanisms in the event of failure. Retention schedules address the maintenance of the data in active and inactive form and the permanence of the storage medium.

A person's identity can be determined by many types of data in addition to common identifiers such as name and number. Universal identifiers or other methods are required for integrating health data of an individual distributed across multiple systems at different sites.

Information Processing. Application functions provide for effective retrieval and processing of data into useful information. These include decision support tools such as alerts and alarms for drug interactions, allergies, and abnormal laboratory results. Reminders can be provided for appointments, critical path actions, medication administration, and other activities. The systems also may provide access to consensus- and evidence-driven diagnostic and treatment guidelines and protocols. The nurse could integrate a standard guideline, protocol, or critical path into a specific individual's CPR/EHR, modify it to meet unique circumstances, and use it as a basis for managing and documenting care. Outcome data communicated from various caregivers and health care recipients themselves also may be analyzed and used for continual improvement of the guidelines and protocols.

Information Communication. Information communication refers to the interoperability of systems and linkages for exchange of data across disparate systems. To integrate health data across multiple systems at different sites, identifier systems (unique numbers or other methodology) for health care recipients, caregivers, providers, payers, and sites are essential. Local, regional, and national health information infrastructures that tie all participants together using standard data communication protocols are key to the linkage function. There are hundreds of types of transactions or messages that must be defined and agreed to by the participating stakeholders. Vocabulary and code systems must permit the exchange and processing of data into meaningful information. CPR/EHR systems must provide access to point-of-care information databases and knowledge sources such as pharmaceutical formularies, referral databases, and reference literature.

Security. Computer-based patient record systems provide better protection of confidential health information than paper-based systems because such systems incorporate controls designed to ensure that only authorized users with legitimate uses have access to health information. Security functions address the confidentiality of private health information and the integrity of the data. Security functions must be designed to ensure compliance with applicable laws, regulations, and standards. Security systems must ensure that access to data is provided only to those who are authorized and have a legitimate purpose for its use. Security functions also must provide a means to audit for inappropriate access. Three important terms must be clearly understood when discussing the issues surrounding access: privacy, confidentiality, and security.

- *Privacy* refers to the right of an individual to keep information about himself or herself from being disclosed to anyone else. If a patient has had an abortion and chooses not to tell a health care provider this fact, the patient would be keeping that information private.
- *Confidentiality* refers to the act of limiting disclosure of private matters. Once a patient has disclosed private information to a health care provider, that provider has a responsibility to maintain the confidentiality of that information.
- *Security* refers to the means to control access and protect information from accidental or intentional disclosure to unauthorized persons and from alteration, destruction, or loss. When private information is placed in a confidential CPR/EHR, the system must have controls in place to maintain the security of the system and not allow unauthorized persons access to the data (CPRI, 1995).

Information Presentation. The wealth of information available through CPR/EHR systems must be managed to ensure that authorized caregivers (including nurses) and others with legitimate uses have the information they need in their preferred presentation form. For example, a nurse may want to see data organized by source, caregiver, encounter, problem, or date.

Data can be presented in detail or summary form. Tables, graphs, narrative, and other forms of information presentation must be accommodated. Some users may need only to know of the presence or absence of certain data, not the nature of the data itself. For example, blood donation centers draw blood for testing for human immunodeficiency virus, hepatitis, and other conditions. If a donor has a positive test result, the center may not be given the specific information regarding the test, but only general information that a test result was abnormal and that the patient should be referred to an appropriate health care provider.

Interface Between the Informatics Nurse and the Clinical Information System

Information demands in health care systems are pushing the development of the CIS and CPR/EHR. The ongoing development of computer technology—smaller, faster machines with extensive storage capabilities and the ability for cross-platform communication—is making the goal of an integrated electronic system a realistic option, not just a long-term dream. As these systems evolve, nurses will play an important role in their development, implementation, and evaluation.

Because of their expertise, nurses in informatics are in an ideal position to assist with the development, implementation, and evaluation of the CIS. Their knowledge of policies, procedures, and clinical care is essential as workflow systems are redesigned within a CIS. It is not unusual for nurses within an institution to have more hands-on interaction with and knowledge of different departments than any other group of employees in an institution. Jenkins (2000) suggests that the process model of nursing (assessment, planning, implementation, and evaluation) works well during a CIS implementation; thus nurses have a familiar framework from which to understand the complexity of a major system change.

TRENDS IN COMPUTING: PAST, PRESENT, AND FUTURE

As noted earlier, computers have moved from the realm of a "nice to know" luxury item to a "need to know" essential resource for professional practice. Nurses are knowledge workers who require accurate and up-to-date information for their professional work. The explosion in information—some estimate that all information is replaced every 9 to 12 months—requires nurses to be on the cutting edge of knowledge to practice ethically and safely. Trends in computing will affect the work of professional nurses in areas beyond the development of the CIS and CPR/EHR. Research advances, new devices, monitoring equipment, sensors, and "smart body parts" will all change the way that health care is conceptualized, practiced, and delivered.

Within this context, not every nurse will need to be an informatics specialist, but every nurse must be computer-literate. *Computer literacy* is defined as the knowledge and understanding of computers, combined with the ability to use them effectively (Joos et al, 1996). Computer literacy may be interpreted as different levels of expertise for different people in various roles. On the least specialized level, computer literacy involves knowing how to turn on a computer, start and stop simple application programs, and save and print information. For health care professionals computer literacy requires having an understanding of systems used in clinical practice, education, and research settings. For example, in clinical practice electronic patient records and clinical information systems are becoming more widely used. The computer-literate nurse is able to use these systems effectively and can address issues discussed earlier, such as confidentiality, security, and privacy. At the same time, the nurse must be able to effectively use applications typically found on personal computers (PCs), such as word processing software, spreadsheets, presentation graphics, and statistics for research. Finally, the computer-literate nurse must know how to access information from a variety of electronic sources and how to evaluate the appropriateness of the information at both the professional and patient level. The remainder of this chapter is designed to help you gain a broader understanding of computer literacy and the computing environment of PCs and the on-line world, along with a discussion of future trends.

The Past and Future

Weiser and Brown (1996) have characterized the history and future of computing in three phases. The first phase is known as the "mainframe era," in which many people share one computer. Computers during this phase were found behind closed doors and run by experts with specialized knowledge and skills. Although we have mostly moved beyond the mainframe era, it still exists in certain health care CIS settings (for instance, in the departmental systems discussed earlier) and other industries that rely on large mainframe systems, such as banking, weather forecasting, and legacy systems in academic institutions.

The archetypal computer of the mainframe era is certainly the Electronic Numerical Integrator and Computer (ENIAC), developed at the University of Pennsylvania in 1945. This system was proposed by John Mauchly, an American physicist, and built at the Moore School of Engineering by Mauchly and J. Presper Eckert, an engineer. It is regarded as the first successful digital computer. It weighed more than 60,000 pounds and contained more than 18,000 vacuum tubes. Roughly 2000 of the computer's vacuum tubes were replaced each month by a team of six technicians. Even though one vacuum tube blew approximately every 15 minutes, the functioning of the ENIAC was still considered to be reliable! Many of the first tasks of the ENIAC were for military purposes, such as calculating ballistic firing tables and designing atomic weapons. Because ENIAC was initially not a stored program machine, it had to be reprogrammed for each task.

Phase II in modern computing is the era of personal computers (PCs), which is characterized by one person (linked) to one computer. In this era the computing relationship is personal and intimate. Similar to how consumers think of a car, perception of a computer is that of a special, relatively expensive item that requires attention but provides a very valuable service in one's life.

The first harbinger of the PC era was in 1948 with the development of the transistor at Bell Telephone Laboratories. The transistor, which could act as an electrical switch, replaced the costly, energy-inefficient, and unreliable vacuum tubes used in computers and other devices, including televisions. By the late 1960s integrated circuits, tiny transistors, and other electrical components arranged on a single chip of silicon replaced individual transistors in computers. Integrated circuits became miniaturized, enabling more components to be designed into a single computer circuit. In the 1970s refinements in integrated circuit technology led to the development of the modern microprocessor, integrated circuits that contained thousands of transistors. Weiser and Brown (1996) date the true start of Phase II as 1984, when the number of people using PCs surpassed the number of people using shared computers.

Manufacturers used integrated circuit technology to build smaller and cheaper computers. The first PCs were sold by Instrumentation Telemetry Systems. The Altair 8800 appeared in 1975. Graphic user interfaces were first designed by the Xerox corporation in a prototype computer, the Alto, developed in 1974. The corporate decision not to pursue commercial development of the PC (Xerox identified its core business strategy as copiers, not computers) has become a bit of a computer history legend (Hiltzik, 2000; Smith and Alexander, 1988). Continuing development of sophisticated operating systems and miniaturization of components (modern microprocessors contain as many as 10 million transistors) have enabled the development of computers that can run programs and manipulate data in ways that were unimaginable in the era of the ENIAC.

Phase III has been dubbed the era of ubiquitous computing (UC), in which there will be many computers to each person. Weiser and Brown (1996) estimate that the crossover of the UC era with the PC era will occur between 2005 to 2020. In this phase computers will be everywhere: in walls, chairs, clothing, light switches, cars, appliances, and so on. Computers will become so fundamental to our human experience that they will "disappear" and we will cease to be aware of them. For those who are skeptical that this will come to pass, consider two other ubiquitous technologies: writing and electricity. In Egyptian times writing was a secret art, known and performed only by specially trained scribes who lived on a level close to royalty. Clay tablets and later papyrus were precious commodities. Many people died without ever having seen a piece of paper in their lives! Now paper and writing are everywhere. Within the course of an average day, most people use and discard hundreds of pieces of paper, never giving them a second thought. Electricity has a similar history. When electricity was first invented in the nineteenth century, entire factories were designed to accommodate the presence of light bulbs and bulky motors. The placement of workers, machines, and parts were all designed around the need of electricity and motors. Today electricity is everywhere. It is hidden in the walls and stored in tiny batteries. The average car has more than 22 motors and 25 solenoids.

One only has to look around a typical house to see how UC is already becoming part of our lives. Microprocessors exist in every room: appliances in the kitchen, remote controls for television and stereo in the family room, and clock radios and cordless phones in the bedroom. And the bathroom? Matsushita of Japan has developed a prototype toilet (dubbed the "smart toilet") that includes an on-line, real-time health monitoring system. It measures the user's weight, fat content, and urine sugar level; plots the recorded data on a graph; and sends it instantaneously to a health care provider for monitoring (Watts, 1999).

Another dimension of UC is the proliferation of personal digital assistants (PDAs). These hand-held devices, made by companies such as Palm and Dell, were first developed primarily to maintain calendars and phone lists. However, since their inception, companies have been busy developing applications that run on these devices for specialized uses. Nurses have embraced this technology. Applications designed specifically for nurses include drug guides, care plans, laboratory reference and results, databases of diseases and therapeutics, and dictionaries of medical terms. These are just a few of the hundreds of applications that have been developed; many of them are available free or at nominal cost. Learn more on-line (www.pdacortex.com).

Finally, the Internet must be considered as an integral component of UC. Each time you connect to the Internet, you are connecting with millions of information resources and hundreds of information delivery systems. A person truly does become one person linked to hundreds of computers. Ironically, the interface to the UC world of the Internet is still through a PC. However, this is changing. Wireless infrared connections will eliminate wires; handheld devices will eliminate the relatively bulky PC. Once we become wireless and mobile, UC will become a reality.

The Present: The Internet

With its presence in both Phase II and Phase III, the Internet is the bridge between the PC era and UC. Applications such as word processing and database management typically reside on a stand-alone PC and are under the purview of one user. However, this is only one dimension of personal computer use. The other major component is the on-line world, commonly called the Internet (with a capital I) and its graphic component, the World Wide Web (www). The exponential growth of the Internet makes it an essential realm for the computer-literate nurse to master. Information and professional resources that cannot be found anywhere else are available on the Internet; this trend shows no sign of slowing. Most people use the Internet for two broad purposes: to communicate with others, either individually or in groups, and to find information. Nurses are no exception, and as knowledge workers they must do both of these tasks for their professional work.

Using the Internet: Communicating With Others

Individual E-Mail. By far the most common use of the Internet is to send electronic mail (e-mail). The fact that sending e-mail is so easy is a major driving force behind its phenomenal growth. In 2000 there were 891 million e-mailboxes, an increase of 63% over 1999 (Year End, 2000). Analysts estimate that by 2005 there will be 1.7 billion on-line mailboxes, outnumbering both televisions and phone lines. Even with this growth, every e-mail journey begins with a single message. For many people, exchanging e-mail with colleagues is their first introduction to the Internet. Since the interaction is limited and often with someone who is known, it is usually a nonthreatening experience.

E-mail tends to be informal, and most recipients are tolerant of "less-than-perfect" communications. Even so, if your mail program includes features such as a spellchecker, it is wise to use it. Another useful feature is to create a signature file. With a signature file, certain information, such as your name, e-mail address, and phone number will be appended to every message you send.

Group E-Mail: Mailing Lists. Another popular feature of the Internet is the mailing list (commonly called a listserv), which provides a forum for groups of people with similar interests to get together and share their information through a mail-based discussion group. These lists can range in size from a few people to thousands, and they can generate anywhere from a few messages a week to a hundred or more in a day. Being on a mailing list can put information and resources literally at your fingertips. Imagine asking 900 fellow students around the world a question concerning a clinical problem and receiving multiple answers within minutes.

To find out about mailing lists, talk to others and find out whether they subscribe. Actual subscribers are the most reliable source of information regarding a listserv (e.g., how active it is, whether the discussions are valuable). Another option is to check an on-line source for nursing discussion forums (http://www.ualberta.ca/~jrnorris/nursinglists/). This website is a "list of lists" specific to nursing and was created by Judy Norris, a faculty member at the University of Alberta. Dr. Norris is also the founder of NURSENET, one of the oldest mailing lists in nursing. At this site there is an alphabetized list with information about each one of the nursing lists and individual instructions on how to subscribe. Finally, another option is to visit a website that provides a generalized list of lists, not just those related to nursing (e.g., www.liszt.com).

Although there are hundreds of mailing lists on the Internet, they all work in a similar fashion. As noted above, each listserv is developed around a particular topic or interest area. One subscribes to a list, but unlike subscribing to a magazine, there is no charge for the service. Once you subscribe to a list, you will receive messages that you can read, reply to, or delete. The communications are asynchronous (i.e., the discussions are not occurring in real time, such as you would have with a personal conversation or in a "chat" forum). Instead the discussions occur via e-mail, with one person asking a question or posting a comment and other members on the list replying. Even though the discussions are not synchronous, they are real discussions which sometimes generate heated debates.

Although all mailing lists work in a similar fashion, each list has its own quirks. Typically, when you successfully subscribe to a mailing list, you will receive a welcome message from the listserv owner. Print this message and save it, because it contains useful information about how to manage your subscription: how to unsubscribe, how to temporarily stop the mail, and how to receive the list in different formats such as digest.

As with individual e-mail, there are some mailing list courtesies to keep in mind. Mailing lists are not anonymous; there are real people behind the messages. These people give the list its personality, and you will get to know the other listserv members through their discussions and comments. Many people choose to "lurk," that is, read messages but not post, when they first subscribe to a list. This gives you a chance to get a feel for the members of the community. When you do decide to post a message, a short introduction is a good idea. Keep it simple: for instance, "Hi, my name is . . . I subscribed to this list because I am interested in . . . ."

When you post a question, be clear and to the point. Tell people what information you want and how you want to receive it. Do you want people to post their replies to the list or reply to you privately? Similarly, if you are replying to a message, know to whom you are replying. By default, all responses go to the whole list.

If the nature of the topic changes, change the subject line. This allows the list members to quickly scan and delete messages that are not of interest.

"Flaming" is not a good idea. A flame is when someone attacks another person, usually in a virulent and violent manner. Remember that the whole point of a list is to have a discussion; it is possible and even likely that you will disagree with someone's ideas, but that does not mean you have to denigrate the person in the process.

Finally, "newbies" (newcomers) are afforded a wide degree of latitude, and mistakes are expected and accepted, but do your best to learn the ropes and manage your subscription in a responsible and professional manner. Although list owners are loathe to do this, they can unsubscribe people who repeatedly post off topic, flame others, send viruses, or mismanage their account. Keep these points in mind when you join a list.

Chatting On-Line. Mailing lists are extremely useful, but what if you want to have a synchronous (real-time) conversation with someone else? To do this, you need to find a way to "chat," which is not too difficult to do since Internet chatting is becoming as popular as e-mail. There are literally hundreds of chat "rooms," scattered all over the Internet, with people talking on every imaginable topic. Chat rooms appeal to some people but not to others. The only way to find out whether this is a communication medium that suits you is to dive in and try it.

To get started, you have two major options: the first is to find a chat room that exists on the Internet. With that, you simply "enter the room" and begin conversing. The second option is to download software that allows you to chat, such as Internet relay chat (IRC) or ICQ ("I seek you"). Many people use both options. People tend to have favorites, so you may find certain friends in ICQ, others on IRC, and yet others in chat rooms on America Online or whatever Internet provider you use.

No matter which option you choose, certain rules of etiquette govern chatting. You should also observe certain precautions to protect yourself. One important rule: never give out personal information in a chat room. Do not give out credit card information or passwords, no matter how the request is made. You might want to investigate using moderated chat rooms initially. In these rooms, moderators are "present" to keep an eye on the content and flow of conversation. They also have the authority to kick out people who are misbehaving. As with mailing lists, rules of common courtesy prevail in chat rooms. Do not harass others, do not flame, and avoid obscene and suggestive language.

If you chat regularly, you may begin to see familiar names and become friends with your fellow chatters. You may fall in love. You may meet someone and get married. I know people who have done all three. You also may find yourself in a difficult and potentially dangerous situation. As with anything in life, be careful. The Internet does have a dark side.

That said, I have met some great people on the Internet, and we have met in person and become good friends. The Internet is making our world smaller and giving all of us the opportunity to meet people we might never have met otherwise. However, I used a good deal of caution and common sense in allowing these friendships to develop. If you do the same, you will go a long way to ensure that your Internet interactive experiences are pleasant and rewarding.

Using the Internet: Finding Information

The other major use of the Internet is finding information. To do so, you must develop skills for searching quickly and efficiently. A variety of strategies can be used for searching, including "quick and dirty searching," "links," and "brute force." Keep in mind that you must be persistent: no one search strategy is going to work all the time, nor is any one search engine inherently more effective than any other. A study published in *Science* in 1998 (Lawrence and Giles, 1998) revealed that the best search engines found approximately 33% of the information available on the Internet. That means, of course, that 67% of useful information is being missed. Search engines are good starting points, but you can augment their effectiveness by adding a few other strategies to your Web exploration toolkit.

First, you should target your search by conducting a "purpose-focus-approach" (PFA) assessment. To determine your purpose, ask yourself why you are doing the search and why you need the information. Consider questions such as the following:

- Is the information for personal interest?
- Do you want to obtain information to share with co-workers or a client?
- Are you verifying information given to you by someone else?
- Are you preparing a report or writing a paper for a class or project?

Based on your purpose, your focus may be:

- Broad and general (basic information for yourself)
- Lay-oriented (to give information to a patient)
- Professionally oriented (for colleagues)
- Narrow and technical with a research orientation

Purpose combined with focus determines your approach. For example, information that is broad and general can be found using brute force methods or quick and dirty searching. Lay information can be quickly accessed at a few key sites, including MEDLINEplus and consumer health organizations. Similarly, professional associations and societies are a good starting point for professionally oriented information. Scientific and research information usually requires literature resources that can be found in databases such as MEDLINE or CINAHL.

Quick and Dirty Searching. Quick and dirty searching is a very simple but surprisingly effective search strategy. First, start with a search engine such as Google (www.google.com). Next, type in the term of interest. At this point, do not worry about being overly broad or general. You will retrieve an enormous number of found references (called "hits"), but you are only interested in the first ten to twenty. Look at the URLs and try to decipher what they mean. URLs usually start with www (for World Wide Web). Next, there is the "thing in the middle" followed by a domain (the "dot" plus suffix). Pay attention to the domains—*.com* is commercial; *.edu* is used by educational institutions; *.gov* is government-affiliated. Quickly visit a few sites. Look for the information you need or useful links. If a site is not relevant, use the "Back" button to return to your search results and go to the next site. Once you find a site that appears to be useful, begin to explore the site. If there are links, click on the links to connect to other relevant sites. This process—quick search, quick review, clicking and linking—can provide a starting point for useful information in a relatively short period of time.

Brute Force. Brute force searching is another alternative. To do this, type in an address (URL) and see what happens. The worst outcome is an annoying error message, but you may land on a site that is exactly what you want. Perhaps you are trying to find a school of nursing at a certain university. What is the common name for the university? For example, to find the website for the University of New Hampshire, www.unh.edu is a very logical choice (and also correct!) Organizations also tend to be quite logical in their choice of URLs: for instance, www.ana.org is the American Nurses Association; www.aone.org is the American Organization of Nurse Executives.

Taking Advantage of Links and Using the Bookmark Feature. Virtually every website has links to other websites of related interest. Take advantage of these links because the site developer has already done some of the work of finding other useful resources. Combine quick and dirty searching or brute force with links to get the information you need. Each site you visit will have more links, and in this way the resources keep building. Visiting a variety of sites will open up the vistas of information that are available. When you find a site of interest, "bookmark" it or add it to your list of favorites. This guarantees you will be able to return to the site quickly and easily in the future.

Resources for Professionals and Consumers. The preceding discussion has focused on strategies to use when you are faced with a "needle in a haystack" searching situation—just dive in and see what you find. The advantage of this method is that it is fast and easy. The disadvantages are that sites of dubious quality may be obtained and the process, although fast, is not terribly efficient.

Another approach is to develop a "short list" of well-known, well-researched sites that can be used as starting points for further exploration. Such a list is useful to share with others so that they can begin their own exploration. These should be sites that you have determined are trustworthy and reliable. Examples of such sites include organizations and associations with which we are all familiar such as the American Cancer Society (ACS). The ACS website (www.cancer.org) has patient education and consumer information materials. In addition to the traditional types of resources available from the ACS, it is also possible from the website to send an e-mail requesting more information, sign up for regular updates and news, read news items, and obtain updated statistical information. The website is truly a "value-added" version of the ACS. Practically any health organization you can think of has created a virtual storefront on the Internet. Professional associations in nursing, medicine, and other disciplines are also becoming comprehensive resource sites on the Internet.

Other resources are U.S. government agencies such as the Agency for Healthcare Research and Quality (AHRQ) (www.ahrq.gov) and the National Institutes of Health (NIH) (www.nih.gov). The AHRQ website is an excellent resource that contains (a) clinical information, including clinical practice guidelines; (b) health care information for consumers and patients; (c) grant funding opportunities; (d) research findings; (e) health care quality information and resources; and (f) information on pubic health preparedness. The NIH website is an equally valuable resource that contains grant funding opportunities, scientific resources such as the Human Embryonic Stem Cell Registry, consumer health information, and links to the Institutes that make up the NIH, including the National Institute for Nursing Research and the National Institute on Aging. Once again, all of these agencies have been busy creating virtual institutes on the Internet. Another useful resource is Healthfinder (www.healthfinder.gov), which can point you to news, information, tools, and databases.

Although these resources are the Internet versions of known and useful organizations, there are also virtual resources that exist only on the Internet. One such site that is particularly impressive is MEDLINEplus (http://www.medlineplus.gov), developed by the National Library of Medicine. A similar resource, specific to oncology, is OncoLink at the University of Pennsylvania (www.oncolink.org). OncoLink was created in 1994 and was the first multimedia oncology information resource placed on the Internet. This resource continues to be true to its original mission to "help cancer patients, families, health care professionals and the general public get accurate cancer-related information at no charge" (About OncoLink, 2003).

Literature Resources. Thinking back to PFA (purpose-focus-approach), if you are searching for scientific, technical, or research-oriented information, you must search literature databases. In this case, the first place to turn is to the National Library of Medicine (NLM), which is the home of the MEDLARS (Medical Literature Analysis and Retrieval System), a computerized system of databases and databanks offered by the NLM. You can search the computer files either to produce a list of publications (bibliographic citations) or to retrieve factual information on a specific question. The most well known of all the databases in the MEDLARS system is MEDLINE, NLM's premier bibliographic database covering the fields of medicine, nursing, dentistry, veterinary medicine, and the preclinical sciences. Journal articles are indexed for MEDLINE, and their citations are searchable, using NLM's controlled vocabulary, MeSH (Medical Subject Headings). MEDLINE contains all citations published in Index Medicus and corresponds in part to the International Nursing Index and the Index to Dental Literature. Citations include the English abstract when published with the article (approximately 76% of the current file). MEDLINE contains over 11 million records from 4600 health science journals. The file is updated daily. An individual can search MEDLINE for free, using the PubMed search engines (http://www.ncbi.nlm.nih.gov/entrez/query.fcgi). There are no fees to the user to access the MEDLINE database.

Another literature resource to investigate is the National Guideline Clearinghouse (NCG) (www.ngc.gov). Whereas MEDLINE includes citations to articles in professional journals, the NGC is a comprehensive database of evidence-based clinical practice guidelines and related documents produced by the Agency for Healthcare Research and Quality in partnership with the American Medical Association and the American Association of Health Plans. The NGC mission is to provide physicians, nurses, other health professionals, health care providers, health plans, integrated delivery systems, and purchasers an accessible mechanism for obtaining objective, detailed information on clinical practice guidelines and to further their dissemination, implementation, and use.

There are also a variety of other literature resources available on the Internet, some of which have fees attached. However, do not automatically assume that you must pay the fee. Your workplace or school may have licensing agreements in place with different vendors, and as an employee or student you may have access to the literature resources. Check with your library or information services department to see whether this applies to you.

The final element of searching literature on-line is finding full text of articles. The databases so far discussed (MEDLINE and others) do not contain full text; they only include literature citations. Finding full text on-line at the present time is an unorganized situation. Some journals provide full text on-line either free or for a fee; in other cases, you may be forced to do things the "old-fashioned way"—that is, by taking a trip to the library and photocopying articles by hand. Always check with your librarian about the availability of full-text articles on-line through the library resources. Another option is to begin exploring, using quick and dirty or brute force methods. You can also visit the publisher's website to see whether access to the journal is available. A final option is to use a document delivery service; this can be quite expensive but may be necessary if you are not able to obtain an article any other way.

Evaluating Information Found on the Internet. Traveling through the Internet, you must always use critical thinking skills to evaluate the information that is found. The "wide open" nature of the Internet means that just about anyone with a computer and on-line access can create a home page and post it for the world to see. Although there are many excellent health- and nursing-related sites, there are others that simply do not measure up in terms of accuracy, content, or currency.

In recent years criteria for website evaluation have proliferated. They range from the simple and cursory to the elaborate and expansive. I have found a simple mnemonic, "Are you PLEASED with the site?" to be very helpful.* The PLEASED mnemonic makes the seven criteria very easy to remember, but as I have found, during hundreds of hours of surfing and evaluating, the criteria are extremely comprehensive (Nicoll, 2000; Nicoll, 2001). To determine whether you are PLEASED, consider the following:

- *P: Purpose.* What is the author's purpose in developing the site? Are the author's objectives clear? Many people will develop a website as a hobby or way of sharing information they have gathered. It should be immediately evident to you what the true purpose of the site is. At the same time, consider *your* purpose (i.e., think back to your PFA assessment). There should be congruence between the author's purpose and yours.
- *L: Links.* Evaluate the links at the site. Are they working? (Links that do not take you anywhere are called "dead links.") Do they link to reliable sites? It is important to critically evaluate the links at sites hosted by organizations, businesses, or institutions because these entities are usually presenting themselves as authorities for the subject at hand. Some pages, such as those created by individuals, are really nothing more than a collection of links. These can be useful as a starting point for a search, but it is still important to evaluate the links that are provided at the site.

*Thanks to Linda Johnson of Excelsior University (formerly Regents College), Albany, NY, for her original suggestion of this mnemonic.

- *E: Editorial (site content).* Is the information contained in the site accurate, comprehensive, and current? Is there a particular bias, or is the information presented in an objective way? Who is the consumer of the site: is it designed for health professionals, patients, consumers, or other audiences? Is the information presented in an appropriate format for the intended audience? Look at details, too. Are there misspellings and grammatical errors? Do you see "under construction" banners that have been there for months? I find that these types of errors can be very telling about the overall quality of the site.

- *A: Author.* Who is the author of the site? Does that person have the appropriate credentials? Is the author clearly identified by name, and is contact information provided? Many times I will double-check an author's credentials by doing a literature search in MEDLINE. When people advertise themselves as "the leading worldwide authority" on such-and-such topic, I figure they should have a few publications to their credit that establish their reputations. It is surprising how many times this search brings up nothing.

  Also be wary of how a person presents his or her credentials. I have seen many sites where "Dr. X" is touted as an expert. On further exploration, I verify that, in fact, Dr. X does have a PhD (or MD or EdD), but the discipline in which this degree was obtained has nothing to do with the subject matter of the site. Remember that there is no universal process of peer review on the Internet and anyone can present himself or herself in any way that he or she wants. Be suspicious.

  Keep in mind that the "webmaster" and the author may be two (or more) different people. The webmaster is the person who designed the site and is responsible for its upkeep. The author is the person who is responsible for the content and is the supposed expert in the subject matter provided. In your evaluation, make sure to determine who these people are.

- *S: Site.* Is the site easy to navigate? Is it attractive? Does it download quickly or have too many graphics and other features that make it inefficient? A site that is pleasing to the eye will invite you to return. Sites that cause my computer to crash go on the "never visit again" list. I am also not fond of sites that have annoying music that cannot be turned off.

- *E: Ethical.* Is there contact information for the site developer and author? Is there full disclosure of who the author is and the purpose of the site? Is this information easy to find, or is it buried deep in the website? There are many commercial services, particularly pharmaceutical companies, that have excellent websites with very useful information. However, others exist only to sell their products, although this is often not immediately evident on evaluation.

- *D: Date.* When was the site last updated? Is it current? Is the information something that needs to be updated regularly? Generally, with health and nursing information, the answer to that last question is yes. I become concerned with sites that have not been updated within the last 12 to 18 months. The date the site was last updated should be prominently displayed on the site. Keep in mind that different pages within the site may be updated at different times. Be sure to check the date on each of the pages that you visit.

As you become more proficient at website evaluation, you may have additional criteria that you would add to this list or criteria that are important to you for a specific purpose.

I have found that this simple group of seven has served me well on countless Internet journeys. Test them for yourself. Do a quick search on a topic of interest, visit a number of sites, and determine just how PLEASED you are with what you find.

S U M M A R Y

Computers have opened for us a world of information; at the same time, they have given us the responsibility to learn how to use them—and use them well. As a nurse, you have the opportunity to specialize in the expanding field of nursing informatics. Within this role, you will provide a vital link between the world of information science and clinical nursing practice. Even if you choose not to specialize in informatics, you will still be using computers on a day-to-day basis and thus must be (or become) computer-literate. It is not enough to know how to turn on the computer and to complete a few simple tasks. A nurse must know generalized applications such as word processing, as well as specialized applications such as clinical information systems. The nurse must also know how to access the on-line world of information and resources and how to critically evaluate the information that is found. This is not going to change. As the Internet continues to grow and as computers become smaller and more powerful, they will continue to have a major impact on how health is conceptualized and delivered.

C R I T I C A L   T H I N K I N G   A C T I V I T I E S

1. Some institutions are reluctant to issue passwords to nursing students allowing them to access the CIS, fearing that this could compromise its security. Is this a legitimate concern? Do you agree with this position? Why or why not?

2. A lifetime patient record, such as the type envisioned in a CPR/EHR, would include all health information from a person's life. Some people have questioned the necessity of this amount of detail. They also are concerned that it would limit the information that a person is able to keep private. Health care providers, on the other hand, argue that they need access to all information to provide appropriate care. Is this always true? Give three examples of health information from the past that might not be relevant to a current problem. What strategies could be used to help patients maintain the privacy of sensitive health data in a lifetime electronic record?

3. A major issue facing the developers of CPR/EHR systems is the patient identifier. Some have suggested using a modified version of the social security number; others have advocated developing a unique patient identifier. In your opinion, why is this a major issue? What suggestions do you have for a patient identifier?

4. Go on-line and find four different types of health-related sites on similar topics, including a nurse's personal home page, a patient's home page, one from a pharmaceutical company, and one from a news agency that reports on health. Using the PLEASED criteria, evaluate the sites. Which sites would you return to for professional information? Which sites would you recommend to a patient? Which sites would you never visit again? Explain your decisions.

5. Interview a person who completed a major project (e.g., thesis or dissertation) in the "precomputer" days. What resources did the person use to prepare the project? If data were analyzed, how was that accomplished? How did the person write the final version of the project? Would availability of computers have made the project easier? Why or why not?

6. Identify a listserv of interest. Subscribe and "lurk" for 3 to 5 days. What type of information is discussed? How active is the list? Is the information that is provided accurate? What is the signal-to-noise ratio?

Additional resources are available on-line at: http://evolve.elsevier.com/Cherry/

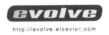

http://evolve.elsevier.com

REFERENCES

About OncoLink: *The Trustees of the University of Pennsylvania,* Philadelphia, December 4, 2003 (http://www.oncolink.com/about/index.cfm).

American Medical Informatics Association: *Education in nursing informatics,* Bethesda, Md, 2003 (http://www.amia.org/working/ni/education/cat3.html).

American Nurses Association: *Scope of practice for nursing informatics,* Washington, DC, 1994, ANA.

American Nurses Association: *NIDSEC: recognized languages for nursing,* Washington, DC, 2003, ANA (www.nursingworld.org/nidsec/classlst.htm).

American Nurses Credentialing Center: *Statement of philosophy,* Washington, DC, 1993, ANA.

American Nurses Credentialing Center: *ANCC certification exam results for ambulatory care nursing, nursing case management, nursing informatics, and nursing administration,* Washington, DC, 2003a, ANA (http://nursingworld.org/ancc/certification/cert/exams/results/others.html).

American Nurses Credentialing Center: *Informatics nurse certification exam,* Washington, DC, 2003b, ANA (http://nursingworld.org/ancc/certification/cert/certs/informatics.html).

Ball MJ, Hannah KJ, Douglas JV: Nursing and informatics. In Ball MJ et al, editors: *Nursing informatics: where caring and technology meet,* ed 3, New York, 2000, Springer-Verlag.

Computer-Based Patient Record Institute: *Guidelines for establishing information security policies at organizations using computer-based patient records: work group on confidentiality, privacy, and security,* Schaumburg, Ill, 1995, CPRI.

Encarta World English Dictionary, 2003 (http://encarta.msn.com/dictionary_/lexicon.html).

Gassert CA: Academic preparation in nursing informatics. In Ball MJ et al, editors: *Nursing informatics: where caring and technology meet,* ed 3, New York, 2000, Springer-Verlag.

Gorn S: Informatics (computer and information science): its ideology, methodology, and sociology. In Machlup F, Mansfield U, editors: *The study of information: interdisciplinary messages,* New York, 1983, John Wiley & Sons.

Hersher BS: New roles for nurses in healthcare information systems. In Ball MJ et al, editors: *Nursing informatics: where caring and technology meet,* ed 3, New York, 2000, Springer-Verlag.

Hiltzik M: *Dealers of lightning: Xerox PARC and the dawn of the computer age,* New York, 2000, Harper Business.

Jenkins S: Nurses' responsibilities in the implementation of information systems. In Ball MJ et al, editors: *Nursing informatics: where caring and technology meet,* ed 3, New York, 2000, Springer-Verlag.

Joos I et al: *Computers in small bytes: the computer workbook,* ed 2, New York, 1996, National League for Nursing Press.

Lawrence S, Giles CL: Searching the world wide web, *Science* 280:98-100, 1998.

Moore-Cox A: Formal education in nursing informatics, *Comput Inform Nurs* 21(5):276-282-284, 2000.

National Institute of Nursing Research: *Nursing informatics: enhancing patient care,* Bethesda, Md, 1993, U.S. Department of Health and Human Services.

Newbold SK: The informatics nurse and the certification process, *Computer Nurs* 14(2):84-85, 88, 1996.

Newbold SK: Nursing informatics organizations: virtual and otherwise, *Comput Inform Nurs* 21(5):275-281, 2003.

Nicoll LH: Quick and effective website evaluation, *CIN Plus* 3(3):9, 12, 2000.

Nicoll LH: *Nurses' guide to the Internet,* ed 3, Philadelphia, 2001, JB Lippincott.

Nicoll LH: Continuing education in nursing informatics, *Comput Inform Nurs* 21(5):277, 284-286, 2003.

Schwirian PM: The NI pyramid—a model for research in nursing informatics, *Computer Nurs* 4(3):134-136, 1986.

Semancik M: *The history of clinical information systems: legacy systems, computer-based patient record and point of care,* Clinical Information Systems, Seattle, 1997, SpaceLabs Medical.

Smith DK, Alexander RC: *Fumbling the future: how Xerox invented, then ignored, the first personal computer* New York, 1988, W Morrow.

Snyder-Halpern R: Letter to the editor, *Comput Inform Nurs* 22(1), 45, 2004.

Styles MM: *On specialization in nursing: toward a new empowerment,* Kansas City, Mo, 1989, American Nurses Foundation

Watts J: The healthy home of the future comes to Japan, *Lancet* 353(9164):1597-1600, 1999.

Weiser M, Brown JS: *The coming age of calm technology,* October 5, 1996 (http://www.ubiq.com/hypertext/weiser/acmfuture2endnote.htm).

Year-end 2000 mailbox report (www.messagingonline.net).

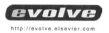

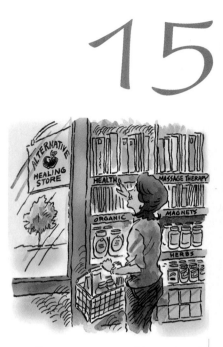

Complementary and Alternative Healing

Charlotte Eliopoulos, PhD, RNC, MPH, ND

15

Consumers are seeking natural remedies; nurses have a responsibility to be aware of the potential effects.

VIGNETTE

Ruth Jeffers is a registered nurse (RN) who works in a rehabilitation unit of a community hospital. Many of the clients on this unit suffer from chronic musculoskeletal pain. Nurse Jeffers has noted that a growing number of clients have a history of independently using acupuncture, nutritional supplements, and other alternative healing therapies to improve their symptoms. Although they report beneficial results, most do not tell their physicians that they are using alternative therapies.

Last year, Nurse Jeffers completed a course in the use of therapeutic touch and has used this therapy to promote relaxation and pain control with friends and family with considerable success. She is aware of many positive reports on the benefits of these unconventional approaches. She believes therapeutic touch and some other alternative healing therapies could benefit clients on the rehabilitation unit and informally introduces the topic to the team with whom she works. With the exception of one nurse who states that she believes these therapies are associated with the occult and wants no part of them, the nursing staff is enthusiastic and eager to implement alternative therapies. The physical and occupational therapists believe that alternative therapies could prove helpful to clients but that only therapists within their departments, not nursing, should provide these. The physician on the team opposes the use of all alternative therapies, claiming he "isn't about to put his license on the line for these unproven ideas."

Additional resources are available on-line at: http://evolve.elsevier.com/Cherry/

Questions to consider while reading this chapter:

1. What is the best course of action for Nurse Jeffers if she really believes that complementary and alternative therapies could benefit clients on the unit?
2. What would a hospital need to do to prepare for the inclusion of complementary and alternative therapies in its existing services?
3. What are some of the obstacles that could be anticipated when introducing complementary and alternative therapies into a conventional setting?
4. What discipline(s) should be responsible for providing and/or coordinating/supervising the practitioners who provide complementary and alternative therapies in the hospital?

KEY TERMS

Alternative medical systems Acupuncture, anthroposophic Ayurvedic medicine, community-based health care practices (e.g., Native American, shamans), environmental medicine, homeopathy, naturopathy, traditional Oriental medicine.

Biologically based treatments Herbal therapies, individual and orthomolecular biologic therapies, special diets.

Complementary and alternative medicine (CAM) Healing philosophies, practices, and products that are outside of what Western society considers mainstream medicine and are not typically taught in the educational programs of physicians, nurses, and other health professionals.

Conventional medicine Western style of medicine practiced in the United States; also called allopathic.

Energy therapies Qigong, Reiki, therapeutic touch, healing touch, bioelectromagnetic-based therapies.

Manipulative and body-based methods Chiropracty, massage and related techniques (e.g., manual lymph drainage, Alexander technique, Feldenkrais method, pressure point therapies, Trager psychophysical integration), osteopathy.

Mind/body interventions Aromatherapy, art therapy, biofeedback, dance therapy, hypnosis, imagery, meditation, music therapy, prayer, relaxation, self-help support groups, tai chi, yoga.

LEARNING OUTCOMES

After studying this chapter, the reader will be able to:

1. Describe various complementary and alternative healing practices.
2. Effectively incorporate pertinent complementary and alternative therapies into patient care.
3. Provide patient education regarding uses, limitations, and precautions associated with complementary and alternative healing practices and products.

CHAPTER OVERVIEW

This chapter presents an overview of complementary and alternative medicine (CAM) therapies and products, which are rapidly gaining popularity in Western society. As increasing numbers of consumers and clinical settings become interested in and actually use CAM therapies, nurses must become knowledgeable about the uses, limitations, and precautions associated with these new practices and products. Professional nurses have an obligation to understand such practices and products in order to advise patients and effectively incorporate pertinent therapies into patients' care. Nurses who have knowledge and skills in this area are in key positions to empower patients for self-care that complements conventional medicine.

USE OF COMPLEMENTARY AND ALTERNATIVE HEALING METHODS

CAM includes healing philosophies, practices, and products that fall outside what Western society considers mainstream (conventional) medicine and that are not typically taught in the educational programs of physicians, nurses, and other health professionals.

The past few decades have witnessed CAM progress from a fringe movement to highly popular, widely used therapies that are being integrated into conventional care. Recent surveys reveal that more than 4 out of every 10 Americans have visited an alternative health care practitioner and most are paying for these services out of their own pockets (Eisenberg et al, 1998).

Rather than emerging from the leadership of health care professionals, the growing popularity of CAM has been consumer-driven. Several factors contribute to consumers' desire for CAM:

- *Dissatisfaction with the conventional health care system:* The impersonal nature of health care has grown with costs. Shorter hospital stays, several months' waiting periods to see a physician, hurried staff that barely have time to provide basic care, and horror stories of the adverse effects of medications are causing consumers to look for alternative approaches that are safer, less costly, and more responsive and personalized than conventional health care.
- *Unwillingness to "grin and bear" the effects of diseases:* Today's consumers are less willing than their parents to live with symptoms that alter their lifestyles or to passively accept a terminal diagnosis and wait to die. They want options and to be empowered to do everything conceivable to promote the best possible quality and quantity of their lives, and they are willing to look to alternative healing measures to do so.
- *Shrinking world:* The rapid pace and ease of information sharing has enabled individuals to learn about practices of people throughout the world.
- *Growing evidence of effectiveness:* The body of research supporting the effectiveness of alternative therapies increases almost daily. People are hearing testimonials from friends and family about the way they have been helped by acupuncture, herbs, and other forms of CAM. In addition, the media regularly reports these findings, contributing to consumers' awareness of the body of evidence.

CAM practices and products are consistent with the values, beliefs, and philosophic orientations toward health held by many people (Astin, 1998). With rare exceptions, consumers prefer natural approaches that afford them an active role in their care over high-tech interventions that relegate them to a passive, obedient role. They want to connect with their health care providers, have their individuality recognized, and gain education and skills to effectively make decisions and direct their care. Increasingly, consumers are seeking measures to enhance not just their bodies, but also their minds and spirits. The quality of their lives is equally, if not more, important to the quantity of years they live. Consumers often discover that CAM promotes many principles of holistic care that they value, such as individual empowerment, self-care, and a high quality of life.

PRINCIPLES UNDERLYING ALTERNATIVE HEALING

A wide range of healing therapies are encompassed in CAM; yet most share some common principles at their core (Eliopoulos, 1999):

- *The body has the ability to heal itself.* Most conventional medicine works from the premise that the elimination of sickness requires an intervention "done to" the body (e.g., giving medications, surgery). In CAM there is the assumption that the body heals itself. Alternative healing therapies enhance the body's ability to self-heal.
- *Health and healing are related to a harmony of mind, body, and spirit.* The mind, body, and spirit are inseparable; what affects one affects all. Healing and the improvement of health demand that all of the facets of a person be addressed, not merely a single symptom or system.
- *Basic, positive health practices build the foundation for healing.* Good nutrition, exercise, rest, stress management, and avoidance of harmful habits (e.g., smoking) are essential ingredients to health maintenance and the improvement of health conditions. Practitioners of healing therapies are more likely than conventional practitioners to look at total lifestyle practices rather than the diseased body part.
- *Approaches to healing are individualized.* The unique composition and dynamics of each person are recognized in CAM. Practitioners of healing therapies explore the underlying cause of a problem and customize approaches accordingly. It is rare in CAM to find a standing protocol that treats all persons with similar conditions similarly.
- *Individuals are responsible for their own healing.* People can use a wide range of therapies, from conventional prescription drugs or herbal remedies, to treat illness. However, it is the responsibility of competent adults to seek health advice, make informed choices, gain necessary knowledge and skills for self-care, engage in practices that promote health and healing, and seek help when needed. Clients are responsible for getting their minds, bodies, and spirits in optimal condition to heal rather than look externally for a doctor or nurse to heal them.

A holistic philosophy, promotion of positive health habits, and the client's responsibility for facilitating his or her own health and healing are common threads among healing therapies.

OVERVIEW OF POPULAR ALTERNATIVE HEALING THERAPIES

Hundreds of healing therapies are practiced throughout the world, with varying degrees of evidence to support their effectiveness. As the use of these therapies grew in the United States, the National Institutes of Health (NIH) established the Office of Alternative Medicine in 1992 to evaluate these complementary and alternative practices and products. In 1998 the Office of Alternative Medicine became a freestanding center within NIH and was named the National Center for Complementary and Alternative Medicine (NCCAM). NCCAM has categorized CAM into five fields of practice (Box 15-1); the Center supports research and serves as a clearinghouse for information on alternative practices and products.

Consumers' growing use and the increased integration of CAM therapies into conventional care place a demand on nurses to become familiar with these therapies. Some of the frequently used CAM therapies are discussed below.

Acupuncture

Practiced in China for over 2000 years, acupuncture is a major therapy within traditional Chinese medicine. It is based on the belief that there are invisible channels throughout the body called meridians, through which energy flows. This energy is called Qi (pronounced chee) and is considered the vital life force. It is believed that illness and symptoms develop when the flow of energy becomes blocked or imbalanced. Health is restored when the energy becomes unblocked; this is achieved by stimulating acupuncture points on the meridian(s) affected (Fig. 15-1).

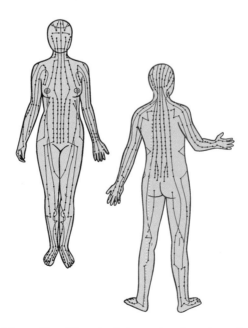

FIG. 15–1 Acupuncture meridians. (From Eliopoulos C: *Integrating alternative and conventional therapies,* St Louis, 1999, Mosby.)

The acupuncturist typically begins the treatment by taking a history, examining the tongue, and evaluating pulses. Based on where the acupuncturist assesses the energy imbalance to be, he or she places needles at specific points. The placement of the needles may have no obvious relationship to the area of the body that is symptomatic. Sometimes the acupuncturist applies heat to the acupoints by burning a dried herb on the top of the needle or skin; this procedure is known as moxibustion. Electro-acupuncture, a process in which a small current of electricity is applied to the tip of the needle, is another means of stimulating acupoints.

Pain relief is the most common reason people seek acupuncture treatment, and research supports its effectiveness for this problem. The use of acupuncture for dental pain and chemotherapy-induced nausea and vomiting also has been supported by research. There is some evidence that acupuncture can be of help for nicotine withdrawal, asthma, stroke rehabilitation, carpal tunnel syndrome, and a growing list of other conditions.

Insurance companies vary in their coverage of acupuncture, so it is best for clients to call their individual insurer for determination of benefits. State health departments can be consulted for licensing requirements for acupuncturists in a given state.

Ayurveda

Although it recently has gained popularity because of the writings and lectures of Deepak Chopra (1993), Ayurveda has existed in India for over 5000 years. Ayurveda means "the science of life" and is a system of care that promotes spiritual, mental, and physical balance. Noninvasive approaches are used to achieve balance and include yoga, massage, diet, purification regimens, breathing exercises, meditation, and herbs.

Individuals are believed to have distinct metabolic body types called doshas, which are vata, pitta, and kapha (Table 15-1). Signs of illness occur when the delicate balance of the doshas is disturbed. The treatment to restore balance is influenced by the body type a client possesses and could include:

- Cleansing and detoxification
- Palliation
- Rejuvenation through special herbs and minerals
- Mental hygiene and spiritual healing

Currently there is no process for licensing or certifying Ayurvedic practitioners. Because some of the treatments have the potential to cause complications (e.g., dehydration from cleansing enemas, herb-drug interactions), finding a reputable trained practitioner is

Table 15-1	**Ayurvedic Metabolic Body Types**
TYPE	CHARACTERISTICS
Vata	Unpredictable, moody, vivacious, hyperactive, imaginative, intuitive, impulsive, fluctuating energy levels, slender, prominent features and joints, eats and sleeps at varying times throughout day, prone to insomnia, PMS, cramps, and constipation
Pitta	Predictable, orderly, efficient, perfectionist, intense, passionate, short-tempered, medium build, follows routine schedule, warm skin, prone to heavy perspiration, thirst, acne, ulcers, hemorrhoids, and stomach problems
Kapha	Relaxed, graceful, tendency toward procrastination, affectionate, forgiving, compassionate, sleeps long and deeply, cool, pale and oily skin, eats slowly, prone to high cholesterol, obesity, allergies, sinusitis

important. The Ayurveda websites listed in Box 15-2 can assist in locating qualified practitioners.

Biofeedback

Biofeedback is a technique in which the client is taught to alter specific bodily functions (e.g., heart rate, blood pressure, muscle tension). The client uses various relaxation and imagery exercises to affect desired responses. Machinery such as electroencephalograms, electromyelograms, and thermistors are used to measure and offer feedback about the function that the client is trying to alter. As the client becomes familiar with ways to successfully alter bodily responses, the equipment may no longer be necessary.

There are many conditions for which biofeedback can offer benefit, including urinary incontinence, anxiety, stress, irritable bowel syndrome, neck and back pain, and cardiac arrhythmias.

Chiropractic Medicine

Chiropractic medicine is a popular and widely accepted CAM therapy in the United States, perhaps because it was developed here and has been practiced for over a century. Chiropractors are licensed in every state, and most insurance companies will pay for chiropractic treatments.

Chiropractic medicine is based on the belief that misalignments of the spine, called subluxations, put pressure on the nerves, leading to pain and disruptions in normal bodily function. The misalignment is treated by manipulation and adjustment of the spine. Typically, the chiropractor's hands do the alignment, although chiropractors increasingly are using heat, electrical stimulation, and other treatments.

Dietary Supplements

The past advice that vitamin and mineral supplements are unnecessary if one is eating well has been replaced with the recommendation that everyone should take a daily vitamin and mineral supplement. This shift in thinking has resulted from the realization that many people do not consume the proper nutrients through their diets. Pollutants, stress, and other factors that are more common today than in previous generations heighten the body's need for added protection. Also, unlike our ancestors, who consumed produce that was picked the same day, we tend to eat more processed foods and produce that may have been in transit for several days before reaching us; therefore the foods we consume contain fewer vitamins and minerals. Given these factors, the National Research Council of the United States National Academy of Sciences is reevaluating the need to increase the Recommended Daily Allowances (RDAs).

Specific dietary supplements are believed to be beneficial for specific health conditions (e.g., vitamin E to improve arthritis and heart disease). However, too much of a good thing could prove harmful, and high doses of vitamins and minerals can lead to serious complications. For example, high doses of folic acid can mask a vitamin B_{12} deficiency (a cause of dementia), and calcium in excess of 2500 mg/day can cause kidney stones and impair the body's ability to absorb other minerals.

Herbs

Plants have been used for medicinal purposes for nearly as long as humans have inhabited the earth. It is estimated that as many as 70,000 plant species have been

BOX 15–2 Helpful Websites

General Information
NCCAM Clearinghouse
www.nccam.nih.gov

Acupuncture
American Academy of Medical Acupuncture
www.medicalacupuncture.org

American Association of Acupuncture and
   Oriental Medicine
www.aaom.org

National Certification Commission for Acupuncture
   and Oriental Medicine
www.nccaom.org

Ayurveda
Ayurvedic Institute
www.ayurveda.com

Ayurveda Holistic Center
http://ayurvedahc.com/index.htm

Biofeedback
Biofeedback Webzine
www.webideas.com/biofeedback/

Biofeedback Certification Institute
www.bcia.org/

Chiropractic Medicine
American Chiropractic Association
www.amerchiro.org

International Chiropractors Association
www.chiropractic.org

Dietary Supplements
NIH Health Office of Dietary Supplements
http://dietary-supplements.info.nih.gov/

FDA Guide to Dietary Supplements
www.vm.cfsan.fda.gov/~dms/supplement.html

Herbs
American Botanical Council
www.herbs.org

FDA's website on recent warnings on herbal products
http://www.cfsan.fda.gov/~dms/aems.html

Herb Net
www.herbnet.com

Homeopathy
National Center for Homeopathy
www.healthy.net/nch

Hypnotherapy
American Institute of Hypnotherapy
www.hypnosis.com/aih

National Guild of Hypnotists
www.ngh.net

Massage
Associated Bodywork and Massage Professionals
www.abmp.com

American Massage Therapy Association
www.amtamassage.org

Naturopathy
American Association of Naturopathic Physicians
www.naturopathic.org

Reflexology
Association of Reflexology
www.reflexology.org

Tai Chi
Qi Journal
www.qi-journal.com/

Touch Therapies
Healing Touch International
www.healingtouch.net

Nurse Healers Professional Associations
www.therapeutic-touch.org

Yoga
American Yoga Association
www.americanyogaasociation.org

Yoga Site
www.yogasite.com

used at one time or another by various cultures for medicinal purposes (Libster, 2002). Botanical medicine was a mainstream practice in the United States until the early nineteenth century, when medicine's shift toward a more scientific approach caused drugs to be viewed more favorably than herbs. But in the 1960s when the movement toward natural health began to grow, interest in herbal products increased. The use and sales of herbal remedies have grown significantly since.

In reality, herbs are not that foreign to conventional medicine. Many modern drugs are derived from plants, including:

- Atropine from *Atropa belladona*.
- Digoxin from *Digitalis purpurea*.
- Ipecac from *Cephaelis ipecacuanha*.
- Reserpine from *Rauwolfia serpentina*.

With more than 20,000 herbs and related products on the market (McCaleb, 2000) staying current of uses, dosage, interactions, and adverse effects is a near impossibility. However, nurses would be wise to become familiar with some of the most commonly used herbs (Box 15-3) and know where to obtain information on other herbs when needed (see Box 15-2). Because of consumers' widespread use of herbs, questions regarding use of all supplements and education to ensure safe use are significant nursing responsibilities.

Homeopathy

Homeopathy is a branch of medicine developed in the late eighteenth century by Samuel Hahnemann. It was widely practiced in the United States until the early 1900s, when modern (i.e., conventional) medicine discredited it as being unscientific and ineffective. Homeopathy remained popular in other parts of the world, however, and recently has regained popularity in our country.

The origin of the word *homeopathy* helps to understand this therapy. In Greek the word *homios* means "similar," and *pathos* means "suffering." The foundation of homeopathy is the Law of Similars and builds on the idea of prescribing remedies that produce symptoms similar to those of the illness being treated. Before judging this theory to be outrageous, note that this is the same principle on which vaccines are based. In homeopathy a dilute preparation is made from a plant or other biologic material; the more dilute the preparation, the higher its potency. The solution typically is added to a sugar tablet or powder for oral use or to a lotion or ointment for external use.

In homeopathy, the Law of Cure is used to evaluate the effectiveness of a remedy. If the treatment is successful, symptoms should travel from vital to less vital organs of the body, move from within the body outward, and disappear in reverse order of appearance. If symptoms do not follow this sequence, a new or additional treatment is used. In homeopathic medicine a worsening of symptoms after a remedy is given is considered a positive sign that healing is taking place.

Although the reason for their effectiveness is not fully understood, homeopathic remedies have been shown to be effective for a variety of conditions; some of the most common conditions for which people use homeopathic medicine are listed in Box 15-4.

The ideal way to use homeopathic remedies is to have a homeopath prescribe a customized remedy based on individual characteristics and symptoms. However, homeopathic practitioners are not plentiful, so the next best thing is to buy over-the-counter preparations that are labeled for their intended purpose (e.g., arthritis, headache, hay fever, cold).

BOX 15–3 *Facts About Commonly Used Herbs*

Chamomile
Uses: Sedative effect, calming upset digestive tract.
Cautions: Because it contains coumarin, it could affect coagulation, although clinical studies have not proven this to date; if client is using an anticoagulant and chamomile, monitor.

Echinacea
Uses: Antimicrobial; stimulates immune system; useful in prevention and treatment of upper respiratory infections.
Cautions: Some persons with ragweed and other environmental allergies may have sensitivity; although immuno-suppressive effects with long-term use are inconclusive at present, best to limit to short-term use.

Feverfew
Use: Relief of migraines.
Cautions: Contraindicated for clients with allergies to ragweed and other members of Compositae family; can affect coagulation so contraindicated in persons on anticoagulant therapy.

Garlic
Uses: Lowers blood pressure; reduces "bad" cholesterol; stimulates immune system; cancer preventive; antioxidant.
Cautions: Close monitoring necessary if taken by person using anticoagulant because it can prolong bleeding time; can potentiate action of hypoglycemic drugs.

Ginger
Use: Antiemetic.
Caution: Regular use can prolong bleeding time, monitor if used with an anticoagulant.

Ginkgo biloba
Use: Improves cognitive performance in persons with dementia.
Cautions: Close monitoring necessary if taken by person using anticoagulant because it can prolong bleeding time; can reduce effectiveness of anticonvulsants.

Ginseng
Uses: Improves resistance to stress, immune stimulant; general stimulant.
Cautions: Raises blood pressure; close monitoring necessary if taken by person using anticoagulant because it can prolong bleeding time; may increase digoxin levels; contraindicated when other stimulants are used; can cause insomnia, headache, epistaxis, vomiting.

Saw palmetto
Uses: Improves symptoms with benign prostatic hypertrophy; diuretic; urinary antiseptic.
Caution: Do not take with hormonal therapies.

St. John's Wort
Uses: Antidepressant; antianxiety.
Cautions: Can cause photosensitivity, particularly in fair-skinned individuals; contraindicated when other antidepressants are used.

Valerian
Use: Sedative.
Caution: Do not use with barbiturates.

BOX 15–4	Ten Most Common Conditions for Which People Use Homeopathic Medicine

Asthma	Neurotic disorders
Depression	Allergy (nonspecific)
Otitis media	Dermatitis
Allergic rhinitis	Arthritis
Headache/migraine	Hypertension

From Jacobs J, Chapman EH, Crothers D: Patient characteristics and practice patterns of physicians using homeopathy. In Fontanarosa PB, editor: *Alternative medicine: an objective assessment,* Dover, Del, 2000, American Medical Association, pp 422-426.

Hypnotherapy

Although the use of trance states for healing purposes dates back to primitive cultures, hypnotherapy was not approved as a valid medical treatment until the 1950s. This mind-body therapy is now widely and successfully used for a wide range of conditions, including chronic pain, migraines, asthma, smoking cessation, and irritable bowel syndrome.

The process of hypnosis begins by the therapist guiding the client into a relaxed state and then creating an image that focuses attention to the specific symptom or problem that needs to be improved. The client must be in a state of deep relaxation to be receptive to a posthypnotic suggestion. Most people are capable of being hypnotized if they are willing.

Imagery

Imagery is the process of creating a "picture" (image) in the mind that can cause a specific bodily response. Although hypnosis uses imagery, in hypnosis an image and suggestion are presented to the person, whereas in imagery the person creates an image on his or her own. The process of imagery begins by the client establishing a desired outcome (e.g., to relieve stress, enhance circulation, reduce blood pressure). The nurse or other practitioner assists the client in creating an image that helps to achieve the outcome (e.g., the nurse may describe how the blood circulates through the body, help the client develop an image of how cancer cells can be eliminated, or suggest that the client think of a peaceful place where cares can "melt away"), and guides the client in reaching a relaxed state. As an alternative to having someone guide him or her through an imagery exercise, a client can learn the process from books or use commercially prepared audiotapes.

Imagery is not a difficult mind-body healing therapy to master and can be easily implemented in virtually every practice setting.

Magnet Therapy

Although a mainstream therapy in Germany and Japan, the use of magnets has only recently become popular in the United States. The most common uses of magnet therapy are for pain and wound healing.

The mechanism by which magnets work is not completely understood and is being investigated at present. It is believed that magnets relieve pain by creating a slight electrical current that stimulates the nervous system and consequently blocks nerve sensations. Magnets are hypothesized to speed wound healing by dilating vessels and increasing circulation to an area. Distributors of magnet products make additional claims about the health benefits of magnets, ranging from improving attention deficit disorder to boosting the immune system, although these benefits are yet to be proven.

Magnets come in a variety of forms, strengths, and prices. There are magnet disks that can be strapped to limbs, magnet mattresses that one can sleep on, and magnet jewelry. To be effective for therapeutic purposes, the magnet should have a strength of at least 500 Gauss (which is about eight times stronger than the magnets used for attaching things to your refrigerator door).

Persons with pacemakers should not use magnets, and, because the effects of magnets on fetal growth are not fully understood, they should not be applied to the abdomen of a pregnant woman.

Massage, Bodywork, and Touch Therapies

Massage for healing purposes has been used for thousands of years to maintain health. Many people today receive regular massages as an important component of their self-care to aid in stress management. In addition to promoting relaxation, massage can be beneficial for reducing edema, promoting circulation and respirations, and relieving pain, anxiety, and depression.

Massage is the manipulation of soft tissue by rubbing, kneading, rolling, pressing, slapping, and tapping movements. The term *bodywork* is applied to the combination of massage with deep tissue manipulation, movement awareness, and energy balancing. Touch therapies include techniques in which the hands of the nurse/therapist are near the body, in the client's energy field. Examples of various types of massage, bodywork, and touch therapies are described in Box 15-5.

Because therapeutic touch (TT) is a popular alternative healing therapy among nurses, it deserves some discussion. TT became popular in nursing in the 1970s with the work and research of Delores Krieger (Krieger, 1979; 1997). Krieger advanced the theory that people are energy fields and that obstructed energy could be responsible for unhealthy states. She proposed that the nurse could draw on the universal field of energy and transfer this energy to the client. This incoming energy could help the client mobilize his or her own inner resources for healing and help unblock the client's obstructed energy.

In TT there is little direct physical contact between the practitioner and the individual being treated. Rather, TT is an energy-based therapy; the nurse enters the client's energy field to assess and treat energy imbalances.

In the first step of TT, the nurse centers herself or himself and focuses on the intent to heal (this is sometimes referred to as healing meditation). During this phase the nurse quiets the mind and prepares physically and psychologically to connect with the client. This is considered a crucial step in the process to enable the nurse to be fully present in the moment with the client. This is followed by the nurse passing his or her hands over the client's body to assess the energy field and mobilizing areas in which energy is blocked or sluggish by directing energies to that area. TT is used to reduce anxiety, relieve pain, and enhance immune function.

Meditation and Progressive Relaxation

Meditation, the act of focusing on the present moment, has been used for centuries throughout the world. This practice gained considerable attention in the United States in the 1970s when Harvard Medical School cardiologist Herbert Benson published research on the "Relaxation Response" (Benson and Beary, 1974). Benson reported that after 20 minutes of meditation, participants' heart rate, respirations, blood pressure, oxygen consumption,

BOX 15-5 Types of Massage, Bodywork, and Touch Therapies

Alexander technique
Teaches improved balanced, posture, and coordination by using gentle hands-on guidance and verbal instruction

Feldenkrais method
Teaches movement reeducation by using gentle manipulations to heighten awareness of the body; believes each person has an individualized optimum style of movement

Healing touch
A multilevel energy healing program that incorporates aspects of therapeutic touch with other healing measures

Reflexology
Application of pressure to pressure points on the hands and feet that correspond to various parts of the body

Reiki
A therapy that uses techniques to direct universal life energy to specific sites

Rolfing (structural integration)
Use of manual manipulation and stretching of body's fascial tissues to establish balance and symmetry

Swedish massage
Most prevalent form of massage that uses long strokes, friction, and kneading of muscles

Trager approach
Use of gentle, rhythmic rocking, and touch to promote relaxation and energy flow

carbon dioxide production, and serum lactic acid levels decreased. This led to meditation being used for a variety of conditions, including stress, anxiety, pain, and high blood pressure.

Progressive relaxation is another exercise that shares some of the same benefits as meditation. Typically a person learns to guide himself or herself through a series of exercises that relax the body, such as tightening and relaxing various muscle groups. Many audiotapes are available in bookstores and health food stores that offer scripts to guide meditation and progressive relaxation exercises.

Naturopathy

An intense interest in natural cures in Europe during the nineteenth century led to the development of spas that offered natural treatments to promote health and healing. Soon the movement spread to the United States, and in 1896 the American School of Naturopathy was founded. Naturopathic physicians and treatment facilities using natural cures became popular in the early part of the twentieth century. For example, John Kellogg ran such a facility in Battle Creek in which he subsequently became famous for the natural breakfast cereals that he used. As time progressed, medications and high-tech interventions caused naturopathy to pale by comparison; however, as consumers are seeking approaches that are more natural, this form of alternative medicine is making a comeback.

Naturopathy is based on the principle that the body has inherent healing abilities that can be stimulated to treat disease. Naturopathic doctors assess and treat the cause of the disease rather than merely alleviate symptoms. They help clients identify unhealthy practices, encourage healthy lifestyle habits, and guide them in managing health problems using natural approaches such as herbs, homeopathic remedies, diet modifications, dietary supplements, and exercise.

There are a limited number of accredited schools of naturopathic medicine (e.g., Bastyr University, Southwest College of Naturopathic Medicine and Health Sciences, and National College of Naturopathic Medicine). A handful of states license naturopaths and require that they must have graduated from an accredited program. However, there are many individuals practicing as naturopaths who have obtained their education and experience through other means or who practice in states that do not require licensure; thus learning about the credentials of naturopath before receiving services is beneficial for clients.

Prayer and Faith

Many people consider their faith to be an integral part of their total being rather than a therapy, but now there is scientific evidence supporting the therapeutic benefits of faith and prayer in health and healing. Hundreds of well-conducted studies have revealed that people who profess a faith, pray, and attend religious services are generally healthier, live longer, have lower rates of disability, recover faster, have lower rates of emotional disorders, and otherwise enjoy better health states than those who do not (Larson, Sawyers, and McCullough, 1998; Wilt and Smucker 2001). Not only do the faith and religious practices of individuals themselves affect health and healing, but research also supports the benefit of intercessory prayer.

Nurses need to appreciate that most people believe in the healing power of prayer and may expect their health care providers to join them in prayer if requested. This does not suggest that nurses or other health professionals should be forced into prayer if it is contrary to their beliefs; rather, if there is no objection from either party, prayer by the client and health care provider can be used as a valuable healing measure.

Tai Chi

Tai chi is another practice from traditional Chinese medicine used to stimulate the flow of Qi, the life energy. It is a combination of exercise and energy work that looks like a slow, graceful dance using continuous, controlled movements of the arms and legs. There is a specific sequence of steps to follow in doing tai chi, but fortunately there are many inexpensive videos that can be used, in addition to classes that are offered to aid people in learning this practice.

Tai chi has some proven benefits, including reduction of falls and improved coordination in older adults (Province, 1995) and improved function in persons with arthritis (Horstman, 1999). Many people find that tai chi helps to reduce stress and promote a general sense of well-being.

Yoga

Yoga has changed from a mystical form of Hindu worship practiced more than 5000 years ago to what is now known as a system of exercises involving various postures, meditation, and deep breathing. The word *yoga* means "union"; the union of body, mind, and spirit is achieved through yoga. This exercise has been found helpful for pain, anxiety, stress, high blood pressure, poor circulation, respiratory and digestive disorders, and carpal tunnel syndrome (Garfinkel et al, 2000). Yoga can be adapted to any level and capability so that it can be easily used.

There are many other alternative healing modalities, and new ones are appearing regularly. Some may be safe and effective but lack sufficient experience or clinical research to support their claims; others may be worthless and merely an attempt to sell a product or service. Discretion is crucial. Assistance in gaining objective information regarding CAM therapies can be obtained from the National Center for Complementary and Alternative Medicine at 888-644-6226 (on-line at nccam.nih.gov/).

NURSING AND COMPLEMENTARY AND ALTERNATIVE MEDICINE THERAPIES
A Holistic Approach

The use of natural or "alternative" healing measures is hardly new to nursing. From Florence Nightingale (1860), who wrote about the importance of creating an environment in which natural healing could occur, through contemporary nurse theorists who discuss human and environmental energy fields (Rogers, 1970), nurses have long realized that healing quite effectively occurs in ways not encompassed within the conventional biomedical system. Nursing also has promoted many of the same principles evident in CAM, particularly care of the body, mind, and spirit. In fact, this is what holistic nursing is all about (Box 15-6). Nurses must ensure that the integration of CAM into their practice is done within a holistic paradigm to truly make them healing therapies and not merely disconnected procedures within an already fragmented health care system.

Facilitating Clients' Use of Complementary and Alternative Medicine

Nurses need to integrate CAM into their nursing practice. This begins during the assessment process by exploring clients' use of CAM practices and products. Because it is not unusual for clients to use these without the knowledge of their physicians, nurses may be the first health professional with whom clients have discussed this issue. Factors to assess include:

- CAM practices and products being used and their sources
- Appropriateness of use of CAM practices and products
- Side effects and risks associated with use of CAM
- Conditions for which CAM currently is not used that could benefit by its use

---

BOX 15-6 *Beliefs Guiding Holistic Nursing Practice*

- The uniqueness of each individual is honored.
- Health is a harmonious balance of body, mind, and spirit.
- The needs of individuals' bodies, minds, and spirits are assessed and addressed in the caregiving process.
- Health and disease are natural parts of the human experience.
- Disease is an opportunity for increased awareness of the interconnectiveness of body, mind, and spirit.
- Individuals have the capacity for self-healing; the nurse facilitates this process.
- Nurses empower individuals for self-care.
- Individuals' cultural values, beliefs, and practices are honored and incorporated into the caregiving process.
- Individuals have a dynamic relationship with their environment; the environment is part of the healing process.
- Nurses, through their presence and being, are tools of the healing process.
- Nurses engage in self-care and an ongoing process of unfolding inner wisdom.
- Nurses can learn about holistic nursing and network with holistic nurses through involvement in the American Holistic Nurses' Association; learn more by visiting the AHNA website (www.ahna.org).

Through the assessment process nurses may identify the need to educate clients about the appropriateness of the CAM products and practices they are using. For example, a client with a pacemaker who uses magnets needs to be advised against continuing this practice; likewise, a client drinking ginseng tea at bedtime requires an explanation that his insomnia may be the result of the stimulant effects of the herb.

There may be situations in which nurses identify that specific conditions could benefit from the use of CAM therapies. As client advocates, nurses would bring this to the attention of the physician and other members of the health care team and make recommendations accordingly.

Nurses traditionally have been responsible for the coordination of client care. As CAM therapies are integrated into conventional care, nurses are the logical professionals to oversee the various parts and ensure that they are working in harmony for the client's benefit.

Nurses can learn to use many alternative healing measures to enhance nursing care. Among these are acupressure, aromatherapy, biofeedback, imagery, massage, and therapeutic touch. Nurses should seek whatever additional education and training required to gain competency in these therapies and ensure compliance with state licensing laws.

Integrating Complementary and Alternative Medicine Into Conventional Settings

Nurses can demonstrate leadership in helping conventional clinical settings integrate CAM therapies. In fact, nursing's holistic orientation and traditional coordination responsibilities make nurses logical for this role. Let us look at the way in which one nurse accomplished this.

CASE STUDY

Becky Blake recently joined the nursing staff in a combined coronary care/step-down unit. It did not take her long to note the expert technical skill of her colleagues, who could read monitors in a flash and respond to emergencies without missing a beat. The skill, efficiency, and organization of the nursing staff were evidenced by the lack of medication errors, infections, and pressure ulcers, coupled with the lowest length of stays of comparable hospital units in the area.

Yet there seemed to be something missing. Clients and their families often showed signs of anxiety and fear that were not addressed. Familiar faces reappeared as some clients were readmitted because they failed to alter lifestyle habits that contributed to their conditions. The same nursing staff who cared for people with hearts damaged by the effects of smoking, poor diet, and stress were guilty of the same practices themselves.

It came to a head for Nurse Blake one morning when she was at a bedside changing an intravenous bag and checking equipment. The client, a man in his 50s, pulled at her arm, looked Nurse Blake in the eyes, and tearfully said, "How do you think I'm going to do? I've been awake all night wondering if I'll be able to do my job, take care of my wife, see my grandkids grow up, do the things I like to do." For the first time, Nurse Blake saw beyond the body in the bed to a human being experiencing considerable emotional distress—distress that was hardly beneficial to his condition. We've managed to get this man's heart repaired, she thought, but we haven't begun to help him heal the emotional and spiritual pain that this illness created. This began a journey for Nurse Blake of discovering measures to help clients that went beyond the conventional treatments that were regularly prescribed.

Nurse Blake found a local network of holistic nurses and began attending their meetings. Through this group she learned of the difference between healing and curing and the importance of addressing the needs of body, mind, and spirit. She also heard nurses discussing their own need to be nurtured and committed to positive self-care practices. She met nurses who shared how they were using alternative healing practices and who led her to resources from which she could learn more.

Continued

CASE STUDY — Cont'd

Within the months that followed, Nurse Blake attended several workshops and learned how progressive relaxation, meditation, therapeutic touch, and aromatherapy could be used to benefit the clients on her unit. As her understanding of holism grew, she recognized that stress reduction and improved health habits for her co-workers were sorely needed.

After planting seeds through informal discussions and sharing of articles, Nurse Blake requested a formal meeting with the interdisciplinary team on the unit. In this meeting she described her areas of concern, which included the need to:

- Address clients' emotional and spiritual needs more effectively.
- Promote improved health habits of the staff.
- Develop practices that would reduce stress for clients, their families, and staff.

The staff concurred with these needs and expressed a desire to take actions to address them. Nurse Blake offered some suggestions:

- Coordinate with the staff development instructor to have classes offered on progressive relaxation, imagery, meditation, therapeutic touch, and stress reduction.
- Form an ad hoc committee to develop guidelines, policies, and procedures on how these healing therapies could be safely and legally implemented.
- Begin to include healing therapies into the care plans.
- Arrange for the nutritionist to offer classes to staff on healthy eating.
- Add healthy snacks to the break room.
- Coordinate with the housekeeping and maintenance departments to introduce aromatherapy diffusers, plants, and piped-in music in the unit.
- Develop a system to remind staff to use stress reduction measures throughout their shift.
- Collaborate with the nutritionist, social worker, spiritual care counselor, and nursing clinical resources to provide group sessions for clients and their families on topics such as coping with illness, stress management, promoting healthy lifestyle habits.
- Request the quality improvement coordinator to monitor and evaluate the impact of these interventions.

It did not take long for the effects of these new approaches to be realized. Clients requested fewer sedatives and analgesics. Surveys of clients and families revealed higher levels of satisfaction. Staff sick days were reduced, and there seemed to be a greater sense of team spirit and cooperation. Soon staff in other parts of the hospital began requesting that similar interventions be implemented in their units.

Using Complementary and Alternative Medicine Competently

As increasing numbers of consumers and clinical settings are interested in or actually using CAM therapies, nurses are challenged to become knowledgeable about the uses, limitations, and precautions associated with these new practices and products. Maintaining a resource library and becoming familiar with websites to stay current are beneficial measures.

Nurses must become familiar with cultural factors that can influence acceptance and use of alternative healing practices. For instance, some individuals may object to therapeutic touch on the grounds that they associate it with occult practices, or they may have anxiety about meditation because they believe evil spirits could invade their minds. As comforting as a massage can be, some people who come from cultures that believe it is inappropriate for someone to touch a person of the opposite sex could become distressed with this measure. Knowledge and sensitivity to personal and cultural preferences are essential.

Legal Considerations

The use of CAM practices could present some legal issues for which nurses need to be concerned. As growing numbers of practitioners of healing therapies advocate for recognition and separate licensure, some of the healing therapies once considered part of nursing care may require separate licensure. Such is the case with massage. In some states nurses may not provide a massage unless they are licensed as massage therapists. Acupressure and biofeedback are among the other areas in which the nurse could be challenged if not licensed. Nurses need to clarify the therapies that fall within the realm of nursing practice and take a proactive role in ensuring that other disciplines do not attempt to limit them.

Another legal concern for nurses in the growing arena of CAM is the question of to whom the nurse is responsible when practicing CAM therapies. New, nonconventional practice settings are developing. For example, a nurse may be employed in a setting in which there is an acupuncturist, hypnotherapist, and homeopath. Here are some questions that could arise: Who supervises the nurse? Can these therapists delegate responsibilities to the nurse? How does the nurse ensure that in such a practice setting diagnoses are not being made or treatments being prescribed that are beyond the scope of the CAM practitioners? Nurses need to begin to consider the implications of new practice models and develop clear practice guidelines that ensure a legally sound practice.

SUMMARY

An opportunity exists for nursing to demonstrate leadership in the integration of CAM with conventional care. Representing the largest number of health care professionals, nurses can have a significant impact on implementing CAM throughout the health care system. Nurses' historical holistic orientation to care enables them to ensure that the integration of CAM and conventional services is done in a manner that addresses the client's body, mind, and spirit. Without such coordinated efforts there is the risk that these new therapies will merely be additional ingredients in an already fragmented system of care. Nurses have proven that they can coordinate and promote comprehensive care like no other discipline. Therefore nursing is the logical discipline to be the hub of the wheel of integrative services.

CRITICAL THINKING ACTIVITIES

1. Develop a care plan that integrates CAM healing therapies with conventional ones for a client who is experiencing pain.
2. Describe some potential constraints to integrating complementary and alternative healing measures into practice.
3. List risks and opportunities to nurses as they use complementary and alternative healing measures.
4. Describe complementary and alternative healing measures that nurses can use as part of their own self-care.

Additional resources are available on-line at: http://evolve.elsevier.com/Cherry/

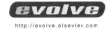

http://evolve.elsevier.com

REFERENCES

Astin JA: Why patients use alternative medicine: results of a national study, *JAMA* 279(19):1548-1553, 1998.

Benson H, Beary JZ: The relaxation response, *Psychiatry* 37:37-46, 1974.

Chopra D: *Ageless body, timeless mind,* New York, 1993, Harmony Books.

Eisenberg DM et al: Trends in alternative medicine use in the United States, 1990-1997: results of a follow-up national survey, *JAMA* 280(18):1569-1575, 1998.

Eliopoulos C: *Integrating conventional and alternative therapies: holistic care for chronic conditions*, St Louis, 1999, Mosby.

Garfinkel MS et al: Yoga-based intervention for carpal tunnel syndrome. In Fontanarosa PB, editor: *Alternative medicine: an objective assessment*, Dover, Del, 2000, American Medical Association.

Horstman J: *The Arthritis Foundation's guide to alternative therapies*, Atlanta, 1999, Arthritis Foundation.

Krieger D: *The therapeutic touch*, Englewood Cliffs, NJ, 1979, Prentice-Hall.

Krieger D: *Therapeutic touch inner workbook*, Santa Fe, NM, 1997, Bear & Co.

Larson DB, Sawyers JP, McCullough ME, editors: *Scientific research on spirituality and health: a report based on the Scientific Progress in Spirituality Conferences*, Rockville, Md, 1998, National Institute for Healthcare Research.

Libster M: *Delmar's integrative herb guide for nurses*, Albany, NY, 2002, Delmar, p 4.

McCaleb RS, Leigh E, Morien K: *The encyclopedia of popular herbs: your complete guide to the leading medicinal plants*, Roseville, Calif, 2000, Prima Publishing.

Nightingale F: *Notes on nursing*, London, 1860, Harrison.

Province MA: The effects of exercise on falls in elderly patients, *JAMA* 273(17):1341-1347, 1995.

Rogers M: *The theoretical basis for nursing,* Philadelphia, 1970, FA Davis.

Wilt DL, Smucker CJ: *Nursing the spirit*, Washington, DC, 2001, American Nurses Publishing.

RECOMMENDED READINGS

Cerrato PL: Complementary therapies update, *RN* 61(6):549-52, 2001.

Earthlink Inc: Alternative healthcare: is it the right alternative for you? *Blink* June/July, p 27, 2000.

Eisenberg DM: Advising patients who seek alternative medical therapies, *Annals Intern Med* 127(1):61-69, 1997.

Fontaine KL: *Healing practices: alternative therapies for nursing*, Upper Saddle River, NJ, 2000, Prentice Hall.

Huebscher R, Shuler PA: *Natural, alternative, and complementary health care practices*, St Louis, 2004, Mosby.

Kirskey KM et al: Complementary therapy use in persons with HIV/AIDS, *J Hol Nurs* 20(3):250-263, 2002.

McGovern K et al, editors: *Nurse's handbook of alternative and complementary therapies*, ed 2, Philadelphia, Pa, 2003, Lippincott Williams & Wilkins.

Olshansky E: *Integrated women's health: holistic approaches for comprehensive care*, Gaithersburg, Md, 2000, Aspen Publications.

Skinner SE: *An introduction to homeopathic medicine in primary care*, Gaithersburg, Md, 2001, Aspen Publishers, Inc.

Smith DW et al: Effects of integrating therapeutic touch into a cognitive behavioral pain treatment program, *J Hol Nurs* 20(4):367-387, 2002.

Stephenson NLN, Dalton J: Using reflexology for pain management, *J Hol Nurs* 21(2):179-191, 2003.

Taylor FA: *Finding the right treatment—modern and alternative medicine: a comprehensive reference guide that will help you get the best of both worlds,* Point Roberts, Wa, 2002, Hartley & Marks Publishers.

Trivieri L, Anderson JW, editors: *Alternative medicine: the definitive guide*, ed 2, Berkeley, Ca, 2002, Celestial Arts.

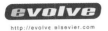
16

Nursing Leadership and Management

Barbara Cherry, MSN, MBA, RN

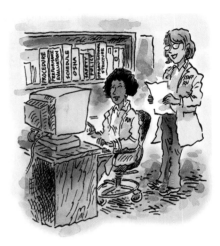

> As a manager, the nurse will coordinate many aspects of care delivery.

VIGNETTE

Nancy Brown, a new registered nurse (RN), has accepted a position in a busy, outpatient dialysis unit. During nursing school Nancy worked in the facility as a patient care technician, and she is confident in her clinical skills because of this previous experience. Mary, the nurse manager of the dialysis unit, has scheduled Nancy to attend the new-nurse orientation. Although Nancy thinks to herself, "I know what the RNs do around here; I'd like to jump right in without attending orientation," she readily accepts the assignment.

The nurse manager begins the orientation program with a discussion about the mission of the organization and the RN's responsibility to ensure that quality patient care is provided in a safe and cost-effective manner. As Nancy progresses through the orientation program, her confidence quickly fades. She becomes overwhelmed as she listens to a description of her new responsibilities as an RN. The RN's duties involve much more than the expected physical assessment, identifying nursing diagnoses, and developing and implementing care plans. Some of Nancy's many new responsibilities as a staff RN are to:

- Supervise patient care technicians and manage the task assignments and supply use for a group of patients
- Meet with the social worker, dietitian, nephrologist, nurse manager, and the patient and family to develop the patient's interdisciplinary care plan and then follow up to coordinate and implement the plan of care

Additional resources are available on-line at: http://evolve.elsevier.com/Cherry/

- Serve on a task force charged to develop and implement a new training and mentoring program for patient care technicians
- Perform chart audits to review patient education documentation, identify problems, develop recommendations, and report to the quality management committee

As Nancy is trying to assimilate the information being presented, she almost fails to hear Mary say that within 6 months of employment, all staff RNs are expected to begin orientation for the charge nurse position to provide back-up coverage. At the end of the orientation, Nancy has a new perspective about professional nursing practice—it seems to be more about managing the delivery of patient care than actually giving the care!

Questions to consider while reading this chapter:

1. What leadership and management skills will assist Nancy as she begins her new role as a staff RN responsible for supervising a group of patient care technicians, managing supply usage, and serving on a task force to implement a new training program?
2. Why is it important for the nursing staff to understand the mission and values of the organization in order to provide direct patient care?
3. What type of team building skills will help Nancy as she learns to work with the interdisciplinary team and coordinate the patient's plan of care with a diverse group of health professionals?
4. What resources are available to help Nancy learn and enhance her management and leadership skills?

KEY TERMS

Budget Financial plan for the allocation of the organization's resources (money) and a control for ensuring that results comply with the plans.

External customers People in need of services from an organization who are not employed by the organization, including patients, family members, physicians, students, payers, discharge planners, and other groups that are a source of patient referrals.

Health care organization Any business, company, institution, or facility (e.g., hospital, home health agency, ambulatory care clinic, health insurance company, nursing home) engaged in providing health care services or products.

Internal customers People who are employed by the organization to provide services to various groups and individuals across the organization (nurses and other patient care staff, administrators, social workers, dietitians, therapists, housekeeping staff, clerical support staff, etc.).

Leadership The act of guiding or influencing people to achieve desired outcomes; occurs any time a person attempts to influence the beliefs, opinions, or behaviors of an individual or group (Hersey and Blanchard, 1988).

Management Coordination of resources such as time, people, and supplies to achieve outcomes; involves problem-solving and decision-making processes.

Organizational chart A visual picture of the organization that identifies lines of communication and authority.

Productivity The amount of output or work produced (e.g., home visits made) by a specific amount of input or resources (e.g., nursing hours worked).

Resources Personnel, time, and supplies needed to accomplish the goals of the organization.

LEARNING OUTCOMES

After studying this chapter, the reader will be able to:

1. Relate leadership and management theory to nursing leadership and management activities.
2. Differentiate among the five functions of management and essential activities related to each function.
3. Integrate principles of the customer service role in professional nursing practice.
4. Implement effective team-building skills as an essential component of nursing practice.
5. Implement the nursing process as a method of problem solving and planning.
6. Apply principles and strategies of change theory in the management role.
7. Integrate knowledge of human behavior and conceptual and technical skills into the role of the nurse leader and manager.

CHAPTER OVERVIEW

During nursing school, students are often more concerned with learning and developing clinical knowledge and skills and are less concerned with management and leadership skills. However, immediately after graduation the new nurse is placed in many situations that require leadership and management skills—managing a group of assigned patients, serving on a task force or committee, acting as team leader or charge nurse, or supervising unlicensed assistive personnel and licensed vocational/practical nurses. In addition to providing safe, evidence-based, high-quality clinical care, the challenges for RNs in the twenty-first century are to manage nursing units that are constantly admitting and discharging higher-acuity patients, motivate and coordinate a variety of diverse health professionals and nonprofessionals, embrace change to develop work environments that are safer and more conducive to professional nursing practice, and manage limited resources and shrinking budgets.

Regardless of which position or area the nurse is employed, the health care organization will expect the professional nurse to have leadership and management skills, including these:

- Making good clinical decisions based on safety, quality, cost, legal, and ethical aspects of care
- Promoting evidence-based practice (see Chapter 21)
- Coordinating patient care activities for the interdisciplinary team
- Promoting staff satisfaction, patient satisfaction, and overall unit productivity
- Creating and sustaining trust between and among managers and staff
- Actively managing the process of change through good communication, staff involvement, training, sustained attention, and measurement and feedback
- Providing leadership to maintain compliance with governmental regulations and accreditation standards

As the reader can easily visualize, leadership and management activities are a primary responsibility for the RN. In fact, it has been suggested that the activities of a professional nurse within the health care organization have more to do with managing the delivery of care rather than actually providing that care (Norman, 1997). This chapter presents key leadership and management concepts that will guide the professional nurse in meeting the employing organization's expectations.

Throughout this chapter the term *organization* will be used to refer to the hospital, home health agency, post-acute care facility, long-term care facility, ambulatory clinic, managed care company, or any other area in which a nurse might be employed to practice professional nursing. Legal and ethical issues are a critical component of nursing management, although it is not within the scope of this chapter to discuss these issues. The reader is encouraged to review Chapter 8 regarding legal issues and Chapter 9 regarding ethical issues.

LEADERSHIP AND MANAGEMENT DEFINED AND DISTINGUISHED

Leadership Defined

Leadership occurs any time a person attempts to influence the beliefs, opinions, or behaviors of a person or group (Hersey and Blanchard, 1988). Leadership is a combination of intrinsic personality traits, learned leadership skills, and characteristics of the situation. The function of a leader is to guide people and groups to accomplish common goals. For example, an effective nurse leader is able to inspire others on the health care team to make patient education an important aspect of all care activities.

It is important to note that leaders may not have formal authority granted by the organization but are still able to influence others. "A job title alone does not make a person a leader. Only a person's behavior determines if he or she occupies a leadership position" (Marquis and Huston, 2003, p. 4). Leadership ability may be related to qualities such as unique personality characteristics, exceptional clinical expertise, or relationships with others in the organization.

Management Defined

Management refers to the activities involved in coordinating people, time, and supplies to achieve desired outcomes and involves problem-solving and decision-making processes. Managers maintain control of the day-to-day operations of a defined area of responsibility to achieve established goals and objectives. Managers plan and organize what is to be done, who is to do it, and how it is to be done. A nurse manager will have the following:

- An appointed management position within the organization with responsibilities to perform administrative tasks such as planning staffing requirements, performing employee performance appraisals, controlling use of supplies and time, and meeting budget and productivity goals
- A formal line of authority and accountability to ensure that safe and effective patient care is delivered in a manner that meets the organization's goals and standards

Leadership Versus Management

Although leadership and management are intertwined concepts and it is difficult to discuss one without the other, these concepts are different. Leadership is the ability to guide or influence others, whereas management is the coordination of resources (time, people, supplies) to achieve outcomes. People are led, whereas activities and things are managed. Leaders are able to motivate and inspire others, whereas managers have assigned responsibility for accomplishing the goals of an organization. A good manager should also be a good leader, but this may not always be the case. A person with good management skills may not have leadership ability. Similarly, a person with leadership abilities may not have good management skills.

Leadership and management skills are complementary; both can be learned and developed through experience, and improving skills in one area will enhance abilities in the other.

Power and Authority

Leadership and management require power and authority to motivate people to act in a certain way. Authority is the legitimate right to direct others and is given to a person by the organization through an authorized position such as nurse manager. For example, a nurse manager has the authority to direct staff nurses to work a specific schedule. Whereas authority is the formal right to direct others granted by the organization, power is the ability to motivate people to get things done with or without the formal right granted by the organization. The primary sources of power identified by Hersey, Blanchard, and Natemeyer (1979) are described as follows:

1. *Reward power* comes from the ability to reward others for complying and may include such rewards as money, desired assignments, or the acknowledgment of accomplishments.
2. *Coercive power*, the opposite of reward power, is based on fear of punishment for failure to comply. Sources of coercive power include withheld pay increases, undesired assignments, verbal and written warnings, and termination.
3. *Legitimate power* is based on an official position in the organization. Through legitimate power, the manager has the right to influence staff members, and staff members have an obligation to accept that influence.
4. *Referent power* comes from the followers' identification with the leader. The admired leader is able to influence others because of the followers desire to be like the leader.
5. *Expert power* is based on knowledge, skills, and information. For example, nurses who have expertise in areas such as physical assessment or technical skills or who keep up with current information on important topics will gain respect and compliance from others.
6. *Information power* is based on a person's possession of information that is needed by others.
7. *Connection power* is based on a person's relationship or affiliation with other people who are perceived as being powerful.

An individual may also have informal power resulting from personal relationships, being in the right place at the right time, or unique personal characteristics such as attractiveness, education, experience, drive, or decisiveness. By understanding the authority of an assigned position and the sources of formal and informal power, the nurse manager will be better able to influence others to accomplish goals.

Formal and Informal Leadership

Both formal and informal leadership can exist in every organization. Formal leadership is practiced by the nurse who is appointed to an approved position (e.g., nurse manager, supervisor, charge nurse, coordinator) and given the authority to act by the organization. Informal leadership is exercised by the person who has no official or appointed authority to act but is able to persuade and influence others. The informal leader, who may or may not be a professional nurse, may have considerable power in the work group and can influence the group's attitude and significantly affect the efficiency and effectiveness of work flow, goal setting, and problem solving.

The nurse manager must learn to recognize and effectively work with informal leaders. Informal leadership may be positive if the informal leader's purpose is congruent with that of the nursing unit and organizational goals. For example, the informal leader of a patient care group may be highly supportive of a new nursing care delivery model being implemented on the unit, and as a result, the other team members will be more willing to accept the change. However, an informal leader who is not supportive of the nursing unit's goals can create an uncomfortable work environment for the nurse manager and the entire team. Following are some strategies the nurse manager can use to work with informal leaders:

1. Identify the informal leaders in the work team and develop an understanding of their source of power.
2. Involve the informal leaders, as well as other staff members, in decision-making and change-implementation processes.
3. Clearly communicate the goals and work expectations to all staff members.
4. Do not ignore an informal leader's attempt to undermine teamwork and change processes. Counseling the person and setting clear expectations may be required.

LEADERSHIP AND MANAGEMENT THEORY

Understanding the development and progression of leadership theory is a necessary building block for developing leadership and management skills. Researchers began to study leadership in the early 1900s in an attempt to describe and understand the nature of leadership. Early leadership theory centered on describing the qualities or traits of leaders and has been commonly referred to as trait theory (Stogdill, 1974).

Leadership Trait Theory

Leadership trait theory sought to describe intrinsic traits of leaders and was based on the assumption that leaders were born with certain leadership characteristics. Traits found to be associated with leadership include intelligence, alertness, dependability, energy, drive, enthusiasm, ambition, decisiveness, self-confidence, cooperativeness, and technical mastery (Stogdill, 1974). Although trait theories have been important in identifying qualities that distinguish today's leaders, these theories have neglected the interaction between other elements of the leadership situation. Trait theories also have failed to recognize the possibility that leadership traits can be learned and developed through experience. However, keeping in mind these traits associated with effective leadership, the new nurse can identify areas in which he or she should improve and develop.

Interactional Leadership Theories

Researchers progressed from developing trait theory to studying the interaction between the leader and other variables of the leadership situation. Contemporary theories of leadership such as situational and behavioral theories have attempted to integrate the dynamics of the interaction between the leader, the worker, and elements of the leadership situation, arguing that effective leadership depends on several variables, including (1) organizational culture, (2) values of the leader and values of the followers, (3) influence of the leader/manager, (4) complexities of the situation, (5) work to be accomplished, and (6) environment (Marquis and Huston, 2003).

Situational leadership theory has explored the impact of the situation on the leadership role and suggests that leadership may vary in relation to the situation. The expectations, needs, attitudes, personalities, and developmental level of the leaders and followers will influence the style and effectiveness of leadership. Other aspects of a situation that influence the leadership role include the degree of interpersonal contact, time constraints, organizational structure, physical environment, and influence of the leader outside of the group. Situational theory suggests that a person may be a leader in one situation and a follower in another situation (Stogdill, 1974). By understanding the various elements that may influence the leadership situation, the nurse can become a more effective leader.

Transformational Leadership

In a contemporary concept of leadership, Burns (1978) identified and defined transformational leadership. Burns contends that there are two types of leaders: (1) The transactional leader, who is concerned with the day-to-day operations of the facility; and (2) the transformational leader, who is committed to organizational goals, has a vision and is able to empower others with that vision. Box 16-1 compares characteristics of Burns' transformational and transactional leadership styles.

Studies have reported that as nurse executives demonstrate more transformational leadership characteristics, they achieve higher levels of staff satisfaction and work group effectiveness. In one large national study of 396 randomly selected hospital nurse executives, Dunham-Taylor (2000) explored nurse executives' leadership characteristics and the relationship to staff satisfaction, work group effectiveness, and the nurse executive's effectiveness as rated by his or her superior. The study results demonstrated that staff satisfaction and work group effectiveness decreased as nurse executives were rated higher on transactional characteristics. The implication for nurse managers is that transformational leadership is very effective in increasing staff satisfaction and work effectiveness. The student is encouraged to read more about transformational leadership and to seek out transformational leaders as mentors. However, it is important to note that even the most effective transformational leader will fail without possessing the day-to-day management skills of transactional leaders (Bass, Avoliio, and Goodheim, 1987).

Management Theory

Behavioral theories emerged to explain aspects of management and leadership based on behaviors of managers/leaders and followers. Three prevalent management behavior styles were identified by Lewin (1951) and White and Lippit (1960): authoritarian, democratic,

---

BOX 16–1   *Comparison of Transformational and Transactional Leaders*

Transformational Leaders	Transactional Leaders
■ Identify and clearly communicate vision and direction	■ Focus on day-to-day operations and are comfortable with the status quo
■ Empower the work group to accomplish goals and achieve the vision; impart meaning and challenge to work	■ Reward staff for desired work ("I'll do *x* in exchange for you doing *y*")
■ Are admired and emulated	■ Monitor work performance and correct as needed *or*
■ Provide mentoring to individual staff members based on need	■ Wait until problems occur and then deal with the problem

and laissez-faire. Box 16-2 presents characteristics of these management styles, which vary in the amount of control exhibited by the manager and the amount of involvement that the staff has in decision making. At one extreme, the autocratic manager makes all decisions with no staff input and uses the authority of the position to accomplish goals. At the opposite extreme is the laissez-faire manager, who provides little direction or guidance and will forgo decision making. Democratic management is also often referred to as participative management because of its basic premise of encouraging staff members to participate in decision making.

Depending on the situation, the nurse manager may need to use different types of management styles. This concept of situational leadership requires consideration of staff members' needs and experiences, the manager's abilities, and the goals and tasks to be accomplished. For example, in a life-threatening situation such as treating a patient in cardiac arrest, autocratic management might be appropriate. However, in structuring the weekend call schedule for a home health agency, a participative style of management would be more effective.

The health care system of the twenty-first century requires the use of a democratic or participative management style that will involve the staff in goal setting, problem solving, and decision making. Health care settings are driven to become increasingly cost-effective while continuing to improve quality, customer satisfaction, and positive patient outcomes. Staff directly involved in the challenges presented by patient care often can suggest the most workable, practical solutions. Problem solving and goal attainment are more likely to be successful when staff are involved in decisions affecting their daily work.

Research has shown that staff nurses' job satisfaction increases as their involvement in decision making and problem solving increase (Sengin, 2003; Moss and Rowles, 1997). The new nurse manager should understand that the nurse's management style is what the staff perceives it to be, not what the manager has decided to practice. Managers have a responsibility to develop astute self-awareness about their intended leadership and management style and the style that the staff perceives.

Organizational Theory

Just as leadership and management theories have evolved to provide a framework for understanding leadership and management, organizational theory has evolved to provide a

---

BOX 16–2 *Management Styles*

Autocratic/Authoritative
- Determines policy and makes all the decisions
- Ignores subordinates' ideas or suggestions
- Dictates the work with much control
- Gives little feedback or recognition for work
- Makes fast decisions
- Successful with employees with little education or training

Democratic/Participative
- Encourages staff participation in decision making
- Involves staff in planning and developing
- Believes in the best in people
- Communicates effectively and provides regular feedback
- Builds responsibility in people
- Works well with competent, highly motivated people

Laissez-faire
- Does not provide guidance or direction
- Unable or unwilling to make decisions
- Does not provide feedback
- Initiates little change
- Rules by memos
- May work well with professional people

framework for understanding complex organizations. A brief review of bureaucracy theory, systems theory, and chaos theory can provide the reader with insight into the value of using organizational theory to understand management process within today's dynamic, complex health care organizations.

Weber's Theory of Bureaucracy. Max Weber, known as the father of organizational theory, began his work in the 1920s when he observed the growth of large organizations and predicted that this growth required a formal set of procedures. Weber, in his classic work on defining the characteristics of bureaucracy, argued that the great benefit of bureaucracy was in its ability to apply general rules to specific cases, making the actions of management fair and predictable. The basis of Weber's concepts of bureaucracy revolves around explaining authority within organizations. He postulated that authority, thus the right to issue commands within an organization, is based on the impersonal rules and rights granted by virtue of the management position rather than related to the person who occupies that position. Weber's conceptualization of bureaucracy emphasized rules instead of individuals and competency instead of favoritism as important for effective organizations. Other characteristics of organizations identified by Weber include the following:

1. Managers are chosen because they have demonstrated knowledge, skill, and ability to fill the position.
2. The division of labor, authority, and responsibility is clearly defined.
3. Impersonal rules govern the actions of superiors over subordinates.
4. All personnel are chosen for their competence and are subject to strict rules that are applied impersonally and uniformly.
5. A system of procedures for dealing with work situations is in place.

Although the structure of bureaucracy described by Weber is still present in most organizations today, his work failed to recognize the complexity of human behavior within organizations and the constantly changing environment of today's organizations. As previously

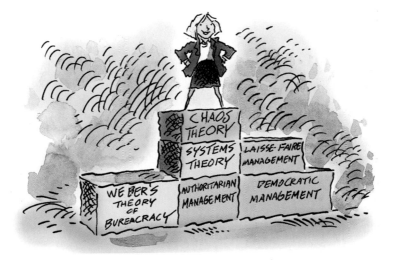

Leadership, management, and organizational theories provide the building blocks for effective nursing management practices.

discussed, current leadership and management theory (participatory management, transformational leadership) recognizes the importance of supportive, respectful relationships between managers and employees, with employees being involved in decision making and problem solving.

Systems Theory. Systems theory views the organization as a set of interdependent parts that together form a whole (Thompson, 1967). The interdependent nature of the parts of the organization suggests that anything that affects the functioning of one aspect of the organization will affect the other parts of the organization. Open systems suggest that the organization is not only affected by internal changes among any of its parts, but also external environmental forces will have a direct influence on the organization and vice versa—the internal forces will impact the external environment. In contrast to open systems theory, closed systems theory views the system as being totally independent of outside influences, which is an unrealistic view for health care organizations. In order to be successful, today's health care organizations must be able to continually adapt to both internal and external changes.

Consider the following example to help explain systems theory. The hospital in which William Scoggins, RN, works has reduced the number of RNs employed by the hospital and now requires that the remaining RNs work overtime "at the request of administration." The quality of patient care, patient safety, and the individual nurses' professional practice and personal health have been negatively affected by this change. William and his fellow RNs seek advice from their State Nurses Association (SNA) about their professional responsibility to work mandatory overtime. The SNA is responding to the situation, which is occurring more frequently across the state and nation, by proposing legislation to mandate nurse/patient ratios, as well as limits to mandatory overtime. The SNA and state government may now require hospital administrators to respond to the need for increased staffing levels.

This example demonstrates open systems theory. As internal forces in one department (hospital administration) mandated changes that affected another area (RNs and patient care), internal forces (RNs) pushed for changes from the external environment (SNA and state government). The external environment may now force changes to the organization (hospital administration).

Systems theory has provided nurse managers with a framework to view nursing services as a subsystem of the larger health care organization and to realize the interrelatedness and interdependence of all the parts of the health care organization. Open systems theory suggests that shared responsibility among all groups is necessary to help patients gain and maintain health and wellness (McGuire, 1999). The nurse manager will be wise to consider open systems theory and the impact a change in one area will have in another area, both internal and external to the organization.

Chaos Theory. Chaos theory is a more recently developed organizational theory that attempts to account for the complexity and randomness in organizations. Despite the implications of the word "chaos," the theory actually suggests that a degree of order can be attained by viewing complicated behaviors and situations as predictable. Nurse managers may wish for balanced and steady work environments, but in reality they are dealing with, what seems at best, a chaotic system. Chaos theory says that variation is a normal part of managing health care systems. Examples of variation in health care are cultural diversity, constantly fluctuating patient census, and staffing shortages. Until nurse managers understand that these variations

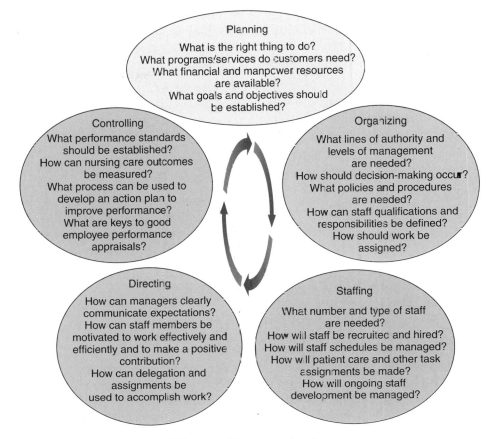

FIG. 16–1 Management functions.

are a normal, predictable state in the organization, they may continue to experience anxiety, discomfort, and dissatisfaction with their role (McGuire, 1999).

MANAGEMENT FUNCTIONS

Classic theories of management suggest that the primary functions of managers are planning, organizing, and controlling (Stogdill, 1974). Leaders in nursing management have added two additional functions to this list and now recognize five major management functions as necessary for the management of nursing organizations: (1) planning, (2) organizing, (3) staffing, (4) directing, and (5) controlling (Marquis and Huston, 2003; Fig. 16-1).

- ■ Planning includes defining goals and objectives, developing policies and procedures, determining resource allocation, and developing evaluation methods.
- ■ Organizing includes identifying the management structure to accomplish work, determining communication processes, and coordinating people, time, and work.
- ■ Staffing includes those activities required to have qualified people accomplish work, such as recruiting, hiring, training, scheduling, and ongoing staff development.

- Directing encourages employees to accomplish goals and objectives and involves communicating, delegating, motivating, and managing conflict.
- Controlling processes include performing employee performance appraisals, analyzing financial activities, and monitoring quality of care.

These management functions are interrelated; different phases of the process occur simultaneously, and the processes should be circular, with the manager always working toward improving the quality of health care, patient safety, and staff and customer satisfaction. Because understanding these five management functions is essential for success as a nurse manager, they will be now be discussed in further detail.

Planning

Planning is the first management function and has been defined as "deciding in advance what to do; who is to do it; and how, when, and where it is to be done" (Marquis and Huston, 2003, p. 55). All management functions are based on planning. Without effective planning, the management process will fail. Effective planning requires the nurse manager to understand the following elements:

- Mission statement and philosophy of the organization
- Organizational strategic plan
- Goals and objectives for the entire organization
- Operational plan for the individual unit or facility

Mission and Philosophy. The mission statement, the foundation of planning for any organization, describes the purpose of the organization and the reason it exists. Most health care organizations exist to provide high-quality patient care, but emphasis may be on different concepts such as research, teaching, preventive care, spiritual care, or community service. The philosophy is the set of values and beliefs that guides the actions of the organization and thus serves as the basis of all planning. The philosophy statement should speak for the primary mission of the organization and reflect the values of the organization, any special approaches to care, and/or any particular beliefs regarding patients and/or employees (Marquis and Huston, 2003). New nurses should be aware of the mission and philosophy of the employing organization and understand the relationship between their own personal value system and that of the organization. Box 16-3 provides an example of an organization's mission and philosophy statement.

Strategic Planning. Strategic planning is long-range planning (extending 3 to 5 years into the future) and results from an in-depth analysis of (1) the business, community, and regulatory and political environment outside the organization (external assessment); (2) customer needs; (3) technologic changes; and (4) strengths, problems, and weaknesses internal to the organization. The purposes of strategic planning are the following:

- Provide direction for the organization.
- Identify strategies to respond to changes in customer needs, technology, health care legislation, the business environment, and the community.
- Dedicate resources to important services.
- Eliminate duplication, waste, and underused services.

The strategic plan is a written document that details organizational goals, allocates resources, assigns responsibilities, and determines time frames. Responsibility for development

BOX 16–3   *Sample Mission, Values, and Philosophy Statement*

The mission of Community Hospital is to provide high-quality, cost-effective health services that patients and their families recommend; physicians prefer; employees, volunteers and board members are proud of; health professional students learn and excel from; and the community values

The Philosophy and Values of Community Hospital are:

- Commitment to professional and individual excellence with support for personal and professional growth within the organization.
- Continuous improvement by identifying the key needs of our customers, assessing how well we meet those needs, continuously improving our services, and measuring our progress.
- Ethical and fair treatment for ALL through a commitment to forming and maintaining relationships of fairness and trust with our patients, purchasers of our services, and our employees. Our business is conducted according to the highest ethical standards.
- Teamwork is consistently demonstrated as we work together to provide ever-improving customer service. People at all levels of the organization will participate in decision making and process improvement.
- Compassion is our highest priority, and we will always provide care and comfort to people in need and our patients and families will receive respectful and dignified treatment from all of our people at all times.
- Innovation in service delivery is accomplished by investing in the development of new and better ways to deliver services.

of the strategic plan rests with upper-level management, although there is increasing emphasis on including employees at all levels in strategic planning processes. Consider the following example.

CASE STUDY

Melanie Clements, an RN employed by the Quality Care Home Health Agency, noticed the office had been receiving several calls per week for skilled nursing care for pediatric oncology patients. The agency did not provide services for pediatric patients. Melanie reported the situation to the administrator. Melanie soon was involved in gathering information about the number of home health agencies that offered pediatric oncology care, the standards of nursing care recommended for pediatric oncology patients, how pediatric oncology patients were currently receiving home care, how many pediatric patients in the area might need such services, and what reimbursement was available for these services. Within the next few months, the administrator for Quality Care Home Health Agency decided that as part of the agency's strategic plan, a program for pediatric oncology services would be developed.

Goals and Objectives. Goals and objectives state the actions necessary to achieve the strategic plan and are central to the entire management process. Goals should be measurable, observable, and realistic. Objectives are more specific and detail how a goal will be accomplished with an established target date.

Goals and objectives serve as the manager's road map; without them it is difficult to know where one is going. Organization-wide goals will be established in the strategic planning process, and then unit goals that support the organization-wide goals should be developed. Every nurse manager should be able to clearly articulate the organization-wide goals, as well as the goals of the nursing unit for which he or she is responsible. Additionally, goals and objectives must be communicated to everyone who is responsible for their attainment. Consider the following case example.

Judy Anderson, RN, recently has been appointed as nurse manager in a 150-bed, long-term care facility. The mission and philosophy of the organization is to "respect the dignity and worth of the individual and to provide care that will help restore the patient to the best possible state of physical, mental, and emotional health while maintaining his or her sense of spiritual and social well-being." Kenneth Cole, the administrator, has asked Judy to develop a set of goals that she views as priorities to accomplish in the next year. After gathering data about patient needs, costs, and staffing levels, and meeting with the medical director and patient care staff members, and rehabilitation therapy, social services, dietary, and maintenance staff, Judy develops the following goals: (1) increase the coordination of care activities between nursing, therapy, and social services to more effectively meet patient care needs for increased emotional well-being and socialization; (2) maintain a safe environment for patients and staff by implementing the patient safety program outlined in the safety manual; and (3) improve the patient care staff's competencies in meeting the needs of the elderly patient. After reviewing Judy's goals, Kenneth agrees that they fit with the overall organizational plan and that the goals addressed needs identified in Judy's facility assessment activities. However, Kenneth poses several questions: What is the specific plan for obtaining goals? What costs are involved? How does the staff feel about these goals? How will goal accomplishment be measured?

Operational Planning. The nurse manager is most likely to be responsible for operational planning, or the short-range planning that encompasses the day-to-day activities of the organization. For example, short-range planning for a medical-surgical unit in a hospital might include maintaining an overall patient-to-staff ratio of 6:1, with 40% of the staff being RNs. As part of accomplishing organizational goals and objectives, the nurse manager involved in operational planning will be concerned with the following:

- Number, type, and location of patients to be cared for
- Qualifications and abilities of nursing and other health care staff
- Type and amount of supplies and other physical resources available
- Allocation of resources (staff, supplies, time) to meet budgetary requirements

The nurse manager also must plan for a variety of other activities, such as staff development, regulatory compliance, and quality improvement projects.

Organizing

Organizing is the second management function. At the organizational level, organizing is necessary to establish a formal structure that defines the lines of authority, communication, and decision making within an organization. The formal organizational structure helps define roles and responsibilities of each level of management. The organizational chart provides a visual picture of the organization and identifies lines of communication and authority. All nurses should be familiar with the organizational chart of their employing institution. Organizing also involves developing policies and procedures to help outline how work will be done and establishing position qualifications and job descriptions to define who will do the work.

At the unit level, the nurse manager must determine how to best organize the work activities to meet organizational goals in an efficient and effective manner. Organizing involves:

- Using resources (people, supplies, time) wisely
- Assigning duties and responsibilities appropriately
- Coordinating activities with other departments
- Effectively communicating with subordinates and superiors to ensure a smooth workflow

Models for organizing the delivery of patient care are discussed in Chapter 19.

Staffing

Staffing is the third management function. The provision of health care is labor-intensive, with a work force composed of people with a variety of education and skill levels (i.e., professional nurses, physicians, pharmacists, social workers, therapists, dietitians, licensed vocational/practical nurses, technicians, and unlicensed assistive personnel). Hiring and managing staff to accomplish the work of the institution is an important function for all levels of managers.

Marquis and Huston (2003) have described steps in the staffing function as follows:

1. Determine the number and type of staff needed based on organizational planning goals and budgetary requirements.
2. Recruit, interview, select, and assign personnel based on job description requirements and performance standards.
3. Use staff development resources to orient, train, socialize, and develop staff members.
4. Develop a staff-education program to assist personal and professional development and enhance knowledge and skill levels.
5. Implement creative and flexible scheduling based on patient care needs, employee needs, and organizational productivity requirements.

The staffing process most likely will prove to be one of the most time-consuming and challenging functions for the nurse manager; however, it is probably the nurse manager's most important job. Little can be accomplished without the right people properly trained to do the work.

Staff schedules are a key element to keeping employees happy and productive, whereas patient assignment schedules are critical to ensure the provision of safe, effective patient care. In addition, the nurse manager has the important responsibility of assigning patients to staff members based on assessed patient needs, patient acuity levels, and the abilities and competencies of the staff members. Staffing and assignments are further discussed in Chapter 19.

While meeting staff and patient scheduling needs, the nurse manager also must meet organizational staffing and productivity goals. Productivity is the amount of work produced through the use of a specific amount of resources and is measured as output divided by input. For example, the number of nursing hours worked over a 24-hour period divided by the patient census is a standard productivity measurement used by many hospitals. Other examples of productivity measurements include number of home visits completed or number of procedures performed.

Directing

Directing is the fourth management function. After managers have planned what to do, organized how to do it, and staffed positions to do the work; they must direct personnel and activities to accomplish goals. Directing involves issuing assignments and instructions that allow workers

BOX 16–4	Factors Influencing Nurses' Job Satisfaction and Dissatisfaction

Sources of Satisfaction	Sources of Dissatisfaction
Sense of achievement	Vague, inconsistent rules and regulations
Thanks and positive recognition	No thanks or recognition
Guidance, mentorship, and opportunities for professional development	No commitment by management to professional development
Open communication/being informed	Not being informed about changes
Challenging work and responsibility	Poor communication, unclear expectations
Advancement potential	Nonnursing duties
Pleasant work environment	Uncooperative physicians
Adequate staffing; help from managers during stressful times	No help from managers during crisis
Supportive managers who demonstrate respect and caring for each individual	Lack of involvement in decision making
Ongoing feedback about performance	Inadequate feedback about performance
Agreeable working hours and flexibility in scheduling when necessary	Excessive workload, negatively affecting quality

Adapted from Marriner-Tomey A: *Nursing management and leadership*, St Louis, 2000, Mosby; and McNeese-Smith D: The influence of manager behavior on nurses' job satisfaction, productivity and commitment, *J Nurs Admin* 27(9):47-55, 1997.

to clearly understand what is expected, as well as guiding and coaching workers to contribute effectively and efficiently to achieve planned goals. Directing requires the nurse manager to:

- Establish a motivating climate and team spirit
- Manage time efficiently
- Manage conflict and facilitate collaboration
- Demonstrate excellent communication skills

Motivation. Motivation is the inner drive that compels a person to act in a certain way. The amount and quality of work accomplished by a person is a direct reflection of his or her motivation. A great deal of research has been undertaken to better understand human motivation. Most researchers will agree that motivation is complex and involves a combination of extrinsic, or external, rewards such as money, benefits, and working conditions; as well as intrinsic, or internal, needs for recognition, self-esteem, and self-actualization. Box 16-4 summarizes factors that influence nurses' job satisfaction, dissatisfaction, and motivation.

Positive Reinforcement. Positive reinforcement is one of the most powerful, yet most often underused resources available to the nurse manager. To be effective, positive reinforcement should (1) be specific with praise given for a particular task done well or goal accomplished; (2) occur as close as possible to the time of the achievement; (3) be spontaneous and unpredictable (praise given routinely tends to lose its value); and (4) be given for a genuine accomplishment (Peters and Waterman, 1982). Furthermore, according to Marquis and Huston, "Managers can also create a motivating climate by being a positive and enthusiastic role model in the clinical setting. Managers who frequently project unhappiness to subordinates contribute greatly to low unit morale" (2003, p. 325).

Several other skills are essential as nurse managers function in the directing role, including effective communication and conflict management skills (discussed in Chapter 17), delegation skills (discussed in Chapter 18) and team building skills (discussed later in this chapter). The nurse manager is challenged to create a climate that will generate worker satisfaction, motivate workers to accomplish goals, and encourage high productivity.

Controlling

The purpose of controlling, the fifth management function, is to ensure that employees accomplish goals while maintaining a high quality of performance. Controlling involves:

- Establishing performance or outcome standards
- Measuring and evaluating performance against established standards
- Determining an action plan to improve performance

Performance Standards. Controlling activities require the nurse manager to maintain a mindset that continually looks for ways to improve individual, team, and organizational performance. Performance standards describe a model of excellence for work activities and serve as the basis of comparison between actual and desired work performance. For example, performance standards in an ambulatory outpatient clinic might include that (1) every patient is informed about all lab results within 48 hours, whether normal or abnormal, and (2) all diabetic patients must remove their shoes and socks for a thorough foot exam each time they come into the clinic. Chapter 20 provides more discussion about performance standards and also presents an excellent process for measuring performance and planning for improvement. The nurse manager can draw on several resources for establishing performance standards, including:

1. Written organizational policies and procedures
2. Standards for the practice of professional nursing developed by the American Nurses Association and published in *Nursing: Scope and Standards of Practice* (ANA, 2004)
3. Standards for professional nursing specialty practices such as the *Scope and Standards of Diabetes Nursing Practice*, ed 2 (ANA, 2003) and *Standards and Scope of Gerontological Nursing Practice* (ANA, 2001)

Employee Feedback. Other important controlling functions are continual employee feedback and employee performance appraisal activities. Employee performance appraisals must be ongoing, objective, and based on established performance standards. A manager should never wait until the "annual performance review" to discuss problems or deficiencies with a staff member. Consistent, day-to-day feedback and coaching about job performance clarifies expectations, improves the quality of work, and allows the manager to correct problems before they become serious. Ongoing documentation about an employee's job performance also is an essential management responsibility. The result of routine performance appraisals should be mutual goal setting designed to meet the employees' training, educational, and work-improvement needs. Box 16-5 presents some useful tips for providing employee feedback, and Box 16-6 presents some useful tips for successful employee performance evaluations.

The management functions of planning, organizing, staffing, directing, and controlling provide the nurse manager with a defined, practical set of skills to guide the implementation

---

BOX 16–5 *Tips for Successful Employee Feedback*

Giving Successful Employee Feedback

- Ask the employee whether they will hear your feedback—it is helpful to ask whether the person is open to your feedback (e.g., "*Can we talk about some good ways to communicate with physicians?*").
- Help employees not to take feedback personally—emphasize that feedback is to improve a process, not to blame for poor performance.
- Be specific and provide clear examples when possible; explain how your feedback can help improve a process or service.
- Focus on work-related outcomes and don't get personal.
- Allow time for a response.
- Thank the employee for listening.
- Ask for feedback from your co-workers, subordinates, and peers and *listen* when it is offered.

Adapted from Grensing-Pophal L: Give-and-take feedback, *Nurs Manage* Feb:27-28, 2000.

---

of management activities. The new nurse manager will be challenged to maintain the different stages of management that occur in the span of just one day. In addition to managing different phases of the process occurring simultaneously, the nurse manager also must function in many different management roles further described in the following section.

ROLES OF THE NURSE MANAGER

Nurse managers must assume various roles as they function in leadership and management positions. A different set of roles and responsibilities will be required in almost any position in any health care setting. Therefore, professional nurses should clearly understand the job

---

BOX 16–6 *Tips for Successful Employee Performance Appraisals*

Giving Effective Performance Appraisals

- Each employee must understand the standard by which his or her work is being evaluated—at a minimum by receiving a copy of the appraisal form and more effectively by being involved in developing the evaluation criteria.
- Conduct the appraisal during a time when there will be no interruptions for either party; select a comfortable seating arrangement that denotes collegiality such as side-by-side chairs.
- Avoid surprises—good leaders/managers will provide feedback and communicate with staff on a continual basis.
- Focus on the employee's performance and work-related outcomes, not on personal characteristics.
- Avoid vague generalities such as "your performance is fine" or "your attitude needs to improve"—give explicit examples; use positive examples liberally and negative examples sparingly (again, nothing should be a surprise!).
- Encourage input from the employee.
- Set goals together for continued growth and improvement; decide how goals will be accomplished and evaluated—then follow up!
- Be sensitive and caring; demonstrate that you value the employee and his or her contribution to the organization.

Adapted from Marquis BL, Huston CJ: *Leadership role and management functions in nursing*, ed 4, Philadelphia, 2003, JB Lippincott.

---

description, roles and responsibilities, and policies and procedures related to the position in which they are employed or assigned. The following discussion will present information about the primary roles that a nurse will assume in any position. By understanding these roles, the nurse can (1) know what is expected to be effective and (2) identify areas that require additional learning and improvement.

Customer Service Provider

Over the past few years, patient satisfaction has moved to the forefront of the nurse manager's agenda. Nursing shortages, reduced length of stay, more complex patient needs, and national concerns about the quality and safety of patient care have all contributed to this growing concern about patient satisfaction and customer service. From how quickly call lights are answered to the extent of family support provided, nurse managers are challenged to meet a wide spectrum of patient needs. The complex health care environment has created a competitive marketplace in which home health agencies, hospitals, ambulatory clinics, and even hospice agencies compete for patients. In order to survive and thrive in this competitive environment, the nurse must keep customer service, which includes safety and quality care, first and foremost as the motivator of all plans and activities.

External and Internal Customers. Effective management requires that the health care organization and the nurse develop a comprehensive view of the term customer. Customers can be categorized as external or internal, depending on their relationship to the organization. External customers are not employed by the organization and include patients and families, as well as physicians and other employees in facilities that serve as referral sources for new patients. For example, home health nurses should view hospital discharge planners as customers and find ways to meet their patients' discharge needs. Physicians will not refer patients to a particular hospital or clinic if they are not happy with the services provided by that facility.

Payers (insurance companies, managed care plans) are also being considered as primary external customers. For example, hospitals seek to contract with managed care plans to gain the plan's covered members as customers. Managed care companies seek to contract with hospitals that can demonstrate outstanding service that will please the plan's members. Thus, the managed care company becomes the hospital's customer.

Internal customers are employed by the organization and may include patient care staff members, staff members of other departments (e.g., laboratory, dietary), faculty, administrators, social workers, dietitians, and therapists. For example, nurse managers should view staff members as "customers" and determine how to meet their needs in order to facilitate effective and efficient work performance. Other departments—social services, laboratory, maintenance, housekeeping—are essential to manage an effective nursing unit, and the needs of these "customers" should be considered. If every department in the organization provided great service to both internal and external customers, imagine how much more effective and efficient the entire organization would be!

Customer Service Standards. The customer will define standards for customer service. "Today's consumers expect to be asked about their individual preferences and to be treated—to the most extreme degree possible—as if those preferences are respected" (McKenna, 1997). Certainly, all customers have a need to be treated with kindness and respect, to have services provided in a timely and cost-effective manner, and to have effective communication about what is or will be occurring. Further service standards can be defined by listening to and

---

BOX 16–7 *Sample Customer Service Commitment for a Health Care Organization*

Community Clinics' Customer Service Commitment
This is our customer service commitment. Translated, it stands for listening, caring, helping, and healing.

- Caring, friendly, professional staff members
- Prompt and personal attention to requests
- Timely, convenient services with reasonable wait times
- Confidentiality and privacy respected and upheld
- Serious responses to concerns and complaints
- Ongoing effotrs to improve our systems and processes

---

observing customers and analyzing customer surveys, customer complaints, and unsolicited comments or letters. A sample customer service commitment for a health care organization is presented in Box 16-7. Meeting customer needs should be the focus in all planning, organizing, staffing, directing, and controlling activities, as well as in all meetings and communications with superiors and subordinates.

Team Builder

A team is a group of people organized to accomplish the necessary work of an organization. Teams have become important in the changing health care environment. Teams bring together a range of people with different knowledge, skills, and experiences to meet customer needs, accomplish tasks, and solve problems. Team members may include unit secretaries, nursing assistants, social workers, dietitians, therapists, physicians, licensed vocational/ practical nurses, and RNs. A team should have clearly defined goals to accomplish work in the health care unit, and should be empowered to make decisions within its realm of responsibility. Team building should create synergy. Synergy is the ability of a group of people working together to accomplish significantly more than each person working individually.

Bringing people together to work as a group does not necessarily make them a team. To create synergy, teams must have defined goals and objectives, a commitment to work together, good communication, and a willingness to cooperate. Team members should be encouraged to communicate with one another to identify effective work division and solutions to problems so that synergy is accomplished. The nurse manager, as team builder, must serve as a role model to encourage and help develop team principles of respect, cooperation, commitment, and a willingness to accomplish shared goals. As a role model for team members, the nurse manager should do the following:

- Show respect for all members of the team and value their input.
- Clearly define team goals ("What do we want to accomplish?").
- Clearly define the decision-making authority within the realm of the team.
- Encourage the team members to develop a sense of stewardship (or ownership) for the success of the team.
- Exhibit a personal commitment to the team goals.
- Encourage team members to willingly help one another.

- Provide the resources necessary to accomplish goals (i.e., time for team meetings, information, supplies).
- Provide relevant and timely feedback to the team.

The leader's behaviors have a significant impact on the behaviors of the team. As Porter-O'Grady stated, "Every moment the leader operates in the leader role, he/she is influencing the roles and actions of other team members" (2003a, p. 105). Thus the nurse manager as leader must have an astute self-awareness of his or her own personal emotional patterns and an understanding that negative moods can have a negative influence on relationships with staff members. Learning to recognize and manage one's emotional patterns and negative moods is an important step in team building. The nurse manager who is enthusiastic, caring, and supportive can generate those same feelings among all team members (Porter-O'Grady, 2003a).

Resource Manager

Resources include the personnel, time, and supplies needed to accomplish the goals of the organization. Resources cost money and always will be in limited supply. Unfortunately no health care organization can afford the luxury of an unlimited number of staff or supplies to accomplish the required work. With health care facilities' current focus on cost-containment, it is essential that nurses develop an understanding of and expertise in resource management. It is the responsibility of the nurse manager to effectively manage resources in order to provide safe, effective patient care in an economic manner.

Budget. Planning resource management begins in the development of the budget, or fiscal planning. According to Marriner-Tomey, a budget is a plan that details how resources will be allocated and that ensures compliance with the plan (2000). Budgets are most often developed for a 1-year time period and are based on predicted amounts of services for the time period involved. For example, hospitals will predict patient census for the coming year and then allocate funds for nursing salaries based on this predicted census.

Historically, nursing has had limited input into fiscal (or financial) planning and development of the organization's budget. Administrators with no nursing background and no understanding of nursing values, beliefs, and care requirements may have made decisions about resource allocation related to nursing. Participating in the budget process to determine resource allocation should be viewed as a fundamental responsibility of the nurse manager. Involving staff nurses in the budgeting process is also appropriate. Managers and staff members who participate in fiscal planning are more likely to be cost-conscious and have a better understanding of how their unit should function to meet the overall financial goals.

The nurse manager will be concerned with three types of budgets: (1) the personnel budget, (2) the operating budget, and (3) the capital budget. In most organizations, these budgets are outlined and explained in budgeting policies and procedures. Fiscal objectives and lines of authority and responsibility for budget and financial management should also be clearly stated. It is the responsibility of the nurse manager to learn about and understand these policies and procedures.

Personnel Budget. The personnel budget represents the funds allocated for employee salaries and benefits and is the largest expense for a health care organization. Factors that affect the personnel budget include salary rates, overtime, benefits (e.g., paid time off, health insurance), staff development and training, and employee turnover. In managing the personnel budget, the nurse manager must be aware of the staffing mix, or the number of varied health care providers (experienced RNs, new graduates, licensed practical/vocational nurses, nursing assistants), required to competently meet patient needs and remain within budgetary guidelines. Chapter 19 will discuss staffing mixes in more detail.

One of the primary difficulties encountered in managing the personnel budget is accurately predicting future staffing needs. Because budgets are based on a predicted amount of services (i.e., patient census), variances between actual staffing levels and budget levels will occur if the facility experiences an unanticipated increase or decrease in patient services. At this point, the nurse manager might be required to complete a budget variance report to explain the difference between the budgeted staffing levels and the actual staffing levels.

Operating Budget. The operating budget represents the funds allocated for daily expenses required to operate the facility, including utilities, repairs, maintenance, and patient care supplies. After personnel costs, the operating budget is the second most important component of the organization's overall costs. Maintaining an effective supply allocation system (how supplies are distributed and accounted for) and an inventory management system are crucial to helping the nurse manager control supply usage. The nurse manager who is able to manage both personnel costs and supply costs effectively will make a major contribution to the cost-containment goals of the organization.

Capital Budget. The capital expenditure budget represents funds allocated for construction projects and/or long-life equipment (e.g., cardiac monitor, defibrillator, computer hardware) that generally is more expensive than operating supplies. Because capital expenditures are associated with long-range planning and may be projected 1 to 3 years in advance, it is important that the nurse manager be aware of the organization's capital expenditure plan to have input about future equipment needs for the unit or facility. The three types of budgets are summarized in Box 16-8.

Financial Reports. To be effective as a resource manager, the nurse should understand the organization's financial goals and how to track expenditures. Each organization should have a reporting mechanism in place to provide nurse managers with financial reports specific to their area of control. The variance report is a monthly or quarterly report that details budgeted expenses compared with actual expenditures for items such as the number of staff hours or cost of supplies per patient service provided. The variance report will provide the

---

BOX 16–8   Three Types of Budgets

Personnel Budget
Allocates funds for salaries, overtime, benefits, staff development and training, and employee turnover costs

Operating Budget
Allocates funds for daily expenses such as utilities, repairs, maintenance, and patient care supplies

Capital Budget
Allocates funds for construction projects and/or long-life equipment such as cardiac monitors, defibrillators, and computer hardware—items that are generally more expensive than operating supplies

nurse manager with valuable information about the unit's financial performance and can be used to compare actual expenditures with predicted levels of service.

Other budget reports that the nurse manager might utilize include overtime, productivity, and supply usage reports. The more frequently the nurse manager analyzes financial reports, the more quickly he or she can make revisions to meet goals. Budget analysis requires the nurse manager to relate expenditures to actual patient care practices and to identify areas, such as staffing levels or supply usage, where adjustments might be necessary.

Each of the management activities of planning, organizing, staffing, directing, and controlling will come into play in the role of resource manager. The nurse manager needs to learn and develop skills in the following areas:

- Planning for the necessary resources to manage the unit
- Organizing the resources to meet identified goals
- Staffing appropriately as determined by patient needs and the budget plan
- Directing to maintain resource allocations within budgetary guidelines
- Controlling by analyzing financial reports and making adjustments where necessary

This author would like to encourage all readers not to be unsettled by financial and budget reports and conversations. Instead, get involved! Don't be afraid to say "I don't understand. Please explain." Review budget and financial reports, ask questions, talk to seasoned nurse managers, talk to the organization's accountants and financial planners and even consider taking an accounting or finance course at the local college. Understanding financial and budget management is one of the most useful and powerful tools you can have as a nurse manager.

Decision Maker and Problem Solver

Problem solving and decision making are essential skills for professional nursing practice. Not only are these skills required in clinical patient care, but they also are vital components of effective leadership and management. As Yoderwise stated, "Decision making is a purposeful and goal-directed effort using a systematic process to choose among options" (2003, p. 76). Decision making is not always related to a problem situation and is required throughout all aspects of the management functions of planning, organizing, staffing, directing, and controlling. Problem solving is focused on solving an immediate problem and includes a decision-making step.

The Nursing Process as a Guide for Decision Making and Problem Solving. The nursing process, familiar to nurses for addressing patient care needs, can be applied to all management activities requiring decision making and problem solving. The nursing process is a problem-solving process that includes assessment, analysis and diagnosis, planning, implementation, and evaluation and has proven to be effective to manage the complex decisions required in nursing practice (Howenstein et al, 1996). Table 16-1 summarizes the decision-making and problem-solving activities in each stage of the nursing process.

Assessment. During the assessment stage it is important for the nurse to separate the problem from the symptom by gathering information about the problem or situation. It often is appropriate to involve others who are knowledgeable of the situation to provide a different viewpoint or information the manager lacks. For example, the nurse manager concerned about increasingly high absenteeism among the patient care staff may consider implementing a strict policy to punish absentee staff members. In this situation the nurse manager may be addressing the symptom instead of the real issue. The following questions should first be

| Table 16-1 | The Nursing Process Applied to Problem Solving | | | |

ASSESSMENT	ANALYSIS AND DIAGNOSIS	PLANNING	IMPLEMENTING	EVALUATION
■ Gather information about the situation	■ Analyze results of information gathering	■ Identify as many solutions as possible	■ Communicate plans to everyone affected	■ Identify evaluation criteria in the planning stage
■ Identify the problem; separate the symptoms	■ Identify, clarify, and prioritize the actual problem(s)	■ Elicit participation from people or groups affected	■ Be sure plans, goals, and objectives are clearly identified	■ Identify who is responsible for evaluation, what will be measured and when it will take place
■ Identify people and groups involved	■ Determine whether intervention is appropriate	■ Review options and consider safety, efficiency, costs, and quality	■ Maintain open, two-way communication with staff	
■ Identify cultural and environmental factors		■ Consider positive and negative outcomes	■ Support and encourage compliance among all staff	■ Maintain open communication with all involved
■ Encourage input from involved parties		■ Remain open-minded and flexible when considering options		■ Was the decision successful?
				■ What might have made it better?

asked: What is causing the absenteeism? Are there problems on the unit creating an unhappy work environment? Are several staff members coincidentally having personal problems? Are absentee policies being unfairly administered? The nurse manager must correctly assess and diagnose the problem before developing solutions.

Analysis and Diagnosis. During the analysis stage, decision makers use information gathered in the assessment phase to identify the specific problem to be solved. At this stage, the manager must also decide whether the situation is important enough to require intervention and whether it is within their authority to intervene. Managers should not attempt to intercede in every situation brought to their attention. Purposeful inaction is an intentional plan on the part of the manager and should not be confused with a "do-nothing approach" taken by a manager who chooses to do nothing when intervention is indicated.

Planning. During the planning stage the goal is to identify as many options as possible and then objectively weigh the options as to possible risks and consequences and positive and negative outcomes, including patient outcomes and staff effectiveness as key considerations. The decision maker should remain flexible, open-minded, and creative when reviewing options and avoid preconceived ideas or rigid thinking (Yoderwise, 2003). "There is only one way to do this job" or "that's the way we have always done it" are examples of rigid thinking. At this stage of the process, it is also important to remember that decisions made with input from those affected are more likely to result in positive outcomes. Cost, quality, and legal and ethical aspects of care also should be carefully considered.

Implementation. The implementation stage should include effective communication, delegation, and supervision. It is important for the manager to show positive support for the decision outcome and encourage compliance among all staff. Persons higher in the organizational structure may mandate some decisions, and although not able to control that decision, the nurse manager can influence a positive outcome.

Evaluation. The evaluation stage is necessary to ensure that the implemented plan effectively resolved the problem or the decision situation. Considerable time and energy may be spent on identifying the problem, generating possible options, and selecting and implementing the best solution. However, time for follow-up evaluation must also be allocated. It is important to establish early (during the planning stage) how and what evaluation and monitoring will take place, who will be responsible, and when it will be accomplished.

Staff input should be included in each stage of the decision-making, problem-solving process. Additionally, the nurse manager might seek help from others who are more experienced and knowledgeable in specific areas. Even the most experienced nurse managers will not be able to effectively solve every problem, nor will any nurse manager have all the answers. The key to being a good manager is to understand and incorporate the decision-making, problem-solving process into all activities; know when and how to access resources; and learn and improve as successes and failures are experienced.

Change Agent

This text frequently has referred to the "changing" health care environment, and true to that concept, change is an inevitable occurrence in health care organizations. Whether working with individuals, groups, or the entire organization, the professional nurse is certain to be involved in managing change. The nurse as the change agent is responsible for guiding people through the change process and must develop an understanding about the nature of change and effective change strategies. To successfully engage in change, the nurse manager must first be willing to confront the demand for change; staff cannot be expected to embrace change if their nurse manager has not done so. The nurse manager must also be willing to help others make the change become an integral part of their work (Porter-O'Grady, 2003b).

People often feel threatened by change and may react, especially at first, with resistance and hostility. Change that is carefully planned and implemented slowly with all people continually informed and involved will be more successful in reaching the desired outcome (or change). As Marquis and Huston have noted, "Regardless of the type of change, all major change brings feelings of achievement, loss, pride, and stress. What differentiates a successful change effort from an unsuccessful one is often the ability of a change agent—a person skilled in theory and implementation of planned changed—to deal appropriately with these very real emotions and to connect and balance all aspects of the organization that will be affected by that change" (2003, p 80). Lewin (1951) has identified several rules that should be followed when change is necessary:

1. Change should be implemented only for good reason.
2. Change should always be planned and implemented gradually.
3. Change should never be unexpected or abrupt.
4. All people who may be affected by the change should be involved in planning for the change.

Change may be indicated for several reasons, including solving an identified problem, implementing a new program, improving work efficiencies, or adjusting to new mandates by regulatory agencies. For example, some states are implementing stricter "patient rights" regulations for long-term care facilities that will require changes to current patient care practices. Even though a strong reason for change may exist, it almost always will be met with some resistance. Resistance is demonstrated by refusing to cooperate with a course of activity or showing active opposition to the change. The effective change agent will recognize that resistance is a natural response to change and will not waste time or energy attempting to eliminate it. Instead the effective change agent will identify and implement effective change strategies that will overcome resistance.

Stages of Change. Effective change strategies can be developed through the three classic stages of change identified by Lewin (1951). These stages are:

1. *Unfreezing stage*—The change agent promotes problem identification and encourages the awareness of the need for change. People must believe that improvement is possible before they are willing to consider change. The change agent's responsibilities during this stage include the following:

   - Gathering information about the problem
   - Accurately assessing the problem
   - Deciding if change is necessary
   - Making others aware of the need for change

2. *Moving stage*—The change agent clarifies the need to change, explores alternatives, defines goals and objectives, plans the change, and implements the change plan. The change agent's responsibilities during this stage include the following:

   - Identifying areas of support and resistance
   - Setting goals and objectives
   - Including everyone affected in the planning
   - Developing an appropriate change plan with target dates
   - Implementing the change plan
   - Being available to help, support, and encourage others through the process
   - Evaluating the change and making modifications if necessary

3. *Refreezing stage*—The change agent integrates the change into the organization so that it becomes recognized as the status quo. If the refreezing stage is not completed, people may drift into old behaviors. The change agent's responsibilities during this stage include the following:

   - Requiring and enforcing compliance with the changed processes
   - Supporting and encouraging others until the change is no longer viewed as new but as part of the status quo

In alignment with Lewin's three stages of change (unfreezing, moving, and refreezing), education and training and involvement of those involved are keys to successful change.

Involvement. The importance of involving all individuals, groups, or departments affected by the change cannot be overstated. Involvement will include clear, two-way communication throughout all phases of the change project and a concerted effort to garner information and feedback from all affected parties about the need for change. The effective change agent will take into consideration the needs of both external and internal customers and understand that a change in one area almost always will affect another group or department. (Remember systems theory?) Consider the following case example.

CASE STUDY

As the number of procedures being performed in an outpatient surgery department continued to increase, Kevin Michaels, RN, nurse manager, recognized the need to extend the hours of the department to relieve the tight surgery schedule. When the staff began to complain about working through lunch and staying late some evenings, Kevin encouraged them to accept the need for a new department schedule. Kevin discussed the situation with the administrator and all nursing, technical, and secretarial staff. He carefully assessed the department's scheduling needs, surveyed the physicians regarding their scheduling preferences, reviewed all options, and finally planned to add a half-day Saturday surgery schedule. Kevin carefully planned the new schedule with the staff and physicians and was pleased that the new plan seemed to be going smoothly. However, Jane Holmes, the housekeeping supervisor, who schedules heavy cleaning duties on Saturday mornings when the department is normally closed, was not informed or involved in the schedule change. Much to her dismay, Jane learned through a hallway conversation that she would have to quickly rearrange cleaning schedules and staff schedules to adjust to the new Saturday morning plan.

Peripheral departments (e.g., housekeeping, maintenance, security) are crucial to safe, efficient operations, but they often are forgotten in the planning activities. The nurse manager as the change agent is responsible for informing and involving *all* individuals and departments to ensure that change is implemented as smoothly as possible.

Education and Training. Education and training also are important components of effective change. People must have appropriate education and training to understand and comply with new policies, procedures, work processes, duties, or responsibilities. Early in the change process, the change agent must consider the training needs of all individuals, groups, and departments. Education and training can reduce fear of the unknown and allow the staff to feel prepared and comfortable with taking on new or different responsibilities.

Other Roles

In addition to the roles of customer service provider, team builder, resource manager, and change agent, nurses in leadership and management positions will find themselves functioning in many other roles. Each of the management roles described in this chapter are equally important to performing effectively as a nurse manager.

Clinical Consultant. Staff members will look to the nurse manager as a resource for clinical advice. For example, the nurse manager will frequently be called on to assess difficult or unusual patient cases and guide the staff nurse to make appropriate nursing judgments. In this role, the nurse manager serves as a role model for excellence in nursing care and provides ongoing staff training and education.

Staff Developer. The nurse manager should be ever mindful of the need for learning and training opportunities to enhance professional and personal growth for all employees he or she supervises. Accessing resources and planning staff development activities that meet the needs of individual staff members, including RNs, LPNs/LVNs, unlicensed assistive personnel, and clerical staff is a very important role for the nurse manager.

Mentor. As the nurse develops into an effective leader and manager, he or she should accept the responsibility to act as a mentor to new nurses, helping them develop effective leadership and management skills. Mentorship is key to developing our future nursing leaders and managers.

Corporate Supporter. The nurse manager, as a corporate supporter, has a responsibility to embrace the mission, goals, and objectives of the employing organization. In this role as corporate supporter, the nurse manager is a professional representative for the organization and is committed to supporting and accomplishing organizational goals.

CREATING A CARING ENVIRONMENT

Perhaps the most important responsibility for the nurse in any leadership or management role is to create an environment of caring—caring for staff members as well as for patients and families. Staff members who feel that their manager sincerely cares about them and the work they do are able to pass that feeling of caring on to their patients and other customers. Caring for the staff members can be demonstrated through the following measures (McNeese-Smith, 1997):

- Offering sincere positive recognition for both individuals and teams
- Praising and giving thanks for a job well done
- Spending time with staff members to reinforce positive work behaviors
- Meeting the staff member's personal needs whenever possible, such as accommodating scheduling needs for family events and being flexible in times of illness
- Providing guidance and support for professional and personal growth
- Maintaining a positive, confident attitude and a pleasant work environment

Staff members who feel that their work is valued and that they are respected and cared about as individuals are able to further contribute to a positive, caring environment in which to provide excellent patient care. Demonstrating respect and concern for every person at every level in the organization is an important leadership quality that the new nurse can use to develop a caring environment.

Creating a caring environment in the highly technical, fast-paced, and extremely stressful environments in which nurses work can be a significant challenge to the nurse manager. However, it is a challenge that is at the heart of nursing if we are to promote the very best in patient care. As Benner has observed, "Failing to attend to caring practices will continue to fuel a technical cure approach to health care rather than attend to illness prevention, care of the chronically ill and health promotion. Sometimes care itself is the most significant outcome, as well as the most significant means to cure, healing and health" (1999, p. 318).

SPECIAL LEADERSHIP AND MANAGEMENT CHALLENGES IN THE TWENTY-FIRST CENTURY

Generational Differences in the Workplace

The two primary generations in today's workplace are "baby boomers" and "gen-Xers." The differences between these two groups in communication styles, motivational needs, and professional goals make the work of today's manager extremely challenging. The 20-something generation is seeking a manager who is approachable, supportive, receptive, and motivating. They want to be taught by and led by someone who serves as a coach, mentor, and guide who gets to know them personally. The young men and women in the emerging workforce are searching for opportunities to gain advanced training, education, and certification; they are seeking feedback on performance to help refine their skills; they expect their managers to take a personal interest in them and to guide them to build a competitive portfolio. This group excels at developing innovative solutions to problems and needs to be challenged with specific time frames and clear and achievable outcomes—but they do not want their manager to interfere with how the job gets done. They will demand a balance between work, family, and friends. Flexible shifts, self-scheduling, cross-training, and educational incentives are appropriate motivators for this group (Wieck, 2000).

The baby boomers, the largest generation currently in the nursing workforce, have also been referred to as the "sandwich generation" because they may be caring simultaneously for their children and their aging parents. As experienced, dedicated workers, they also have heavy family responsibilities, as well as goals for healthy living; thus they set a grueling work pace and may be running from morning until night (Cordeniz, 2002). Baby boomers highly value group participation and consensus; recognition is highly valued, and they care about what others think (Cordeniz, 2002). Having time to meet their extensive family obligations is important to baby boomers.

Understanding and learning to handle these generational differences is an emerging skill for the nurse manager. Approaches suggested to draw the generations together include (1) teaching the generations about their differences and how to honor and respect those differences; (2) having the groups actively participate in identifying values that can be supported by all; and (3) having the groups participate in problem solving, moving towards consensus whenever possible (Kowalski, 2001).

Patient Safety and the Nurse's Work Environment

Most practicing nurses and students are now aware of the Institute of Medicine's (IOM) landmark report *To Err Is Human: Building Safer Healthcare Systems* (2000), which reported that up to 98,000 people die each year in our nation's hospitals as a result of medical errors. In follow-up to this landmark report, the IOM's most recent report, entitled *Keeping Patients Safe: Transforming the Work Environment of Nurses* (2003), has made a strong connection between the nurse's work environment and medical errors. As the scientific evidence that nurses are essential to patient safety and improved outcomes continues to grow, nurse leaders and managers are challenged to actually implement changes and impart significant improvements in hospitals, nursing homes, home health agencies, ambulatory clinics, and all other settings across the continuum of care. Although the IOM report has provided guidance and recommendations to improve nurses' work environments, it is now up to nurse leaders at all levels, including those in direct patient care, to turn these recommendations into action. Following is a short summary of the IOM's (2003) recommendations for improving the work environment of nurses.

Transformational Leadership and Evidence-Based Management. Acquire nurse leaders at all levels in the organization who will:

- Participate in executive decision making.
- Facilitate mutual trust among management and nursing staff.
- Achieve effective communication among nursing and other clinical leaders.
- Facilitate input from direct-care staff into decision making.
- Actively manage the process of change.
- Have available necessary resources to support and develop staff nurses' knowledge in clinical decision making.

Maximize Workforce Capability. Achieve appropriate staffing levels with nursing staff who have the required clinical knowledge and skills to keep patients safe. Although recommendations for specific nurse/patient ratios were not made (except for hospital intensive care units and nursing homes), the IOM did recommend further research on hospital staffing to better identify staffing needs. Specific recommendations to maximize workforce capabilities included:

- Incorporate patient volume estimates that count all admissions and discharges rather than a patient census at one point of time.
- Involve direct-care staff in identifying appropriate staffing levels, causes of nursing staff turnover, and methods to improve retention.
- Provide for staffing flexibility in each shift's schedule to accommodate variations in patient volume.
- Avoid the use of "agency" nurses.
- Empower nursing unit staff to set criteria for closing the unit to new admissions as necessitated by workload.
- Ensure that adequate financial and other resources are dedicated to support nursing staff in the acquisition and maintenance of new knowledge and skills.
- Promote interdisciplinary collaboration through such activities as interdisciplinary rounds and formal education and training in interdisciplinary collaboration.

Work Redesign to Prevent Errors. Nurses' work processes and work environments need to be more conducive to detecting and preventing errors. Fatigue has been particularly addressed as a threat to patient safety. Following are some specific recommendations in the area of work redesign:

- Prohibit nursing staff from providing patient care in excess of 12 hours in any given 24-hour period or in excess of 60 hours in a 7-day period.
- Enable nursing staff to collaborate with other health care personnel to identify and redesign high-risk and inefficient work processes to make them safe and efficient.
- Redesign documentation practices with assistance from regulators and oversight organizations (i.e., JCAHO, state licensing agencies).
- Address handwashing and medication administration among the first work redesign initiatives.

Create and Sustain a Culture of Safety. Patient safety requires a vigilant and strong organizational commitment to prevent errors and to detect, analyze, and rectify errors when they do occur, with organizations placing as high a priority on safety as they do on financial management and revenue generation. To this end, the IOM makes the following recommendations:

- Specify short- and long-term safety objectives.
- Continuously review success in meeting these objectives and provide feedback at all levels.
- Conduct an annual confidential survey of nursing and other health care workers to assess the extent to which a culture of safety exists.
- Institute a fair, just, and blameless reporting system for errors and near misses.
- Engage in ongoing employee training in error detection, analysis, and reduction.
- Implement procedures for analyzing errors and providing feedback to direct-care workers.
- Institute rewards and incentives for error reduction.

The IOM report emphasizes that a "piecemeal" approach to improve patient safety and the work environment of nurses will not work—all of the areas described above must be addressed if we are to create a safe and effective health care system in which nurses feel very good about the care they are able to provide to patients. It will be up to nurse leaders at all levels of health care organizations to begin this long, yet exciting, process of redesigning work environments. Copies of the IOM's *Keeping Patients Safe* can be obtained on-line (www.nap.edu).

LEADERSHIP AND MANAGEMENT SKILLS AND BEHAVIORS

Hersey and Blanchard (1988) have identified that effective leadership and management requires skills in three major areas.

- Technical skills—including clinical expertise and nursing knowledge
- Human skills—the ability and judgment to work with people in an effective leadership role
- Conceptual skills—the ability to understand the complexities of the overall organization and to recognize how and where one's own area of management fits into the overall organization

At the staff nurse level of management, a considerable amount of technical skill and clinical expertise is needed, because the nurse generally is involved in direct supervision of patient care and may be required to help train and mentor nurses and other health care providers. As one advances from lower levels to higher levels in the organization, more conceptual skills are needed. The common denominator at any level of management is the ability to work with people and provide effective leadership (Hersey and Blanchard, 1988).

Box 16-9 summarizes behaviors and practices that are essential to any nurse who strives to become an effective leader and manager. Notice that human—or caring—skills encompass the largest portion of the behaviors and practices identified.

SUMMARY

In every area of health care, the professional nurse is expected to provide leadership and management expertise to help manage complex and ever-changing health care organizations. The multifaceted set of theories, functions, roles, and skills presented in this chapter may at first seem overwhelming to the novice nurse. However, by learning and understanding the principles and concepts involved, the graduate nurse can become a successful nurse leader and manager.

Leadership, management and organizational theories provide a framework on which to build effective nursing management practices. Although there is no one "best" leadership theory, professional nurses should maintain an awareness of their own behavior and how the key elements of the leadership situation influence outcomes.

The management functions of planning, organizing, staffing, directing, and controlling provide the nurse manager with a defined, practical set of skills to guide management activities. Professional nurses can apply these management functions to perform effectively in various management roles, including customer service provider, team builder, resource manager, change agent, clinical consultant, staff developer, mentor, and corporate supporter. The professional nurse should use conceptual, caring, and technical skills in all leadership and management activities.

BOX 16–9   *Effective Leading and Managing: Conceptual, Human, and Clinical Practices Required*

Conceptual Practices

■ Make a commitment to support the mission, vision, and goals of the organization.
■ Accept the realities of the complex health care system. All health care organizations are under pressure to improve productivity, enhance quality, and cut costs—to "do more with less."
■ Understand the needs of external customers (patients, families, physicians, referring facilities) and internal customers (staff, administrators, executives, and other departments).
■ Incorporate legal, ethical, and nursing practice standards into all management functions and activities.

Caring Practices

■ Maintain honesty and integrity in work and relationships—Trust is an essential requirement for effective leadership.
■ Create a teaching and learning environment—Earn a reputation for exceptional training and mentoring for everyone on the team.
■ Model the behavior desired—Develop and exhibit a commitment to excellence.
■ Create an open, nonthreatening environment—Share information, keep staff informed and encourage them to discuss issues.
■ Make an emotional investment—Give of yourself in a way that the staff understands your commitment to quality patient care. Care as much as one would like others to care.
■ Humanize the work environment—Understand and respect both organizational and staff problems. Respect superiors. Coach, counsel, and correct subordinates in private; praise them in public.
■ Communicate effectively—Develop good listening skills; listen more than you talk and clarify areas of potential misunderstanding.
■ Give frequent feedback—All staff should know when their performance is excellent or needs improvement.
■ Become a proactive problem solver—Knowing *how* to solve problems is more important than knowing all the answers.
■ Get out of the office and into the patient care areas—*Listen* to patients and staff.
■ Maintain a confident, positive outlook—Identify areas in which you are weak and seek help to learn and grow.

Clinical Practices

■ Keep your own clinical skills and knowledge current.
■ Train staff members adequately—Be certain they are competent to perform their assigned responsibilities.
■ Know the organization's policies and procedures well—Ensure that all staff members maintain compliance at all times.
■ Become results-oriented and outcomes-focused in all patient care activities—Resource utilization (staff, time, supplies) is more effective when done with the end results in mind.
■ Act as a willing consultant for clinical problems—Perform patient assessments, contribute to sound nursing judgments, and teach others.

Developing effective leadership and management skills is an ongoing process that will continue throughout one's career as a professional nurse. (Box 16-10 provides some nursing leadership and management resources.) Nurses in management positions should routinely analyze personal strengths and weaknesses in each of these management roles and identify areas in which learning and development is needed. Modeling effective nurse managers and reading relevant professional journal articles and books are ways to increase leadership and management knowledge and skills. Management and leadership roles are challenging and exciting and present a wonderful opportunity to grow professionally as well as personally.

BOX 16–10   *Nursing Leadership and Management Resources*

Nursing Leadership and Management On-Line Resources
American Organization of Nurse Executives
http://www.aone.org/

American Nurses Association
http://www.nursingworld.org/

National Academy Press (copies of the IOM's *Keeping Patients Safe* available)
www.nap.edu

The National Database of Nursing Quality Indicators (NDNQI) is a project of ANA's Safety & Quality Initiative, which addresses the issues of patient safety and quality of care arising from changes in health care delivery. NDNQI advances this initiative by developing an information resource that will be used to quantify the specific role of nursing interventions in patient outcomes. Data are being collected from hospitals across the United States for the NDNQI database.
http://nursingworld.org/quality/

College of Business, University of Missouri–Columbia: Provides good information about behavioral interviewing, the latest interview style that more and more companies are using in their hiring processes
http://business.missouri.edu/Career+Services/Resources/Interviews/Interview+Styles/default.aspx

Nursing Management and Leadership Journals
American Journal of Nursing (http://www.nursingworld.org/ajn/)
Journal of Nursing Administration Quarterly
Nursing Management
Journal of Nursing Administration
Nursing & Health Care Perspectives
The Journal of Clinical Systems Management

CRITICAL THINKING ACTIVITIES

1. Obtain a copy of the mission, values, philosophy, and goals of a nursing unit. How is the mission communicated to staff members? How are the goals accomplished? Identify and list behaviors that you observe on the unit that are not consistent with beliefs, values, and activities expressed in the document. If you were the nurse manager, how would you handle those behaviors that are inconsistent with the mission, values, philosophy and goals of the nursing unit?

2. Identify experienced nurses who seem to be efficient at accomplishing their daily work. How do these nurses plan and organize their daily assignments? How do the experienced nurses interact with other members of the health care team? Identify and list several management skills that help the nurses accomplish their work more efficiently.

3. Think about a situation in the nursing unit in which an unsatisfactory management decision was made. Was the decision based on inaccurate or incomplete information or an incorrectly identified problem? How could this situation have been avoided? What would you recommend to prevent a similar circumstance from occurring in the future?

4. Identifying and meeting customer (patients, clients, families) needs are important management functions. Identify and describe how an organization gathers and uses input from customers. What follow-up evaluation is done by the organization in response to positive and negative comments by customers? that incorporates four or five of the trends described in the chapter.

Additional resources are available on-line at: http://evolve.elsevier.com/Cherry/

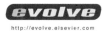

http://evolve.elsevier.com

REFERENCES

American Nurses Association: *Standards and scope of gerontological nursing practice*, Washington, DC, 2001, ANA.

American Nurses Association: *The scope and standards of diabetes nursing practice*, Washington, DC, 2003, ANA.

American Nurses Association: *Nursing: scope and standards of practice*, Washington, DC, 2004, ANA.

Bass BM, Avoliio BJ, Goodheim L: Biography and the assessment of transformational leadership at the world-class level, *J Manage* Jan:7-19, 1987.

Benner P: Nursing leadership for the new millennium: claiming the wisdom and worth of clinical practice, *Nurs Healthcare Perspect* 20(6):312-319, 1999.

Burns J: *Leadership*, New York, 1978, Harper and Row.

Cordeniz JA: Recruitment, retention and management of generation X: a focus on nursing professionals, *J Healthcare Manage* 47(4):237-245, 2002.

Dunham-Taylor J: Nurse executive transformational leadership found in participative organizations, *J Nurs Admin* 30(5):241-250, 2000.

Grensing-Pophal L: Give-and-take feedback, *Nurs Manage* Feb:27-28, 2000.

Hersey P, Blanchard K: *Management of organizational behavior: utilizing human resources*, ed 4, Englewood Cliffs, NJ, 1988, Prentice-Hall.

Hersey P, Blanchard K, Natemeyer W: Situational leadership, perception and impact of power, *Group Organization Studies* 4:418-428, 1979.

Howenstein MA et al: Factors associated with critical thinking among nurses, *J Contin Ed Nurs* 27(3):100-103, 1996.

Institute of Medicine: *To err is human: building a safer health system*, Kohn L, Corrigan J, Donaldson M, editors: Washington, DC, 2000, National Academy Press.

Institute of Medicine: *Keeping patients safe: transforming the work environment of nurses*, Page A, editor: Washington, DC, 2003, National Academy Press.

Kowalski K: Nursing work force of the future: the administrative perspective, *J Perinat Neonat Nurs* 15(1):8-15, 2001.

Lewin K: *Field theory in social sciences*, New York, 1951, Harper & Row.

Marquis BL, Huston CJ: *Leadership roles and management functions in nursing*, ed 4, Philadelphia, 2003, Lippincott.

Marriner-Tomey A: *Nursing management and leadership*, St Louis, 2000, Mosby.

McGuire E: Chaos theory: learning a new science, *J Nurs Admin* 29(2):8-9, 1999.

McKenna R: Real time, *Inc.* 19(12):87-90, 1997.

McNeese-Smith D: The influence of manager behavior on nurses' job satisfaction, productivity and commitment, *J Nurs Admin* 27(9):47-55, 1997.

Moss R, Rowles C: Staff nurse job satisfaction and management style, *Nurs Manage* 28(1):32-34, 1997.

Norman L: Continuous improvement in nursing education, *Quality Connection* 6(20):4, 1997.

Peters T, Waterman RH: *In search of excellence*, New York, 1982, Harper & Row.

Porter-O'Grady T: A different age for leadership, part 1: new context, new content, *J Nurs Admin* 33(2):105-110, 2003a.

Porter-O'Grady T: A different age for leadership, part 2: new rules, new roles, *J Nurs Admin* 33(3):173-178, 2003b.

Sengin KK: Work-related attributes of RN job satisfaction in acute care hospitals, *J Nurs Admin* 33(6):317-320, 2003.

Stogdill RM: *Handbook of leadership: a survey of theory and research*, New York, 1974, The Free Press.

Thompson JD: *Organizations in action*, New York, 1967, McGraw-Hill.

White RK, Lippit R: *Autocracy and democracy: an experimental inquiry*, New York, 1960, Harper & Row.

Wieck L: Tomorrow's nurses: are we ready for them? *Texas Nurs* June-July:1-4, 2000.

Yoderwise P: *Leading and managing in nursing*, St Louis, 2003, Mosby.

SUGGESTED READINGS

Covey S: *The seven habits of highly effective people*, New York, 1990, Simon & Schuster.

McElhaney RM: Conflict management in nursing administration, *Nurs Manage* 27(3):49-50, 1996.

Scholtes PR, Joiner BL, Streibel BJ: *The team handbook*, Madison, Wisc, 1996, Joiner Associates.

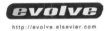
Effective Communication and Conflict Resolution

Anna Sallee, PhD(C), RN, CCRN, and
Sandy Forrest, PhD, RN

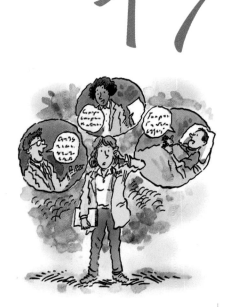

Effective communication
is a major component of
successful nursing practice.

The greatest problem of communication is the illusion that it has been accomplished.

— **GEORGE BERNARD SHAW**

VIGNETTE

Christy Shannon, RN, the charge nurse on 4-East, receives a phone call from the secretary in the emergency room (ER) informing her that a patient is ready for transfer. Christy was expecting this patient but had not anticipated the transfer would occur so soon and had not yet informed the nurse who would be assigned to the patient. The ER secretary explains that there are many patients waiting to be seen in the ER and it is becoming increasingly chaotic. Christy replies that she will locate the nurse who will be assigned to the patient and facilitate the transfer as soon as possible. As Christy goes down the hallway to locate this particular nurse, she learns that the nurse has left the unit on a short break and is expected back within 10 minutes.

Christy calls the ER secretary to arrange for the transfer to occur in 20 minutes. To her surprise, she finds out that the patient has left the department and is being brought to 4-East immediately. Within a few moments the patient and ER nurse arrive. The ER nurse states that he wants to give report on this patient quickly because he needs to return to the ER right away. Christy assists him in transferring the patient to a bed and making the patient as comfortable as possible.

Additional resources are available on-line at: http://evolve.elsevier.com/Cherry/

As Christy completes this process, the nurse who was on break returns to the unit, learns that she has a new patient she did not expect, and immediately has to receive report from the ER nurse. Christy notes through both body language and tone of voice that the interaction between the two nurses is less than cordial.

Within 10 minutes Christy receives a phone call from the ER charge nurse wanting to discuss this incident. Negative comments are made about the 4-E nurse who left the unit "unannounced" and that "there is a concern for patient safety." How can Christy best facilitate a positive outcome in this situation?

Questions to consider while reading this chapter:

1. What communication strategies should Christy use to respond to the accusations being made by the ER charge nurse and to help resolve the conflict?
2. What strategies can Christy use to build a trusting relationship between herself and the ER charge nurse?
3. What positive communication techniques could have prevented this situation from occurring?
4. What nonverbal cues might Christy have observed between the two nurses during the report exchange?
5. Should Christy have intervened when she observed the interaction between the two nurses? If so, how?
6. What strategies can Christy implement to increase the communication skills of her staff?

KEY TERMS

Active communication A participatory form of communication that promotes change.

Active listening The process of hearing what others are saying with a sense of seriousness and discrimination.

Aggressive communication A manner of communicating that limits the focus on, or understanding of, the opinions, values, or beliefs of others.

Assertive communication A form of communication that enables a person to act in his or her own best interest without denying or infringing on the rights of others.

Blocking Obstructing communication through noncommittal answers, generalization, or other techniques that hamper continued interaction.

Communication A process of relaying information between or among people by the use of words, letters, symbols, or body language.

Conflict An experience in which there is simultaneous arousal of two or more incompatible motives.

Decode A process whereby the receiver takes the message and interprets its meaning.

Empathy An attempt to experience another person's point of view without losing one's own identity.

Encode A process of translating an idea already conceived into a message suitable for transmission.

Equality An attitude that relays acceptance and approval of another person.

Feedback Response from the receiver, which can be verbal or nonverbal.

Filtration Unconscious exclusion of extraneous stimuli.

Information The data that are meaningful and have an effect on the receiver's understanding.

Interpretation Receiver's understanding of the meaning of the communication.

Negative communication techniques Behaviors that block or impair effective communication.

Nonassertive communication A timid and reserved manner of communication that results in limited concern for one's own rights regardless of the situation.

Nonverbal communication Unspoken cues (intentional or unintentional) from the communicant, such as body positioning, facial expression, or lack of attention.

Openness An attitude of willingness to self-disclose, react honestly to the messages of others, and own one's feelings and thoughts.

Passive communication A form of communication in which the sender fails to say what is meant.

Perception The manner is which one sees reality.

Positive Communication Techniques Behaviors that enhance effective communication.

Receiver The destination for or receptor of a message.

Sender Anyone who wishes to convey an idea or concept to others, to seek information, or to express a thought or emotion.

Supportiveness The concern that is fostered by being descriptive rather than evaluative and being provisional rather than certain.

LEARNING OUTCOMES

After studying this chapter, the reader will be able to:

1. Outline factors that can influence the communication process.
2. Communicate effectively with diverse intergenerational and interdisciplinary team members.
3. Apply positive communication techniques in diverse situations.
4. Recognize negative communication techniques.
5. Evaluate conflicting verbal and nonverbal communication cues.
6. Examine constructive methods of communicating in conflict situations.

CHAPTER OVERVIEW

Effective communication is the essence of professional nursing. Understanding communication processes and principles is required for nurses to interact professionally with patients, families and significant others, nursing peers, managers, student nurses, physicians, other members of the interdisciplinary team, and the public. Nurses communicate through a variety of media, including the spoken and written word, demonstration, role modeling, and on occasion, public appearances. The exchange of ideas and feelings is not limited to verbal communication. There are many types of nonverbal communication that often are as meaningful as, and in some instances more meaningful than, audible expression. Because communication is such a complex process, there are infinite opportunities for sending or receiving incorrect messages. All too frequently, communication is faulty, resulting in misperceptions and misunderstandings.

This chapter will review the key components of the communication process, communication styles, and principles of effective communication in professional nursing, including special communication issues related to documentation, cultural diversity, gender, generational differences and interdisciplinary teams. A major focus of the chapter is effective, positive communication techniques that can prevent or reduce conflict. The chapter also provides techniques that can be used to effectively manage conflict situations when they do occur.

THE COMMUNICATION PROCESS

The communication process contains five elements: who relays what, in what way, to whom, and with what effect (Burley-Allen, 1982) (Fig. 17-1). During this process the sender encodes

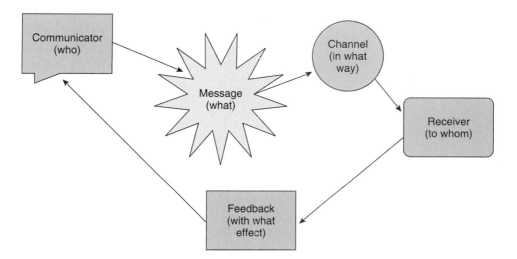

FIG. 17–1 The communication process.

the intention of the desired message and the receiver decodes the message to gain meaning. As a dynamic process, communication is cyclic so that the receiver becomes the sender when responding. When communication with another person occurs, verbally or nonverbally, a typical pattern occurs that includes the actual message being sent, the receiver's belief about or interpretation of that message, and the reaction to the message.

Think about nurse-patient, nurse-nurse, or nurse-physician interaction. Often there is much to communicate within a limited period of time. Personal goals or hidden agendas can influence the communication process. One may be unaware of the intent of the communication at the time of the encounter, and in fact, parties involved can disagree as to why the interaction is occurring. While the sender is attempting to convey a precise message, words have specific meanings in relation to the environment in which they are placed (Burley-Allen, 1982). Often it is the unspoken message that has a deeper meaning than the message being articulated. Thus it becomes important to understand the countless elements that influence the communication process. These elements will be discussed in relation to the communication components of interpretation, filtration, and feedback.

Interpretation

Interpretation of information can be influenced by such factors as context, environment, precipitating event, preconceived ideas, personal perceptions, style of transmission, and past experiences. Because of the interaction of these factors, the sender's message may mean to the receiver something that was entirely unplanned or unexpected by the sender (Fig. 17-2).

Context and Environment. Context refers to the entire situation relevant to the communication, such as the environment, the background, and the particular circumstances that lead to the discussion. Environment can denote physical surroundings and happenings and the emotional conditions involved in the communication.

Precipitating Event. Precipitating event refers specifically to the event or situation that prompted the communication. Precipitating event refers to a specific single event, whereas

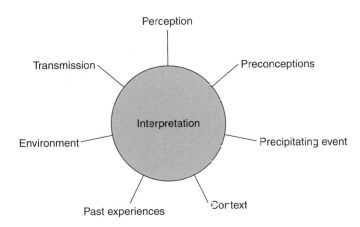

FIG. 17–2 Factors influencing interpretation of messages.

context describes the whole ambiance of the situation with the inclusion of multiple circumstances that have led to the precipitating event.

Preconceived Ideas. Preconceived ideas are conceptions, opinions, or thoughts that the receiver has developed before the encounter. Such ideas can dramatically affect the receiver's acceptance and understanding of the message.

Style of Transmission. Style of transmission involves many aspects of the manner of conveyance of the message. Transmission styles include aspects such as open or closed statements or questions, body language, method of organizing the message, degree of attention to the topic or to the receiver, vocabulary chosen (professional jargon versus language a layperson could easily understand), and intonation.

Past Experiences. Each person comes to any type of communication, whether it is friendly conversation, informational lecture, staff meeting, performance evaluation, or any other possible scenario, with baggage in terms of past experiences. Because past experiences will be a variety of positive, neutral, and negative events, the influence that the experiences can and will have on communication may be positive, neutral, or negative. The importance of recognizing that any reaction from the receiver may be biased by previous experiences cannot be overstated. An astute sender will begin to investigate such a possibility if the receiver reacts in an unexpected or inappropriate manner to information that was not expected to produce such a response, which may range from nonresponse to overly vehement response.

Personal Perceptions. Personal perceptions can have a profound effect on the quality of communication. Perception is awareness through the excitation of all the senses. Perception can be described as all that the person knows about a situation or circumstance based on what each of the senses—taste, smell, sight, sound, touch, and intuition—discover and interpret.

Filtration

The most concise delivery of information is subject to some amount of filtration. Think of the process as similar to washing vegetables in a colander. A large amount of water is poured over the produce. Some of the water comes quickly through the colander holes; some water drips through more slowly; and some water hangs on the contents or settles in the solid portions of the colander and never filters through. If people were not able to filter out a portion of the stimuli that bombard them daily, the clutter would be unmanageable! At the same time, however, it is possible to filter out some part of intended communication that is essential to facilitate understanding.

Feedback

Feedback, simply put, is the response from the receiver. However, as with all communication, feedback is a dynamic process. As the receiver interprets and responds to the original message, the sender begins the same process of feedback to the receiver. Because of this circular property, the process frequently is referred to as the "feedback loop" (van Servellen, 1997). As with the original message, feedback is not confined to verbal responses alone. Both communicants constantly assess nonverbal communication as well. Feedback is formed based on all the components of interpretation and filtration.

VERBAL VERSUS NONVERBAL COMMUNICATION

Verbal Communication

Verbal communication is the most common form of interpersonal communication and involves talking and listening. An important clue to verbal communication is the tone or inflection with which the words are spoken and the general attitude used when speaking. Suzette Haden Elgin refers to the "tune the words are set to" (1993, p. 186). More of Elgin's work is available on-line (www.sfwa.org/members/elgin/). The key to the true meaning of a statement may be contained in the emphasis placed on a specific word. Consider how differently the following phrase could be perceived based on the inflection or the emphasis on the wording:

- You are going to *bed*.
- *You* are going to bed.
- You *are going* to bed.

With an emphasis on *bed,* the first phrase most likely will be perceived as an inquiry. The second phrase might imply that *you* are going to bed, but no one else is. The last phrase, an imperative (or command), gives the impression of increased emotion, such as anger or frustration.

Another element central to verbal interaction is the concept of attitude. Being aware of and learning to understand the concept of attitude is key to effective communication. Attitude involves a predisposition or tendency to respond in one way or another. Often the attitude that accompanies a verbal interaction, which can be positive or negative, is much more meaningful than the actual words spoken. Although we may hear "attitude" in a person's tone of voice, it is most often communicated loud and clear through nonverbal communication.

Nonverbal Communication

Nonverbal communication involves many factors that either confirm or deny the spoken word. Facial expression, the presence or absence of eye contact, posture, and body movement all project a direct message. Indirect nonverbal messages might include dressing style, lifestyle, or material possessions. Never presume that external trappings and physical presentation do not influence the quality of communication. Preconceived ideas and expectations interpret input from all such sources, often on an almost subconscious level.

Consider the following scenario: Rhonda, a young wife and mother, was admitted through the emergency department with significant abdominal pain. As the nurse inquires about her symptoms, Rhonda repeatedly glances at her husband, Tommy, before she answers. Although she denies any pain at this time, you observe that she guards her stomach, has a "clenched" jaw line, and does not make eye contact with you. As you assess and question Rhonda, Tommy often interrupts with comments such as, "She's just fine. It was only a stomach ache, and it's gone this morning, isn't it, dear?" Which message seems more likely to be true—the verbal or the nonverbal? How will you address the nonverbal cues? What strategies will you use to enhance communication with this couple?

The inability to make eye contact may be construed to mean that the speaker is shy, scared, or not telling the truth. The judgment of which condition is the correct one is based on all the factors that feed into the receiver's interpretation—perception, preconceptions, precipitating event, context, past experiences, environment, and transmission. Faced with the many opportunities for incorrect interpretation, is it any wonder that misunderstandings occur?

An important concept to remember is that when the verbal message and the nonverbal message do not agree, the receiver is more likely to believe the nonverbal message. Jan Hargrave (2001) tells us that our bodies give "hidden messages" all the time. We can't get away from what our bodies say; they don't lie!

An understanding of the importance prescribed to body language and other nonverbal clues to the intent of the message explains the advantage of face-to-face communication whenever possible. Although a telephone conversation supplies verbal messages, intonation, and feedback, other signals are missing such as facial expression, body position, and environmental clues. The perils inherent in written communication will be discussed later in this chapter.

POSITIVE COMMUNICATION TECHNIQUES

Effective, positive communication is characterized by (1) openness—a willingness to self-disclose, react honestly to incoming stimuli, acknowledge, and assume responsibility for one's own thoughts and actions; (2) empathy—experiencing another person's point of view without judgment or losing one's own identity; (3) supportiveness—maintaining a nonthreatening, nonjudgmental attitude; (4) positiveness—affirmative regard for self, others, and the interaction; and (5) equality—acknowledging that each individual is valuable and should be heard (Gibb, 1961). Following are techniques that the nurse can use to put positive communication into practice.

Developing Trust

Trust between the nurse and the patient is essential to good communication and often must be cultivated. Factors that enhance the development of trust include openness on the part of the nurse, honesty, integrity, and dependability. These can be achieved by:

- Communicating clearly in language that laypersons can understand
- Keeping promises
- Protecting confidentiality
- Avoiding negative communication techniques such as blocking and false reassurance
- Being available to the patient

The need for trust is not limited to the nurse-patient relationship, but rather pervades all associations. Care is more effective when the nursing team and the interdisciplinary team share the essential element of trust.

Using "I Messages"

The use of "I messages" is a fundamental component in acceptable communication. Consider the following exchange.

> Laura: You make me so mad, Donald.
>
> Donald: I don't mean to make you mad.
>
> Laura: Well, you do. You never think about how I feel. You know I hate it when you leave a patient's room as cluttered as 103.
>
> Donald: You don't have the vaguest idea what went on here last night! That's what I hate about you—always so quick to judge. You are so critical. You must think that you are perfect!

When a comment starts with "you," most commonly the receiver's defenses will promptly go on alert. The use of "you" in such a context sounds—and most probably is meant to be—accusatory. Notice how the emotions quickly escalate to anger. Also notice that although the receiver initially tries to sound conciliatory, he soon begins to respond in a similar accusatory form. Instead of using accusatory and defensive language, the sender should frame the comment in terms of how it makes her or him feel. Consider this alternative:

> Laura: Donald, I feel so upset when I find a cluttered room like 103 at the beginning of my shift. I feel as if I am behind when I start.

The difference is obvious. When "I messages" are used, they become less likely to sound accusatory. By using such an opening, the sender allows the receiver to respond to the true message rather than start to mount a defense. It allows for more effective communication because the receiver is more likely to offer an explanation such as the following:

> Donald: I'm really sorry about Room 103, Laura. I guess the wheel that doesn't squeak doesn't get oiled, as they say. Our shift started last night with a patient coding right after he arrived from the emergency room. There was no family here. It took forever to find them and then to support them through the shock. About the time things settled down, the patient in Room 110 coded. It was quite a night.

In this instance, the "I message" enhances communication by giving Donald the opportunity to address the real concern. In addition, if Laura is truly astute, she has a wonderful opportunity to support her colleague by voicing appreciation for the working circumstances of his shift. Most people respond gratefully to recognition and commiseration. The exchange could build collegiality between the two coworkers and perhaps between the two shifts.

Establishing Eye Contact

As mentioned previously, the avoidance of eye contact can be interpreted in a number of different ways. A person who does not make eye contact may be thought to be shy, scared, insecure, preoccupied, unprepared, dishonest—the list could go on and on. None of these qualities is likely to be appreciated in a primary caregiver. By making direct eye contact, the nurse gives undivided attention to the patient, and the patient is likely to feel valued and understood by the nurse. Eye contact in essence says, "I am wholly available to you. What you are saying is important to me."

Eye contact is equally important in communication with coworkers and other members of the interdisciplinary team. This quality is lost in telephone conversations or written communications.

Keep in mind, however, that the use of direct eye contact is a Western value. In some cultures avoidance of eye contact is considered more appropriate social behavior. By careful observation, the nurse quickly will recognize whether direct eye contact is interpreted as inappropriate or disrespectful. Nurses must make every effort to be sensitive to the cultural values of the client and their coworkers to enhance effective communication.

Keeping Promises

Little else can destroy the fragile trust developing in any interpersonal relationship as quickly as making and then breaking promises. Inherent in the concept of promise keeping are the qualities of honesty and integrity. Once a commitment is made, every effort must be expended to fulfill the expectation. Sometimes the request is impossible to satisfy. If this happens, the nurse must explain the situation or circumstances. The fact that the patient understands the nurse has made an effort to meet his or her needs or desires often is more important than whether the goal is accomplished. If the nurse responds, "I'll check on that," and then finds the request impossible to fulfill, but never returns with an explanation, the lack of dependability perceived by the patient (or colleague) will surely drive a wedge into the relationship.

Expressing Empathy

Empathy is the ability to mentally place oneself in another person's situation to better understand the person and to share the emotions or feelings of the person. Empathy is not feeling sorry for another; it is understanding the experiences of the other person, and it is integral to the therapeutic relationship. The nurse is able to perceive and address the needs of the patient without emotional involvement to the point of becoming inappropriately immersed in the situation.

Using Open Communication

Certain styles of phrasing questions and statements lend themselves to obtaining more information. For example, suppose Chris asks Mr. Barrow, "Do you know where you are?" and Mr. Barrow responds, "Yes." Can Chris assume that Mr. Barrow knows he is in the hospital? Not necessarily. Chris may be surprised to hear a completely unexpected response if he rephrases the inquiry:

Chris: Mr. Barrow, tell me where you are.
Mr. Barrow: Why, I'm in the honeymoon berth of the Titanic, of course. Have you seen my lovely bride?

Using open-ended questions or statements that require more information than "yes" or "no" can help gather enough facts to build a more complete picture of the circumstances. Questions or statements that are phrased to require only one- or two-word responses may miss the mark entirely.

Clarifying Information

Both communicants have a responsibility to clarify anything not understood. The sender should ask for feedback to be certain the receiver is correctly interpreting what is being said.

The receiver should stop the sender anytime the message becomes unclear and should provide feedback regularly so that misinterpretation can be identified quickly. Such phrases as "What I hear you saying is . . ." or "I understand you to mean . . ." help to communicate to the sender what is being perceived. Other techniques of clarification include using easily understood language, giving examples, drawing a picture, making a list, and finding ways to stimulate all the senses to enhance the ability to understand.

Being Aware of Body Language

Body positioning and movement send loud messages to others. The nurse can imply openness that facilitates effective communication by awareness of body position and movement. In addition to eye contact, effective communication is enriched through an open stance, such as holding one's arms at the side or out toward the patient, rather than crossed, or leaning toward the patient as if to hear more clearly, rather than away from the patient.

Using Touch

Most people have a fairly well-defined personal space. It is important for the nurse to be sensitive to each patient's personal preference and cultural differences in terms of touch. However, for many people, a gentle touch can scale mountains in terms of demonstrating genuine interest and concern. A pat on the back, a hand held, a touch on the shoulder—these are all behaviors that indicate availability and accessibility on the part of the nurse.

NEGATIVE COMMUNICATION TECHNIQUES

Several negative communication techniques have been alluded to in the previous discussion. Closed communication styles, such as asking yes-or-no questions or making inquiries or statements that require other single-word answers, potentially limit the response of the person and may prevent the discovery of pertinent facts. Closed body language also can hinder effective communication. Crossed arms, hands on the hips, avoidance of eye contact, turning away from the person, and moving away from the person all impose a sense of distance in the relationship. Three other techniques that are detrimental to good communication are termed *blocking, false assurances,* and *conflicting messages.*

Blocking

Blocking occurs when the nurse responds with noncommittal or generalized answers. For example:

"Nurse, I've never had surgery before. I'm afraid I might not ever wake up." Mr. Clayton is twisting the bed sheet as he speaks. "Oh, Mr. Clayton, many people feel that way. It'll be okay." Amanda Butler, RN, smiles brightly, pats his hand, picks up the dirty linen bag, and bounces out of the room.

Does Mr. Clayton feel reassured? Not likely. Will he be inclined to broach the subject with Amanda again? Probably not. Amanda has incorporated some important aspects of positive communication into her response—cheerfulness and touch—but she has not truly communicated. She has effectively blocked Mr. Clayton's attempt to get the reassurance he wanted from her. He may be too intimidated to ask anyone else, assuming that his fear is invalid.

By generalizing in this way, Amanda has trivialized Mr. Clayton's concerns. He is not "many people." He needs to be validated as an individual experiencing a legitimate feeling.

Amanda can validate his fear and put it into perspective at the same time with a different approach.

> Amanda: What makes you think you might not wake up, Mr. Clayton?
>
> Mr. Clayton: Well, my wife's cousin's husband had surgery about 25 years ago, and he never woke up.
>
> Amanda: What kind of surgery did he have?
>
> Mr. Clayton: Uh, it was some kind of heart surgery, and he had another heart attack on the table and died right there.
>
> Amanda: It sounds like his condition was critical going into surgery.
>
> Mr. Clayton: Yes, ma'am. He'd been sick for a long time.
>
> Amanda: It's not uncommon to feel afraid of having anesthesia, especially if you have never had surgery before. There are rare cases in which complications do occur during surgery. That's why we put the disclosures on the consent form, so that you will know just what the risks are. Thankfully, though, most surgeries are without such drastic problems. Although your gallbladder certainly has made you uncomfortable, you are otherwise in good health. The tests that were done before surgery, like the chest radiograph and the laboratory work, show that you are healthy and should do well with the anesthesia. That drastically decreases the chance for complications in your case. I would be glad to answer any other questions you have or to ask the anesthetist to come and talk with you some more.

Amanda has validated Mr. Clayton's feeling as legitimate, provided an explanation with reasonable reassurances, and offered to explore the issue with him further or to have someone else talk with him.

Some things are difficult to talk about with another person. The dying patient may want to talk about how he or she feels, ask questions, or perform a life review. A nurse who is uncomfortable with such topics may consciously or unconsciously block communication through generalizations or closed responses. Avoidance of the blocking technique requires a good understanding of oneself. If unable to provide the open communication the patient obviously needs, the nurse should access other personnel who are more comfortable in the situation.

False Assurances

False assurances are similar to blocking and have about the same effect. When someone is trying to get real answers or express serious concerns, an answer such as "Don't worry" or "It'll be okay" sends several unintended messages. Such answers can be interpreted by the patient as placating or showing a lack of concern or a lack of knowledge. The patient might even conclude that the nurse is being neglectful through trivialization of an issue that is important to him or her. At the very least, the nurse has neither recognized the need the patient has expressed nor provided validation.

Conflicting Messages

Conflicting messages also have been alluded to in the previous discussion. If a person professes pleasure at seeing someone but draws back when that person extends a hand of greeting, the nonverbal message speaks more loudly than the words spoken. If a nurse enters a room and goes through the routine greeting by rote (even with a smiling face and a bouncing step), a patient can quickly perceive this and consider the nurse less approachable.

The nurse's statement that the patient's condition is important to the nurse followed by failing to answer the call bell in a timely manner or by forgetting to bring items promised to the patient sends a double message. Such behavior can leave the patient confused, frustrated, or angry. Carrying through with a commitment, no matter how unimportant it may seem, is a premier method of saying to the person, "You are important to me."

COGNITIVE DISTORTIONS AND LOGICAL FALLACIES

Cognitive distortions and logical fallacies are related to an individual's culture, gender, background, and personal experiences and are barriers to meaningful communication. Individuals often cannot separate moods, thoughts, and perceptions, for they become interconnected in one continuous evaluation process, involving feeling, thinking, and responding. In times of increased stress, as is common in health care settings, it is more likely that people will employ faulty thinking that affects the communication process. Recognition of distortions and faulty logic will promote effective communication and reduce confusion or even prevent conflict. Box 17-1 present examples of common cognitive distortions; you can find more information about logical fallacies on-line (www.nizkor.org/features/fallacies/ or www.datanation.com/fallacies/index.htm). Following are examples of logical fallacies that are frequently encountered.

BOX 17–1 *Cognitive Distortions (Beck, 1988; Burns, 1999)*

All-or-nothing thinking: Dichotomous thinking; seeing things as black-and-white.
- "I missed delivering that medication on time. I am an inadequate nurse."

Catastrophizing: Exaggerates the harmful effects of a disappointing event.
- "I didn't react very well with that doctor the other day. She probably thinks I am very incompetent."

Disqualifying the positive: Rejects positive experiences by insisting they are not relevant, thus maintaining a negative belief that is contradicted by reality.
- A peer praises your ability to work with a difficult patient. You respond, "It really wasn't that difficult, and besides, my patient load was light so I had extra time others did not have."

Emotional reasoning: Assumes that your negative emotions necessarily reflect the way things really are.
- "I have one admission and two discharges scheduled during this shift. I know that I will be unable to accomplish everything."

Filtering: Focuses on the negative aspects of an experience while ignoring the positive side.
- "I can't believe that patient liked his bed bath. I felt so rushed."

Mind reader: Arbitrarily concludes that someone is reacting negatively to you without bothering to check this out.
- "I know that my care coordinator thinks that I am stupid and slow."

Fortune teller: Anticipates how things will turn out as if it is an established fact.
- "I didn't sleep well last night, and I'm going to make mistakes today."

Labeling or mislabeling: An occasional characteristic becomes magnified globally to encompass the entire person.
- "I had trouble understanding what that patient wanted. I am really stupid."

Magnification or minimization: Exaggerating or diminishing the importance of actions.
- "I did not anticipate that patient's need for pain medication. I am not a good nurse."

Ad Hominem Abusive

Ad hominem abusive is an argument that attacks the person instead of the issue. The speaker hopes to discredit the other person by calling attention to some irrelevant fact about that person. Perhaps a nurse has just had a disagreement with a physician about lab results that were not properly reported. The nurse makes the following comment to colleagues: "She thinks she's so smart just because she's a doctor." What does that have to do with the disagreement? Nothing. It is an unwarranted attack on the doctor. Does it accomplish the purpose? Very likely, the group will be influenced by the disparaging comment. They may also become angry at the physician, who had legitimate cause to be upset about not receiving lab results. Ultimately, the issue of unreported lab values is lost in the personal attack against the doctor.

Appeal to Common Practice

Appeal to common practice occurs when the argument is made that something is okay because most people do it. This logic is likely to be faulty in two ways: (1) Do "most" people really do it? (2) Does common practice really make an action okay? It's easy to imagine a situation in which using an explanation that you did something because you'd seen someone else do it that way, rather than checking the organization policy and procedure manual, could lead to significant professional and legal problems.

Appeal to Emotion

Appeal to emotion is an attempt to manipulate other people's emotions in order to avoid the real issue. For example, consider Deb, RN, who has repeatedly failed to document patient care properly. She has been called into the nurse manager's office to discuss the incident and receives a written warning. She comes out tearful. It is obvious to her colleagues that she has been reprimanded. She begins to discuss the problem and makes the following statements: "I am the first person in my family to even go to college. I'm a single parent, and I've worked so hard to get where I am. Our manager doesn't care anything about that. She just wants to pass out written warnings to cover herself. She doesn't care about us as individuals." After a bit of this type of talk, the entire staff is probably becoming angry with the nurse manager—who may feel bad that she had to give the written warning because she does indeed care about her staff. However, Deb has successfully deflected the attention away from the real issue, failure to document properly, which was legitimately addressed.

Appeal to Tradition

Appeal to tradition is the argument that doing things a certain way is best because they've always been done that way. This argument is often expressed as "that's just how it's done here." Another version would be, "Oh, we tried that once and it didn't work so we went back to the old way." Change always brings some uncertainty, but choosing to continue a practice just because "that's the way we've always done it" is not very sound reasoning. Health care is a very dynamic arena. The old ways of doing things seldom work out to be the best in this time of rapid change.

Red Herring

Red herring is the introduction of an irrelevant topic in order to divert attention away from the real issue. Two nurses, Brian and Nikoah, are having an argument regarding Brian's failure to complete his assigned tasks. Brian states, "It's not my work that you're really mad about.

It's that I'm a guy. You just don't like male nurses." Nikoah then begins to defend herself, denying any prejudice against male nurses. The focus of the argument has been turned from the real issue, Brian's failure to complete his assigned tasks, to a situation in which Nikoah is on the defensive about her opinion of male nurses.

Slippery Slope

Slippery slope is the belief that one event will inevitably follow another without any real support for that belief. In fact, this type of logic often leads from a fairly harmless situation to an assumption akin to the notion that the sky is falling. Kathy and Janet are talking in the nurses' lounge over lunch. Kathy is upset over the recent announcement that the unit is going to convert to computerized bedside charting. Kathy makes the following statement: "It was bad enough having to chart all we do. Now, we have to learn to use computers and make all kinds of entries. We'll probably have just as much paperwork. We'll end up spending even less time with the patients. The next thing you know, nurses will be sitting at a computer terminal and someone else will be taking care of patients. Then, they'll decide they don't really need nurses at all!" Kathy's logic takes her from a simple unit change to the end of nursing as we know it! All too frequently we hear this kind of "escalating disaster" logic when change is introduced.

Understanding cognitive distortions and logical fallacies should help the nurse recognize the difference between legitimate and faulty reasoning. A clear understanding and use of sound logic will help health care providers resolve problems and stay focused on the true issues.

LISTENING

Listening is certainly as important an element in clear and effective communication as any other component. Many distracters contribute to poor listening habits. Framing an answer while the other person is still talking interferes with receiving the entire message. Environmental disturbances can provide major disruption. A crying baby, a call light buzzing, or multiple concurrent conversations in a busy nurses' station are a few of the interruptions that jumble the simplest of instructions. Preexisting concerns or worries can block absorption of conversation because of the preoccupation. Attempts to continue work in progress leads to inattention. Ineffective engagement or peculiar mannerisms on the part of the speaker can be distracting. A person who does not make eye contact, shuffles through papers while talking, or overuses hand movements can also deter communication.

A number of techniques can be used by the receiver to facilitate the ability to listen:

- Give undivided attention to the sender by moving to a quieter area and stopping the speaker to clarify any points not understood.
- Provide feedback in terms of perceived meaning of the message rephrased in the receiver's own words.
- Give attention to positioning by facing the sender and making eye contact.
- Note nonverbal messages such as body language and respond to them.

Active listening will dramatically improve the likelihood of receiving the correct message. Equally important, active listening implies a respect for the speaker and communicates a regard for what the speaker has to offer. The nonverbal message that active listening delivers is, "I value you, and what you have to say is important to me."

WRITTEN COMMUNICATION

The professional nurse must interface with many forms of written communication on a daily basis. Nursing documentation includes a variety of reports, such as the nurse's notes in patient charts, memos, e-mails, kardexes, incident reports, discharge teaching forms, and written shift reports, to name a few. Many of the forms that nurses use for documentation are part of the legal record and require careful consideration. Unclear instructions or reports by the nurse, either written or read, can lead to misunderstandings, errors, and the potential for litigation. Most profoundly, misinformation potentially can lead to patient harm or injury. Therefore special attention must be paid to communicating effectively in writing.

Accuracy

Absolute accuracy is paramount in recording legal documentation. For the nurse, this most specifically applies to the nursing notes or any other entry in the patient's chart. Every effort should be made to report concisely, descriptively, and truthfully. To write "Patient walked today" is not adequate. A more concise and descriptive entry reads, "Patient walked to the nurses' station and back three times this shift, a total distance of 96 yards." (Many hospitals have distance measures marked in the hallway for this purpose.)

Consider the following scenario: Cody Johnson, RN, entered the patient's room and found the patient agitated and speaking loudly into the phone as she twisted her hair with her free hand. She was crying and periodically pounded the bedside table with her fist. Later the patient told Cody that she had been talking with her mother. Would it be appropriate for Cody to chart, "Patient became very angry with her mother while talking on the phone." No! The nurse must be diligent not to include personal judgments or quantify the patient's emotional state in such terms.

More accurately, Cody could chart, "Patient found crying while talking on the phone in a loud tone to her mother. Patient was twisting her hair and hitting bedside table with her fist." The information is descriptive and states exactly what Cody observed factually without any judgmental conclusions. If, however, the patient had said, "My mother makes me so mad," Cody could have charted the statement as a direct quote (enclosed in quotation marks).

Attention to Detail

In addition to absolute accuracy, written documents should be descriptive. As mentioned in the previous section, information should be quantified whenever possible. How many feet did the patient walk? How many times was the patient out of bed? How many mL of fluid did the patient drink? Precisely what did the patient say?

Words can be used to depict a verbal picture of a wound, rash, bruise, or any type of injury or situation. Illustrative terms can create a mental image for the person reading the notes, memo, or other communication. Descriptive categories can include measurement, color, position, location, drainage, or condition when speaking of a physical condition, or time, setting, people present, issues or goals discussed, or direct quotes when speaking of a meeting, conference, evaluation, or other interchange. Consider the differences between the following written communications:

"1000: Dressing change completed. Site healthy."
"1000: Dressing change completed. Edges of 4-inch surgical wound approximated, no drainage noted. Skin pink without any redness or edema."

BOX 17–2 *Incomplete Memo*

Anecdotal Report
Memo
To: Bonnie Thompson, RN, BSN, Nurse Manager
From: Jessica Lindsay, RN, BSN, Charge Nurse
Date: August 18
Subject: Lucas Alfred, RN

I have had lots of complaints about Lucas Alfred's treatment of students. I do not think he should be assigned as a preceptor anymore and do not plan to do so from now on.

The second entry allows the reader to "see" the wound mentally and follow the progress of healing even when unable to be present at the time of the dressing change. A good rule when describing any kind of break in skin integrity—whether from a stabbing, a surgical wound, or an intravenous line—is to describe color, drainage, and presence or absence of edema.

Consider the memo written in Box 17-2. What does this memo really tell the nurse manager? Not much—only that there is some kind of perceived problem between Lucas and the students. The nurse manager does not know based on the information provided whether the problem is "real," whether it is based on a bias of Jessica's or a student bias, whether the problem has occurred more than once, whether an interpersonal communication problem or misunderstanding exists, or whether obvious mistreatment of a student or students has occurred.

Now consider the memo written in Box 17-3. Carefully constructing a factual memo of this length is more time-consuming initially, but it will save a lot of confusion and misinterpretation in the long run. The nurse manager now has a clear picture of what has occurred and knows that an ongoing problem exists. Most appropriately, Jessica will speak to Bonnie about the problem, even if only briefly, when she delivers the memo. However, a written account of the incident must be submitted and should be composed promptly while the facts are freshly remembered. Additionally, written communication often is the first source of contact because the nurse manager is not likely to be immediately available on all shifts.

The skill of writing concisely yet descriptively must be developed. Over time, nurses build a repertoire of phrases and illustrative terminology that are useful and effective. Often, when a nurse is stumped as to how to express a situation, she or he will ask a colleague, "How would you write . . . ?" Accessing the experience and expertise of nursing peers is productive in terms of problem solving while also demonstrating respect for the colleague.

Thoroughness

The memo examples in the previous section also illustrate the need for thoroughness. In addition to being descriptive in terms of the incident, Jessica's memo in Box 17-3 reported her interview with other nursing students. By doing so, Jessica has been thorough in describing and reporting the extent of the problem she has discovered. Providing such completeness of information helps to avoid communication breakdown. Anticipating and

BOX 17–3   *Descriptive, Thorough Memo*

Anecdotal Report
Memo
To: Bonnie Thompson, RN, BSN, Nurse Manager
From: Jessica Lindsay, RN, BSN, Charge Nurse
Date: August 18
Subject: Student Precepting

Today (Monday, August 18) at 0710 I observed what appeared to be an animated conversation between Lucas Alfred, RN, and John Roberts, SN, a student nurse from North Hills University. As I moved toward them, I heard Lucas say loudly, "Well, you better stay with me because I am not going to come looking for you all day. I know how lazy students are." I asked Lucas, "Is there a problem?" He replied, "Oh, no problem. I just hate having students, that's all. They're more trouble than they're worth." I asked Lucas, "Would you prefer that I reassign the student?" He shrugged his shoulders and walked away. I suggested to the student that I assign him to another nurse for the day. He responded, "I'd really appreciate that. Mr. Alfred has let me know since I arrived that he didn't want to work with me."

Because this group of students has been on the unit 2 days a week for the past 3 weeks, I spoke to the other students who had worked with Lucas and asked them how things had gone. The other three students who have worked with Lucas reported similar experiences.

I would like to arrange a time to meet with you and Lucas to address this problem.

answering relevant questions before they are asked exemplifies thoroughness and clarifies communication.

Conciseness

Written communication must be concise. The message must state the necessary information as clearly and as briefly as possible. Consider the memo written in Box 17-4.

Whew! Extraneous details tend to confuse more than clarify. An inherent dilemma often develops as the nurse attempts to determine how to be descriptive and concise at the same time. One must determine what facts are pertinent to enable the reader to understand the true message. When in doubt and when appropriate, the writer can ask another party to read the message and provide feedback to the writer as to what the reader believes the message means. However, the right to confidentiality and privacy of the people involved must be observed. This basic principle applies to patients, families, students, members of the health care team—to all persons. Consequently, the nurse must be as judicious in handling written material in a confidential matter as with any other form of communication.

Electronic Communication

More and more communication is computer-based, using e-mail, chat rooms, attachments, and other electronic modes. The computer-based written record may be somewhat more transient than other written documents. For example, emails are often read and then deleted. However, remember that communication via the computer can be saved and is often retrievable even after deletion. As with any form of written communication, computer-based interaction loses nonverbal cues. Therefore, it is important for the sender to elicit feedback and/or for the receiver to ask for clarification if the meaning of the communication is not clear. Box 17-5 offers guidelines for using e-mail as an effective, time-saving communication tool.

BOX 17–4 *Anecdotal Note*

Subject: Student Precepting

Today at about 0730 (it may have been earlier, because I don't remember whether the breakfast trays had been served or not), I observed what appeared to be an animated conversation between Lucas Alfred, RN, and John Roberts, SN, a student nurse from North Hills University. I thought they might be arguing, but I couldn't tell for sure, so I decided to go over and see what the conversation was about. It really seemed like Lucas was angry because he was talking loudly and not smiling, and neither was the student smiling, and I heard Lucas say, "Well, you better stay with me because I am not going to come looking for you all day. I know how lazy students are." Well, I could just imagine how that made the student feel, so I asked, "Is there a problem?" even though it was pretty obvious that something was wrong. Lucas said, "Oh, no problem. I just hate having students, that's all. They're more trouble than they're worth." I asked Lucas, "Would you prefer that I reassign the student?" He shrugged his shoulders and walked away. Well, I don't know for sure about the student, but I really thought that was rude. I suggested to the student that I assign him to another nurse for the day. He responded, "I'd really appreciate that. He has let me know since I arrived that he didn't want to work with me." Well, I know how that would make me feel—to be a student and be treated that way.

The same group of students has been on the unit 2 days a week for the past 3 weeks (maybe a month, I'm not sure, and some of them may have been here on make-up days too), so I talked to other students who had worked with Lucas and asked them how things had been going. They said he'd acted the same way to them. We need to talk to him.

BOX 17–5 *Tips on Using E-Mail Effectively*

The subject line should be meaningful and clear and get the receiver's attention. For example: "Draft Delegation Policy Attached."

Remember, e-mail is meant to be quick; an important point or question may be lost in a long message.

When sending an e-mail with specific questions to be answered, write each question on its own individual line so it stands out clearly to the reader; questions risk getting lost if placed among long lines of text.

Use the "Reply to All" option only when necessary.

Do not overuse the high-priority option.

If a timely response is important, pick up the phone and call the person or leave a voice message (e.g., "Jane, this is Tom. I just sent you an important e-mail. I hope you can read it and respond by early afternoon. Thank you.").

When replying to a message, include enough of the original message to provide a context.

Do not write in ALL CAPITALS. This may be interpreted as shouting.

Use common courtesies such as "please" and "thank you."

Use proper grammar, spelling, and punctuation; most e-mail programs can be set up to spell-check before sending the message.

Attach files only when necessary. Do not overwhelm the receiver with many files that may not be needed.

When first establishing relationships with co-workers, colleagues, or friends, verify whether e-mail is a good way to communicate. Many people may not use or check e-mail regularly.

Do not copy or forward a message or attachment without permission.

Do not use e-mail to discuss confidential information.

Do not send personal or sensitive information by e-mail; remember, there is no such thing as a "secure" mail system; e-mail can be forwarded without your knowledge, and delicate or embarrassing messages may fall into the wrong hands.

Use the e-mail auto reply function if you are unable to respond to messages within 24 hours.

Always provide your name and contact information at the bottom of each message.

Review the message and be certain it is appropriate before clicking "Send".

COMMUNICATION STYLES

Communication occurs as a continuous transaction, with no clear-cut beginning or end. Because communication has content and relationship dimensions, problems occur when people fail to recognize the distinction between what is being said and the relationship within which it is occurring (DeVito, 1992). As previously discussed, the factors that can influence an individual's communication style are numerous and varied depending on the content and type of interaction that is occurring.

Although individuals may use various communication styles, as described in Box 17-6, there are three basic communication styles: assertive, nonassertive, and aggressive (DeVito, 1978). It is important for the nurse to understand the clear distinctions between these types of communication, with the goal of becoming adept at assertive communication.

BOX 17–6 *Communication Styles (Alder & Elmhorst, 2002; Satir, 1972)*

- Blamers—Blamers are faultfinders; they act superior, believing that no one else can do things correctly. Their tone of voice is high, shrill, and loud, because they want others to believe that they are strong.
- Computers—Computers are always correct and rarely show any emotion; they appear cool and calculated. Their voice is monotonous, and they may seem disassociated. They attempt to deal with a threat as though it is harmless, employing words to establish self-worth.
- Directors—Directors can be aggressive and competitive; they see things from their viewpoint and do not like idle chitchat.
- Distracters—Distracters say or do things that are irrelevant to the situation and seem unaware of the point of the interaction; the may become panicked as they attempt to ignore the perceived threat by behaving as though it was not really there.
- Levelors—Levelors perceive few threats to their self-esteem, and relationships tend to be free and easy. Although their communication is open and honest, levelors seem to need approval from others rather than from themselves.
- Open communicators—Open communicators express a willingness to disclose, responding spontaneously without subterfuge to the communications and the feedback of others. These individuals own their feelings and thoughts and bear responsibility for the messages that they send.
- Placaters—Placaters speak in an ingratiating way. They apologize for their actions with the goal of pleasing others at any cost.
- Provincial communicators—Provincial communicators have a tentative, open-minded attitude and a willingness to hear opposing points of view. They will change their opinions when warranted.
- Regulators—Regulators monitor, maintain, or control the speaking of others. They will shake their head to show disbelief or lean forward in their chair to show that they want to hear more.
- Relators—Relators communicate in a slow, precise manner. They are concerned with the feelings of others and do not respond well to aggressive communicators.
- Reserved communicators—Reserved individuals tend to hold back on disclosing anything that might give clues to their nature; they are more comfortable with indirect eye contact and maintaining distance between themselves and other people.
- Socializers—Socializers enjoy interaction and are quite talkative; they have a need for personal prestige and will act on intuition.
- Thinkers—Thinkers view themselves as efficient and place a high regard on thoroughness and precision. Approach thinkers with facts and data.

Assertive Communication

Assertive individuals pronounce their basic rights without violating the rights of others. They state their wants, needs, desires, and feelings using objective, direct comments. Assertiveness connotes a style of positive declaration and a persistent demonstration of confidence. To speak assertively, the person must be sure of the facts, have carefully considered the options, and exude confidence while making the observation, request, or point.

Nonassertive Communication

Nonassertive communication is characterized by timid and reserved behaviors, regardless of the specifics of the situation. Nonassertive individuals do what others tell them to do without questioning and without concern for what is best for them.

Aggressive Communication

People who claim their basic rights in ways that violate the rights and the well-being of others communicate in an aggressive manner. These individuals use commanding, dominant, superior, or loaded words and make accusations that blame or put-down others. Aggressiveness conveys dominance and implies an inclination to start quarrels or fights. Aggressive behavior often leads to conflict and seldom leads to resolution or effective communication.

Active or Passive Communication

Within the framework of assertive, nonassertive and aggressive styles, communication can also be described as active or passive. People who communicate in an active manner are participating in the conversation and are causing motion, action, or change. Passive communicators appear to be influenced or acted upon without acting in return. They use apologetic words with hidden meanings, seem disconnected, and fail to say what is meant. All of the positive communication techniques and styles that have been discussed must be used to produce assertive and active rather than nonassertive, passive, or aggressive communication.

SPECIAL INFLUENCES ON COMMUNICATION

Development of truly effective communication necessitates understanding various circumstances that influence communication. In addition to the concepts discussed up to this point, characteristics exist that might impede efficacious exchange of information. Issues such as gender differences, generational differences, cultural diversity, and dissimilarities in the professional approach of the various health care disciplines all contribute to disparate understandings and interpretations.

Communication and Gender Differences

A significant clarification must be made regarding communication between men and women. The information about gender differences resulting from socialization, although based on research and many years of observations and writings, are still generalizations and should be viewed from that perspective. Attributes described do not necessarily apply to all persons or all of the time. Nevertheless, a multitude of observations indicate that men and women solve problems, make decisions, and communicate from different perspectives based on socialization that begins shortly after birth (Cummings, 1995; Elgin, 1993; Heim, 1995). Typically, boys are taught to be tough and competitive; girls are taught to be nice and to avoid conflict.

Dr. Pat Heim (1995) suggests, "Playing team sports boys learn to compete, be aggressive, play to win, strategize, take risks, mask emotions, and focus on the goal line." Regarding girls' play, Dr. Heim comments, "Relationships are central in girls' culture and therefore they learn to negotiate differences, seek win-win solutions, and focus on what is fair for all instead of winning."

Clearly, learning to approach life on such different terms—with different rules—can lead to frustration, sometimes a sense of total defeat in the communication arena! For the most part, women work toward compromise even when it means relinquishing some of the original goal. Preserving relationships is usually of paramount importance to women. The role of peacemaker and nurturer has been a traditional expectation of women throughout the ages.

Generally, men work toward winning. Traditional role expectations of men have included provider and protector. Men learn early in life how to focus on goals and move aggressively toward accomplishment. Team sports teach men that relationships are not destroyed in the "battle" (Heim, 1995). Consequently, men have been socialized to behave assertively when such performance is needed in pursuit of the goal and then move on without loss of friendships. Women have been socialized that assertive behavior will endanger relationships and that conflict should be avoided in order to preserve friendships.

Men typically use communication as a tool to deliver information, whereas women value the process of communication itself as an important part of the relationship. Therefore in an effort to improve communication, men might try spending more time in discussion, and women might try to phrase comments more succinctly. Consider the following conversation.

> Nurse: Dr. Vernon, this is Holly Michaels, RN. I'm calling to talk to you about Mrs. Guevara. She says she's having more pain and feels a little dizzy. I've given her pain medicine as soon as I can each time. She says she's a little nauseated. Her husband's in the room, and he says she feels worse too. She did not sleep much last night and has not been able to nap today.
>
> Doctor: I have patients to see! Just give me the facts.
>
> Nurse: Okay, she has received her medication every 4 to 5 hours this shift. I do not know if she needs a higher dose or just needs the medication more frequently, or maybe we should try a different medicine.
>
> Doctor: What are her vitals? Does she have any drug allergies?
>
> Nurse: Just a second, and I'll get the chart.
>
> Doctor: Confound it, when you get your act together, call me back!
>
> Dr. Vernon slams down the phone.

Consider the many communication styles and concepts illustrated by the previous conversation. Preparedness, conciseness, contributing environmental conditions (patients waiting), and even courtesy are issues that could be more competently addressed. The fact that the conversation is occurring by telephone instead of in person also is a factor, responsible for the lack of eye contact and the lost potential for additional information through other body language. Telephone conversations are a fact of life in health care. Careful planning and preparation of what will be said will facilitate effective information exchange. In the professional setting especially, men are more prone to favor brief, concise information exchange. In the professional setting, women still tend to prefer verbal problem-solving as the situation is discussed. Knowledge of the gender differences in communication style could have altered the nurse's telephone call in the following manner.

"Dr. Vernon, this is Holly Michaels, RN, from Fairmont Genera calling about Mrs. Guevara in room 496. She has been receiving her pain medication exactly every 4 hours and continues to complain of incisional pain. She currently is complaining of slight dizziness and nausea, although she has had no emesis. Her blood pressure is 135/86; pulse 112; and respirations 24, which are higher than they have been running. Her temperature is 98.8°. She has no drug allergies. How would you like to change her orders?"

In this example, Holly has prepared the information the physician will need and communicates it in an orderly fashion.

Communication and Generational Differences

An awareness of generational differences can help facilitate communication and prevent conflict (Lancaster and Stillman, 2002; Williams and Nussbaum, 2001). Traditionalists, for whom the Great Depression and World War II were critical events, place a high premium on formality and the top-down chain of command. These individuals are more likely to write a memo to relay their thoughts or opinions and can become offended by a direct, immediate approach. Respect from others is preferred, including the use of formal titles as opposed to first names and scheduling a meeting rather than dropping by unannounced. Putting things in historical perspective is important because traditionalists are comfortable making decisions based on what worked favorably in the past.

"Baby boomers" experienced the reshaping of corporate culture. As a group, boomers are considered to be highly competitive people who are willing to sacrifice their own personal interests and needs in order to achieve success. Boomers strive for recognition and desire a personable style of communication that builds rapport. Like traditionalists, they desire a top-down organizational approach that places value on earning respect.

On the other hand, "generation Xers" (or "gen-Xers") are associated with a high divorce rate among their parents, working mothers, and the latch-key phenomenon. Their parents sacrificed for the companies and their careers, but many were then laid off during the recession of the 1980s. Gen-Xers are characterized as skeptics who value a balance in their work and personal life. Most of these individuals would choose to be rewarded with extra time off as opposed to a promotion. However, they value efficiency and may agree to working extra hours if the reason is deemed beneficial. Expectations are immediate and instantaneous, and the chosen communication pattern includes brevity and directness.

"Millennials" are the newest members of the workforce. They are highly collaborative and optimistic, and they strive for a balance between work and home life. It is important that they have a voice in organizational decision making and prefer communication that is framed in a positive manner.

As health professionals from different generations struggle to work collaboratively under stressful conditions, being aware of their various differences can certainly help improve communication and the work environment.

Communication and Cultural Diversity

Although Chapter 11 is devoted to cultural and social issues, it is important here to highlight cultural issues specific to communication. Sensitivity to cultural differences is an integral part of the nurse's responsibility. Many cultural beliefs are tightly interwoven with strong religious convictions. Societies throughout the world depend as strongly, or even more strongly, on a variety of alternative healing sources as on medical science. Some people rarely have an opportunity to interface with medical science as it is known in the "developed" countries.

The obvious difficulty is a potential language barrier. Even if the person speaks English as a second language, the preponderance of slang terms and colloquialisms can confound a literal translation. Additionally, the stress associated with illness and possible hospitalization only adds to the potential for misunderstanding and frustration. Fortunately, most communities have interpreters willing to translate in the health care setting. The variety of language interpreters (including sign language for the deaf) available even in smaller communities is surprising. Keep in mind, however, that even though a translator may ensure accuracy of the message, his or her presence creates "distance" between the nurse and the patient—and some essential aspects of the communication process may be lost in the translation.

Many forms of communication do not carry the same meanings in various cultures. In some instances, direct eye contact is to be avoided if possible. Touch, also considered a positive communication technique in Western culture, may be perceived as a serious invasion of privacy by members of other cultures. Gestures considered innocuous in one culture may represent vulgarity in another. Some cultures strictly adhere to paternalism—unless the male head of the family agrees to a procedure or treatment, the patient may refuse under any circumstance. Although many people share a sense of modesty, some cultures experience a greater feeling of violation at having to expose certain body parts than do others. The consumption of certain foods, the use of blood or blood products—the possibilities of culturally diverse practices are endless. The prudent nurse must become knowledgeable of the specific cultural practices in the region of her or his employment.

Interdisciplinary Team Communication

The interdisciplinary team is composed of a variety of disciplines, each approaching health care from the unique perspective of the theories and therapies of that individual profession. Consider the variety represented by nurses, physicians, dietitians, respiratory therapists, pharmacists, occupational therapists, physical therapists, psychologists, and social workers. Then add to the mosaic the sublevel of specialists: cardiologists, endocrinologists, oncologists, orthopedists, clinical nurse specialists, recreational therapists, nurse anesthetists, nurse practitioners, and nurse scientists. RNs with varied educational backgrounds (diploma, associate degree, bachelor or master of science in nursing) and licensed vocational nurses are often found in the same unit with similar assignments. Now add managers, administrators, unlicensed assistive personnel, clerical staff, accountants, and housekeeping personnel, to name just a few. Also consider cultural and generational differences among these health care professionals and workers. Is it any wonder that communication disasters occur?

All of the positive communication techniques must be used to clearly understand another's perception. Listening is an essential tool for determination of the intended message as seen from the unique perspective of the other discipline. Frequent clarification and a sense of "safety" are paramount as people explore the meanings that each person attributes to the situation and the discipline-specific suggested solutions. Realization that the fundamental goal of all health care professionals and of ancillary staff is to provide quality patient care should facilitate positive communication.

UNDERSTANDING AND MANAGING CONFLICT
The Nature of Conflict

A major goal of communication is to establish understanding and cooperation with others. However, much of our social environment is characterized by interactions that involve conflict, misunderstanding, and a failure to communicate. When more than one person is involved in the interaction, a potential exists for disagreement and misunderstanding. When the interaction becomes stressful, taking on a competitive, hostile, or oppositional nature, it can be classified as conflict (Mayer, 2000). Conflicts stemming from differences in goals or desires are not good or bad. The two fundamental bases for conflict are information (one person has information that another doesn't have or two individuals have different sets of information) and perception (people see things differently based on their unique belief systems). Despite the potential discomfort, disparate points of view can result in constructive behavior and positive outcomes.

Conflict, like stress, can have both beneficial and detrimental consequences to an individual. Some of the benefits that may arise from conflict include (1) recognizing talents and innovative abilities, (2) identifying an outlet for expression of aggressive urges, (3) introducing innovation and change, (4) diagnosing problems or areas of concern, and (5) establishing unity (Mayer, 2000). Harmful consequences of prolonged conflict can include a negative effect on emotional and physical well-being, an emphasis on personal welfare over that of the group, a diversion of time and energy from important goals, financial and emotional costs, and personal fatigue.

Most of us experience abundant opportunities for conflict, which may be related to the fact that we bring to our relationships an accumulation of attitudes, beliefs, opinions, and habits. Thus, conflict is normal and isn't necessarily something to avoid. Although often uncomfortable, conflict signals the presence of diverse points of view, which can spark creativity, nourish growth, and strengthen relationships. Maintaining an environment supportive of professional, clear and sensitive communication enables individuals to disagree more productively, with less hurt, and with a greater chance of resolving differences and disagreements. Characteristics of environments that support professional communication include the following:

- Empathy: Feeling what the other person is feeling and seeing the situation as the other person sees it; entails believing that the other person's feelings are valid, legitimate, and justified.
- Equality: All participants in the process are equal; respect for individual differences is apparent, and people are comfortable expressing themselves freely and openly.
- Openness: Feelings and thoughts are stated directly and honestly; no attempt is made to hide or disguise the real object of disagreement.
- Positiveness: Entails capitalizing on agreements and using them as a basis for approaching disagreements and impasses; conflict is viewed as positive and individuals involved express positive feelings for each other and the relationship.
- Supportiveness: Feelings are expressed with spontaneity rather than with strategy; requires flexibility and a willingness to change personal opinions and positions (Gibb, 1961).

Adopting these communication attitudes, as well as using the positive communication strategies previously discussed, can prevent most episodes of conflict in the workplace. However, situations are bound to arise in which the nurse will need to know how to handle a conflict situation and achieve a positive resolution.

Conflict Resolution

People's ability to connect with one another, especially during times of conflict, depends on their capacity to tune in to the subtle clues that reveal how a message is actually being received. We seldom create conflict intentionally. Rather, it occurs because we may not be aware of how our own behavior contributes to interpersonal problems. Because interpersonal communication is fragile, there may be barriers to an effectual and meaningful process. Successful resolution to conflict begins to occur when people are aware of their own and others' feelings and emotions and believe that these concerns are relevant and should be respected.

The first step in conflict resolution is to recognize how individuals manage conflict. The most common conflict resolution styles include the following:

- Avoidance: One person uses passive behaviors and withdraws from the conflict; neither person is able to pursue goals.
- Accommodation: One person puts aside his or her goals in order to satisfy the other person's desires.
- Force: One person achieves his or her own goals at the expense of the other person.
- Compromise: Both people give up something to get partial goal attainment.
- Collaboration: Both people actively try to find solutions that will satisfy them both.

Self-awareness of one's usual conflict resolution style will go far in helping to understand how one's own behavior contributes to disagreements. For example, if an individual nurse recognizes avoidance as his or her common style of dealing with conflict, then it would be important for that nurse to review the communication strategies presented in this chapter to identify specific techniques that can be used to develop a more collaborative style of conflict resolution.

The second—and very important—step in conflict resolution is active listening (Axelrod and Johnson, 2003). Although many of us are apprehensive or reticent when communicating during times of conflict, active listening can reduce the emotional charge from the situation so that both parties can deal with their differences and assist in resolving the conflict. Some excellent active listening techniques and examples are provided in Table 17-1.

Finally, the principle that underscores all successful conflict resolution is that all people involved must view their conflict as a problem to be solved mutually so that each has a sense of winning or discovering options that are acceptable to all. Although this is an easy principle to understand, it can be challenging to put into practice. If all participants can remain open, honest, and respectful of one another's positions, feelings of resentment may be minimized. Box 17-7 presents some basic strategies that can augment a professional response to conflict. The principles listed are remarkably effective in cases of conflict and will help the nurse present herself or himself as a confident and competent professional who will not react to inappropriate behavior in like form but also will not withdraw from the issues. As always, the focus should be kept on the delivery of quality patient care.

SUMMARY

In today's health care environment, where high stress levels are all too common and patient safety, quality care, and financial constraints are everyday concerns, nurses play a vital role in promoting a productive work environment in which trust and rapport among the health care team members are common and all are working towards the same goal—delivery of safe, timely, efficient, effective, and patient-centered health care. Professional, clear, and sensitive communication provides the foundation for creating such supportive, effective health care environments.

Table 17-1	Active Listening Techniques		
TECHNIQUE	**WHY DONE**	**HOW DONE**	**EXAMPLE**
Paraphrase the content of the message	Shows that you are listening, checking meaning, and interpreting the content	Restate basic ideas and facts in your own words	"What I hear you saying is that you weren't consulted" or "So, you weren't consulted about this?"
Reflect the emotion of the message	Shows understanding of how the person feels; reflects what is observed rather than what is heard; helps the other person evaluate his or her own feelings after hearing them expressed by someone else	Listen to voice tone and watch for nonverbal cues that indicate feelings; listen to what the person tells you they are feeling; state back how you perceive the feeling	"So you are angry about what happened?"
Open questioning	Results in more information and avoids any assumptions about what the other person is thinking; encourages the other person to talk	Ask questions that begin with what, how, when, and where; use questions that begin with "why" cautiously	"What happened after you spoke with her?"
Acknowledging	Conveys that you appreciate the other person's perspective; acknowledges his or her worth and actions	Acknowledge the value of the person's issues and feelings; show appreciation for his or her efforts and actions	"That must be very frustrating".
Summarize	Reviews progress; pulls together important ideas and information; establishes a foundation for further discussion	Restate the central ideas and feelings you have heard	"So basically what is most important to you is . . . "
Framing	Communicates your message in a way the other person will be more open to hearing; increases the opportunity of meeting his or her goals	Present your message in a hopeful, nonjudgmental, and open-ended way; point to common ground and away from differences	"I think it would be best to speak to your supervisor directly about these issues, because she is more directly involved with implementation than I am. What do you think about this idea?"
Reframe	Helps others see their concerns in a new light; broadens the meaning of an issue to identify needs or interests; diffuses negative feelings; establishes a focus for resolution	Recognize underlying needs; reword concerns from negative to neutral or positive, from past to future, from problem to opportunity	"It sounds as if you would like more direct communication to resolve these concerns."

Used with permission from Axelrod L, Johnson R: *Successful resolution,* Vancouver, BC, 2003, The Neutral Zone.

The first step toward developing a professional communication style is understanding the many complex and varied factors that influence the communication process, such as gender, cultural, generational, and interdisciplinary differences, each of which presents many challenges for the nurse who must strive to understand and to be understood. The second step is adopting positive communication techniques, which include developing trust, using "I" messages, establishing eye contact, keeping promises, expressing empathy, using an open

BOX 17–7 Professional Response to Verbal Conflict

- Maintain an open and empathetic tone of voice.
- Maintain eye contact (keeping cultural differences in mind). This may be difficult, but it conveys to the other party that you are confident and competent.
- Maintain an open body stance with your hands at your side or open toward the person (but not invading the other person's space). Do not cross your arms, tap your toe, wag or point your finger, or perform any body language that is commonly associated with anger.
- Do not physically back away unless you perceive you actually are in physical danger. By standing your ground, your carriage will convey the message of assurance.
- Be aware of your own values, beliefs, and cultural perspectives.
- When a conversation is obviously escalating, move to a more private location.
- Listen actively and carefully without criticizing or being defensive.
- Focus on the problem or issue, not the person(s) involved.
- Use "I" messages that state your thoughts, feelings, and beliefs in an open and clear manner.
- Use nonjudgmental, noninflammatory language such as "It seems to me . . ."
- Establish ground rules to maintain a safe environment for dialogue (e.g., only one person speaks at a time while the other listens).
- Offer explanations, but do not make excuses.
- Be redundant, summarize, and convey the same idea in more than one way.
- Try to understand the intended meaning of what other people are saying.
- Identify ideas that clarify your own issues and concerns and are helpful to identify solutions.
- Avoid unhelpful responses to conflict, such as arguing, sarcasm, moralizing, disbelief, contradiction, criticism, ridicule, and threats.
- Use metaphors and analogies as subtle ways to create and maintain rapport.
- Maintain a positive context by stating what you want and avoid stating what you don't want.
- Repeat, or play back, what you believe you are hearing.
- If you say you will take care of something, report something, or change something, do it! Then seek out the person to whom you made the commitment and report your action and the result. Little else will go as far as demonstrating that you are dependable and want to work toward a solution.

communication style, clarifying information, and being aware of body language. The third step is for each nurse to reflect on his or her use of negative communication techniques, such as blocking, false assurances, conflicting messages, logical fallacies, and cognitive distortions, which may interfere with effective relationships with patients and coworkers. Recognizing, then avoiding, the use of these negative communication techniques is essential if the nurse is to move toward a more professional communication style.

The next step in developing a professional communication style is learning to address and resolve conflict in a positive way. Role playing with trusted colleagues using the conflict resolution techniques discussed in this chapter can help the nurse become more adept at managing conflict. Finally, the nurse's professional communication style can be further developed and enhanced through ongoing study, using the various web resources suggested in Box 17-8 and elsewhere in this chapter.

Demonstrating a professional, clear, and sensitive communication style is essential to the professional nursing skill set. As the foundation for effective, supportive work environments and excellent patient care, professional communication must be one goal every nurse strives to achieve.

| BOX 17–8 | *Useful Websites Related to Communication and Conflict Resolution* |

Be effective in your communication style!
http://jenniferwebb.com/bureau/influence.html

Communication style test
http://rabbitbrush.com/personality/

Learning healthier thought patterns
www.freemindware.net

Success tips
http://www.mlmsuccesstips.com/4types.html

Avoiding and resolving conflicts
http://para.unl.edu/para/Communication/lesson5.html

Surviving and thriving with conflict
http://nsweb.nursingspectrum.com/ce/ce112.html

C R I T I C A L   T H I N K I N G   A C T I V I T I E S

1. Listen attentively to your own conversations over the course of the next few days. Focus on your use of questions. This awareness can prove valuable in improving your communication skills.
2. Make a list of the negative messages you frequently hear yourself making. Realize how these are affecting the ways in which you view your world. Assess how these messages affect your daily communication.
3. To explore your ease in sharing your ideas and speaking for yourself, complete the following sentences:
   a. "I would like to talk to you about . . . "
   b. "You and I need to discuss . . ."
   c. "I need you to . . ."
   d. "Let me clarify by saying . . ."
   e. "I want to know that . . ."
4. Dr. Blademan, whom you recently paged to report an abnormal laboratory result, approaches you and shouts angrily, "Why did you page me with that report? You know I make rounds in the evenings, and I would have been here soon." You attempt to explain that the client was symptomatic, that the abnormal laboratory result was high enough to be labeled a critical value, and that you believed prompt reporting was in the best interest of the client. You also are thinking about the fact that "in the evening" could be anytime from 6:00 p.m. to 11:00 p.m. for this particular physician. Nothing you say in defense of your decision appeases the physician, who has digressed to making general statements about the lack of consideration that nurses give doctors. What do you perceive to be the true message here? How will you respond to the physician's comments? What techniques can you use to prevent the situation from escalating? If the situation continues to escalate, what would be your next course of action?

5. You are talking with Mr. Phillips about his new diagnosis of diabetes mellitus. You state, "Mr. Phillips, I noticed that the diabetic educator was in to talk with you this morning. What did you talk about?" His response is, "Oh, she told me about the special diet . . . you know . . . no sugar and that stuff. But I'm going to tell you now that I drink sodas, and nobody is going to take those away from me!" You comment, "Have you tried diet sodas?" to which he responds, "Are you kidding? That stuff tastes like crank case oil! I'm not using any of that sweetener stuff!" The conversation continues along the same lines, indicating a lack of commitment to healthy self-regulation on his part. What will you do? It appears that Mr. Phillips is resistant to the restrictions of his new diagnosis. What additional resources can you use to help interpret his health beliefs? What techniques will you use to clarify the issues he must address?

6. Choose a partner and formulate questions related to delegation of patient care assignments. Summarize for one another the positive and negative aspects of each question. An example for phrasing each question is provided:
   a. Close-ended question (limits the answer to "yes" or "no"): "Did you . . ."
   b. Open-ended question (allows the responder total freedom in answering): "What happened when you . . ."
   c. Direct question (asks for specific information; limits answers to brief fact statements): "Which action did you . . ."
   d. Probing question (follows up on related questions to solicit additional information): "Can you tell me more about . . ."
   e. Hypothetical question (presents a theoretical situation to which the receiver responds): "What would you have done if . . ."

7. Take a few moments to write down your thoughts about constructive feedback that focuses on facts, not people; solving problems instead of placing blame; and strengthening relationships instead of being right. Why is it necessary to give constructive feedback to others? What makes it hard to give this type of feedback? What are obstacles to receiving this type of communication? Share your thoughts with the class.

8. Nonverbal communication or body language sends positive and negative signals. What message are you sending if:
   a. Someone is presenting a new idea and you are frowning?
   b. You are dressed casually at an important meeting?
   c. You are looking at other things in a room when someone is speaking to you?
   d. You keep moving closer to a person who is backing away from you?
   e. During a disagreement you start speaking loudly?

9. Questioning is an effective tool to facilitate purposeful communication and problem solving. Complete the following examples and formulate an additional question for each situation.
   a. Energize the patient's thoughts with new treatment alternatives
      "Had you considered . . . ?"
   b. Elicit the patient's feelings
      "What is happening that is making you angry?"
   c. Redirect the patient's ideas
      "Could we talk about . . . now?"
   d. Link subjects discussed in an earlier conversation
      "So, I notice your comments today are similar to . . . ?"
   e. Ask for clarification and additional information
      "When you said . . . did you mean . . . ?"

Additional resources are available on-line at: http://evolve.elsevier.com/Cherry/

http://evolve.elsevier.com

REFERENCES

Alder R, Elmhorst JM: *Communicating at work,* New York, 2002, McGraw Hill.

Axelrod L, Johnson R: *Successful resolution,* Vancouver, BC, 2003, The Neutral Zone.

Beck AA: *Love is never enough,* New York, 1988, Harper and Row.

Burley-Allen M: *Listening: the forgotten skill,* New York, 1982, Wiley.

Burns DD: *Feeling good: the new mood therapy,* New York, 1999, Avon.

Cummings SH: Attila the Hun versus Attila the hen: gender socialization of the American nurse, *Nurs Admin Q* 19(2):19-29, 1995.

DeVito JR: *Communicology: an introduction to the study of communication,* New York, 1978, Harper and Row.

DeVito JR: *The interpersonal communication book,* ed 6, New York, 1992, Harper Collins.

Elgin SH: *Genderspeak: men, women, and the gentle art of verbal self-defense,* New York, 1993, John Wiley & Sons.

Gibb, J: Defensive communication, *J Commun* 11:141-148, 1961.

Hargrave J: *Nonverbal communication.* Available on-line (http://www.janhargrave.com/index.html).

Heim P: Getting beyond "she said, he said," *Nurs Admin Q* 19(2):6-13, 1995.

Lancaster LL, Stillman D: *When generations collide,* 2002, Boston, Harvard Business.

Mayer B: *The dynamics of conflict resolution,* San Francisco, 2000, Jossey-Bass.

van Servellen G: *Communication skills for the healthcare professional: concepts and techniques,* Gaithersburg, Md, 1997, Aspen Publishers.

Satir V: *Peoplemaking,* Palo Alto, 1972, Science and Behavior.

Williams A, Nussbaum JF: *Intergenerational communication across the lifespan,* Mahwah, NJ, 2001, Lawrence Erlbaum.

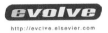
Effective Delegation and Supervision

Barbara Cherry, MSN, MBA, RN, and
Margaret Elizabeth Strong, MSN, RN, CNA

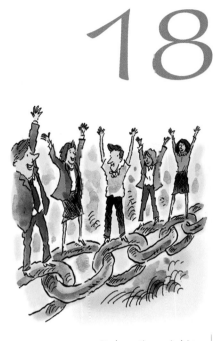

Delegation: linking together for better patient care.

VIGNETTE

Glenda Miller, RN, works on a medical-surgical floor of a small hospital. She has just received report from the 11 p.m. to 7 a.m. shift and is about to make assignments for the 7 a.m. to 3 p.m. shift. The philosophy of the unit is that the RN coordinates all patient care. Today on this 12-bed unit there are eight patients and four empty beds. The nursing staff consists of Glenda, one licensed practical nurse, 1 nursing assistant, and one unit secretary. The following members of the interdisciplinary health care team are available to help with patient care needs: one respiratory therapist, one physical therapist, one occupational therapist, one speech therapist, one medical social worker, one nutritional support nurse and one chaplain. The patients are medically complex, many tasks are required to complete their care, and they need a great deal of emotional support. The patients are described to Glenda as follows:

502: Mr. A is ventilator-dependent with an infection that requires IV antibiotics every 12 hours. He needs to be OOB in a chair BID. He has a stage I sacral decubitus ulcer and a PEG tube with bolus feedings. He is very hard of hearing, tries to speak, and becomes very frustrated and uncooperative.

503: Mrs. B is on day 2 of 40 days of antibiotics for osteomyelitis. She is dehydrated with a central line in her right subclavian and on TPN. She needs to be OOB and AMB in the room. She receives a respiratory treatment every 4 hours and needs assistance with AM care. Her daughter is at her bedside and very upset that her mother may need to go to a nursing home.

504: Mr. C is to be discharged to a rehabilitation hospital today. His chart needs to be copied. The family is at his bedside and extremely anxious.

Additional resources are available on-line at: http://evolve.elsevier.com/Cherry/

507: Mr. D has TPN infusing into his left subclavian and is on multiple antibiotics. He has vancomycin-resistant *Enterococcus* in his urine and a stasis ulcer on his left leg that requires pulsavac every day.

508: Mr. E is a ventilator-dependent patient who will start weaning this AM. He is on continuous tube feedings and IV antibiotics and needs to be assessed for a PICC line. He is to ambulate in the hall twice a day per doctor's orders. He also needs to have a pharyngeal speech evaluation scheduled.

509: Mrs. F is 3 days post-CVA and unable to move her right extremities. She has an IV infusing via her left arm. Her blood pressure is 170/100. She needs total care with personal hygiene and feeding. The doctor just ordered ROM exercises every day. Her husband is at her bedside crying continuously and asking, "What am I going to do now?"

510: Mr. G has been off the ventilator for the past 24 hours and is doing very well. He continues on respiratory treatments q4h. His TPN is being decreased, and his PEG feedings are increasing. He has accuchecks ordered q4h, a Foley to straight drainage, and IV antibiotics q12h. He needs to be out of bed, ambulating in the hall with assistance. If he stays off the ventilator, he will be discharged in 5 days. The family needs to find a nursing home for him; however, the family has not visited Mr. G since his admission 18 days ago.

511: Mr. H is a new admission that will be coming from ICU sometime during your shift.

In addition to the tasks mentioned, routine activities of taking vital signs, giving scheduled medications, updating care plans, and answering call lights must be assigned. When reviewing the tasks to be accomplished, Glenda must consider several issues in order to make safe and effective delegation and supervision decisions.

Questions to consider while reading this chapter:

1. Which of the above tasks must the RN perform as required by your state's Nursing Practice Act?
2. Which of the above tasks can be delegated to the nursing assistant?
3. How can the training, skills, and competencies of the licensed practical nurse (LPN)/licensed vocational nurse (LVN) and nursing assistant be determined?
4. How can other members of the interdisciplinary health care team contribute most effectively to meet patients' needs?

K E Y   T E R M S

Accountability In the context of delegation, accountability means bearing responsibility for both the action and inaction of the nurse and those to whom he or she delegates tasks (Fisher, 1999).

Assignment The downward or lateral transfer of both the responsibility and accountability of an activity from one individual to another. The transfer must be made to an individual of appropriate skill, knowledge, and judgment, and the assigned activity must be within the individual's scope of practice (ANA, 1997).

Competency Determination of an individual's capability to perform up to defined expectations (Joint Commission on Accreditation of Healthcare Organizations, 2000).

Delegation Transferring to a competent individual the authority to perform a selected nursing task in a selected situation; the nurse retains accountability for the delegated task (National Council of State Boards of Nursing, 1995).

Supervision The active process of directing, guiding, and influencing the outcome of an individual's performance of an activity or task (ANA, 1997).

Unlicensed assistive personnel An unlicensed individual who is trained to function in an assistive role to the RN by performing patient care activities as delegated by the nurse (ANA, 1997).

LEARNING OUTCOMES

After studying this chapter, the reader will be able to:

1. Evaluate the impact of changes in the current health care system on nurse staffing patterns and responsibilities.
2. Apply principles of delegation and supervision to specific examples of professional nursing practice.
3. Incorporate principles of delegation and supervision in professional nursing practice to ensure safe and legal patient care.

CHAPTER OVERVIEW

The delivery of patient care is the fundamental goal of every health care organization. To accomplish this goal in a cost-effective manner, teams of diverse professionals and assistants are used to deliver care. Because the RN is most often responsible for coordinating care provided by the various team members, he or she must clearly understand and be able to effectively use the management processes of delegation and supervision to ensure high-quality, safe patient care. This chapter highlights current issues that are influencing staffing patterns and delegation and supervision processes. The chapter also discusses the RN's role and responsibility in delegating to and supervising unlicensed assistive personnel (UAP) and LPNs/LVNs and provides useful guidelines for establishing a safe and effective delegation and supervision practice.

DELEGATION AND SUPERVISION IN THE HEALTH CARE SYSTEM

Several factors affecting the health care industry have influenced staffing patterns and the provision of patient care. First, the prospective payment system and reduced reimbursement from Medicare, Medicaid, and private insurance companies to health care organizations have led to cost-cutting measures and restructuring of health care systems. Second, the growing uninsured population is forcing health care organizations to provide care in the most cost-efficient manner possible. Third, the rapid advances in medical technology are causing a sharp increase in the cost of providing care. Finally, the current nursing shortage has affected staffing patterns and will continue to do so for at least the next decade. The employment of UAP such as nursing assistants, patient care technicians, and medical office assistants is one strategy used by health care facilities to increase the cost-effectiveness of providing patient care.

As the use of UAP increases, the RN is forced to delegate more tasks to a person who does not have clearly defined parameters for education, training, job responsibilities and role limitations. Therefore it is up to the RN to know the laws and regulations that govern nursing practice. It is also important that the RN work closely with nonclinical administrators and managers to make sure they understand the assessment and decision-making activities that must be performed by the RN according to state law.

There is also a growing concern that the roles and responsibilities of care providers, including RNs, LPNs/LVNs, and UAP are significantly overlapping. In some practice settings LPNs/LVNs are functioning as managers and supervisors and are performing more complex and invasive procedures. In some states UAP are trained to perform complex procedures such as venipunctures and catheter insertions. This trend has prompted many nurses, nursing organizations, and state boards of nursing to reexamine the scope of nursing practice and the nurses' delegation and supervision responsibilities.

More recently, the issue of health care errors and the RN's essential role in keeping patients safe has been brought to the nation's attention through the Institute of Medicine's (IOM) report *Keeping Patients Safe: Transforming the Work Environment of Nurses* (2003). This report very effectively highlights how nurses improve patient outcomes through the ongoing monitoring of patients' health status, coordinating care, educating patients and families, providing essential therapeutic care, and intercepting health care errors before they can adversely affect patients (IOM, 2003). RNs must learn to delegate nursing tasks safely and effectively so that they will be available to deliver these most important aspects of professional nursing care.

In support of the role of UAPs and LPNs/LVNs in delivering patient care, the National Council of State Boards of Nursing (1995) states, "there is a need and a place for competent, appropriately supervised, unlicensed assistive personnel in the delivery of affordable, quality health care. However, it must be remembered that unlicensed assistive personnel are equipped to assist—not replace—the nurse" (p. 2). As the nursing shortage continues to worsen and health care facilities continue to seek more cost-effective ways to provide care, RNs will remain in short supply. Thus it is imperative that nurses learn new ways of managing care and delegating tasks. This requires nurses to understand the importance of "nursing presence" with the patient, value what nurses know, and delegate effectively (Boucher, 1998). Benner (1984) defines *nursing presence* as focusing on the patient's responses to interventions, not on the skills used during interventions.

Because the use of UAPs and LPNs/LVNs has increased dramatically in today's health care system, the reality exists that RNs are becoming increasingly responsible for delegation and supervision. Therefore it is imperative that RNs have confidence with delegation skills and understand the legal responsibility that they assume when delegating to and supervising licensed personnel and UAPs. RNs should know what aspects of nursing and health care can be delegated and what level of supervision is required to ensure that the patient receives safe, competent, and effective care.

WHAT IS DELEGATION?

Delegation, as defined by the American Nurses Association (ANA) (1997), is "the transfer of responsibility for the performance of an activity from one individual to another while retaining accountability for the outcome" (p. 4). Although RNs can transfer the responsibility and authority for the performance of an activity, they remain accountable for the overall nursing care. The essential aspects of delegation—nursing process, task identification and transfer, communication, supervision, and accountability for outcomes—are incorporated into the following comprehensive definition of delegation:

Delegation is a legal and management concept and a process that involves assessment, planning, intervention, and evaluation in which selected nursing tasks are transferred from one person in authority to another person, involving trust, empowerment, and the responsibility and authority to perform the task. In delegation, communication is succinct, guidelines are clearly delineated in advance and progress is constantly monitored in which the person in authority remains accountable for the final outcomes (Timm, 2003).

Delegation is a two-way process in which the RN requests that a qualified staff member (UAP, LPN/LVN) perform a specific task. When a task is delegated, the delegator shares with the delegatee the ultimate responsibility and authority for the accomplishment and outcome of the task. However, the RN delegator remains accountable for the nursing care outcomes. When delegating, the RN delegator is accountable for:

- The act of delegation
- Supervising the performance of the delegated task
- Assessment and follow-up evaluation
- Any intervention or corrective actions that may be required to ensure safe and effective care

The delegatee (i.e., LPN/LVN or UAP) is accountable for:

- His or her own actions
- Accepting delegation within the parameters of his or her training and education
- Communicating the appropriate information to the delegator
- Completing the task

Delegation is a management strategy that, when used effectively, can ensure the accomplishment of cost-effective health care services.

WHAT SHOULD AND SHOULD NOT BE DELEGATED?

Unfortunately, there is no easy answer as to what can and cannot be delegated. The answer varies, depending on the (1) Nursing Practice Acts and other applicable state laws, (2) patient needs, (3) job descriptions and competencies of the UAP and LPNs/LVNs, (4) policies and procedures of the health care organization, (5) clinical situation, and (6) professional standards of nursing practice. To establish a safe, effective delegation practice, the RN must seek guidance and integrate information regarding each of these areas as discussed in the following paragraphs (Fig. 18-1).

State Nursing Practice Acts

Each state's Nursing Practice Act provides the legal authority for nursing practice, including delegation (Hutcherson, Sheets, and Williamson, 1998). However, each state's Nursing Practice Act expresses delegation criteria differently, and the criteria often are not clearly spelled out in the act, or they may be presented in various parts of the act. It is absolutely essential that every RN be familiar with his or her state Nursing Practice Act and know the delegation criteria contained within the act. Johnson (1996) has identified 10 essential elements related to delegation criteria in nursing practice acts, as follows.

1. Definition of delegation
2. Items that cannot be delegated
3. Items that cannot be routinely delegated
4. Guidelines for the RN about what can be delegated
5. Description of professional nursing practice
6. Description of LPN/LVN and unlicensed nursing assistant roles
7. Degree of supervision required
8. Guidelines for decreasing the risks associated with delegation
9. Warnings about inappropriate delegation
10. Restricted use of the word *nurse* to licensed nurses only

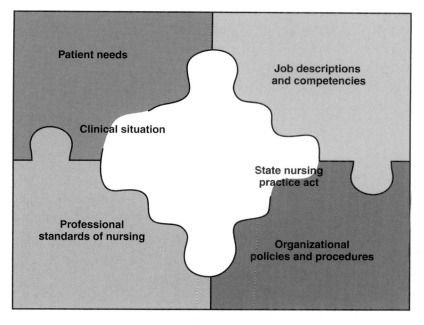

FIG. 18–1 Solving the delegation puzzle.

Although not every state's Nursing Practice Act contains all 10 elements, the RN can use this list to assist in understanding delegation criteria in his or her own Nursing Practice Act and to apply the information to enhance delegation activities. Box 18-1 presents policies common to many nursing practice acts.

If the Nursing Practice Act does not provide clear direction regarding delegation, the state board of nursing may be able to offer guidance. The board of nursing may have developed definitions, rulings, advisory opinions, or interpretations of the law to provide guidance regarding delegation activities. Many state boards of nursing may also have practical tools available such as delegation decision trees or delegation checklists. Fig. 18-2 is a delegation decision tree recommended by the National Council of State Boards of Nursing and provides an excellent framework for making delegation decisions.

Most states also have a practice act to govern practice by LPNs/LVNs. Because the practice of LPNs/LVNs varies significantly from state to state, RNs should know the LPN/LVN practice act in the state in which they practice and understand the LPN/LVN's legal scope of practice. State law generally does not define practice by UAP, although such practice should be governed by the health care organization's standards.

Patient Needs

When deciding to delegate, the RN must remember that tasks can be delegated, but nursing practice cannot. The functions of assessment, evaluation, and nursing judgment cannot be delegated. Generally, the more stable the patient, the more likely delegation is to be safe. However, it also is important to remember that many tasks that can be delegated may also carry with them a nursing responsibility. Taking vital signs on a physiologically stable,

| BOX 18–1 | Policies Common to Many State Nursing Practice Acts |

- Only nursing tasks can be delegated, not nursing practice.
- The RN must perform the patient assessment to determine what can be delegated.
- The LPN/LVN and UAP do not practice professional nursing.
- The RN can delegate only what is within the scope of nursing practice.
- The LPN/LVN works under the direction and supervision of the RN.
- The RN delegates based on the knowledge and skill of the person selected to perform the tasks.
- The RN determines the competency of the person to whom he or she delegates.
- The RN cannot delegate an activity that requires the RN's professional skill and knowledge.
- The RN is accountable and responsible for the delegated task.
- The RN must evaluate patient outcomes resulting from the delegated activity.
- Health care facilities can develop specific delegation protocols, provided they meet the state board delegation guidelines.
- Delegation requires critical thinking by the RN.

From Johnson SH: Teaching nursing delegation: analyzing nurse practice acts, *J Cont Educ Nurs* 27(2):52-58, 1996.

post-CVA patient could be delegated to UAP, but the task presents an opportunity for the RN to assess the patient's cognitive functioning. In the vignette presented at the opening of this chapter, Glenda cannot delegate any care on the newly admitted patient until the nursing assessment is complete and the plan of care is developed.

Job Descriptions and Competencies

The RN who is delegating also has the responsibility of knowing the background, skill level, training received, and job requirements of each person to whom tasks are delegated. The job description provides important information about what a staff member is allowed to do and delineates the specific tasks, duties, and responsibilities required of the person as a condition of employment. Job descriptions generally comply with state laws and the health care organization's standards of care. However, in all cases, legal requirements related to delegation supersede any organizational requirement or policy. The RN should be aware of what type of education and training the person received to function as described in the job description. The RN should also know what kind of orientation is provided to new employees and be part of the orientation process. In the opening vignette, the LPN's job description most likely would include duties such as "perform dressing changes" and "administer oral medications," but Glenda also should know the LPN's knowledge and skill level for the patient population being cared for.

In addition to requiring job descriptions for care providers, health care organizations also require employees to demonstrate that they are competent to perform certain technical procedures and to apply specific knowledge to safely care for patients. Written documentation of those skills and knowledge for which the employee has demonstrated competency is maintained in the employee's personnel file. Most health care organizations require employees to undergo annual competency training for aspects of care unique to the population of patients generally being cared for. Box 18-2 provides an example of annual competencies to

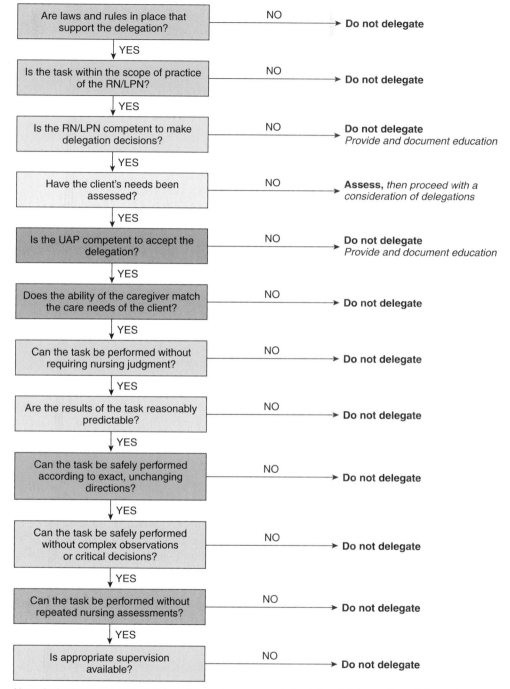

Note: Authority to delegate varies, so licensed nurses must check the statutes and regulations of the jurisdiction. RNs may need to delegate to the LPN the authority to delegate to the UAP.

FIG. 18–2 **Delegation decision-making tree.** (Used with permission from the National Council of State Boards of Nursing, 1997.)

<table>
<tr><td colspan="2">BOX 18–2 Annual Competencies to Be Demonstrated by RNs and LVNs in a Family Practice Ambulatory Care Clinic</td></tr>
</table>

Safety rules and regulations
HIPPA policies and procedures
Patient safety goals
Infection control
Telephone triage
Glucose testing

Patient education and health literacy
Medication management
Reporting abuse and neglect
Documentation in the medical record
Handling emergencies in the outpatient setting

be demonstrated by nurses in a family practice ambulatory care clinic. Various regulatory and accrediting agencies such as the Joint Commission on Accreditation of Healthcare Organizations (JCAHO) require written documentation of staff competencies. It is important for the RN to be aware of the documented competencies for all staff members whom he or she supervises.

Organizational Policies and Procedures

When delegating, the RN should comply with the specific skill requirements designated in the organization's written policies and procedures, which usually describe the supervision required for a specific task and how problems or incidents should be reported and documented. Again, it is important for the nurse to remember that the legal requirements related to delegation supersede any organizational requirement or policy. The RN should also know the organization's general standards of care, such as infection control, and ensure that the delegatee has the necessary knowledge and skills to comply with the standards. In the previous vignette Glenda should be aware of the hospital's policy regarding the orientation process. All the clinical staff members should have received training about the unit's infection control, emergency, and safety procedures.

Clinical Situation

Each delegation opportunity presents the RN with a variety of considerations, including the delegatee's current workload and the complexity of the task in relationship to the patient. Does the staff member realistically have time to accomplish the task? Is the staff member familiar with characteristics of the patient population (i.e., pediatrics or geriatrics) and with the task to be performed? Is the RN able to provide the appropriate level of supervision? Other considerations include the availability of resources such as supplies and equipment.

Professional Standards of Nursing Practice

Professional standards of nursing practice as established by professional nursing organizations exist to guide the RN in providing patient care. According to the ANA, "A standard is a model of established practice which has general recognition and acceptance among registered professional nurses and is commonly accepted as correct. Standards of practice are agreed-on levels of competence as determined by the ANA and specialty nursing organizations" (1996). To practice safe delegation, the RN should be familiar with the standards of practice outlined in the ANA's *Nursing Scope and Standards of Practice* (2004) and with the standards for any specialty area in which the RN practices. (Refer to Appendix A on the EVOLVE website for a list of most of the specialty nursing organizations in the United States.)

The ANA has addressed delegation directly in its position statement *Registered Nurse Utilization of Unlicensed Assistive Personnel* (1997). As an accepted standard of care, the RN should use professional judgment to determine activities that are appropriate to delegate based on the concept of providing safe and effective patient care and protecting the public. In delegation the RN will consider the following:

- Assessment of the patient condition
- Capabilities of the nursing and assistive staff
- Complexity of the task to be delegated
- Amount of clinical oversight (supervision) the RN will be able to provide
- Staff workload

The RN cannot delegate activities that include the core of the nursing process and require specialized knowledge, judgment, and/or skill (ANA, 1996).

The ANA (1997) has also delineated activities that *can* be delegated by the nurse. The RN may delegate direct or indirect patient care activities. Direct-care activities assist the patient to meet basic human needs and include activities related to feeding, drinking, positioning, ambulating, grooming, toileting, dressing, and socializing. They may involve the collecting, reporting, and documenting of data related to these activities. The patient-related data are reported to the RN, who uses the information to make clinical judgments about patient care. Indirect care activities that may be delegated focus on maintaining a clean, safe, efficient environment in which to practice nursing. Indirect care activities, which only incidentally involve patient contact, include activities involved in housekeeping, transporting, record keeping, stocking, and maintaining supplies. Activities that the nurse may not delegate include the following:

- Initial nursing assessment and any subsequent assessment that requires professional nursing knowledge, judgment, and skill
- Determination of nursing diagnoses, establishment of nursing care goals, development of the nursing plan of care, and evaluation of the patient's progress with the nursing plan of care
- Any nursing intervention that requires professional knowledge, judgment, and skill (ANA, 1996)

Box 18-3 presents a list of questions to assist the nurse in making delegation decisions.

DEVELOPING SAFE DELEGATION PRACTICES

For the RN to make safe, effective delegation decisions and develop a sound delegation practice, he or she must have a strong foundation of knowledge related to the legal criteria and standards of practice governing delegation decisions. In addition to having a good understanding of what should and should not be delegated based on the previous discussion, the RN also must know the patient, the staff members to whom he or she is delegating, and the tasks to be performed. The RN must provide for effective outcomes by clearly communicating expectations, supporting and appropriately supervising the delegatee, evaluating the outcomes, and reassessing the patient after the delegated task is completed. Following is a brief discussion about these essential requirements for safe and effective delegation.

BOX 18–3 *Questions to Guide Delegation Decision Making*

A. State Nursing Practice Act
   1. Is the task within the RN's scope of practice?
   2. Does the Nursing Practice Act address delegation of the task?
   3. Does the task to be delegated require the exercising of nursing judgment?
   4. Is the RN delegator willing to accept accountability for the performance of the delegated task?
B. Job description and competencies
   1. Does the RN delegator understand the nature of the task and have the knowledge, skills, and competency required to perform the task?
   2. Does the delegatee have the appropriate education, training, skills, and experience to perform the task?
   3. Is there documented or demonstrated evidence that the delegatee is competent to perform the task?
   4. Does the delegatee perform the task on a routine basis?
   5. Is the delegatee familiar with the patient population?
C. Organizational policies and procedures
   1. What skill level and level of supervision are required for the task as stated in the procedure manual?
   2. What is the policy or procedure for documenting tasks and reporting results, observations, problems, or unusual incidents?
   3. Does the delegatee have the necessary knowledge and skills to comply with general standards of care such as infection control?
D. Clinical situation and task
   1. Is adequate supervision by the delegator available?
   2. Are adequate resources available, including supplies and equipment, to the delegatee?
   3. What is the delegatee's current workload? Does the person realistically have time to perform the task?
   4. How complex is the task? Does it frequently reoccur in the daily care of patients? Does it follow a standard and unchanging procedure?
E. Patient needs
   1. Has the nursing assessment and plan of care been completed by the RN?
   2. What is the patient's clinical, physiologic, emotional, cognitive, and spiritual status?
   3. Is the patient's condition considered stable?
   4. What is the potential for change in the patient's condition as a result of the delegated task?
   5. Can the patient's safety be maintained with delegated care?
F. Professional Standards of Nursing Practice
   1. What specific standards of nursing practice apply to the specific situation?
   2. Does the delegated task include health counseling, teaching, or other activities that require specialized nursing knowledge, skill, or judgment?

Know the Patient

A nursing assessment must be completed before delegation—know the level of care required by the patient, considering the clinical, physiologic, emotional, cognitive, and spiritual status. Is the patient's condition considered stable? Generally, the more stable the patient, the more likely delegation is to be safe. What is the potential for change in the patient's condition as a result of the delegated task? If there is moderate-to-high risk that the task will result in a change in the patient's condition, delegation should not be considered. Can the patient's safety be maintained with delegated care? The answer to this question must be a firm "Yes" for delegation to be considered.

Know the Staff Member

Before the task is delegated, the delegatee must have the skills and knowledge necessary to perform it, as evidenced by the person's job description, training program, and documented competencies. Experience and past job performance should also be considerations. Is the staff member knowledgeable and trained to perform the task? Does the staff member perform the task on a routine basis? Select the right person for the right task. It is very helpful for the RN to be involved in development of job descriptions, training programs, and competency documentation for UAPs and LPNs/LVNs.

Know the Task(s) to be Delegated

The RN delegator must be competent and skilled in performing any task he or she is considering delegating, and the task must be in the RN's scope of practice. Routine, standardized tasks that are performed according to a standard and unchanging procedure and have predictable outcomes are the safest to delegate. These routine tasks are most likely to have been documented in the staff member's competencies and may require fewer directions and less supervision. Complex tasks or activities that pose high risk for patient complications or unpredictable outcomes should be examined closely before delegation is considered.

Explain the Task and Expected Outcomes

The RN should explain the delegated task, what must be done, and the expected outcomes. If necessary, outline the task in writing. Failure to effectively communicate what is expected may result in unsatisfactory performance, errors, and possible harm to the patient. Directions should be provided in a clear, concise manner. Demonstration and return demonstration by the delegatee or other inservice education may be required. The delegated task is acceptable only when the staff member understands the task and is adequately prepared to carry it out.

Expect Responsible Action From the Delegatee

When the staff member accepts and understands the task, he or she should then be allowed to perform the task. The staff member becomes responsible for his or her own actions and is obligated to complete the task as mutually agreed. The RN should provide appropriate supervision but should not intervene in task performance unless assistance is requested or an unsafe situation is recognized. Interfering with the delegatee's task will negate his or her responsibility and obligation. The RN should expect responsible actions, give authority, and retain accountability.

Assess and Supervise Job Performance

Supervising job performance provides a mechanism for feedback and control. Job performance is assessed by making frequent rounds, observing, and communicating (ask about progress and determine whether there are any questions or concerns). Determine the appropriate level of supervision. The RN should be available to the delegatee if there are any questions or unexpected problems. Supervise in a positive and supportive manner to reassure the staff member that his or her work is important and appreciated. Intervene immediately if the task is not being performed in a safe and appropriate manner. Poor performance must be documented and reported to the nurse manager. Never ignore poor performance! When a mistake is made, use it as a learning opportunity for the staff member involved.

Evaluate and Follow-Up

Once the task is complete, evaluate the staff member's performance and reassess the patient to ensure that the expected outcomes were achieved. Follow up with any interventions that may be required based on the patient's care outcomes or the delegatee's job performance. Review and document the skills that were learned. Appropriate evaluation and follow-up will ensure a positive outcome for both patient and staff member. Box 18-4 presents some important steps to remember after the decision to delegate has been made.

High-Risk Delegation

The RN often expresses concern about legal liability—"putting my license on the line" —when delegating to UAPs and LPNs/LVNs. How does the RN know whether he or she might be at risk when delegating tasks to the UAP or LPN/LVN? The RN may be at risk if the (ANA, 1996):

- Delegated task can be performed only by the RN according to law, organizational policies and procedures, or professional standards of nursing practice.
- Delegated task could involve substantial risk or harm to a patient.
- RN knowingly delegates a task to a person who has not had the appropriate training or orientation.
- RN fails to adequately supervise the delegated activity and does not evaluate the delegated action by reassessing the patient.

RNs can avoid being placed into unsafe, risky delegation situations by adhering to the safe delegation practices recommended in this chapter. Box 18-5 presents a case study demonstrating excellence in delegation practice in a home health setting.

BOX 18–4 *From Deciding to Delegate to Actual Delegating: Steps to Remember*

A. Communicate effectively.
   1. The delegatee accepts the delegation and accountability for carrying out the task correctly.
   2. The RN delegator provides clear directions to the delegatee, including what specific task is to be performed, for whom is the task to be done, when is the task to be done, how is the task to be performed, what data are to be collected, and any patient-specific instructions.
   3. The RN delegator clearly communicates expected outcomes and timelines for reporting results.
B. Provide appropriate supervision.
   1. Monitor performance to ensure compliance with established standards of practice, policies, and procedures.
   2. Obtain and provide feedback.
   3. Intervene if necessary.
   4. Ensure proper documentation.
C. Evaluate and reassess.
   1. Reassess the patient.
   2. Evaluate the performance of the task and the delegatee's experience.
   3. Reassess and adjust the overall plan of care as needed.

BOX 18–5 *Excellence in Delegation Practice*

Amy Laurence, RN, works for a home health care agency. Amy manages a caseload of 35 patients and makes between eight and ten skilled nursing visits a day. Several of Amy's patients need assistance with activities of daily living such as personal hygiene and mobility. Amy assigns these tasks to the home health aides (HHA) that she has worked with over the last 6 months. From her ongoing evaluation of patient outcomes and supervision of these aides, she knows they are skilled and proficient in performing their assigned tasks.

Five of Amy's patients are newly diagnosed with diabetes and need extensive assistance with monitoring blood glucose levels and administering insulin. The home health agency where Amy works has recently adopted a "Diabetic Delegation Policy." This policy allows HHAs that have been specifically trained and certified to perform glucose testing and give insulin from prefilled, labeled syringes. Amy actively participates in the training classes to certify HHAs in diabetic care.

In caring for her patients with diabetes, Amy does extensive diabetic teaching with each of her patients and sees them weekly to assess their learning, monitor their physiologic status, evaluate and adjust their individualized plans of care and provide ongoing education and support as needed. During the weekly visits, Amy fills and labels the exact number of insulin syringes with the correct doses of insulin to last the week. Amy is then able to delegate the daily insulin administration and glucose monitoring to the HHAs certified in diabetic care. During the initial delegation process, Amy makes supervisory visits to each patient's home to ensure that the HHA is performing the tasks correctly and has been carrying them out according to the patient's plan of care. In order to provide appropriate supervision of these delegated tasks, Amy plans her weekly skilled nursing visits to coincide with the HHA's daily visit. During these visits, Amy observes each HHA perform the glucose testing and insulin administration and reinforces any specific training needed. Following these supervisory visits Amy is confident that the HHAs are competent to perform the delegated tasks.

In this case, Amy is following all of the criteria essential for safe delegation. She is adhering to the agency's policy, which also is in line with the State Board of Nursing rules for delegation in a home setting. She has actively participated in the training programs for the HHAs and provided clear direction during the initial delegation process. Amy provides ongoing patient assessment, care evaluation and supervision of the HHAs. In performing appropriate delegation, Amy is able to focus her energy on skilled nursing services, such as providing patient education, assessing and monitoring patients' physiologic condition, and coordinating the care for the interdisciplinary home health team.

Delegation and the Nursing Process

Understanding safe delegation practices may seem overwhelming for the novice nurse, although the components of the delegation process become familiar when compared with the nursing process. After assessing the patient and planning the care, the RN identifies tasks that someone else can perform. Implementing the plan of care includes assigning and supervising task performance. Finally, evaluating the delegatee's performance, planned outcomes, and patient response completes the process.

Another method to simplify the delegation process has been recommended by the National Council of State Boards of Nursing (1995) and is referred to as the "Five Rights of Delegation":

1. *The right task*: Delegated tasks must conform to the established guidelines.
2. *The right circumstances*: Delegate tasks that do not require independent nursing judgment.
3. *The right person*: Delegate to someone who is qualified and competent.
4. *The right direction and communication*: Give clear explanation about the task and expected outcomes and indicate when the delegatee should report back to the RN.

5. *The right supervision and evaluation*: Invite feedback to assess how the process is working and how to improve the process. Also evaluate the patient's outcomes and results of the tasks.

Box 18-6 provides a list of on-line resources related to delegation and supervision.

SUPERVISION

Supervision is defined by the ANA (1997) as "the active process of directing, guiding and influencing the outcome of an individual's performance of an activity" (p. 20). Supervision may be categorized as on-site, in which the nurse is physically present or immediately available while the activity is being performed, or off-site, in which the nurse has the ability to provide direction through various means of written, verbal, and electronic communication (ANA, 1997). On-site supervision generally occurs in the acute care or ambulatory care settings where the RN is immediately available. Off-site supervision may occur in home health practice, community settings, and long-term care facilities.

As a result of the rapidly increasing use of telecommunication technologies, the distinction between on-site and off-site supervision has become unclear. Some operational guidelines of supervision are (ANA, 1996):

1. *Who is in control of the activity?* If the nurse is responsible, he or she should incorporate measures to determine whether an activity or task has been completed to meet the expectations.
2. *How should controls be instituted?* Controls must be in place that allow the person delegating an activity or task to stop the task when inappropriately done, review the measures taken, and take back control of the task.

The necessary frequency of periodic instruction dictates the level of supervision required. Hansten and Washburn (1998) have identified three levels of supervision based on the task delegated and the education, experience, competency, and working relationship of the people involved.

1. *Unsupervised*: One RN is working with another RN in a collegial relationship, and neither RN is in the position of supervising the other. Each RN is responsible and

accountable for his or her own practice. However, the RN in a supervisory or management position (e.g., team leader, charge nurse, nurse manager) as defined by the health care organization will be in a position to supervise other RNs.

2. *Initial direction/periodic inspection*: The RN supervises a licensed or unlicensed caregiver, knows the person's training and competencies, and has developed a working relationship with the staff member. For example, the RN has been working with the nursing assistant for 6 months and is comfortable in giving initial directions to ambulate two new postoperative patients and following up with the assistant once during the shift.

3. *Continuous supervision*: The RN has determined that the delegatee will need frequent to continual support and assistance. This level of supervision is required when the working relationship is new, the task is complex, or the delegatee is inexperienced or has not demonstrated an acceptable level of competence.

It is absolutely essential that the RN understands and provides the appropriate level of supervision whenever tasks are delegated.

ASSIGNING VERSUS DELEGATING

Assigning tasks is not the same as delegating tasks. Assignment, as defined by ANA, is "the downward or lateral transfer of both the responsibility and accountability of an activity from one individual to another" (1997, p. 4). An assignment designates those activities that a staff member is responsible for performing as a condition of employment and is consistent with the staff member's job position and description, legal scope of practice, and training and educational background. The staff member—RN, LPN/LVN, or UAP—assumes responsibility and is accountable for completing the assignment.

Assignment Considerations

Assigning groups of patients to various care providers, including UAP and LPNs/ LVNs, is not appropriate. For example, UAP cannot be assigned to a patient or group of patients but rather should be assigned to an RN. Typical assignments for UAP would include passing trays, assisting with transfers, transporting patients, and stocking supplies. The LPN/LVN may be assigned specific patients for whom to perform care, but the RN remains responsible for all nursing practice activities, including patient assessment, care planning, and patient teaching.

The RN is also responsible for assignments made to personnel in the clinical setting. Several factors should be considered when making assignments.

1. *Patient's physiologic status and complexity of care*: Are vital signs unstable? Is the patient's condition changing rapidly? Does the patient have multisystem involvement? Does the patient need extensive health education? Does the patient need extensive emotional support? What technology is involved in the care (e.g., cardiac monitor, intravenous pump, and patient-controlled analgesic pump)? Patients with more unstable physiologic status or complex care requirements need a higher level of skilled care.

2. *Infection control*: To what extent are isolation procedures required? Which patients could be adversely affected as a result of cross-contamination? For example, a new patient is admitted with a history of night sweats and chronic cough. The results of a sputum culture are pending. Another patient on the unit was admitted with complications resulting from chemotherapy. The same caregiver should not be assigned to a potentially infectious patient and an immunosuppressed patient.

3. *Degree of supervision*: What level of supervision, direct or indirect, is required based on the staff member's education, experience, skill level, and competence? Is the appropriate supervision available? The "on-call" RN who works an occasional weekend may require more supervision than the LPN who has worked in the unit full-time and has demonstrated competence in caring for the population of patients on the unit.

Note that the most experienced skilled staff members should not be exclusively assigned to the most complex, difficult cases. Assignments should be used as a staff development tool. Assigning a less experienced nurse to a more complex patient, but at the same time increasing the level of supervision, increases that nurse's skill level, competence, and confidence while maintaining safe, effective patient care.

Working With Interdisciplinary Health Care Team Members

Other health professionals who are members of the interdisciplinary health care team, including respiratory therapists, physical therapists, occupational therapists, speech therapists, nutritionists, medical social workers, and chaplains, are very valuable in helping meet patient care needs. In the vignette Glenda will need to coordinate the efforts of each of the interdisciplinary team members available to her unit to accomplish the many and varied tasks needed by the patients for whom she is responsible and accountable.

The RN must be knowledgeable about the scope of practice and training background of the interdisciplinary team members in order to ensure the very best care for patients. The RN also needs to understand how the work is delegated or assigned to the team members and where they fit in the organizational structure of the unit. In some organizations some or all of the interdisciplinary team members report to the RN, and it is the RN who is responsible for assigning and delegating patient care tasks to the team members. In other organizations

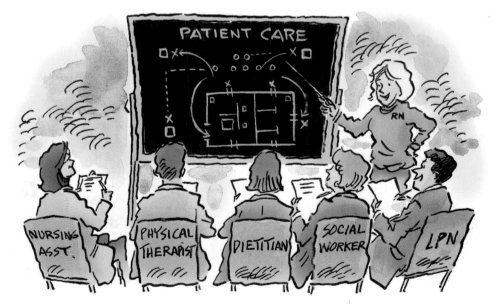

The nurse is responsible for coordinating the efforts of the interdisciplinary team.

the interdisciplinary team members report to supervisors in their individual disciplines and work in a collaborative manner with the RN to provide patient care based on their individual legal scope of practice, knowledge, and experience.

In the opening vignette the interdisciplinary team members do not report directly to Glenda but to a supervisor in their respective disciplines. However, each of the team members is available and willing to work collaboratively with Glenda to meet the needs of the patients on the unit. For example, the respiratory therapist monitors all patients on ventilators and assists in the weaning process. The medical social worker provides valuable assistance to identify family support and assists with nursing home placement for Mr. G. The speech therapist can work on communication techniques with Mr. A, the ventilator-dependent patient who becomes very frustrated when he tries to speak.

BUILDING DELEGATION AND SUPERVISION SKILLS

Effective delegation is an underlying quality for the success of working with others efficiently and cost-effectively. Delegating can be very difficult, especially for the novice nurse. Some of the struggles the nurse has are the fear of being disliked, losing control, taking risks, making mistakes, lack of confidence, and lack of knowledge of the delegation process itself. Because delegation and supervision involve interactions between two people, the RN needs to develop strong interpersonal skills and a supportive work environment to guarantee an effective delegation situation. Following are management skills RNs need to develop to become proficient at delegation and supervision.

Communicate Effectively

Clear communication is the key to successful delegation. The first step toward effective communication is for the RN to know exactly what needs to be done and what outcomes are expected. What is the specific task to be done? For whom is the task to be done? When is the task to be done? How is the task to be performed? What is the expected outcome? What feedback is expected? Why does the task need to be done in a certain way?

Maintaining self-control and confidence is an important communication skill. New RNs often have expressed concern about delegating to more seasoned LPNs/LVNs or UAP. "I have been working here for 12 years, and I do not need you telling me what to do" might be a typical response directed to the new RN. The RN's correct response is to maintain composure and confidence and remain positive. "I appreciate your experience and knowledge, but I need you to . . . (describe the task clearly)."

It also is important to listen carefully to the delegatee's response. Did the delegatee appear to listen and understand the directions? Did he or she appear to be hesitant to accept the task? Angry? Uninterested? Frustrated? If a delegation action elicits a negative response from the delegatee, ask for feedback using open-ended, nonthreatening statements, such as, "You seem unsure about performing this task." Always provide an opportunity for the delegatee to ask questions. The positive communication techniques discussed in Chapter 17 provide additional guidelines for the reader to enhance delegation skills.

Create an Environment of Trust and Cooperation

Staff members will report problems more quickly if they know that the reaction from the supervisor will be nonthreatening and nonjudgmental. When mistakes occur, the person should not be blamed or criticized, but rather the supervisor should look for root causes such as inadequate training or an overly heavy workload. Encourage staff members to report and discuss problems as a method of improving patient care and maintaining a helpful, supportive attitude. Just as the RN establishes trust and rapport with patients, he or she should strive for the same type of supportive relationships with staff members.

Create an Environment of Teaching and Learning

Inadequate training is a common cause for poor performance in the work setting. RNs should identify the learning needs of the staff members with whom they work and either directly or indirectly provide educational programs aimed at building skills and competencies. Parkman (1996) has identified the following areas in which UAP need training and skill development:

- Basic care procedures, including vital sign measurement, transfer and body mechanics, infection control procedures, basic emergency procedures, privacy and confidentiality, and documenting care activities
- Communication skills, including greeting patients and families, handling complaints, resolving conflicts, and reporting to the supervisor
- Decision-making skills, including prioritizing tasks and deciding when and what to report
- Critical thinking skills, including recognizing abnormal vital signs, identifying risks to patient safety, and reporting appropriately to the RN

By creating an environment that encourages teaching and learning, the RN will enhance the quality of care in the nursing unit. The RN should be willing to teach and demonstrate how to perform a task rather than merely telling how it should be done. The RN should strive to earn a reputation for exceptional training and mentoring, involving everyone on the health care team, including LPNs/LVNs and UAP, in educational and staff development activities.

Promote Patient Satisfaction

Patients need and want to know who their caregivers are and what qualifications they have. In this day, when a variety of nursing apparel is acceptable in the clinical setting, it often is difficult to tell the RN from the housekeeper. The RN is responsible for describing the health care team to the patient. For example, "Hello, my name is Marjorie Will. I am a registered nurse, and I will be responsible for your care until 11 p.m. tonight. Mary James, a nursing assistant, is working with me and will be in to take your vital signs and help with your meal tray. Also John Howle, the physical therapist, will be in to work with you on your knee exercises. Please call me if you have any questions."

Provide Feedback and Follow-Up Evaluation

The delegation process is not complete until the RN reassesses the patient and adjusts the plan of care as indicated. The RN also should provide honest feedback to the delegatee about his or her performance. An easy, although often overlooked, delegation skill is to praise good performance. Often more difficult for the RN, and sometimes ignored, is the duty to address poor job performance.

The RN should tell the staff member about mistakes in a supportive manner—in private—with a focus on "learning from mistakes." However, if the LPN/LVN or UAP performs in an inappropriate, unsafe, or incompetent manner, the RN must intervene immediately and stop the unsafe activity, document the facts of the performance, and report to the nurse manager or supervisor. In addition, the RN should request additional training or other appropriate action for the staff member to ensure that patient safety is protected. The RN has a professional responsibility to intervene appropriately when poor performance is observed.

SUMMARY

Effective delegation and supervision are essential skills for the professional nurse in any practice role or setting, especially with the increased use of UAP to provide health care services. Although there is no definitive list of what can and cannot be delegated, the RN is guided to safe, effective delegation and supervision through an assessment of (1) the clinical situation; (2) patient needs; (3) the job descriptions and competencies of the assistive and vocational/practical nursing personnel; (4) the health care organization's policies and procedures; (5) nursing practice acts and other regulations and applicable state laws; and (6) professional standards of nursing practice. This chapter presents information to assist the RN with delegation decisions and also discusses effective delegation and supervision skills, including communicating effectively, creating an environment of trust and cooperation, creating an environment of teaching and learning, promoting customer or patient satisfaction, and providing feedback and follow-up evaluation. These activities and skills provide the tools the RN needs to develop a safe and legal delegation practice.

CRITICAL THINKING ACTIVITIES

1. Review the tasks to be accomplished that are described in the opening vignette. Analyze the factors that Glenda should consider when deciding which tasks can and cannot be delegated. Develop a plan for delegating these activities and explain the rationale for each delegation decision.
2. Analyze the delegation criteria contained in your state's Nursing Practice Act. Explain how delegation practices in a selected clinical site are influenced by the delegation criteria in the Nursing Practice Act.
3. Request to view copies of job descriptions for RNs and LVNs/LPNs and for UAP at a selected clinical site. Compare and contrast the responsibilities and duties described in each job description and analyze how delegation decisions would be influenced by information contained in the job descriptions.
4. Compare and contrast the levels of supervision you have received as a student. How have these supervision levels changed as you progressed from a beginning to a senior nursing student?
5. Consider this scenario and answer the questions that follow: One registered nurse is assigned to care for six medical-surgical patients, with the help of one nursing assistant. The tasks that need to be performed include giving a bed bath, setting up a tray for eating, feeding a patient, Foley catheter insertion, bolus PEG feeding, administering IV antibiotics, getting a patient out of bed and into a chair, teaching a family about dressing changes, performing accuchecks on a patient ever 4 hours with sliding scale insulin, and providing frequent skin care and linen changes for a patient who is incontinent of stool.
   a. Which tasks can be done by the nursing assistant?
   b. What additional information does the RN need to make the best delegation decision?
   c. When the RN delegates the tasks, who is accountable for the nursing care outcomes?
   d. Once the RN delegates the tasks, does the RN need to follow-up? If so, why and how?
6. Consider this scenario and answer the questions that follow: You arrive at work today and are told that one of the RNs scheduled to work has called in sick. The staffing office has called and said they have an extra nurse on another unit who is willing to work with you today. The only issue is that this RN has never worked on a medical-surgical unit in your hospital. The RN has always worked in labor and delivery.

a. What standard care do patients require that the reassigned nurse could perform safely?

b. What type and amount of supervision will the reassigned nurse need?

c. Would safer patient care be provided by working with one less nurse or with a nurse who has never worked on your unit? Explain your answer.

7. Consider this scenario and answer the questions that follow: Today you are the charge nurse, and part of your responsibility is to make patient assignments. There are 18 patients on the unit as well as 2 RNs, 1 LPN, and 3 nursing assistants. You make the following assignments: 1 charge nurse will give the IV medications for the LPN and help as needed; 2 RNs will take 6 patients; 1 LPN will take 6 patients, and 3 nursing assistants will each take 6 patients.

a. Should the nursing assistants be assigned to patients or should they be assigned to a nurse? Why?

b. When assigning patients to the RNs, should you consider the patient's physiologic status and complexity of care? Give examples of patients with more unstable physiologic status or complex care requirements.

c. When making assignments, how should you consider infection control issues? Would you assign one nurse an infectious patient and an immunosuppressed patient?

d. When assigning patients to the LPN, would you consider the level of supervision required by the LPN? Explain.

8. You are a novice nurse, and today you are assigned to care for 6 patients and to supervise a nursing assistant who has worked on this unit for 15 years. At the beginning of the shift you approach the nursing assistant in order to plan the day so that the patients receive the care they need. The nursing assistant tells you she has worked on this unit for 15 years and does not need you to tell her what she is to do today. What is your response? How do you plan to communicate your needs and the patients' needs? How will you create an environment of trust and cooperation and also promote patient satisfaction?

Additional resources are available on-line at: http://evolve.elsevier.com/Cherry/

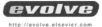

http://evolve.elsevier.com

REFERENCES

American Nurses Association: *Nursing: scope and standards of practice,* Washington, DC, 2004, ANA.

American Nurses Association: *Registered professional nurses and unlicensed assistive personnel,* ed 2, Washington, DC, 1996, ANA.

American Nurses Association: Position statement: registered nurse utilization of unlicensed assistive personnel, *NursingWorld,* 1997 (www.nursingworld.org/readroom/position/uap/uapuse.htm).

Benner PE: *From novice to expert: excellence and power in clinical nursing,* Menlo Park, Calif, 1984, Addison-Wesley.

Boucher M: Delegation alert! *Am J Nurs* 98(2):26-33, 1998.

Fisher M: Do your nurses delegate effectively? *Nurs Manage* 99(5):23-25, 1999.

Hansten RI, Washburn MJ: *Clinical delegation skills: a handbook for professional practice,* ed 2, Gaithersburg, Md, 1998, Aspen Publishers.

Hutcherson C, Sheets V, Williamson S: What five regulatory trends mean to you, *Nursing* 98(5):54-57, 1998.

Institute of Medicine: *Keeping patients safe: transforming the work environment of nurses,* Washington, DC, 2003, National Academy Press.

Johnson SH: Teaching nursing delegation: analyzing nurse practice acts, *J Contin Educ Nurs* 27(2):52-58, 1996.

Joint Commission on Accreditation of Healthcare Organizations: *Hospital accreditation standards,* Oakbrook Terrace, Ill, 2000, JCAHCO.

National Council of State Boards of Nursing: *Delegation: concepts and decision-making process,* Chicago, 1995, Author (www.ncsbn.org/files/publications/positions/delegati.asp).

Parkman CA: Delegation: are you doing it right? *Am J Nurs* 96(9):46-48, 1996.

Timm SE: Effectively delegating nursing activities in home care, *Home Healthcare Nurse* 21(4), 260-265, 2003.

SUGGESTED READINGS

Canavan K: Combating dangerous delegation, *Am J Nurs* 97(5):57-58, 1997.

Fisher M: Do you have delegation savvy, *Nursing* 30(12): 58-59, 2000.

Parsons L: Building RN confidence for delegation decision-making skills in practice, *J Nurse Staff Dev* 15(6):263-269, 1999.

VanCura B, Gunchick D: Five key components for effectively working with unlicensed assistive personnel, *Medsurg Nurs* 6(5):270-274, 1997.

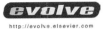

19

Staffing and Nursing Care Delivery Models

Barbara Cherry, MSN, MBA, RN, and
Ruth Ann Bridges, MSN, RN, BC

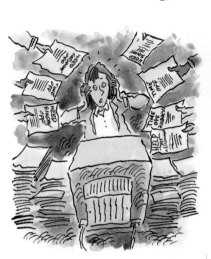

Staffing and assigning work are two of the nurse manager's most important and challenging roles.

VIGNETTE

As a student nurse John Knox noticed that during rotations through the different clinical areas the registered nurses (RNs) had various types of responsibilities and duties. On the medical-surgical units, RNs supervised a group of licensed practical nurses (LPNs) and nursing assistants who provided direct patient care and the RNs performed patient assessments, care planning, and education. In the critical care unit RNs provided all the care required by the patient with little help from any other caregivers. In the obstetric unit two RNs worked as a team to provide care to laboring mothers. In the outpatient health clinic each RN was assigned to perform specific tasks. For example, one nurse was assigned to do all diabetic teaching and another nurse was assigned to triage all telephone calls from patients. John had many questions about why care delivery was very different in the different clinical sites where he worked as a student.

Questions to consider while reading this chapter:

1. Why is the RN's work assignment different in different units—obstetrics, critical care, medical-surgical, and the outpatient clinic?
2. How do nurse managers on nursing units decide how assignments will be made?
3. Who has responsibility and authority for making patient care assignments?

Additional resources are available on-line at: http://evolve.elsevier.com/Cherry/

KEY TERMS

Clinical pathway Also called critical path, practice protocol, or care map; delineates a predetermined, written plan of care and specifies the desired outcomes and interdisciplinary intervention required within a specified time period for a particular health problem (Birdsall and Sperry, 1997).

Multiskilled worker Unlicensed caregiver trained to perform multiple tasks such as phlebotomy, vital signs, housekeeping, and assisting patients with hygiene and ambulation.

Nursing care delivery model Also called care delivery system or patient care delivery model; details the way work assignments, responsibility, and authority are structured to accomplish patient care; depicts which health care worker is going to perform what tasks, who is responsible, and who has the authority to make decisions.

Patient classification system Method used to group or categorize patients according to specific criteria and care requirements and thus help quantify the amount and level of nursing care needed.

Staff mix Combination of categories of workers employed to provide patient care—e.g., RNs, LPNs/licensed vocational nurses (LVNs), nursing assistants, multiskilled workers, or unlicensed assistive personnel (UAP).

Staffing Ensuring that an adequate number and mix of health care team members (e.g., RNs, LPNs/LVNs, unlicensed assistive personnel, clerical support) are available to provide safe, quality patient care; usually a primary responsibility of the nurse manager.

Unlicensed assistive personnel Unlicensed individuals who are trained to function in an assistive role to the RN by performing patient care activities as delegated by the nurse (American Nurses Association [ANA], 1997).

LEARNING OUTCOMES

After studying this chapter, the reader will be able to:

1. Outline key issues surrounding staffing for a health care organization.
2. Evaluate lines of responsibility and accountability associated with various types of nursing care delivery models.
3. Analyze the advantages and disadvantages of nursing care delivery models in relation to patient care in various settings.
4. Integrate essential components of the critical pathway model into patient care planning.
5. Differentiate among several nursing care delivery models by evaluating their defining characteristics.
6. Explain the purpose and components of nursing case management.
7. Summarize criteria to be considered in developing future models of nursing care delivery.

CHAPTER OVERVIEW

Of all the nurse manager's varied and complex roles, staffing and assigning work is probably the most challenging and certainly the most important to the delivery of safe, quality patient care. Staffing ensures that an appropriate number and level of staff members are available to provide care; assigning is the method used to divide work tasks among the various staff members. This chapter presents a brief introduction to staffing and its surrounding issues such as acuity levels and staff satisfaction. A description follows of various nursing care delivery models, which details how work assignments are structured. Also discussed are telehealth and case management as nursing care delivery models, as well as the use of clinical pathways. The chapter attempts to answer the following questions related to staffing and nursing care delivery models:

1. How does staffing affect patient care, staff satisfaction, and the organization's financial status?
2. What staff mix (e.g., combination of RNs, LVNs/LPNs, UAP, technicians) is required to provide quality patient care?
3. Who is responsible for making work assignments?
4. What factors should be considered when making patient care and other work assignments?
5. Is the work assigned by task or by patient?
6. How is communication about patient issues managed?
7. What factors are considered when choosing a nursing care delivery model?
8. What is case management, and how is it used to provide patient care?

STAFFING

Staffing can be defined as the activities required to ensure that an adequate number and mix of health care team members (e.g., RNs, LVNs/LPNs, UAP, clerical support) are available to meet patient needs and provide safe, quality care. Important research is validating the contribution and value of RNs to improving patient outcomes (Needleman et al, 2002) and preventing premature mortality (Aiken et al, 2002). The Institute of Medicine's recent report entitled *Keeping Patients Safe: Transforming the Work Environment of Nurses* (2004) is an extensive analysis of nurses' work environments and staffing issues; this report strongly affirms nurses' essential role in achieving quality patient care and safety. While appreciating the overall value of the RN in providing patient care, several specific considerations regarding staffing will be reviewed in this chapter. They can be categorized in three general areas: (1) patient needs, (2) staff satisfaction, and (3) organizational needs.

Staffing and Patient Needs

The primary considerations for staffing a specific nursing unit are the number of patients, the level of intensity of care required by those patients, and the level of preparation and experience of the staff members providing the care (ANA, 1999). Knowing only the number of patients that require care is an ineffective way to plan staffing because of the wide range of care requirements needed by individual patients. To account for the diverse care needs and quantify the intensity of care required by a group of patients, nurse managers responsible for staffing use various patient classification systems.

Patient Classification Systems. Patient classification systems group or categorize patients according to specific criteria and care needs and thus help quantify the amount and level of care needed. This may be referred to as the "acuity level." The higher the acuity level, the more intense the patient's nursing care needs. For example, patients may be grouped in such categories as "uncomplicated postpartum" or "ventilator-dependent." As the reader can easily visualize, these two groups of patients would require very different levels and amounts of care and therefore would be categorized at different acuity levels. Imagine the many different kinds of patients treated by a health care facility and you can begin to picture the complexity of patient classification systems.

Because of this complexity and the differences in patient populations across different health care facilities, patient classification systems vary from organization to organization. However, the ANA has recommended in its publication *Principles for Nurse Staffing* (ANA, 1999) that the following physical and psychosocial factors be considered when determining the intensity of care required for any group of patients:

- Age and functional ability
- Communication skills
- Cultural and linguistic diversities
- Severity and urgency of the admitting condition
- Scheduled procedures
- Ability to meet health care requisites
- Availability of social supports
- Other specific needs identified by the patient and by the RN

Understanding the intensity of care required by individual patients and groups of patients based on these factors is the first step in developing effective patient classification systems and planning for appropriate staffing levels. The second step is knowing the level of preparation, skill, and experience of the staff members who are available to provide patient care.

Level of Staff Preparation and Experience. It is of critical importance that the staff members available to provide patient care have the educational preparation, skill, and experience necessary to meet patient care needs. Recent research has demonstrated that in hospitals with higher proportions of nurses educated at the baccalaureate level or higher, surgical patients experienced lower mortality rates and fewer deaths from complications (Aiken et al, 2003). Another consideration in staffing is the clinical competencies that are required to care for the population being served. The nurse manager who is responsible for making staffing decisions must be aware of each individual staff member's educational level, competencies, experience, skill, and training. Ideally, clinical support from experienced RNs should be readily available to support and advance the skills of those RNs and other staff members with less experience. Unfortunately, this is not always possible in this time of nursing shortages. If the nurse manager does not believe that adequate numbers of appropriately skilled and experienced staff members are available to provide safe patient care, the nurse manager should immediately address those concerns with the executive level managers.

Staffing and Staff Satisfaction

Nurses who are satisfied with their work generally provide higher-quality, more cost-effective care. In fact, "it has been shown that the quality of work life has an impact on the quality of care delivered" (ANA, 1999, p. 5). Marquis and Houston (2003) report that staff scheduling "factors significantly in promoting job dissatisfaction or job satisfaction and subsequent nurse retention" (p. 295). However, because of the requirements for 24 hours/day, 365 days/year staffing needs in many health care facilities, meshing staffing needs with each nurse's personal needs is often very difficult. Creative staffing options are available to meet the varied needs of staff members, including:

- 10-hour shifts/4 days per week
- 12-hour shifts/3 days per week
- Premium pay or part-time staff for weekend work

- Job sharing, flextime, and/or staff self-scheduling
- Use of supplemental, or agency, staffing

Each of these options has various advantages and disadvantages. For example, long shifts over consecutive days may result in clinical errors when nurses become fatigued (IOM, 2004; Narumi et al, 1999). The excessive use of part-time or supplemental nurses can result in poor continuity of care (Marquis and Huston, 2003). Self-scheduling is a popular staffing technique in which the responsibility for staffing the unit is delegated to the employees on the unit who work collectively to design the schedule based on preestablished staffing criteria and some guidance from the manager. No one scheduling system has proven to be best overall for staff satisfaction. However, staffing methods that gain staff input and enhance staff autonomy seem to be the key to staff satisfaction (Davidhizar, Dowd, and Brownson, 1998).

Staffing and Organizational Needs

The three basic organizational needs that are significantly affected by staffing are (1) financial resources, (2) licensing regulations and Joint Commission on Accreditation of Healthcare Organizations (JCAHO) standards, and (3) customer satisfaction.

Financial Resources. Productivity, the ratio of the amount of outputs produced (i.e., home visits) to the specific amount of input (nursing hours worked), is the measure of staffing efficiency. Because staff salaries are by far the largest expense for any health care organization, productivity—or the efficient use of staff—will have a direct effect on the organization's bottom line. Fortunately, even though RNs represent the highest-paid staff in a facility, research has yet again demonstrated the value of RNs in improving patient outcomes and increasing hospital profitability (McCue et al, 2003). However, it is important to remember that most health care organizations continue to function under tight financial constraints, making efficient management of staff essential to ensure the organization's financial solvency. The nurse manager is accountable for appropriately managing staffing to stay within budgetary guidelines for the following:

- Numbers of staff working at any given time to provide care to a given number of patients
- Staff mix, the combination of types of workers present to provide patient care (e.g., RNs, LVNs/LPNs, nursing assistants, multiskilled workers, or UAP)

Licensing Regulations and Accreditation. Health care facility licensing agencies such as a state's department of health and accreditation agencies such as JCAHO address minimum staffing levels. However, JCAHO and state licensing agencies do not impose mandatory staffing ratios (with the exception of California, which recently enacted legislation mandating specific nurse-patient ratios). Licensing regulations for long-term care facilities stipulate minimum RN coverage for the unit but do not mandate specific nurse-to-patient ratios. However, these agencies do look for evidence that patients receive adequate care, which can only occur with adequate staffing. They also require documentation of staff training and competency to care for the organization's specific patient population.

Customer Satisfaction. Perhaps most critical to an organization's success in a competitive health care environment is customer (patient) satisfaction. The key to customer satisfaction is the patient's personal interaction with the organization's employees. According to Kenagy,

BOX 19–1   *Helpful Staffing Websites*

ANA's Principles for Nurse Staffing
http://www.nursingworld.org/readroom/staffprnc.htm

Nursing-Sensitive Quality Indicators for Acute Care Settings and ANA's Safety and Quality Initiative
http://www.nursingworld.org/readroom/fssafe99.htm

ANA's Nationwide State Legislative Agenda on Nurse Staffing
http://www.nursingworld.org/gova/state/2001/agstaff.htm

Analysis of ANA's Staffing Survey
http://www.nursingworld.org/staffing/

Berwick, and Shore (1999), "interactions with patients and their families . . . have remarkably strong effects on clinical outcomes, functional status and even physiologic measures of health" (p. 663). Appropriate staffing within budget constraints with well-trained, competent, professional staff members who are committed to providing safe, high-quality care is the nurse manager's number-one challenge.

This section has provided the reader with a very brief introduction to staffing issues such as scheduling options, patient classification systems, productivity and staff mix, and the RNs contribution to improved patient outcomes. These issues related to staffing in a health care organization are much more complex than may appear from this introduction. The reader, especially the person interested in entering nursing management, is encouraged to learn more about staffing and these related issues. See Box 19-1 for on-line learning resources related to staffing.

NURSING CARE DELIVERY MODELS

Nursing care delivery models, also called care delivery systems or patient care delivery models, detail the way task assignments, responsibility, and authority are structured to accomplish patient care. The nursing care delivery model describes which health care worker is going to perform what tasks, who is responsible, and who has the authority to make decisions. The basic premise of nursing care delivery models is that the number and type of caregivers are closely matched to patient care needs to provide safe, quality care in the most cost-effective manner possible.

The four classic nursing care delivery models used during the past five decades are (1) total patient care, (2) functional nursing, (3) team nursing, and (4) primary nursing. During the 1990s, in an effort to continually improve both the quality and cost-effectiveness of patient care, variations of these four classic models have been adopted, including modular nursing, partnership model (or co-primary nursing), patient-centered (or patient-focused) care, tele-health nursing, and case management. As the health care system continues to evolve in the twenty-first century with a focus on rapid patient turnover in acute care settings, extensive use of outpatient and community-based settings, and evidence of the RNs valuable role in patient safety and improved outcomes, the need for new models of nursing care delivery is emerging. Thus, considerations for future care delivery models will also be presented.

Total Patient Care

The oldest method of organizing patient care is total patient care, sometimes referred to as case nursing. In total patient care nurses are responsible for planning, organizing, and performing all care, including personal hygiene, medications, treatments, emotional support, and education required for their assigned group of patients during the assigned shift. A diagram of the total patient care model is shown in Fig. 19-1.

Advantages of the Total Patient Care Model

1. The patient receives holistic, unfragmented care by only one nurse per shift.
2. At shift change the RN who has provided care and the RN assuming care can easily communicate about the patient's condition and collaborate about the plan of care to ensure continuity because so few caregivers are involved.
3. The nurse maintains a high degree of practice autonomy.
4. Lines of responsibility and accountability are clear.

Disadvantages of the Total Patient Care Model

1. The number of RNs required to provide total patient care may simply not be available because of the nursing shortage.
2. The RN performs many tasks that could be performed by a caregiver with less training at a lower cost.

Today the total patient care method is commonly used in the hospital's critical care areas such as intensive care units and postanesthesia care units, where continuous assessment and a high degree of clinical expertise are required at all times. This method is less widely used in other patient care settings as health care organizations move to more efficient, interdisciplinary team approaches to patient care, allowing RNs to concentrate on aspects of care essential to good patient outcomes such as providing patient teaching and evaluating the patient's response to the plan of care. However, variations of the total patient care method exist. When reviewing other methods of nursing care delivery, you may see similarities to the total patient care model.

Functional Nursing

In the functional nursing method of patient care delivery, staff members are assigned to complete certain tasks for a group of patients rather than care for specific patients. For example, the RN

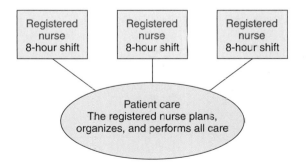

FIG. 19–1 The total patient care (case method) delivery model.

performs all assessments and administers all intravenous medications; the LVN/LPN gives all oral medications; and the assistant performs hygiene tasks and takes vital signs. A charge nurse makes the assignments and coordinates the care. A diagram of the functional nursing model is shown in Fig. 19-2.

Advantages of the Functional Nursing Model

1. Patient care is provided in an economic and efficient manner because less-skilled, lower-cost workers are used in areas where task completion is the focus.
2. A minimum number of RNs is required to supervise and to perform strictly nursing duties.
3. Tasks are completed quickly, and there is little confusion about job responsibilities.

Disadvantages of the Functional Nursing Model

1. Care may be fragmented, and the possibility of overlooking priority patient needs exists because several different workers focus only on performing specific patient care tasks.
2. The patient may feel confused because of the many different individuals providing different aspects of care.
3. Caregivers may feel unchallenged and unmotivated when performing repetitive functions.

Although the functional model is considered efficient and economical, the patient is treated by many caregivers who are not able to give personalized care because they are focused on performing a task—not on meeting patient needs. This model may not fit well in the new health care system, which focuses on customer service. However, functional nursing care delivery is still appropriate in some care settings and often is used in the operating room.

Team Nursing

In team nursing the RN functions as a team leader and coordinates a small group (no more than four or five) of ancillary personnel to provide care to a small group of patients. As coordinator of the team, the RN must know the condition and needs of all the patients assigned to

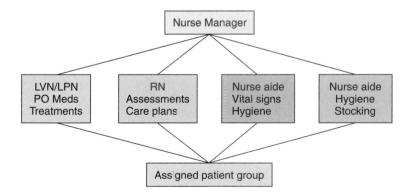

FIG. 19–2 The functional nursing care delivery model.

the team and plan for individualized care for each patient (Marquis and Huston, 2003). The team leader also is responsible for encouraging a cooperative environment and maintaining clear communication among all team members. The team leader's duties include planning care, assigning duties, directing and assisting team members, giving direct patient care, teaching, and coordinating patient activities. A diagram of the team-nursing model is shown in Fig. 19-3.

Advantages of the Team Nursing Model (Marquis and Huston, 2003)

1. High-quality, comprehensive care can be provided with a relatively high proportion of ancillary staff.
2. Each member of the team is able to participate in decision making and problem solving.
3. Each team member is able to contribute his or her own special expertise or skills in caring for the patient.

Disadvantages of the Team Nursing Model

1. Continuity of care may suffer if the daily team assignments vary and the patient is confronted with many different caregivers.
2. The team leader may not have the leadership skills required to effectively direct the team and create a "team spirit."
3. Insufficient time for care planning and communication may lead to unclear goals. Therefore responsibilities and care may become fragmented.

Team nursing is an effective, efficient method of patient care delivery and has been used in most inpatient and outpatient health care settings. However, for team nursing to succeed, the team leader must have strong clinical skills, good communication skills, delegation ability, decision-making ability, and the ability to create a cooperative working environment. In an attempt to overcome some of its disadvantages, the team nursing design has been modified many times since its original inception, and variations of the model are evident in other methods of nursing care delivery, such as modular nursing.

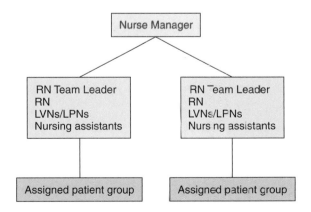

FIG. 19–3 Team nursing model.

Modular Nursing

Modular nursing is a modification of team nursing and focuses on the patient's geographic location for staff assignments. The patient unit is divided into modules or districts, and the same team of caregivers is assigned consistently to the same geographic location. Each location, or module, has an RN assigned as the team leader, and the other team members may include LVNs/LPNs and UAP (Yoder Wise, 2003).

The concept of modular nursing calls for a smaller group of staff providing care for a smaller group of patients. The goal is to increase the involvement of the RN in planning and coordinating care. Communication is more efficient among a smaller group of team members (Marquis and Huston, 2003). To maximize efficiency, each designated module should contain all the supplies needed by the staff to perform patient care. A diagram of the modular nursing model is shown in Fig. 19-4.

Advantages of the Modular Nursing Model (Yoder Wise, 2003)

1. Continuity of care is improved when staff members are consistently assigned to the same module.
2. The RN as team leader is able to be more involved in planning and coordinating care.
3. Geographic closeness and more efficient communication save staff time.

Disadvantages of the Modular Nursing Model (Yoder Wise, 2003)

1. Costs may be increased to stock each module with the necessary patient care supplies (medication cart, linens, and dressings).
2. Long corridors, common in many hospitals, are not conducive to modular nursing.

Just as in team nursing, the team leader in the modular model is accountable for all patient care and is responsible for providing leadership for the team members and creating a cooperative work environment. The success of modular nursing depends greatly on the leadership abilities of the team leader.

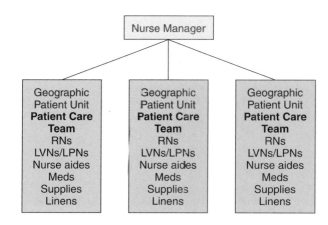

FIG. 19-4 Modular nursing model.

Primary Nursing

In primary nursing the RN, or "primary" nurse, assumes 24-hour responsibility for planning, directing, and evaluating the patient's care from admission through discharge. This model differs significantly from the total patient care model in that the "primary nurse" assumes 24-hour responsibility for directing the patient's plan of care. While on duty, the primary nurse may provide total patient care or he or she may delegate some patient care tasks to LPN/LVNs or UAP. When the primary nurse is off duty, care is provided by an associate nurse who follows the care plan established by the primary nurse. The primary nurse, who has 24-hour responsibility, is notified if any problems or complications develop and directs alterations in the plan of care. A fundamental responsibility for the nurse in the primary nursing model is to maintain clear communication among all members of the health care team, including the patient, family, physician, associate nurses, and any other members of the health care team. A diagram of the primary nursing model is shown in Fig. 19-5.

Advantages of the Primary Nursing Model

1. Direct patient care provided by a few nurses allows for high-quality, holistic patient care (Marquis and Huston, 2003).
2. The patient is able to establish a rapport with the primary nurse, and patient satisfaction is increased (Yoder Wise, 2003).
3. Job satisfaction is high because nurses are able to practice with a high degree of autonomy and feel challenged and rewarded (Marquis and Huston, 2003).

Disadvantages of the Primary Nursing Model (Marquis and Huston, 2003)

1. Implementation may be difficult because the primary nurse is required to practice with a high degree of responsibility and autonomy.
2. An inadequately prepared primary nurse may not be able to make the necessary clinical decisions or communicate effectively with the health care team.
3. The RN may not be willing to accept the 24-hour responsibility required in primary nursing.
4. The number of nurses required for this method of care may be difficult to recruit and train, especially with the current nursing shortage.

The primary care nursing model lends itself well to home health nursing, hospice nursing, and long-term care settings in which the patient requires nursing care for an extended

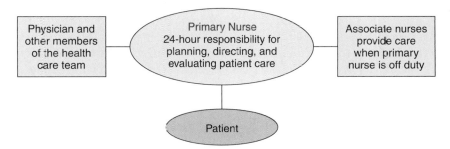

FIG. 19–5 Primary nursing model.

time period. Primary nursing may be more difficult to provide in acute care settings where stays are short and the nurse may see the patient for only 1 or 2 days. Because the concept of primary nursing is sound, some organizations have modified this nursing care model and implemented partnership models that use a wider staff mix.

Partnership Model

The partnership model, sometimes referred to as co-primary nursing, is a modification of primary nursing and was designed to make more efficient use of the RN. In the partnership model the RN is partnered with an LVN/LPN or UAP, and the pair work together consistently to care for an assigned group of patients.

Advantages of the Partnership Model

1. The model is more cost-effective than the true primary care nursing system because fewer RNs are needed.
2. The RN can encourage the training and growth of his or her partner.
3. The RN can perform the nursing duties while the partner can perform the nonnursing tasks.

Disadvantages of the Partnership Model

1. The RN may have difficulty delegating to the partner.
2. Consistent partnerships are difficult to maintain based on varied staff schedules.

Patient-Centered Care

Patient-centered care, sometimes referred to as patient-focused care, is a more recent development in nursing care delivery models and is a result of work redesign in health care organizations in an effort to become more patient-oriented rather than hospital- or department-oriented. This patient-centered care model is a concept in which cross-functional teams of professionals and assistive personnel from nursing and other departments become partners to provide care to a given group of patients. A core component of patient-centered care models is that the patient and family or significant others are integral members of this partnership. From negotiating care plans and discharge plans with patients—to including patients in shift change reports—to establishing "family advisory councils" (Ponte et al, 2003), patients become the focus of all care and decision making in the organization.

Patient-centered care involves all departments and disciplines that provide care to the patient and is truly an interdisciplinary approach to patient care. Patient care functions such as diet teaching, phlebotomy, housekeeping, transportation, and respiratory and therapy treatments, which at one time had no relationship to the nursing department, now are centralized in a patient care unit under the direction of a nurse manager. The ancillary workers who once performed only one function, such as phlebotomy, may be cross-trained to increase their level of productivity. A diagram of a typical patient-centered care model is shown in Fig. 19-6.

Advantages of the Patient-Centered Care Model

1. Making patients an integral part of their care leads to both higher levels of quality and increased patient satisfaction (Ponte et al, 2003).

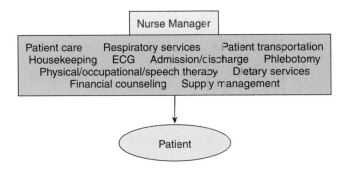

FIG. 19-6 Patient-centered care model.

2. The RN is accountable for a wider range of services to the patient and thus is able to ensure more consistent patient care.
3. The model is cost-effective for the health care organization.

Disadvantages of the Patient-Centered Care Model

1. Nurses may view such models as economic tools for productivity rather than offering opportunities for true patient-centered care (Hagenow, 2003).
2. Significant organizational culture change is necessary, requiring all care providers to commit to a personal mission of patient-centered care (Hagenow, 2003; Ponte et al, 2003).
3. Major change is required not only in the structure of the health care organization, but also in the roles of the nurse manager and the team members.
4. Because many different types of workers and disciplines are involved as a team, new and different issues arise, involving team conflict, problem resolution, and multiple standards of care.

The patient-centered model is appropriate in any health care setting. The RN, as coordinator of the interdisciplinary team, is responsible for making the patient an integral part of the team, keeping the patient involved in decision making, encouraging a cooperative environment, and maintaining clear communication among all team members.

TELEHEALTH NURSING

Telehealth—or telephone nursing—is quickly emerging as an important method of providing nursing care to clients in ambulatory settings. Nurses began to formally use the telephone to interact with patients in the early 1970s. As the efforts of health care organizations to balance quality care with cost control have increased, the use of telehealth and telephone nursing services has increased as well. These services may be referred to as telephone triage, telephone nursing, or telehealth, a term that encompasses all telecommunication methods, including e-mail, Internet, facsimile, and telephone nursing practice. Nurses' roles in telehealth nursing include triage, interventions, consultation, surveillance, and follow-up.

The American Academy of Ambulatory Care Nursing (AAACN) first published practice standards for telehealth nursing practice in 1997 and revised them in 2001. The AAACN has defined the following criteria for telehealth nursing practice (AAACN, 2001a):

- Using protocols, algorithms, or guidelines to systematically assess and address patient needs
- Prioritizing the urgency of patient needs
- Developing a collaborative plan of care with the patient and his or her support systems, which may include wellness promotion, prevention education, care counseling, disease state management, and care coordination
- Evaluating outcomes of practice and care

The AAACN (2001b) has also produced the core course curriculum to educate telehealth nurses, which includes such topics as roles, customer service, communication principles and techniques, legal aspects, and documentation. Any nurse involved in providing nursing care through telehealth methods should review this curriculum. The AAACN can be accessed on-line (aaacn.org).

Telephone nursing may be an integral part of an outpatient clinic practice or the function of a centralized call center. Centralized telephone services are typically used by managed care groups, and operate to provide nursing advice after clinic hours. This centralized service uses nursing time efficiently and facilitates appropriate management of the services; however, processes must be carefully evaluated to ensure nurses are able to practice as intended to meet patient needs (Valanis et al, 2003). Telephone nursing in medical offices may be enhanced by the availability of interaction with the medical professional.

To guide interventions with callers, telephone nurses may use standardized protocols or protocols developed for their particular setting. Many times nurses feel unable to use their nursing judgment when using mandated protocols because they may interfere with interpersonal communication between the caller and the nurse (Valanis et al, 2003). Optimal outcomes are fostered when nurses are involved in decisions about telehealth practices and protocols, have communication with other telephone nurses, and can educate health care providers about their role and function (Valanis et al, 2003).

The ANA has sponsored the formation of the Nursing Organization Telehealth Committee. This committee serves as a forum for groups involved in telehealth practice to address emerging issues from a multidisciplinary perspective. Nurses in telehealth will find ever-increasing roles and opportunities to influence the quality of care during the twenty-first century.

CASE MANAGEMENT
Evolution of Case Management

Case management is a model of care delivery in which an RN case manager coordinates the patient's care throughout the course of an illness. The concept of case management was first introduced in the 1970s by insurance companies as a method to monitor and control expensive health insurance claims, usually created by a catastrophic accident or illness. Today, virtually every major health insurance company has a case management program to direct and manage the use of health care services for their clients. Case management by payer organizations (e.g., health insurance companies, health maintenance organizations [HMOs]) is known as external case management.

By the mid-1980s hospitals had recognized the need for a case management model to manage the treatment plans and lengths of stay of hospitalized patients. When the Medicare prospective payment program was implemented in 1983, hospitals were reimbursed a set payment based on the patient's diagnosis, or diagnosis-related group (DRG), regardless of how long the patient was hospitalized or what treatment was provided. To keep costs lower than the diagnosis-related payment, the hospitals had to efficiently manage the treatment provided to a patient and reduce the patient's length of stay. Thus internal case management, or case management "within the walls" of the health care facility, was created to maintain quality care while streamlining costs. Several studies have since demonstrated the value of case management in both improving patient health outcomes and reducing costs (Galvin and Baudendistel, 1998; Huggins and Lehman, 1997; Gonzalez-Calvo et al, 1997).

Definition of Case Management

The ANA has defined nursing case management as "a dynamic and systematic collaborative approach to providing and coordinating health care services to a defined population. It is a participative process to identify and facilitate options and services for meeting individuals' health needs, while decreasing fragmentation and duplication of care and enhancing quality, cost-effective clinical outcomes. The framework for nursing care management includes five components: assessment, planning, implementation, evaluation, and interaction" (ANCC, 2001, p. 1).

Nursing case management is clinically oriented and business-oriented, and it is based on achieving specified patient outcomes. Patient outcomes should be achieved within a specified time frame while using available resources as efficiently as possible to decrease costs. Preestablished patient outcomes may be designated in critical pathways, which are discussed in the following section of this chapter.

Other disciplines, most notably social work, have been involved in developing case management programs and have identified themselves as case managers. It is common to see the term *case manager* used for many types of caregivers in many different health care settings. However, when clinical knowledge and experience is required, the RN is most effective in the case management role.

The ANA recommends that the case manager be a baccalaureate-prepared RN who preferably has a master's degree and advanced clinical and managerial skills: "Professional nurses are uniquely prepared to be case managers by virtue of their broad-based education in the life, social, and nursing sciences; their experiences in arranging and providing patient education and referrals; their awareness of the vital link between health and environment; and their orientation toward holistic health and its promotion" (ANCC, 2001, p. 2). Variations of case management models now are found in almost all health care organizations, including home health agencies, rehabilitation and long-term care facilities, hospitals, and ambulatory care organizations. A nursing case management model is shown in Fig. 19-7.

Components of Case Management

The nurse case manager "manages" a "caseload" of patients from preadmission (or onset of illness) to discharge (or resolution of illness). Although case managers generally do not perform direct care duties, they assume a planning and evaluative role and collaborate with the interdisciplinary health care team to ensure that goals are met, quality is maintained, and progress toward discharge is made. The goal of case management, whether internal or external, is to focus attention on the quality, outcomes, and cost of care throughout the patient's episode of illness and to assist the patient to move through the continuum of care. For example,

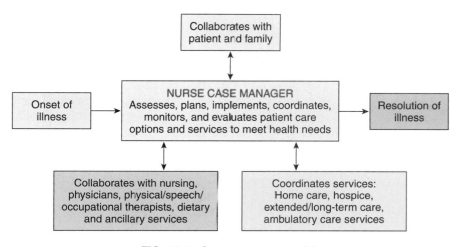

FIG. 19–7 Case management model.

the nurse case manager coordinates arrangements to move the patient from acute care to rehabilitation to home health to independent living, as determined by patient needs. Case managers meet patient needs through assessment, planning, implementation, evaluation, and interaction.

Assessment. The first role of the case manager is to collect and analyze comprehensive information about the client, his or her significant others, and available health care resources. The comprehensive assessment includes collecting and analyzing information in the following areas: physiologic status, psychologic status, cognitive and functional abilities, sociocultural factors and lifestyle, spiritual beliefs, and financial resources. The nurse case manager may also find, appraise, and use research findings as the basis for clinical treatment decisions to ensure evidence-based practice. During the assessment phase the nurse case manager interacts with the client, his or her significant others, physicians and other health care providers, and representatives from the health insurance company to gather detailed information.

Planning. The plan of care is developed based on a comprehensive analysis of information obtained in the assessment phase and delineates desired, realistic patient goals and outcomes. The care plan, which should be client-centered, evidence-based, and interdisciplinary, is developed in collaboration with the client, family members and/or significant others, health care team members, employers, and payers. A primary responsibility of the nurse case manager is to ensure that all parties have had a part in developing the plan of care and are in agreement with the final established plan.

Implementation. During this stage the nurse care manager becomes involved in actual implementation of the plan of care. The nurse case manager's responsibilities might include performing care or, more often, delegating care activities and facilitating and coordinating various aspects of the plan of care. Communication and documentation about progress toward desired outcomes are of primary importance to the case manager, as is ensuring that interventions are consistent with the established plan of care and are implemented in a safe, timely, and cost-effective manner.

The internal case manager assumes an important responsibility for understanding and monitoring the patient's payment source (e.g., private insurance, Medicare, or Medicaid). Not only will case managers confirm payment rates for the facility and initiate treatment preauthorization when required, they also will keep the patient and family members informed about available insurance benefits and how much out-of-pocket expense the patient may expect. For example, the discharge plan for a patient might include home health care. However, if the patient does not have health insurance coverage for home health services and if the patient is not able to pay for the home health services, a different plan of care may have to be developed.

Evaluation. The evaluation process is important to monitor the client's progress toward accomplishing established goals and outcomes, as well as evaluating the components of the case management process. Evaluation can be accomplished through (1) direct observation; (2) interviews, surveys, and/or verbal feedback from the client, significant others, and members of the health care team; (3) documentation review and/or chart audits; and (4) cost-benefit analysis of the client's treatment plan. "Nurse case managers continually evaluate each individual's health plan and challenge and attempt to overcome those obstacles that affect outcomes. Such obstacles may require the nurse case manager to reassess and revise the plan of care" (ANCC, 2001, p. 4).

Interaction. Ongoing interaction and collaboration with all members of the health care team, the client, the family and significant others, and the payer representatives are key responsibilities of the nurse case manager and inherent in all phases of the nursing case management process. To effectively interact and collaborate with all parties involved in the client's care, the nurse case manager needs good communication skills and the ability to motivate a diverse group of individuals to cooperate and collaborate to meet client needs.

Case Management Example. Following is an example to demonstrate the functions of the case manager.

CASE STUDY

Mr. Smith, a 58-year-old man, was diagnosed with lung cancer one year ago. He has been in Medical Center Hospital with multiple complications for more than three weeks. Debra Welch, RN, the internal case manager assigned to Mr. Smith's case, is working with the patient, family, physician, other members of the health care team, and the insurance company to determine a timely, cost-effective discharge plan. Debra has performed a comprehensive health assessment and understands the patient's condition and the available support systems. The physician, patient, family, and health care team agree that Mr. Smith's prognosis is grave and the treatment plan should be for palliative care only. Pain management is most important at this stage of the disease. Mr. Smith has a strong desire to go home, and his wife and adult daughter are willing to share the responsibility for home care. Debra also has identified the family's need for emotional support to deal effectively with the terminal illness.

After contacting Mr. Smith's insurance company, Debra learns that the company does not provide home health or hospice benefits but that the patient could be transferred to a subacute facility for continued care. Knowing Mr. Smith's strong desire to go home and the support systems in place, Debra identifies all the costs for home care (hospital bed, bedside commode, oxygen, wheelchair, and hospice support with pain management) and reports the comparative costs of home care versus subacute care to the insurance company. By demonstrating that home care is slightly less expensive than inpatient, subacute care, Debra is able to negotiate successfully a payment for home care from Mr. Smith's insurance company.

Continued

CASE STUDY—Cont'd

As case manager, Debra's next responsibilities are to coordinate Mr. Smith's discharge and to arrange for home services needed, including hospice care and medical equipment. The home plan of care is developed by the health care team and approved by the physician. Debra communicates the plan of care to the home care providers to ensure unfragmented care. As a result of case management, Mr. Smith and his family are able to go home with continued support and a smooth transition of care.

Box 19-2 presents a review of the components of the nursing case management process and related activities.

Case Management Related to Other Nursing Care Delivery Models

Nursing case management in a health care facility supplements nursing care and does not take the place of the nursing care delivery model in place to provide direct patient care. For example, if a hospital's medical-surgical unit uses a team nursing approach to patient care, a system of case management also might be in place to assist with coordinating the patient's total care through discharge. Case management is not needed for every patient in a health care facility and generally is reserved for the chronically ill, seriously ill or injured, and long-term, high-cost cases. Box 19-3 offers on-line resources for case management.

CLINICAL PATHWAYS

Clinical pathways, also called critical paths, practice protocols, clinical practice guidelines, patient care protocols, or care maps, delineate a predetermined written plan of care for a particular health problem (Birdsall and Sperry, 1997). Clinical pathways specify the desired outcomes and interdisciplinary intervention required within a specified time period for a specified diagnosis or health problem. Clinical pathways were developed in response to the need to identify quality, cost-effective care plans to reduce the patient's length of stay in the hospital. The JCAHO now stipulates that health care facilities use clinical pathways to meet accreditation standards (JCAHO, 2000). Clinical pathways dictate the type and amount of care given and therefore have financial implications for the health care facility.

In essence, the "pathway" can be viewed as a road map the patient and health care team should follow to guide the patient's care management and recovery. As the patient progresses along the path, specified goals should be accomplished. If a patient's progress deviates or leaves the planned path, a variance has occurred. A positive variance means that the patient has progressed ahead of schedule, and a negative variance means that the identified goals are not accomplished as planned. The RN generally identifies that a variance has occurred and mobilizes the interdisciplinary team members to create an action plan to address the problem or issue.

Clinical Pathway Terminology

- *Patient outcomes* are the end result of intervention by the health care team.
- *Interdisciplinary intervention* is the collaborative effort by all disciplines (e.g., nursing, physician, dietitian, physical therapy, occupational therapy, pharmacy), along with the patient and the family, to help the patient reach the desired health outcomes.
- *Variance* is any event that may alter the patient's progress through the clinical pathway.
- *Triggers* alert the caregiver that an unexpected event has occurred and identifies potential and actual variations in the patient's response to the planned intervention (Birdsall and Sperry, 1997).

BOX 19–2 | *Components of Nursing Case Management and Related Activities*

Assessment
- Review the client's history and current status
- Perform comprehensive health assessment
- Identify available resources and support system (e.g., individual, family, financial, health insurance, community)
- Identify barriers to accessing necessary treatment (e.g., lack of health insurance coverage; no family support)
- Identify health promotion and disease prevention opportunities
- Identify adherence patterns, educational needs, and ability to learn
- Determine potential for overuse or underuse of resources
- Find, appraise, and use research findings as the basis for treatment decisions (evidence-based practice)

Planning
- Prioritize needs and set realistic, measurable goals and outcomes
- Identify realistic treatment options
- Coordinate various providers involved in the plan of care (e.g., physician, physical therapist, dietitian)
- Determine appropriate levels of care and realistic treatment settings (e.g., home, long-term care, rehabilitation facility)
- Identify and address gaps in care
- Ensure continuity of care
- Negotiate and manage financial aspects of care

Implementation
- Ensure implementation of the care plan in a safe, timely, and cost-effective manner
- Coordinate services and referrals to providers or agencies
- Ensure compliance with federal, state, and local regulations and standards
- Use appropriate community resources
- Document progress toward achieving goals and outcomes
- Accept accountability for implementation of the care plan

Evaluation
- Measure clinical goals, functional improvement, satisfaction with services, and cost-benefit of treatment plan
- Is/was the plan of care realistic, collaborative, and mutually beneficial to all involved?
- Are/were the established time frames realistic?
- Are/were the best possible and most cost-effective treatments used?
- Are/were individual educational opportunities maximized?

Interaction
- Interact on a daily basis with diverse groups of people: client, family members, and significant others; health care team members; payer representatives; representatives from other health care agencies and community organizations
- Motivate diverse groups to cooperate, collaborate, and work in the best interest of the client
- Use good communication, negotiation, facilitation, and documentation skills

BOX 19–3 *Helpful Case Management Resources*

On-Line Resources

Case Management Society of America website
http://www.cmsa.org

Case management resource guide with searchable listings of over 110,000 health care facilities and companies from the following categories: home care, rehabilitation, subacute care, nursing facilities, assisted living facilities, hospice, long-term acute hospitals, psychiatric and addiction treatment facilities
http://www.cmrg.com/guide.htm

Case management resource guide with links to disease management resources for the following diseases: acquired immunodeficiency syndrome/human immunodeficiency virus, asthma, bone stimulation/healing therapies, bone marrow transplant, burn care, cancer/oncology, cardiovascular disease, diabetes, end-stage renal disease
http://www.cmrg.com/guide.htm

American Nurses Credentialing Center, a division of the ANA, has information on case management and certification as a nurse case manager
http://www.nursingworld.org/ancc/

Journals

Nursing Case Management
Lippincott's Case Management: Managing the Process of Patient Care

Books

Cohen E, Cesta T: *Nursing Case Management: From Essentials to Advanced Practice,* St Louis, 2001, Mosby.
Powell SK: *CMSA Core Curriculum for Case Management,* Philadelphia, 2001, JB Lippincott.

Clinical Pathway Components

Components of a clinical pathway include (1) consultations, (2) laboratory and diagnostic tests, (3) treatments and medications, (4) safety and self-care activities, (5) nutrition, and (6) discharge planning (Yoder Wise, 2003). Many clinical pathways also address triggers (potential negative variances from the path) in addition to patient and family education needs. The most commonly used clinical paths in acute care settings are for treatment of community-acquired pneumonia, total hip or knee replacement, and stroke or transient ischemic attack (Darer et al, 2002).

Developing Clinical Pathways

Clinical pathways should be based on accepted standards of practice. The ANA and specialty nursing organizations publish standards of practice for professional nursing. For example, the American Nephrology Nursing Association publishes standards of practice for nursing care of the patient with end-stage renal disease. Medical specialty boards also recommend standards of practice and actually have developed clinical practice guidelines for a variety of conditions. The American Academy of Pediatrics recommends several practice guidelines, including one entitled "Managing Otitis Media With Effusion in Young Children." This guideline can be found on-line (www.aap.org/policy/otitis.htm).

The Agency for Healthcare Research and Quality (AHRQ), formerly know as the Agency for Health Care Policy and Research, in conjunction with medical specialty associations, professional societies, and various other health care organizations, has developed a series of clinical practice guidelines. The reader is strongly encouraged to view current clinical practice guidelines on-line (www.ahcpr.gov/clinic/cpgonline.htm). Additional information about clinical practice guidelines is also available through the National Guideline Clearinghouse (www.guideline.gov).

Clinical pathways most often are developed for the health care organization's most common or costly diagnoses. For example, a general hospital may develop pathways for the treatment of congestive heart failure from admission in the Emergency Department—to care in the coronary care unit—to care on the general floor—to discharge home. It is important that the clinical pathway be individualized to meet unique patient needs.

A team supported by management, with representatives from various disciplines, including nursing, medicine, therapy, pharmacy, and dietary, develops clinical pathways for the organization. As a starting point, samples of clinical pathways can be found in the literature. In addition, professional medical associations and the AHRQ are excellent sources for currently recommended clinical guidelines. Although these resources provide a place to start, pathways developed by the health care organization's own team result in an individualized plan of care supported by all team members and avoid a "cookbook" approach to care. An excellent, easy-to-follow process for guideline development and implementation can be found in the JCAHO Accreditation Manual (2000). The success of clinical pathway development and implementation depends on input and support from all disciplines, including physicians, involved in using the pathway and caring for the patient.

CHOOSING A NURSING CARE DELIVERY MODEL

The nursing care delivery models presented in this chapter can be integrated into a variety of health care settings, including acute care, long-term care, ambulatory care, home care, and hospice. The organizational structure, patient needs, and staff availability influence which delivery system will be used.

Acute care settings may use different types of care delivery models for various patient care units. Emergency departments often use functional approaches to care because emphasis is on efficient assessment and immediate treatment. Team nursing frequently is used in medical-surgical units, whereas total patient care is common in critical care units. As identified in this chapter's opening vignette, acute care hospitals demand that the RN understand and be able to function in the diverse patterns of care that are in place throughout the organization.

In long-term care settings, such as nursing homes, skilled nursing facilities, and rehabilitation settings, patients remain in the care settings for extended time periods. Therefore the care delivery models may be structured differently than in the acute setting. Because of its economy and efficiency, functional nursing may be used for daily care tasks, whereas a form of primary care nursing is used for assessment and care planning.

The variety of ambulatory care settings continues to grow as health care moves out of the more expensive inpatient settings to the less costly outpatient settings. Outpatient surgery centers, minor emergency clinics, outpatient cancer centers, outpatient dialysis units, outpatient birthing centers, health clinics, and physicians' offices are examples of ambulatory care settings. The nursing care delivery model in ambulatory settings varies widely, depending on the type of patients being treated and their particular needs. For example, in outpatient dialysis units a combination of functional and primary care nursing usually works well. Patient care technicians are assigned to perform specific patient care functions such as dialysis machine set-up, whereas the RN is assigned primary nurse responsibilities for a group of patients to ensure effective assessment, care planning, and care coordination with the interdisciplinary team. Telephone nursing is becoming increasingly important as a method of care delivery in ambulatory settings.

Home health agencies often use a variation of the total patient care model. Although in home care the RN does not provide 24-hour care, he or she is responsible for the patient's needs for a 24-hour period and will coordinate intermittent care provided by others, including the home health aide and therapists involved in the patient's care. In the home health setting the RN may also function in the role of case manager for his or her assigned patients.

In every care setting the nurse manager must carefully evaluate the nursing care delivery model to ensure safe, efficient, and effective patient care. When evaluating nursing care delivery models, the following questions should be asked:

- Are optimal patient outcomes being achieved in a timely, cost-effective manner?
- Are patients and families happy with the care they are receiving?
- Are nurses, physicians, and other health team members satisfied with the safety and quality of care they are able to provide?
- Does the system allow for implementation of the nursing process in a timely and efficient manner?
- Does the system facilitate communication among all members of the health care team?

FUTURE NURSING CARE DELIVERY MODELS

Without a doubt, the ways in which nursing care is delivered over the next 20 years will change dramatically as a result of the following factors:

- Rapid technologic advances in medical care with less invasive procedures for disease treatments becoming available
- Fast-paced patient turnover in acute care settings
- Evidence of the RN's value in promoting patient safety and quality of care
- Ongoing shortages of nurses and other health professionals
- Strong focus on outcomes of care
- Consumers' demands for instant access to care and information
- Need to focus on the underlying determinants of health that are affected by lifestyle and personal choice

As acute care settings now admit only the most seriously ill or injured individuals with a focus on stabilization and transition, the traditional models of nursing care may no longer apply. In the past, nurses provided care based on comprehensive knowledge of the patients needs, which were learned by caring for the patients over an extended period of time. Now, nurses may have an entirely new group of patient to care for every shift, or even more than once during a shift. Nurses of the future must learn to conduct focused assessments and set priorities to be resolved before the patient is quickly transitioned to another level of care (Deutschendorf, 2003).

Nurses in outpatient and community-based settings are challenged with similar problems in attempting to address (1) patients' demands for instant access to care and information and (2) patients' needs for support and education to address lifestyle and personal choices that may affect their health. These challenges in both acute and outpatient settings are further complicated by the nursing shortage, which is only expected to worsen over the next decade.

As health care organizations begin to develop new methods of nursing care delivery, Deutschendorf (2003) has recommended several criteria that should be considered; these criteria include nursing education and experience, availability of expert resources, technology level, patient education needs, symptom management and medication administration, and availability of support personnel. Following are some specific examples of how these criteria might be considered when developing new models of care delivery (Deutschendorf, 2003):

A clinical unit with a high percentage of novice nurses should consider a nursing care model that makes available a higher level of clinical supervision and expert support than a unit with more experienced staff.

A unit for oncology patients and patients with end-stage renal disease will require a nursing care model that incorporates extensive resources for patient education and discharge planning.

A unit in which patients are discharged rapidly—sometimes even within a few hours—will require models of care to support ongoing education and support for patients and families who may be responsible for more complex care in the home.

In high-tech fast-paced environments where nurses struggle to provide care that is consistent with nursing values and to meet their responsibility to provide humane, sensitive, and intelligent care, relationship-based nursing practice should become part of every nurses' model of care (Manthey, 2003). Manthey translated relationship-based care to mean that "regardless of how high-tech, short-term, or financially driven the health system becomes, no one can tell nurses they cannot practice within a conceptual framework of 'intentional presence in a therapeutic relationship with the patient,' where the outcome is competent care that is oriented toward empowering patients to accept responsibility for living their lives with maximum health" (p. 370). Nurse leaders will be challenged to identify new methods of care delivery that are cost-effective and will improve both the quality and safety of care provided—and will facilitate the practice of relationship-based nursing.

Summary

Managers of health care organizations are concerned that patient care is delivered in the most efficient and cost-effective method possible and that staffing is appropriate to ensure safe, high-quality care and contribute to staff satisfaction. For this reason, nursing care delivery models have undergone tremendous changes throughout the past decade and will continue to evolve as organizations look for ways to improve patient outcomes in complex health care systems that are challenged by nursing shortages, reduced reimbursement, rapidly advancing technology, rapid patient turnover, and consumer demand for instant access and information. Regardless of changes that are certain to occur, the RN will retain responsibility to evaluate nursing care delivery models to ensure that patient care is delivered safely and efficiently, that caregivers are competent and legally qualified to perform the duties they have been assigned, and that safe, quality care and staff satisfaction are maintained.

CRITICAL THINKING ACTIVITIES

1. Describe the nursing care delivery models you have observed in the clinical setting. List the advantages and disadvantages of each one, and note the delivery models you liked best and why.
2. Review a critical pathway from a selected clinical setting. How is patient care based on the critical pathway implemented in the facility? How is the patient's progress through the critical pathway

communicated to the entire health care team and documented in the chart? What action does the nurse take if the patient "falls off" the pathway?

3. Your nurse manager has asked you to serve on a committee to review the nursing care delivery system currently in place on the nursing unit and to make recommendations to improve the current system. What factors should you consider when evaluating the current system and reviewing new systems?

Additional resources are available on-line at: http://evolve.elsevier.com/Cherry/

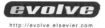

http://evolve.elsevier.com

REFERENCES

Aiken L et al: Hospital nurse staffing and patient mortality, nurse burnout, and job dissatisfaction, *J Am Med Assoc* 288(16):1987-1993, 2002.

Aiken L et al: Educational levels of hospital nurses and surgical patient mortality, *J Am Med Assoc* 290(12): 1617-1623, 2003.

American Academy of Ambulatory Care Nursing: *Telehealth nursing practice administration and practice standards,* Pitman, NJ, 2001a, Author.

American Academy of Ambulatory Care Nursing: *Telehealth nursing practice core course manual,* Pitman, NJ, 2001b, Author.

American Nurses Association: Position statement: registered nurse utilization of unlicensed assistive personnel, *NursingWorld,* 1997 (http://www.nursingworld.org/readroom/position/uap/uapuse.htm).

American Nurses Association: *Principles for nurse staffing, 1999* (http://www.nursingworld.org/readroom/stffprnc.htm).

American Nurses Credentialing Center: *Modular certification: basic eligibility requirements,* 2001 (http://nursingworld.org/ancc/).

Birdsall C, Sperry SP: *Clinical paths in medical-surgical practice,* St Louis, 1997, Mosby.

Darer J, Pronovost P, Bass EB: Use and evaluation of critical pathways in hospitals, *Effect Clin Pract* 5(3):114-119, 2002.

Davidhizar R, Dowd SB, Brownson K: An equitable nursing assignment structure, *Nurs Manage* 29(4):33-35, 1998.

Deutschendorf AL: From past paradigms to future frontiers: unique care delivery models to facilitate nursing work and quality outcomes, *J Nurs Admin* 33(1):52-59, 2003.

Galvin LG, Baudendistel D: Case management: a team approach, *Nurs Manage* 29(1):28-31, 1998.

Gonzalez-Calvo J et al: Nursing case management and its role in perinatal risk reduction: development, implementation, and evaluation of a culturally competent model for African American women, *Public Health Nurs* 14(4):190-206, 1997.

Hagenow NR: Why not person-centered care? The challenges of implementation, *Nurs Admin Q* 27(3):203-207, 2003.

Huggins D, Lehman K: Reducing costs through case management, *Nurs Manage* 28(12):34-37, 1997.

Institute of Medicine, Page A, editor: *Keeping patients safe: transforming the work environments of nurses,* Washington, DC, 2004, The National Academics Press.

Joint Commission on Accreditation of Healthcare Organizations: *2000-2001 Comprehensive accreditation manual for ambulatory care,* Oakbrook Terrace, Ill, 2000, JCAHO.

Kenagy JW, Berwick DM, Shore MF: Service quality in health care, *JAMA* 281(7):661-665, 1999.

Manthey M: aka Primary nursing, *J Nurs Admin* 33(7/8): 369-370, 2003.

Marquis BL, Huston CJ: *Leadership roles and management functions in nursing,* ed 4, Philadelphia, 2003, JB Lippincott.

McCue M, Mark B, Harless D: Nurse staffing, financial performance, and quality of care, *J Health Care Fin* 29(4): 54-76, 2003.

Narumi J et al: Analysis of human error in nursing care, *Accid Anal Prev* 31(6):625-629, 1999.

Needleman J et al: Nurse-staffing levels and the quality of care in hospitals, *N Engl J Med* 346(22):1715-1722, 2002.

Ponte PR et al: Making patient-centered care come alive: achieving full integration of the patient's perspective, *J Nurs Admin* 33(2):82-90, 2003.

Valanis B et al: Making it work: organization and processes of telephone nursing advice services, *J Nurs Admin* 33(4):216-223, 2003.

Yoder Wise P: *Leading and managing in nursing,* ed 3, St Louis, 2003, Mosby.

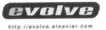

20

Nursing's Role in Improving the Quality of Health Care

Kathleen M. Werner, MS, BSN, RN

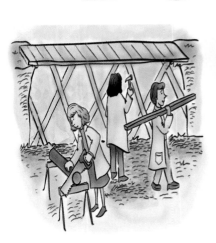

Nurses are building the bridge to patient safety and quality care.

VIGNETTE

It was a typical day on 4 East, a busy med-surg unit in General Hospital. Patients were being admitted, discharged, and transported to surgery at a brisk pace. For Maureen Harper, RN, the day was like most others, until one of her patients was to be discharged. All of the necessary paperwork was completed, the patient's belongings were packed, and all discharge instructions were completed. But Maureen's patient could not be discharged until the pharmacy delivered the newly prescribed medication that was to be taken at home. This was not the first time a patient had to wait for a prescription, and for Maureen it was becoming a repeated pattern in the normal course of discharge preparations. The patient eventually received the medication after an hour's wait and was sent home, but Maureen began to ponder the impact of this repeating set of circumstances.

Maureen calculated the additional cost that resulted from this patient's delayed discharge. This 1-hour delay meant an extra hour of hospital care, an extra hour of nursing care, and because this occurred during lunch time, it also meant that an extra meal needed to be served to the patient while he waited. Although each of these individual costs were small, Maureen began to think of the implications of these costs as they multiplied across dozens of patients throughout the many different nursing units at General Hospital. More important, Maureen was beginning to see the impact this delay had on patients' perceptions of the hospital. Family members often arrived early in the morning to take patients home, only to find they had to wait. Likewise, patients were not pleased when told they would need to wait. An entire positive hospital stay could be tainted with the experience of having to wait for discharge medication. Would that perception stay with them as they spoke to other friends and family about their hospitalization? Maureen began to feel more pressed to do something about the situation.

The next week, Maureen approached her nurse manager and expressed concern about delayed discharges. Maureen's manager thanked her for the feedback and expressed similar interest in resolving this problem. Pharmacy staff members already had been in preliminary conversations with Maureen's manager about the discharge medication process and were willing to work collaboratively with the nursing staff to find a solution to this problem. Maureen eagerly volunteered to participate in a work group that was charged with understanding the common causes of delays in filling discharge medication prescriptions and implementing key changes to eliminate delays. The team met regularly for several weeks and gained a clear understanding of what was contributing to medication delays. This was accomplished through creation of a detailed "picture" of what typically happened in filling discharge medication prescriptions and working on constructive ways to prevent breakdowns in this process. The project involved data collection to validate the sources of the breakdowns; what surfaced were surprises for staff members in each of the major departments involved, who always thought that "someone else" was to blame for the problems. In reality, the interaction of multiple departments led to delays. Over time, with constant monitoring of the turnaround time between the writing of the discharge medication order and delivery of drugs back to the units, progress toward reducing the delays was demonstrated. Maureen now knows that the proper steps are in place to guarantee an efficient way for medication orders to be tracked and filled. When her patients are ready for discharge, so are their medications, and Maureen feels like she is a vested part of this success!

Questions to consider while reading this chapter:
1. What key principles of quality improvement are demonstrated in the vignette?
2. What quality improvement tools did Maureen and the team most likely use to identify the causes for delays in filling discharge medications?
3. What resources are available to help Maureen and others in her organization learn more about improving the quality of health care?

KEY TERMS

Cause-and-effect diagram Tool that is used for identifying and organizing possible causes of a problem in a structured format. It is sometimes called a "fishbone" diagram because it looks like the skeleton of a fish.

Clinical indicators Measurable items that reflect the quality of care provided and demonstrate the degree to which desired clinical outcomes are accomplished; clinical indicators help identify the goals of quality improvement.

Customer Individual or group who relies on an organization to provide a product or service to meet some need or expectation. It is these customer needs and expectations that determine quality.

Flowchart Picture of the sequence of steps in a process. Different steps or actions are represented by boxes or other symbols. A top-down flowchart shows the sequence of steps in a job or process. It can have different levels of detail. A deployment flowchart shows the detailed steps in a process and the people or departments that are involved in each step.

JCAHO Joint Commission on the Accreditation of Healthcare Organizations; a national agency that conducts surveys of inpatient and ambulatory facilities and certifies their compliance with established quality standards.

IOM National Academy of Sciences Institute of Medicine; a nonprofit organization with a mission of advancing and disseminating scientific knowledge to improve human health. The Institute provides objective, timely, authoritative information and advice concerning health and science policy to government, the corporate sector, the professions, and the public.

ISMP Institute for Safe Medication Practices; a nonprofit organization that is well known as an education resource for the prevention of medication errors.

NCQA National Committee for Quality Assurance; an accreditation body that has become the primary group that accredits health maintenance organizations.

Pareto chart A graphic tool that helps break a big problem down into its parts and then identifies which parts are the most important.

Process Series of linked steps necessary to accomplish work. A process turns inputs, such as information or raw materials, into outputs, like products, services, and reports. Clinical processes are a series of linked steps necessary for the provision of patient care. It is through the improvement of processes that an organization improves its work and sustains itself.

Process variation The differences in how the steps in a work process might be accomplished and/or the variables that may affect each step in the process. Variation results from the lack of perfect uniformity in the performance of any process. Understanding variation in a process is necessary to determine the direction that improvement efforts must take.

Quality management (QM) Philosophic framework for managing organizations that recognizes that quality is determined by customer needs and expectations. Attention is paid to how the work is done, with an emphasis on involving the people who best understand the detail of the work processes with which they are involved. Health care quality management (QM) is specifically related to the quality of health care services provided.

Root cause analysis Defined by the JCAHO (2000) as a process for identifying the basic or causal factors that underlie variation in performance, including the occurrence or possible occurrence of a sentinel event. A root cause analysis focuses primarily on systems and processes, not individual performance. It progresses from special causes in clinical processes to common causes in organizational processes and identifies potential improvements in processes or systems that would tend to decrease the likelihood of such events in the future, or determines, after analysis, that no such improvement opportunities exist.

Run chart Graph of data in time order that helps identify any changes that occur over time; also called a *time plot*. A run chart that has a centerline and statistical control limits added is known as a *control chart*. Control limits help detect specific types of change in a process.

Sentinel event Defined by the JCAHO (2000) as an unexpected occurrence involving patient death or serious physical or psychologic injury or the risk thereof. Serious injury specifically includes loss of limb or function. The phrase "or the risk thereof" includes any process variation for which a recurrence would carry a significant chance of a serious adverse outcome. Such events are called "sentinel" because they signal the need for immediate investigation and response.

Standardization Approach to process improvement that involves developing and adhering to best known methods and repeating key tasks in the same way, time and time again, until a better way is found, thereby creating exceptional service with maximum efficiency.

LEARNING OUTCOMES

After studying this chapter, the reader will be able to:

1. Apply principles of QM to the role of the professional nurse.
2. Analyze the basis for the increasing emphasis on health care quality and medical errors.
3. Analyze the role of health care regulatory agencies and how they have embodied the principles of QM.
4. Critique key evolutionary facts that led to the development of QM in health care.
5. Discuss the role process improvement can play in ensuring patient safety and improving quality in the health care system.
6. Describe the tools and skills necessary for successful QM activities.
7. Discuss the professional nurse's role in reducing medical errors and improving health care quality.

CHAPTER OVERVIEW

Although Maureen Harper's story depicted in the vignette seems credible and would be a logical way for any organization to begin addressing customer concerns, far too often that has not been the case. Hospitals and health care organizations have been slow to recognize the necessity of a true customer perspective and to emphasize quality in a proactive manner. Donald Berwick (1990) wrote, "The paradox is infuriating. In some ways, it is the best of times for American health care. . . . But in equally striking ways, it is the worst of times for American health care, at least since it entered the scientific era of twentieth-century practice. Almost no one is happy with the health care system. It costs too much; it excludes too many; it fails too often; and it knows too little about its own effectiveness" (Berwick, Godfrey, and Roessner, 1990, p. xv). Although Dr. Berwick made this statement 15 years ago, it is still timely because, unfortunately, we have documented little progress in addressing the quality issues that continue to plague the U.S. health care system.

The intention of this chapter is make the reader aware of the pressing nature of the nation's quality health care crisis and to address the following questions:

- What is quality in health care?
- Who determines the degree to which quality is evident in our health care system?
- How should the health care system be redesigned to improve quality?
- What do the potential answers to the first three questions mean in relationship to professional nursing accountability?

The responses to these questions, particularly in relation to nursing's commitment to become involved with QM and to participate in its implementation, provide the elements of hope in determining and implementing sustainable, positive improvements in the design and delivery of health care.

THE URGENT CASE FOR QUALITY IMPROVEMENT IN THE U.S. HEALTH CARE SYSTEM

In an alarming 2000 report by the National Academy of Science's Institute of Medicine (IOM) entitled *Too Err Is Human: Building a Safer Health System*, authors extrapolated and summarized data from two major studies and concluded that up to 98,000 patients are killed each year from medical errors, confirming that poor quality of health care is a major problem in the United States (IOM, 2000). Contributing factors cited in the report included the following:

- Overuse of expensive invasive technology
- Underuse of inexpensive care services
- Error-prone implementation of care that could potentially harm patients and waste money

Following this 1999 report on medical errors, The IOM released *Crossing the Quality Chasm: A New Health System for the 21st Century* (2001) to define a vision for improving the quality of our nation's health care. The 2001 IOM report states:

The U.S. health care delivery system does not provide consistent, high quality medical care to all people. Americans should be able to count on receiving care that meets their needs and is based on the best scientific knowledge—yet this frequently is not the case. Health care harms too frequently and routinely fails to deliver its potential benefits. Indeed, between the health care that we now have and the health care that we could have lies not just a gap, but a chasm (p. 1).

The *Quality Chasm* report details a number of factors that have contributed to this chasm, including the unprecedented advancement of science and technology, growing complexity of health care, changing public health care needs, and a poorly organized and uncoordinated health care delivery system. Following are selected indicators from recent IOM reports that indicate just how wide the quality chasm is between what we know is good care and what is current practice:

- Between 44,000 and 98,000 Americans die from medical errors annually (IOM, 2000; Thomas et al, 1999; Thomas et al, 2000).
- Medication-related errors for hospitalized patients cost roughly $2 billion annually (Bates et al, 1997; IOM, 2000).
- 41 million uninsured Americans exhibit consistently worse clinical outcomes than the insured and are at increased risk for dying prematurely (Institute of Medicine, 2002; Institute of Medicine, 2003a).
- The lag between the discovery of more effective forms of treatment and their incorporation into routine patient care averages 17 years (Balas, 2001; Institute of Medicine, 2003b).
- Only 55% of patients in a recent random sample of adults received recommended care, with little difference found among care recommended for prevention, to address acute episodes, or to treat chronic conditions (McGlynn et al, 2003).
- 18,000 Americans die each year from heart attacks because they did not receive preventive medications, although they were eligible for them (Chassin, 1997; Institute of Medicine, 2003a).
- Medical errors kill more people per year than breast cancer, AIDS, or motor vehicle accidents (Institute of Medicine, 2000; Centers for Disease Control and Prevention; National Center for Health Statistics: Preliminary Data for 1998, 1999).
- More than 50% of patients with diabetes, hypertension, tobacco addiction, hyperlipidemia, congestive heart failure, asthma, depression, and chronic atrial fibrillation are currently managed inadequately (Clark et al, 2000; Legorreta et al, 2000; Institute of Medicine, 2003c; McBride et al, 1998; Ni et al, 1998; Perez-Stable and Fuentes-Afflick, 1998; Samsa et al, 2000; Young et al, 2001).

The *Quality Chasm* report details six guiding aims for improvement that should be adopted by every individual and group involved in the provision of health care, including health care professionals, public and private health care organizations, purchasers of health care, regulatory agencies and organizations, and state and federal policy makers. These six guiding aims are collectively referred to by the acronym *STEEEP.* Individually, these aims are for health care to be (IOM, 2001):

Safe: Avoiding injuries to patients from the care that is intended to help them

Timely: Reducing waits and sometimes harmful delays for both those who receive and those who give care

Effective: Providing services based on scientific knowledge to all who could benefit and refraining from providing services to those not likely to benefit

Efficient: Avoiding waste, including waste of equipment, supplies, ideas, and energy

Equitable: Providing care that does not vary in quality because of personal characteristics such as gender, ethnicity, geographic location, and socioeconomic status

Patient-centered: Providing care that is respectful of and responsive to individual patient preferences, needs, and values and ensuring that patient values guide all clinical decisions

To help establish a framework for accomplishing the significant redesign of the health care system, the authors of the *Quality Chasm* report formulated a set of ten simple rules to guide improvement initiatives. Professional nurses must serve as role models for all health care professionals, caregivers, and administrators in practicing these ten rules:

1. *Care is based on continuous healing relationships.* Patients should receive care whenever they need it and in many forms, including face-to-face visits, over the Internet, by telephone, and by other means as needed.
2. *Care is customized according to patient needs and values.* The system should be designed to meet the most common needs but should also be responsive to individual choices and preferences.
3. *The patient is the source of control.* Patients should be given the necessary information and opportunity to exercise the degree of control they choose over health care decisions that affect them.
4. *Knowledge is shared and information flows freely.* Patients should have unfettered access to their own medical information and to clinical knowledge with clinicians communicating effectively and sharing information.
5. *Decision making is evidence-based.* Patients should receive care based on the best available scientific knowledge and care should not vary illogically from clinician to clinician or place to place.
6. *Safety is a system property.* Patients should be safe, reducing risk and ensuring safety require greater attention to systems that help prevent and mitigate errors.
7. *Transparency is necessary.* The system should make available to patients and families information that allows them to make informed decisions, including information describing the system's performance on safety, evidence-based practice, and patient satisfaction.
8. *Needs are anticipated.* The system should anticipate patient needs rather than simply react to events.
9. *Waste is continuously decreased.* The system should not waste resources or patient time.

10. *Cooperation among clinicians is a priority.* Actively engage in collaboration and communication to ensure an appropriate exchange of information and coordination of care.

The remainder of this chapter will provide the reader with a set of principles and skills necessary to implement improvements and move towards a system of health care that is safe, timely, effective, efficient, equitable, and patient-centered.

QUALITY MANAGEMENT PRINCIPLES

There are many buzzwords meant to describe activities associated with QM. The most prevalent are total quality management (TQM), continuous quality improvement (CQI), continuous process improvement, statistical process control, and performance improvement. The terms themselves are not as important as the principles they embody: that of assessment and improvement of work processes while focusing on what customers want and need. In the example of Maureen and her patient waiting for discharge medication, the work process would be that of filling discharge prescription medication orders. The customer in this situation would be Maureen's patient, who wants to receive the medication quickly so that he can go home as soon as possible. Essentially the cornerstones of QM include the following.

1. Recognition and understanding by all who serve a customer that it is the customer who defines quality. In health care, primary customers are patients, and they are the ones who determine what quality is, not those who are in the position of providing the care and service. Historically, caregivers frequently have assumed the role of determining "what is best for the patient."

2. Organizational support for all employees to develop quality knowledge and skills and to begin thinking of their work as a series of processes that can be more deeply understood and improved through data measurements. As employees within an organization work to improve their work processes, they begin to understand the interrelationship and impact of process work across departments, such that ultimately the final product or service offered to the customer can be vastly improved. This chapter's vignette demonstrated this concept through Maureen's participation on a work team in which pharmacy and nursing both studied their contribution to the discharge medication process and found ways to better meet the patients' expectations of timeliness.

3. Belief in the people who are working to serve the customer. By recognizing the insight and knowledge held by those who are closest to the work and allowing them to be involved with the study and improvement of their own work, the potential for dramatic improvements can be realized.

Brian Joiner (1994) refers to these cornerstones of QM graphically in what he terms the "Joiner Triangle," labeling each point respectively as "quality," "scientific approach," and "all one team." He compares this model to a three-legged stool: All legs are necessary for the stool to stand. Remove any leg, and the stool falls. Maureen's example is one that demonstrates these three principles of QM.

1. *Customer defines quality*: Maureen began to consider the patient as the one who would define the quality of his hospital stay. She recognized that the perceived quality of the entire hospital stay could suffer if the timeliness of delivering discharge medications could not be improved.

2. *Organizational support*: Maureen was supported organizationally by her manager, who provided the opportunity for Maureen to collaborate with other key department employees to better understand the current series of processes that were in place for medication delivery. This group's work led to a clearer understanding of the interrelationship of the processes across multiple departments, which together affected the overall timeliness of medication delivery and enabled the group to make the necessary improvements to achieve the desired result.

3. *Belief in the people serving the customer*: There was faith in the people who were working on the medication delivery team. These people were recognized as those who had the best understanding of how the medication delivery "work" was happening and where the system was breaking down.

Quality

To provide a better appreciation of the importance of these three QM cornerstones, Joiner (1994) elaborates on what quality means to customers, noting that customers pay attention to all personal interactions that they may have with an organization and do not just focus on the characteristics of the product or service they receive. The products or services provided to the customer are not made up of just the physical items or a one-time experience that the customer encounters but rather of all the services that go with it. Organizations actually provide a "bundle" of products and services to customers to satisfy some need. If the service and product or outcome together are perceived as a good value, a loyal customer following will be established. Or, as in the case presented in the vignette, Maureen's patient might view the entire hospital stay negatively because of the delay in receiving the medications before discharge.

Scientific Approach

The scientific approach, the second leg of Joiner's three-legged stool of QM, emphasizes that to make significant improvements in an organization's processes, decisions must be based on sound, valid data, and the people managing the processes must have a clear understanding of the nature of variation in processes. Remember, a process is a series of linked steps necessary to accomplish work. For example, the steps necessary to complete a new medication order from the time the order is received until the medication is administered to a patient is a process. Understanding variation—the differences in how the steps in the process might be accomplished and/or the variables that may affect each step in the process—is necessary to identify the direction that improvement efforts must take.

Two types of variation in processes can occur: common cause variation and special cause variation. Processes that demonstrate common cause variation are stable, predictable, and statistically in control. Processes that demonstrate both common cause and special cause variation are unstable, unpredictable, and not in statistical control. The actions that should be taken to implement improvements under each type of variation are significantly different.

The best way to understand common cause and special cause variation is to use Maureen's example again. Maureen's team members collected data over time regarding the length of time it took from the writing of the discharge medication order to delivery of the drugs back to the clinical unit. Overall the time interval showed variability because of numerous factors associated with this process, one example being the total volume of orders written on any given day. The team recognized the total volume of orders written as common cause variation and realized that, to minimize the degree of this variation, the overall process would need to be studied to determine the best ways to change the medication delivery system, regardless of the total order volume.

The team was aware of a significant time delay in medication delivery during the week of the computer system conversion. This variation was special cause, one of extreme impact but related to a clearly identified single source. If the team had modified the overall medication delivery process based solely on the special cause factor, the computer conversion, the underlying problem most likely would not have been improved for the long term.

"All One Team"

The "all one team" concept, the third leg of Joiner's three-legged QM stool, embodies the principles of believing in people; treating everyone in the workplace with dignity, trust, and respect; and working toward win-win situations for all customers, employees, shareholders, suppliers, and perhaps even the broader community as a whole. The team referred to here is not an individual team, a project team, or even a cross-functional team. Joiner (1994) uses the term *team* to mean an organizational environment in which everyone from the front lines, or the direct care provider level in health care, to the executive level understands and acts as if they are all on the same team, working together to continually enhance customer satisfaction. For people to work this way, they must believe it is in their best interest to cooperate; they need to be more concerned with how the system as a whole operates rather than optimizing their own contributing area. In other words, all team members must rely more on cooperation and less on competition.

QUALITY MANAGEMENT IN HEALTH CARE AND THE ROLE OF REGULATORY AGENCIES

TQM in the United States did not begin to grow until well after World War II following Dr. W. Edwards Deming's work with the Japanese in their postwar reconstruction efforts (Neave, 1990). The Western business world was slow to embrace Dr. Deming's philosophy, but by the time of his death, it was evident that quality efforts in U.S. industry were more than a passing fad. As QM moved from manufacturing to service industries, penetration into the health care environment began.

From Quality Assurance to Quality Management

Initially hospitals were some of the first health-related organizations to seriously explore the potential value in adopting a total quality mindset in the 1980s and wrestled with more traditional models of quality assurance versus those of quality improvement. Health care leaders began to recognize that quality improvement was not necessarily a replacement for existing quality assurance activities but rather an approach that broadened perspectives on quality, and therefore they introduced tools that helped facilitate the improvement process previously lacking in quality assurance (Box 20-1).

Another way to think about this shift from quality assurance to QM is that health care quality was historically gauged through "inspection" methods, frequently relying on retrospective reviews of patient incidences or adverse outcomes. For example, an adverse patient response to a medication would have been reviewed through quality assurance auditing with a review of the circumstances surrounding this one particular adverse event. This historical approach focused

BOX 20–1 *Quality Assurance Versus Quality Improvement*

Quality Assurance	Quality Improvement
Inspection-oriented (detection)	Planning-oriented (prevention)
Reaction	Proactive
Correction of special causes	Correction of common causes
Responsibility of few people	Responsibility of all involved with the work
Narrow focus	Cross-functional
Leadership may not be vested	Leadership actively leading
Problem solving by authority	Problem solving by employees at all levels

From Koch MW, Fairly TM: *Integrated quality management: the key to improving nursing care quality*, St Louis, 1993, Mosby.

on specific incidents rather than on widely sweeping improvements that could address the more common causes of declining quality care and lead to preventing problems and improving care.

Regulatory Agencies

Equally important in driving this movement from quality assurance to QM was the incorporation of quality principles into health care regulatory standards and requirements (Bliersbach, 1992). Almost all regulatory and voluntary accrediting agencies now require QM in some form. The Centers for Medicare and Medicaid Services (CMS) (formerly the Health Care Financing Administration [HCFA]), which administers the U.S. Medicare program, has "Conditions of Participation" for its quality foundation, and many state licensing authorities also have required QM standards.

Voluntary accrediting organizations such as the Commission on Accreditation of Rehabilitation Facilities and the Accreditation Council of Developmental Disabilities promote QM requirements primarily for community-based providers serving various populations. The National Committee for Quality Assurance (NCQA) is becoming the primary voluntary accreditation body for managed care organizations, including outpatient clinic and medical practice group settings. This committee's emphasis revolves around performance measures of patient outcomes and results of practice patterns. The NCQA has grown significantly during the 1990s and now surveys at least half of the U.S. health maintenance organizations (HMOs).

Joint Commission on Accreditation of Healthcare Organizations. The Joint Commission on Accreditation of Healthcare Organizations (JCAHO) was one of the first regulatory agencies to embrace quality improvement principles in hospital-based settings. JCAHO standards address the organization's level of performance in key functional areas including patient rights, patient treatment, and infection control. The JCAHO accreditation system not only focuses on an organization's *ability* to provide safe, high-quality care, but now also requires evidence of *actual* performance and continued improvement.

The 2000 JCAHO Accreditation Manual reflected even more clearly the emphasis on actual performance and improvement, with a change in the quality chapter titled, "Improving Organization Performance." The chapter overview emphasizes that the goal of improving organization performance is to ensure that processes are well-designed and that the organization systematically monitors, analyzes, and improves its performance to improve patient outcomes while balancing excellent care, service, and cost (JCAHO, 2000). JCAHO continually updates and revises its accreditation standards and survey process to reflect the most current knowledge about the health care system. For example, in response to the increasing emphasis on patient safety, JCAHO established its Sentinel Event Standard (discussed in a later section in this chapter).

It cannot be emphasized enough that professional nurses are key in enabling an organization to successfully meet the established regulatory standards. Nurses have the unique position of supporting the overall management of patient care throughout the length of stay in the facility, working collaboratively with other health care professionals to initiate changes, and monitoring ongoing effectiveness of the care provided.

CLINICAL INDICATORS AND PROCESS IMPROVEMENT TOOLS AND SKILLS

The basic foundation of the monitoring and evaluation process required by QM principles is in the use of clinical indicators, measurable items that reflect the quality of care. Clinical indicators are aspects of clinical care that can be measured to show the degree to which care is or is not carried out as it should be. Indicators focus on clinical actions, or outcomes of clinical care; indicators should not focus on procedures that support clinical care. For example, replacing the intravenous (IV) solutions on the IV supply cart as they are used is a procedure that supports clinical care. Administering the correct IV solution at the correct rate as prescribed is appropriate clinical care. Both items are measurable, but only the latter is truly a clinical indicator. Indicators are not meant to define quality but rather to point the way to assessment of areas in which quality issues may be present.

How do process improvement skills and tools fit with clinical indicators? Clinical indicators help to identify the goals of quality improvement, whereas process improvement skills and tools support the quantitative understanding of key work processes. There are many process improvement models that incorporate these principles, but each of them has the following in common:

1. Analyzing and clearly understanding the process
2. Selecting key aspects of the process to improve
3. Establishing "trial" targets to guide improvement measures
4. Collecting and plotting data
5. Interpreting results
6. Implementing improvement actions and evaluating effectiveness

Various tools such as flowcharts, Pareto charts, cause-and-effect diagrams, and run charts may be used to accomplish each of these six steps (Joiner Associates, 1995), and it will become increasingly necessary for professional nurses to understand and apply these tools.

Flowcharts

The analysis of a work process usually is initiated through construction of some sort of flowchart or flow diagram. These are indispensable tools in mapping out what actually occurs during the process versus what is intended. There are several different types of flowcharts, each of which is valuable in its own way. A top-down flowchart simply lists the main steps and substeps of a process in a linear fashion (Fig. 20-1). A deployment flowchart maps out the steps of a process

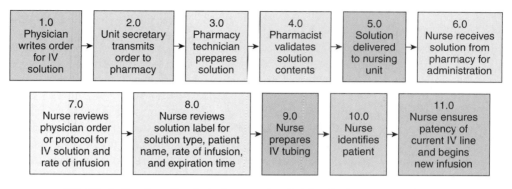

FIG. 20–1 Top-down flowchart of process for administering intravenous solutions.

under headings designating people or departments who actually carry out each step. This type is especially helpful when dealing with processes that cross multiple caregivers or areas and when there is a need for common understanding of what the process is doing as a whole (Fig. 20-2). As illustrated in Figs. 20-1 and 20-2, both a top-down and deployment flowchart can be used to view the process of administering the correct intravenous solution at the correct rate.

Pareto Charts

In selecting key aspects on which to focus within the process, a Pareto chart may be an appropriate tool. By collecting data on presumed or known problems in a given process, areas of focus or concentration can be achieved. This tool itself is a type of bar graph, with the height of bars reflecting the frequency with which events occur or the impact events have on a process problem. The bars are arranged in descending order, so that the most commonly occurring problems are readily visible. Fig. 20-3 is based on the Pareto principle, which proposes that 80% of process or system problems are generated from only 20% of the possible causal factors. Therefore, by focusing on the significant few causes, a much broader impact can be achieved in improvement efforts (Fig. 20-3).

Cause-and-Effect Diagrams

Cause-and-effect diagrams are other worthy tools that can help determine the potential sources of a problem. These diagrams essentially are lists of potential causes, arranged by categories to show their potential impact on a problem. The categories usually are broad, with subsequent levels of detail pursued under each as the "might cause" question is asked of each subsequent level of detail. This diagram sometimes is referred to as a "fishbone" diagram because it resembles a fish skeleton when complete. Cause-and-effect diagrams (Fig. 20-4) are useful when the major problem areas have been localized using the Pareto chart.

Run Charts

Measuring data over time to evaluate patterns in process variation typically is suited for tools such as run charts and control charts. Run charts, also known as "time plots," are graphs of data points as they occur over time. Valuable information can be obtained regarding process variation by studying the trends in the run chart. A control chart is a slightly more sophisticated tool in helping distinguish between common and special cause variation. A control chart is basically a run chart with statistical control limits added (Fig. 20-5).

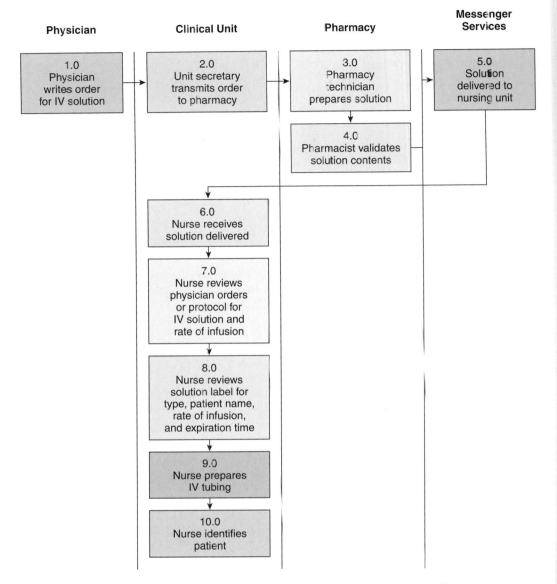

FIG. 20–2 Deployment flowchart of process for administering intravenous solutions.

Through use of these tools, results can be analyzed with interpretations subsequently guiding appropriate improvement actions. Once improvements are initiated, ongoing monitoring follows to evaluate the effectiveness of the changes implemented.

UNDERSTANDING, IMPROVING, AND STANDARDIZING CARE PROCESSES

Standardized processes, otherwise referred to as "best known methods" or "best practices," when effectively managed, have shown themselves to be the foundation for improvements in all areas of business today, but especially in the clinical care setting. There is a typical

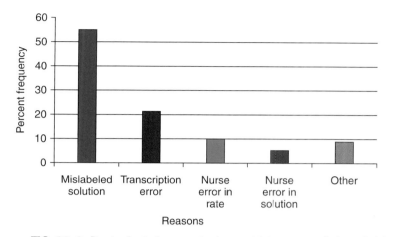

FIG. 20–3 Pareto chart of reasons for incorrect intravenous solution administration.

resistance to standardizing practices, especially when they involve providing patient care and services, but the realistic impact of care without standardization must be considered in the following context as described by Joiner (1994):

- "Management has never effectively emphasized the use of documented standards.
- Few employees have experienced the benefits of effective standardization; many have been subject to rigid implementation of arbitrary rules.
- Virtually no one sees the need for standards.
- Most employees receive little training on how to do their jobs. Instead, the majority are left to learn by watching a more experienced employee.
- Most employees have developed their own unique versions of any general procedures they witnessed or were taught. They think, 'my way is the best way.'
- Changes to procedures happen haphazardly; individuals constantly change details to counteract problems that arise or in hopes of discovering a better method. Tampering is rampant." (p. 191)

Each of Joiner's points could easily be applied to caregiver situations. At first glance it would be assumed that all care practices are based on scientific evidence and research, and

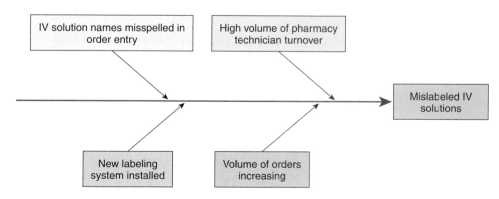

FIG. 20–4 Cause-and-effect diagram of mislabeled intravenous solutions.

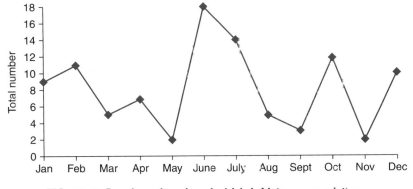

FIG. 20–5 Run chart of number of mislabeled intravenous solutions.

although many are, others exist simply because that was how the practitioner originally was educated. Those practices that are research-based, even though they represent "best known methods," may still not be widely practiced and therefore result in lack of standardization.

During the past few years a number of methods have been used in health care settings for the purpose of supporting standardization of care processes. Clinical guidelines, critical pathways, and case management are standardization methods that are more prevalent and familiar. Although these terms sometimes are used interchangeably, the following is offered as a context in which to understand their potential differences.

Clinical Guidelines or Critical Pathways

A clinical guideline or critical pathway typically defines the optimal sequencing and timing of interventions by physicians, nurses, and other interdisciplinary team members for a particular diagnosis or procedure. These guidelines typically are developed through collaborative efforts of the interdisciplinary team that includes physicians, nurses, pharmacists, and others to improve the quality and value of the patient care provided. Among the most obvious benefits of using clinical guidelines are (1) reduction in variation of the care provided, (2) facilitation and achievement of expected clinical outcomes, (3) reduction in care delays and ultimately lengths of stay in the inpatient setting, and (4) improvements in cost-effectiveness of the care delivered while maintaining or increasing patient and family satisfaction.

One model (Owen, 1996) suggests that the effectiveness of clinical guidelines should be monitored through review of data in three major areas:

1. Patient health outcomes—the actual results of the treatment and care provided in terms of health status
2. Patient satisfaction outcomes—the perceptions that patients have of the care and treatment they received
3. Financial outcomes—the overall charges the patient or payer bears for all aspects of care

All three areas are important and must be appropriately managed to achieve the desired overall outcomes.

Clinical Protocols or Algorithms

Other tools and methods may be used to standardize clinical practice. Examples are clinical protocols or algorithms, which are different from clinical guidelines because they represent

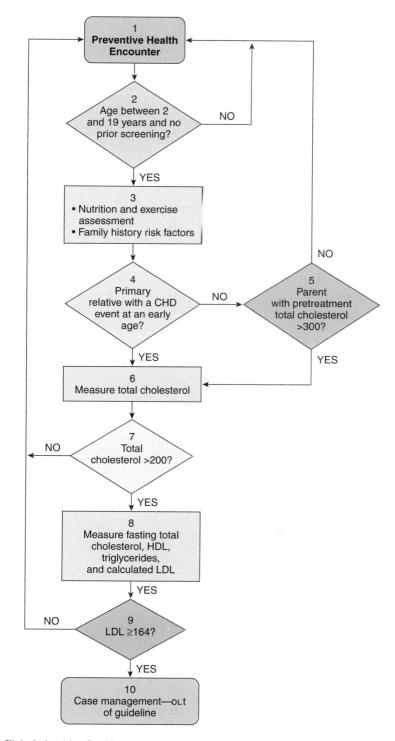

FIG. 20–6 Clinical algorithm/health care guideline: lipid screening in children and adolescents. (From Institute for Clinical Systems Integration: *1996 Health care guidelines*, vol 1, Bloomington, Minn, 1996, ICSI, p. 141.)

more of a decision path that a practitioner might take during a particular episode or need. For example, common algorithms exist for treatment of hypertension, provision of both basic and advanced life support, and general diagnostic screening (Fig. 20-6).

Case Management

Case management embraces somewhat different elements of professional caregiving. Traditionally case management has been provided by professional registered nurses and physicians, although there are appropriate settings in which psychologists or social workers may assume the role. The original intent of case management was to match the most appropriate services to the patient's care needs in the most efficient, effective manner. This potentially could result in reduced costs and lengths of stay, particularly in inpatient settings. Case management is discussed in more detail in Chapter 19.

BREAKTHROUGH THINKING

Just as standardization is critical to the foundation of health care improvement, so is the notion of breakthrough thinking. The premise behind breakthrough thinking and its resulting action is threefold: (1) substantial knowledge exists about how to achieve better performance than currently prevails; (2) strong examples already exist of organizations that have applied that knowledge and "broken through" to substantial results; and (3) the stakes are high and relevant to the most crucial strategic needs of health care (Berwick, 1997).

The Institute for Healthcare Improvement (IHI), a voluntary organization formed to assist leaders in all health care settings actively involved in improving quality, has established and teaches a results methodology that begins with what they term "change concepts." A list of change concepts has been developed by a planning group of national experts in several topic areas such as reducing cesarean deliveries, reducing patient delays and waiting times, and reducing adverse drug events and medical errors. Organizations use these change concepts to develop specific changes that they test, refine, and implement. For example, hospital systems have tested, refined, and implemented changes that have effectively reduced cesarean section rates while maintaining maternal and infant outcomes.

The model that IHI proposes for improvement essentially is composed of two parts. Part one asks three fundamental questions:

1. What are we trying to accomplish?
2. How will we know that a change is an improvement?
3. What changes can we make that will result in improvement?

Part two uses a sequence of steps, starting with developing an action plan based on the three questions, taking actions to test the action plan, making refinements as needed, and finally, implementing the resulting changes in real work settings. This also is known as a "plan-do-check-act" cycle, or PDCA (Fig. 20-7). Organizations are supported in determining measurements that provide guidance for further action.

PROCESS IMPROVEMENT AND PATIENT SAFETY

Nowhere is the need for quality improvement more evident than in the area of health care errors. As discussed previously in the chapter, the IOM report *To Err Is Human: Building a Safer Health System* (Kohn, Corrigan, and Donaldson, 2000) placed the issue of medical mistakes and patient safety on the pages of many national newspapers, on the agendas of

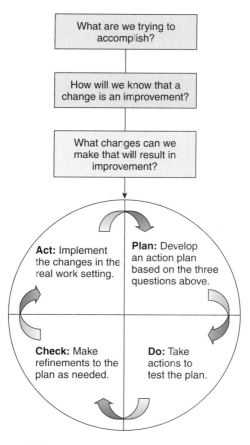

FIG. 20–7 IHI quality improvement model.

health care governing boards, and at the forefront of federal government legislation. The report, which concluded that up to 98,000 patients die each year as a result of medical errors, went on to promote the following recommendations:

1. A national center for patient safety should be developed.
2. A nationwide mandatory, state-based error-reporting system should be established.
3. Systems should be implemented that do not blame individuals but rather look at processes.
4. Safety performance standards for health care organizations should be established.
5. Proven medication safety systems and practices should be implemented.

Building upon this initial report, the IOM's newest report in its quality initiative series is *Keeping Patients Safe: Transforming the Work Environment of Nurses* (Page, 2004). In this report, the following five items surface as practices that are repeatedly linked with successful implementation of process improvements and behavior changes that assist in achieving safety targets in spite of high risks for errors:

1. Organizations need to balance the tension between production efficiency and reliability (safety).

2. Organizations need to support the development and maintenance of trusting relationships throughout the functioning work areas.
3. Organizations must actively manage the process of change.
4. Organizations must involve workers in decision making pertaining to work design and work flow.
5. Organizations need to use knowledge management practices to establish the organization as a "learning organization."

Other credible sources for patient safety improvements mirrored the initial IOM report, *To Err Is Human*. The Risk Management Foundation of the Harvard Medical Institutions (2000) summarized the following themes based on reviews of numerous patient care cases reported within its respective organizations:

1. It is critical to look beyond individual performance to the systems that underlie events, including human, team, organizational, and cultural factors.
2. Active and latent failures in care systems must be identified and addressed and are the basis for effective error reduction efforts.
3. By analyzing details about the process of work and the reasons people sometimes fail, significant flaws in care that affects patients, families, and providers are discovered.
4. By constantly adapting to demanding, complex, and fragmented systems, the clinician's struggle to reach the elusive goal of providing safe care is heroic.
5. Because barriers to communication and teamwork are significant, improvements must be focused in this area to protect patients and providers from the inevitability of error.
6. Health care providers whose mistakes cause or contribute to patient injury are the "second victims" and are often blamed, instead of being viewed as part of the larger system of care.
7. Increasing patient involvement is fundamental to building safer care systems.

To more clearly understand which systems should be of priority concern and what actions should be taken for safety improvements, comprehensive and comparable data must be tracked and made available to all health care organizations. The Institute for Safe Medication Practices (ISMP) is a nonprofit organization that is well known as an education resource for the prevention of medication errors. The ISMP provides independent, multidisciplinary, expert review of errors reported through the U.S. Pharmacopeia-ISMP Medication Errors Reporting Program (MERP). Through MERP, health care professionals across the nation voluntarily and confidentially report medication errors and hazardous conditions that could lead to errors. The reporting process is simple and easily accessible by clinicians. All resulting information and error prevention strategies are shared with the Federal Food and Drug Administration (FDA).

The ISMP has also developed a self-assessment tool for hospitals, which is designed to "heighten awareness of distinguishing characteristics of a safe hospital medication system and create a baseline of hospital efforts to enhance the safety of medication and evaluate these efforts over time" (Medication Safety Self-Assessment, 2000, p. 1).

Role of Regulatory Agencies and Patient Safety

The leaders of regulatory agencies (i.e., the Centers for Medicare and Medicaid Services [CMS]) and accrediting agencies (i.e., JCAHO) are trying to develop new accountability models, emphasizing their consulting role and, when possible, collaborating with the organizations and individuals they oversee. Because these regulators and accreditors remain ultimately responsible to the public they serve, they implement their functions under extreme scrutiny by the media. Accreditors and regulators are continually developing ways to migrate through these tensions while trying to forge successful partnerships with health care organizations and other provider groups.

As one response to the increasing emphasis on patient safety, JCAHO established its Sentinel Event Standard. This standard requires organizations to carry out designated steps in order to fully understand the factors and systems associated with adverse patient events, given that certain defining characteristics have been confirmed. The steps revolve around a "root cause analysis," which is a direct application of the quality improvement principles and methods defined earlier in this chapter. The intention behind the root cause analysis is to understand the systems at fault within the organization so that improvements can be determined and implemented to prevent any future occurrences. The JCAHO allows organizations a degree of latitude in determining the policy for disclosure of these events to the commission. The commission does validate that organizations have policies and systems in place to address sentinel events (O'Leary, 2000).

In February 2002, the Sentinel Event Alert Advisory Group was formed to advise JCAHO in the development of its national safety goals. These goals were to be based on ongoing analyses of reported sentinel events and assessment of the responding recommendations for correcting the identified root causes of these events. The Advisory Group was also directed to consider the practicality and cost-effectiveness of implementing the recommendations. Six national patient safety goals were established in 2003 with one more being added and approved for 2004 by the Joint Commission's Board of Commissioners (Box 20-2). As of January 1, 2004, all JCAHO accredited health care organizations will be surveyed for implementation of these patient safety goals and requirements or acceptable alternatives as appropriate to the services the organization provides.

The Professional Nurse and Patient Safety

Many experts argue that the answers for improved patient safety cannot lie within regulatory agencies alone. The answers reside in care providers pulling together to review critical circumstances and learning from key events. Basic improvement principles can help direct possible solutions within an organization by pinpointing warning flags through analyzing data, applying tools and methods to address the concerns, and continually evaluating the resulting patient outcomes. For nurses, the challenge starts with making patient safety improvement and reducing errors not just an organizational priority, but a personal one as well. This means buying into a state of mind that recognizes the complexity and high-risk nature of modern health care and subscribing to implementing standardized "best practices" and eliminating "never do" events. Specific steps that can be taken by nurses include the following:

- Educating patients and family members about their medications
- Implementing mechanisms with primary care providers to ensure follow-up
- Prominently displaying critical, patient-specific information on every record
- Questioning accessibility to high-hazard drugs such as potassium chloride and epinephrine if limitations have not already been instituted
- Insisting on the use of protocols for highly toxic drugs or those with a narrow therapeutic range
- Acknowledging errors and reporting them immediately in error tracking systems
- Seeking restorative or remedial care immediately when warranted
- Participating in improvement strategies including root cause analyses
- Apologizing to those impacted when appropriate

BOX 20–2 *The 2004 National Patient Safety Goals*

1. *Improve the accuracy of patient identification.* (a) Use at least two patient identifiers (neither to be the patient's room number) whenever taking blood samples or administering medications or blood products. (b) Prior to the start of any surgical or invasive procedure, conduct a final verification process, such as a "time out," to confirm the correct patient, procedure and site, using active-not passive-communication techniques.

2. *Improve the effectiveness of communication among caregivers.* (a) Implement a process for taking verbal or telephone orders or critical test results that require a verification "read-back" of the complete order or test result by the person receiving the order or test result. (b) Standardize the abbreviations, acronyms, and symbols used throughout the organization, including a list of abbreviations, acronyms and symbols not to use.

3. *Improve the safety of using high-alert medications.* (a) Remove concentrated electrolytes (including, but not limited to, potassium chloride, potassium phosphate, sodium chloride >0.9%) from patient care units. (b) Standardize and limit the number of drug concentrations available in the organization.

4. *Eliminate wrong-site, wrong-patient, wrong-procedure surgery.* (a) Create and use a preoperative verification process, such as a checklist, to confirm that appropriate documents (e.g., medical records, imaging studies) are available. (b) Implement a process to mark the surgical site and involve the patient in the marking process.

5. *Improve the safety of using infusion pumps.* (a) Ensure free-flow protection on all general-use and PCA (patient-controlled analgesia) intravenous infusion pumps used in the organization.

6. *Improve the effectiveness of clinical alarm systems.* (a) Implement regular preventive maintenance and testing of alarm systems. (b) Ensure that alarms are activated with appropriate settings and are sufficiently audible with respect to distances and competing noise within the unit.

7. *Reduce the risk for health care–acquired infections.* (a) Comply with current CDC hand hygiene guidelines. (b) Manage as sentinel events all identified cases of unanticipated death or major permanent loss of function associated with a health care–acquired infection.

Approved by the Board of Commissioners of the Joint Commission on Accreditation of Healthcare Organizations. Available on-line at www.jcaho.org/accredited+organizations/hospitals/npsg/04_npsg.htm.

ROLE OF PROFESSIONAL NURSES IN QUALITY IMPROVEMENT

There are lessons for all nurses from one of the original patient safety and quality improvement mentors, Florence Nightingale. Ms. Nightingale used data to support her efforts to reduce the incidence and spread of infections in the patient wards she was accountable for during the Crimean War. What resulted from Ms. Nightingale's work was a broader shift in the culture of health care at that time. *Culture* is defined as a system of shared beliefs, values, customs, behaviors, and material objects that members of a society use to cope with their world and with each other that is passed on from generation to generation through learning. Culture may be viewed as almost any form of behavior that is "learned" rather than instinctive or inherited (Bates and Fratkin, 1999). What can result from the current emphasis on patient safety is a shift in the health care culture of today. "Building health care systems that do no harm" will increasingly be the shared value and goal of all those involved in patient care delivery. Nurses are in the perfect position to lead this cultural change!

Quality improvement should not be considered a separate function within the role of care provider but rather an ongoing part of the professional role for all health care professionals. Box 20-3 presents a list of on-line resources to help the professional nurse seek more information about how to improve the quality of care for all patients.

BOX 20–3 *Organizations Dedicated to Quality Improvement*

The Institute for Healthcare Improvement (IHI)
www.ihi.org

IHI was established in 1991 as an independent not-for-profit organization working to accelerate improvement in health care systems in the United States, Canada, and Europe by fostering collaboration rather than competition among health care organizations. IHI provides bridges connecting people and organizations that are committed to real health care reform and who believe they can accomplish more by working together than they can separately.

"We envision a system of care in which those who give care can boast about their work and those who receive care can feel total trust and confidence in the care they are receiving."—Donald M. Berwick, M.D., MPP President and CEO, Institute for Healthcare Improvement

The Agency for Healthcare Research and Quality (AHRQ)
www.ahcpr.gov

AHRQ supports research to provide evidence-based information on health care outcomes, quality, cost, use, and access. Information from AHRQ's research helps people make more informed decisions and improve the quality of health care services. AHRQ is funded by the federal government and was formerly known as the Agency for Health Care Policy and Research.

National Association for Healthcare Quality (NAHQ)
www.nahq.org

The NAHQ is dedicated to improving the quality of health care and to supporting the development of professionals in health care quality by providing educational and development opportunities for professionals at all management levels and within all health care settings. NAHQ is the nation's leading organization for health care quality professionals and comprises more than 6000 individual members and 100 institutional members.

Joint Commission on Accreditation of Healthcare Organizations (JCAHO)
www.jcaho.org

The JCAHO is an independent not-for-profit organization whose mission is to continuously improve the safety and quality of care provided to the public through the provision of health care accreditation and related services that support performance improvement in health care organizations. JCAHO is the nation's predominant standards-setting and accrediting body in health care and evaluates and accredits nearly 19,000 health care organizations and programs in the United States.

The Institute for Safe Medication Practices (ISMP)
www.ismp.org

The ISMP is a not-for-profit organization that works closely with health care practitioners and institutions, regulatory agencies, professional organizations, and the pharmaceutical industry to provide education about adverse drug events and their prevention. ISMP is dedicated to the safe use of medications through improvements in drug distribution, naming, packaging, labeling, and delivery system design. The Institute provides an independent review of medication errors that have been voluntarily submitted by practitioners to a national medication errors reporting program (MERP) operated by the United States Pharmacopeia in the United States. All information derived from the MERP is shared with the U.S. Food and Drug Administration and pharmaceutical companies whose products are mentioned in reports.

American Society for Quality (ASQ)
www.asq.org

The ASQ is dedicated to the ongoing development, advancement, and promotion of quality concepts, principles, and techniques and offers products, services, and information to help people in all walks of life grapple with

BOX 20-3 —cont'd

perplexing issues such as total QM, benchmarking, and productivity. ASQ has more than 120,000 individual and 1100 organizational members.

Picker Institute
www.picker.org
The Picker Institute offers a variety of products and services for health care providers and organizations seeking to develop practical approaches for improving care through the eyes of the patient.

Partnership for Patient Safety (p4ps)
www.p4ps.com
p4ps is a collaborative network of people and organizations dedicated to reducing the harm caused by health care errors. Within the existing network, p4ps is developing a responsive portfolio of services and products that will enable creation of a continuously safer health care system.

SUMMARY

For today's graduating nurses, the challenge is to find whatever means are available to refine the knowledge and skills fundamentally necessary to enter into partnership with all other interdisciplinary team members in the ongoing improvement of health care. Just as essential to professional nursing practice as knowing, for instance, the symptoms of diabetic ketoacidosis or how to give an injection are understanding the basic principles of quality management, process improvement and variation; using clinical indicators, process improvement tools and standardized care processes; and addressing patient safety in every aspect of care. Every nurse should enter into practice accepting accountability for the quality of care provided by the health care organization and taking a leadership role to implement improvements to achieve health care that is safe, timely, effective, efficient, equitable and patient-centered.

CRITICAL THINKING ACTIVITIES

1. Interview a nurse manager in a clinical setting. What type of QM program is in place in the facility? How are staff members involved in the QM program? How are patient care needs addressed through the QM program? How does the QM process in the selected clinical site relate to the principles presented in this chapter?
2. Think about a situation in the clinical setting that may cause the patient frustration and possibly interfere with nursing care. What areas in the clinical setting does the situation affect (e.g., patient and family perception of care, nursing time, supply costs)? Describe the processes involved in the situation from beginning to end.
3. A staff RN has been appointed to serve on a committee to identify causes for nursing staff not receiving laboratory results in a timely manner. What tool or tools should he or she suggest to help create a picture of the processes involved in obtaining laboratory results?
4. The staff RN is assessing his patient's medication schedule, ordered therapies, and current infusion pump settings when he realizes that the continuous heparin solution the patient is receiving has been administered incorrectly, resulting in a dosage twice what should be prescribed according to the existing protocol. It appears that this occurred during the preceding shift. What actions would the nurse take?

Additional resources are available on-line at: http://evolve.elsevier.com/Cherry/

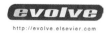

http://evolve.elsevier.com

REFERENCES

Balas EA: Information systems can prevent errors and improve quality [Comment], *J Am Med Inform Assoc* 8(4):398-399, 2001.

Batalden P: Continuous improvement in health professions education, *Qual Connect* 6(2):1, 1997.

Bates D, Fratkin E: *Cultural anthropology,* ed 2, Toronto, 1999, Prentice Hall, Canada.

Bates DW et al: The costs of adverse drug events in hospitalized patients, Adverse Drug Events Prevention Study Group, *JAMA* 277(4):307-311, 1997.

Berwick D: The breakthrough series, *Qual Connect* 6(2):11, 1997.

Berwick D, Godfrey AB, Roessner J: *Curing health care,* San Francisco, 1990, Jossey-Bass.

Bliersbach CM: *Guide to QM,* Skokie, Ill, 1992, The National Association for Healthcare Quality.

Centers for Disease Control and Prevention (National Center for Health Statistics): Births and deaths: preliminary data for 1998, *National Vital Statistics Reports,* Washington, DC, 1999, Department of Health and Human Services.

Chassin MR: Assessing strategies for quality improvement, *Health Aff (Millwood)* 16(3):151-161, 1997.

Clark CM et al: Promoting early diagnosis and treatment of type 2 diabetes: The National Diabetes Education Program, *JAMA* 284(3):363-365, 2000.

Institute of Medicine: *To err is human: building a safer health system,* Kohn L, Corrigan J, Donaldson M, editors, Washington, DC, 2000, National Academy Press.

Institute of Medicine: *Report brief: crossing the quality chasm: a new health system for the 21st century, 2001.* Available on-line (http://www.iom.edu/file.asp?id=4124).

Institute of Medicine: *Care without coverage: too little, too late,* Washington, DC, 2002, National Academy Press.

Institute of Medicine: *Fostering rapid advances in health care: learning from system demonstrations,* Corrigan JM, Greiner A, Erickson SM, editors, Washington, DC, 2003a, National Academy Press.

Institute of Medicine: *Health professions education: a bridge to quality,* Greiner AC, Knebel E, editors, Washington, DC, 2003b, National Academy Press.

Institute of Medicine: *Priority areas for national action: transforming health care quality,* Adams K, Corrigan JM, editors, Washington, DC, 2003c, National Academy Press.

Joiner BL: *Fourth generation management,* New York, 1994, McGraw-Hill.

Joiner Associates: *Plain and simple: introduction to the tools,* Madison, Wisc, 1995, Joiner Associates.

Joint Commission on Accreditation of Healthcare Organizations: *Comprehensive accreditation manual for hospitals: the official handbook,* Oakbrook Terrace, Ill, 2000, JCAHO.

Joint Commission on Accreditation of Healthcare Organizations: Special report! 2004 JCAHO national patient safety goals: practical strategies and helpful solutions for meeting these goals, *Joint Com Perspect Patient Safety* 3(9):2, 2003.

Legorreta AP et al: Variation in managing asthma: experience at the medical group level in California, *Am J Manag Care* 6(4):445-453, 2000.

McBride P et al: Primary care practice adherence to National Cholesterol Education Program guidelines for patients with coronary heart disease, *Arch Intern Med* 158(11):1238-1244, 1998.

McGlynn EA et al: The quality of health care delivered to adults in the united states [Comment], *N Engl J Med* 348(26):2635-2645, 2003.

Medication Safety Self-Assessment, Huntingdon Valley, Pa, 2000, Institute for Safe Medicine Practices (www. ismp.org).

Neave HR: *The Deming dimension,* Knoxville, Tenn, 1990, SPC Press.

Ni H, Nauman DJ, Hershberger RE: Managed care and outcomes of hospitalization among elderly patients with congestive heart failure, *Arch Intern Med* 158(11):1231-1236, 1998.

Norman L: Continuous improvement in nursing education, *Qual Connect* 6(2):4, 1997.

O'Leary D: Accreditation's role in reducing medical errors, *West J Med* 6(172):357, 2000.

Owen L: *CMGs: clinical management guidelines,* unpublished manuscript, Madison, Wisc, 1996, Meriter Hospital.

Page A, editor: *Keeping patients safe: transforming the work environment of nurses,* Washington, DC, 2004, The National Academies Press.

Perez-Stable EJ, Fuentes-Afflick, E: Role of clinicians in cigarette smoking prevention, *West J Med* 169(1): 23-29, 1998.

Pyatt R: Improvement in health care continuing education, *Qual Connect* 6(2):7, 1997.

Risk Management Foundation of the Harvard Medical Institutions: *Case study: key themes,* unpublished paper, Cambridge, Mass, 2000, RMF.

Samsa GP et al: Quality of anticoagulation management among patients with atrial fibrillation: results of a review of medical records from two communities, *Arch Intern Med* 160(7):967-973, 2000.

Thomas EJ et al: Incidence and types of adverse events and negligent care in Utah and Colorado [Comment], *Medical Care* 38(3):261-271, 2000.

Thomas EJ et al: Costs of medical injuries in Utah and Colorado, *Inquiry* 36(3):255-264, 1999.

Young AS et al: The quality of care for depressive and anxiety disorders in the United States, *Arch Gen Psychiat* 58(1):55-61, 2001.

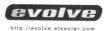

21

Nursing Research

Jill J. Webb, PhD, MSN, BSN, RN

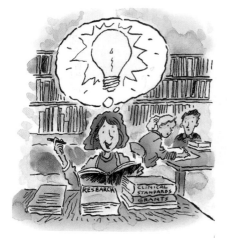

Nursing research
provides the foundation for
evidence-based nursing practice.

VIGNETTE

I didn't understand why I had to take a research class when all I wanted to do was be a staff nurse in a critical care unit. I thought I would never need to know anything about research. However, now that I've taken the course, I have an entirely different way of addressing clinical questions. I have an appreciation for research journals, and I see how important it is to read nursing research reports. I have discovered by reading widely and critically that research reports contain many implications that will apply to my practice in the critical care unit. Now I understand that, by keeping up with the latest research in my practice area, I will provide better care to patients.

Questions to consider while reading this chapter:
1. How can faculty encourage students to read research journals?
2. How does research affect nursing practice?
3. How can nurses motivate colleagues to base their practice on research?

KEY TERMS

Clinical nurse researcher An advanced practice nurse who is doctorally prepared and directs and participates in clinical research.

Additional resources are available on-line at: http://evolve.elsevier.com/Cherry/

Clinical nurse specialist An advanced practice nurse who provides direct care to clients and participates in health education and research.

Control group Subjects in an experiment who do not receive the experimental treatment and whose performance provides a baseline against which the effects of the treatment can be measured. When a true experimental design is not used, this group is usually called a comparison group.

Data collection The process of acquiring existing information or developing new information.

Empirical Having a foundation based on data gathered through the senses (for example, observation or experience) rather than purely through theorizing or logic.

Ethnography A qualitative research method for the purpose of investigating cultures that involves data collection, description, and analysis of data to develop a theory of cultural behavior.

Evidence-based practice The process of systematically finding, appraising, and using research findings as the basis for clinical practice.

Experimental design A design that includes randomization, a control group, and manipulation between or among variables to examine probability and causality among selected variables for the purpose of predicting and controlling phenomena.

Generalizability The inference that findings can be generalized from the sample to the entire population.

Grant Proposal developed to seek research funding from private or public agencies.

Grounded theory A qualitative research design used to collect and analyze data with the aim of developing theories grounded in real world observations. This method is used to study a social process.

Meta-analysis Quantitative merging of findings from several studies to determine what is known about a phenomenon.

Methodologic design A research design used to develop the validity and reliability of instruments that measure research concepts and variables.

Naturalistic paradigm A holistic view of nature and the direction of science that guides qualitative research.

Needs assessment A study in which the researcher collects data for estimating the needs of a group, usually for resource allocation.

Phenomenology A qualitative research design that uses inductive descriptive methodology to describe the lived experiences of study participants.

Pilot study A smaller version of a proposed study conducted to develop or refine methodology such as treatment, instruments, or data collection process to be used in a larger study.

Qualitative research A systematic, subjective approach used to describe life experiences and give them meaning.

Quantitative research A formal, objective, systematic process used to describe and test relationships, and examine cause-and-effect interactions among variables.

Quasi-experimental research A type of quantitative research study design that lacks one of the components (randomization, control group, manipulation of one or more variables) of an experimental design.

Randomization The assignment of subjects to treatment conditions in a random manner (determined by chance alone).

Secondary analysis A research design in which data previously collected in another study are analyzed.

State-of-the-science summary A merging of findings from several studies concerning the same topic. Examples include meta-analysis with a quantitative approach and integrative review with a descriptive approach.

Survey A nonexperimental research design that focuses on obtaining information regarding the status quo of some situation, often through direct questioning of participants.

Triangulation The use of a variety of methods to collect data on the same concept.

LEARNING OUTCOMES

After studying this chapter, the reader will be able to:

1. Summarize major points in the evolution of nursing research in relation to contemporary nursing.
2. Evaluate the influence of nursing research on current nursing and health care practices.
3. Differentiate among nursing research methods.
4. Evaluate the quality of research studies using established criteria.
5. Participate in the research process.
6. Use research findings to improve nursing practice.

CHAPTER OVERVIEW

This chapter provides basic knowledge regarding the research process and the ultimate importance of evidence-based nursing practice. The intent is to inspire an appreciation for nursing research and to show how it can improve nursing practice and how results can be translated into health policy. Nursing research is defined as a systematic approach used to examine phenomena important to nursing and nurses. A summary of major points in the evolution of nursing research in relation to contemporary nursing is presented. A description of private and public organizations that fund research is given, and their research priorities are listed. Major research designs are briefly described, and examples of each are given. Nurses of all educational levels are encouraged to participate in and promote nursing research at varying degrees. The process of locating research is reviewed. Students are introduced to the research process and guided through the process of critically appraising published research. Ethical issues related to research are examined, and historical examples of unethical research are given. The functions of the Institutional Review Board (IRB) and the use of informed consent in protecting the rights of human subjects are emphasized.

DEFINITION OF NURSING RESEARCH

Research is a process of systematic inquiry or study to build knowledge in a discipline. The purpose of research is to develop an empirical body of knowledge for a discipline or profession. (Burns and Grove, 2003, p. 3). Specifically, research validates and refines existing knowledge and develops new knowledge (Burns and Grove, 2003, p. 3). The results of research process provide a foundation on which practice decisions and behaviors are laid. Research results can create a strong scientific base for nursing practice (Mateo and Kirchoff, 1999), and application of results demonstrates professional accountability to insurers and health care consumers (Fain, 2004). In recent decades the nursing discipline has begun to pay much greater attention to the necessity of participating in research.

Nursing research is a systematic approach used to examine phenomena important to nursing and nurses. Because nursing is a practice profession, it is important that clinical practice be based on scientific knowledge. Evidence generated by nursing research provides support for the quality and cost-effectiveness of nursing interventions. Thus recipients of health care—and particularly nursing care—reap benefits when nurses attend to research evidence and introduce change based on that evidence into nursing practice. The introduction of evidence-based change into the direct provision of nursing care may occur at the individual level of a particular nurse or at varied organizational or social levels.

In addition to nursing research aimed at impacting the direct provision of nursing and health care to recipients of nursing care, nursing research also is needed to generate knowledge in areas that affect nursing care processes indirectly. Research within the realms of nursing education, nursing administration, health services, characteristics of nurses, and nursing roles provides evidence for effectively changing these supporting areas of nursing knowledge (Burns and Grove, 2003). Today the importance of nursing research to the discipline is recognized. But much nursing history underlies the current state of acceptance.

EVOLUTION OF NURSING RESEARCH

Nursing research began with the work of Florence Nightingale during the Crimean War. After Florence Nightingale's work, the pattern that nursing research followed was closely related to the problems confronting nurses. For example, nursing education was the focus of most research studies between 1900 and 1940. As more nurses received their education in a university setting, studies regarding student characteristics and satisfactions were conducted. As more nurses pursued a college education, staffing patterns in hospitals changed because students were not as readily available as when more students were enrolled in hospital-affiliated diploma programs. During this period researchers became interested in studying nurses. Questions such as, "What type person enters nursing?" and "How are nurses perceived by other groups?" guided research investigations. Areas such as teaching, administration, and curriculum were studies that dominated nursing research until the 1970s. By the 1970s more doctoral-prepared nurses were conducting research, and there was a shift to studies that focused on the improvement of patient care.

The 1980s brought nursing research to a new stage of development. There were many more qualified nurse researchers than ever before, widespread availability of computers for collection and analysis of data, and a realization that research is a vital part of professional nursing (Polit, Beck, and Hungler, 2001). Nurse researchers began conducting studies based on the naturalistic paradigm. These studies were qualitative rather than quantitative. In addition, instead of many small, unrelated research studies being conducted, teams of researchers, often interdisciplinary, began conducting programs of research to build bodies of knowledge related to specific topics such as urinary incontinence, decubitus ulcers, pain, and quality of life. The 1990s brought increasing concern about health care reform, and now in the twenty-first century research studies that focus on important health care delivery issues such as cost, quality, and access are being conducted.

Research findings are being used increasingly as the basis for clinical decisions. Evidence-based practice can be defined as the process of systematically finding, appraising, and using research findings as a basis for making decisions about patient care. The rise of technology and the worldwide access and flow of information have transformed the decision-making processes of practitioners. No longer do nurses simply compare outcomes of patient care with other units in the same hospital. Nurses and other health care professionals are more likely to look for solutions, choices, and outcomes for patients that represent the best available knowledge internationally (Hamer and Collinson, 1999). To implement clinical practice based on evidence such as legitimate research findings, nurses must ask the question, "Is this treatment effective?" The next step would be to break that question down into something that is answerable. The revised question might contain information about the disease and the patient

BOX 21–1   Helpful Websites

National Guidelines Clearing House—resource for evidence-based clinical practice guidelines:
www.guidelines.gov/

US National Institute for Health Consensus Statements:
http://consensus.nih.gov/cons/cons.htm

Centre for Evidence-based Nursing, based at University of York—United Kingdom:
www.york.ac.uk/healthsciences/centres/evidence/cebn

Cochrane Center—Resource for evidence-based clinical practice guidelines:
www.cochrane.org

such as the specific diagnosis and the patient's age. Evidence might be found in published research journals, in presentations at research conferences (Dawes et al, 1999), or through on-line sources (Box 21-1).

RESEARCH PRIORITIES

Why set priorities for research in the nursing discipline? Can't nurses do research in areas that match personal areas of interest? The answer to the second question is, yes, certainly! But nursing exists to provide high-quality nursing care to individuals in need of health-promoting, health-sustaining, and health-restoring strategies. The main outcome of research activity for a nurse is to eventually put the knowledge gained to work in health care delivery. Research priorities, often set by groups that fund research, encourage nurse researchers to invest effort and money into those areas of research likely to generate the most benefit to recipients of care. Of course, the funding opportunities offered by such groups don't hurt the research enterprise either. Research costs money! Thus nurses engaged in research often match personal interests with funding opportunities that are available during the planning phase for a proposed investigation. Two major sources of funding for nursing research are the National Institute for Nursing Research (NINR) and the Agency for Healthcare Research and Quality (AHRQ) (formerly known as the Agency for Healthcare Policy and Research [AHCPR] and reauthorized as AHRQ by Congress in 1999). Both of these organizations are funded by federal congressional appropriations. Private foundations and nursing organizations also provide funding for nursing research.

The National Institute for Nursing Research

As part of the National Institutes of Health (NIH), the NINR supports research on the biologic and behavioral aspects of critical health problems that confront the nation. The NINR seeks to:

1. Understand and ease the symptoms of acute and chronic illness.
2. Prevent or delay the onset of disease or disability or slow its progression.
3. Find effective approaches to achieving and sustaining good health.
4. Improve clinical settings in which care is provided (NINR Mission Statement, 2003).

With major emphases on at-risk, underserved populations and on high-quality, cost-effective health care, the NINR promotes and supports research in universities, research centers, and at the NINR research campus in Bethesda, Maryland. Objectives of the NINR address the following six broad science areas:

1. *Chronic conditions*—arthritis, diabetes, urinary incontinence, long-term care, and caregiving
2. *Health promotion and risk behaviors*—women's health, adolescence, menopause, environmental health, exercise, nutrition, and smoking cessation
3. *Cardiopulmonary health*—prevention and care of persons with cardiac or respiratory conditions, including research in critical care, trauma, wound healing, and organ transplantation
4. *Neurofunction and sensory conditions*—pain management, sleep disorders, and symptom management in persons with cognitive impairment and chronic neurologic conditions
5. *Immune and neoplastic diseases*—symptoms primarily associated with cancer and acquired immune deficiency syndrome, such as fatigue, nausea and vomiting, and cachexia, as well as risk-factor prevention research
6. *Reproductive and infant health*—prevention of premature labor, reduction of health-risk factors during pregnancy, delivery of prenatal care, care of neonates, infant growth and development, and fertility issues

These areas are not considered to be prescriptive in nature. NINR accepts funding proposals from investigators with unique interests, as well as those specifically detailed in NINR priority research lists.

Annually, the NINR conducts a roundtable discussion with multiple nursing organizations to obtain the feedback of the disciplines regarding the need for continued or new research emphases. In addition, NINR listens to discussions at regional nursing research meetings across the nation to get a grassroots look at ongoing nursing research initiatives (O'Neil, 2001). Information obtained is used in setting future research agendas and making decisions about funding of proposals submitted by researchers. NINR provides a website detailing current announcements regarding research priorities (www.nih.gov/ninr/research.html).

The Agency for Healthcare Research and Quality (AHRQ)

As an agency of the Department of Health and Human Services, AHRQ aims to improve the outcomes and quality of health care, reduce its costs, address patient safety and medical errors, and broaden access to effective services (AHRQ, 2003). The AHRQ broadly defines its function as the provision of evidence-based information to health care decision makers to improve the quality of health care in the nation. Since the inception of the agency in 1989, strategic goals have centered on supporting improvements in health outcomes, strengthening measurement of health care quality indicators, and fostering access to and cost-effectiveness of health care. The 1999 reauthorizing legislation expanded the role of the agency by directing the AHRQ to:

- Improve the quality of health care through scientific inquiry, dissemination of findings, and facilitation of public access to information.
- Promote patient safety and reduce medical errors through scientific inquiry, building partnerships with health care providers, and establishment of Centers for Education and Research on Therapeutics (CERTs).
- Advance the use of information technology for coordinating patient care and conducting quality and outcomes research.

■ Establish an Office on Priority Populations to ensure that the needs of low-income groups, minorities, women, children, the elderly, and individuals with special health care needs are addressed by the agency's research efforts.

The research-related activities of the AHRQ are quite varied. In a process similar to that used by the NIH, investigators are invited to submit research proposals for possible funding through grant announcements. A listing of current areas of the agency's research interests can be found on-line (www.ahrq.gov/fund/grantix).

The AHRQ actively promotes evidence-based practice, partially through the establishment of 13 evidence-based practice centers (EPCs) in the United States and Canada. EPCs conduct research on assigned clinical care topics and generate reports on the effectiveness of health care methodologies. Health care providers may then use the evidence in developing site-specific guidelines that direct clinical practice. AHRQ also actively maintains the National Guideline Clearinghouse (www.guidelines.gov), an Internet site that makes available to health care professionals a wide array of clinical practice guidelines that may be considered in health care decision making. Although most AHRQ activities are intended to support health care professionals and institutions, the agency supports health care recipients by designing some information specifically for dissemination to the lay public. In addition, AHRQ supports the design and development of databases for use in outcomes research (AHRQ, 2003).

Private Foundations

Federal funding is available through the NIH and the AHRQ. However, because obtaining money for research is becoming increasingly competitive, voluntary foundations and private and community-based organizations should be investigated as possible funding sources. Many foundations and corporate direct-giving programs are interested in funding health care projects and research. Computer databases and guides to funding are available in local libraries.

Private foundations such as the Robert Wood Johnson Foundation (2003a, 2003b) or the WK Kellogg Foundation (2001) are sources that offer program funding for health-related research. Investigators should be encouraged to pursue funding for small projects through local sources or private foundations until a track record is established in research design and implementation. After several years of experience in the research arena, investigators are more likely to be successful in securing funding through federal sources such as the NIH.

Nursing Organizations

Nursing organizations such as Sigma Theta Tau International (STTI), the American Nurses Association (ANA), and the Oncology Nurses Society (ONS) are the few of the nursing organizations that fund research studies.

STTI makes research grant awards to increase scientific knowledge related to nursing practice. STTI supports creative interdisciplinary research and places importance on identifying "best practices" and benchmark innovations. Awards are made at the international and local chapter levels.

The ANA awards small grants through the American Nurses Foundation. Specialty nursing organizations offer grants to support research related to their specialty. For example, the ONS awards grants that focus on issues related to oncology.

To summarize, multiple potential sources of funding are available for research projects. The individual or group wishing to conduct research will need to carefully develop a proposal, search for a possible funding source, and submit the proposal. Libraries and the

Internet provide ample information about the many foundations and organizations interested in funding research endeavors. Most research institutions establish offices that help in the search and procurement of funding. Thus researchers are supported in their work of knowledge building.

COMPONENTS OF THE RESEARCH PROCESS

The research process involves conceptualizing a research study, planning and implementing that study, and communicating the findings. The process involves a logical flow as each step builds on the previous steps. These steps should be included in published research reports so that the reader has a basis for understanding and critiquing the study (Box 21-2).

STUDY DESIGNS

Study designs are plans that tell a researcher how data are to be collected, from whom data are to be collected, and how data will be analyzed to answer specific research questions. Research studies are classified into two basic methods: quantitative and qualitative. Quantitative and qualitative research are two distinctly different approaches to conducting research. The researcher chooses the method based on the research question and the current level of knowledge about the phenomena and the problem to be studied. Quantitative research is a formal, objective, systematic process in which numeric data are used. Qualitative research is a systematic approach used to describe and promote understanding of human experiences such as pain. Human experiences related to health (such as caring, caregiving, depression, and pain) are of primary importance to nursing (Struebert and Carpenter, 1999); thus qualitative research design provides a dimension of understanding to nursing science that adds to traditional quantitative methodology.

Quantitative Designs

Arising from early scientific models for doing research, the nursing discipline directly adopted the quantitative method of conducting research. Thus, quantitative design has traditionally been prevalent in nursing research studies. Deriving meaning from the statistical analysis of

---

BOX 21–2 *Components of the Research Process*

Research is a process that takes place in a series of steps:

1. Formulating the research question or problem
2. Defining the purpose of the study
3. Reviewing related literature
4. Formulating hypotheses and defining variables
5. Selecting the research design
6. Selecting the population, sample, and setting
7. Conducting a pilot study
8. Collecting the data
9. Analyzing the data
10. Communicating conclusions

numerical data obtained from samples and populations has yielded significant contributions to nursing knowledge. The usual intent of quantitative study is to apply or generalize knowledge from a smaller sample of subjects to a larger population. Quantitative studies usually produce knowledge about very precise topics, creating a need for multiple studies over multiple years before conclusive knowledge is yielded. The most common quantitative designs used in health care research are case study, survey, needs assessment, experimental, quasiexperimental, methodologic, meta-analysis, and secondary analysis. A brief overview of these predominantly quantitative study designs is given in Table 21-1. For in-depth understanding of particular methods and their suitability for studying particular phenomena, consult research methods texts.

Table 21-1 A Sample of Quantitative Research Methodologies

METHOD	DESCRIPTION
Case study	Case study designs are used to present an in-depth analysis of a single subject, group, institution, or other social unit. The purpose is to gain insight and provide background information for more controlled broader studies.
Survey	Survey research designs are popular in nursing research studies that are designed to obtain information regarding the prevalence, distribution, and interrelationships of variables within a population. Surveys are a good design to use when collecting demographic information, social characteristics, behavioral patterns, and information bases.
Needs assessment	Needs assessments are used to determine what is most beneficial to a specific aggregate group. This design can be used by organizations, communities, or groups to establish priorities for their respective client groups (Polit and Beck, 2004).
Methodologic	Methodologic research focuses on the development of data collection instruments such as surveys or questionnaires. The goal is to improve the reliability and validity of instruments. This work is time-consuming and tedious but necessary for the implementation of research studies. However, when quality instruments are developed, they can be used in multiple studies.
Meta-analysis	Meta-analysis is an advanced process whereby multiple research studies on a specific topic are reviewed and the findings of these multiple studies are statistically analyzed. Meta-analysis synthesizes quantitative data from the different studies, thus enlarging the power of the results and allowing more confident generalizations than a single study.
Experimental study	Experimental studies, having several subtypes, include the manipulation of one or more independent variables, random assignment to either a control or treatment group, and observation of the outcome or effect that is presumably a result of the independent variable. Rigor and control of extraneous variables allow researchers to establish cause-and-effect relationships, testing causal relationships (Polit, Beck, and Hungler, 2001).
Quasi-experimental design	A quasi-experimental design lacking one of the required components of the experimental design. When randomization, a control group, or the manipulation of one or more variables is not possible, this is a useful design. Several subtypes exist.
Secondary analysis	Secondary analysis involves asking new questions of data collected previously. The data may have been generated from previous formal research or may have resulted from any prior systematic collection of data. Examples of prior nonresearch data would include the many inevitable records generated as a by-product of health care delivery systems.

Qualitative Designs

Qualitative research is a method of research designed for discovery rather than verification. It is used to explore little-known or ambiguous phenomena. The researcher is looking to explain a phenomena or process rather than to verify a cause and effect. Qualitative methods can be important to the complex study of humans. Concepts that are important to health care professionals often are difficult to reduce in a quantitative way. Interviewing is the main technique used in qualitative methods to explore the meaning of certain experiences to individuals. This method is time-consuming and costly and uses small samples; therefore generalizations cannot be made from findings. However, when exploring issues such as caregiver strain or hardiness, it might be more appropriate to interview participants to get their perspective than to send out a standard questionnaire that might not encompass everything the researcher would discover from personally interviewing the participant. The main types of qualitative research designs include phenomenology, ethnography, and grounded theory. Table 21-2 provides brief descriptions of these methods. For more complete understanding, refer to qualitative research texts.

Although there is a need for qualitative research studies in health care research, qualitative methods are time-consuming and costly. One-on-one interviews take time; and the interviews must be recorded, typed, transcribed, and analyzed. Data analysis is conducted by the researcher, who reviews each transcribed interview line by line to group common conceptual meanings. Concepts are combined to describe the experience for the particular group being studied. Qualitative studies usually have small samples, and results are not generalizable to the whole population. The researcher cannot assert that findings from a small unique sample would be the same in a large heterogeneous population. However, findings should be transferable. The researcher should give a thorough description of the sample and setting so that findings could be expected to occur in similar individuals in a similar setting. In addition, triangulation studies that involve both quantitative and qualitative methods might provide the strength needed to recommend change based on qualitative research findings.

Triangulation

Triangulation is the use of various research methods or different data collection techniques in the same study. Triangulation commonly refers to the use of qualitative and quantitative methods in the same study. This method can be useful when data from multiple sources and methods are needed to provide a relatively complete understanding of the subject matter.

Table 21-2	*A Sample of Qualitative Research Methodologies*
METHOD	**DESCRIPTION**
Phenomenology	Phenomenology is designed to provide understanding of the participants' "lived experience." Phenomenology is a valuable approach for studying intangible experiences such as grief, hope, and risk-taking.
Ethnography	Ethnography is a method used to study phenomena from a cultural perspective. Ethnographers spend time in the cultural setting with the research participants to observe and better understand their experience.
Grounded theory	Grounded theory is designed to explore and describe a social process. It is a method utilized to explore a process that people use to deal with problematic areas of their lives, such as coping with a terminal illness or adjusting to bereavement.

Pilot Studies

Pilot studies are small-scale studies often referred to as feasibility studies. The purpose of the pilot study is to identify the strengths and limitations of a planned larger-scale study. Pilot work is preliminary research that can be used to assess the design, methodology, and feasibility of a study and typically includes participants who are similar to those who will be used in the larger research study. By performing each step of the procedures to be used in a planned larger-scale study, the researcher can evaluate the effectiveness of the proposed data collection methods. Information can be gained that will aid the improvement of the study, as well as help assess the feasibility of the study (Polit, Beck, and Hungler, 2001).

Before the initiation of a 3-year longitudinal study designed to examine the effectiveness of a small, structured, nurse-led support group on grief reconciliation and health of bereaved older adults whose spouses had hospice care, a smaller-scale pilot study was conducted (Jacob, 1997). Procedures for recruitment of participants were refined during the pilot study. Relationships were established with five different hospice programs, and bereavement coordinators were educated regarding the aims and value of the study. The pilot study involved the facilitation of four groups of bereaved adults, whereas the larger-scale study involved nine groups. Four groups were sufficient to test the methods of facilitation and the clinical model of grief support that was used. A pretest and posttest design was used so that the instruments could be tested, even though the larger-scale study included a pretest and posttests at 6 weeks, 6 months, and 12 months. The methods for collecting, coding, and analyzing the data also were refined during the pilot study. Based on the outcomes of the pilot study, changes were made that facilitated the effectiveness of the 3-year study. It was cost-effective to conduct the smaller scale study before the large study because the most efficient methods were determined in advance.

Pilot studies can serve to determine the feasibility of using interventions and to discover preliminary trends in outcomes for a particular agency, personnel, and clients. Most funding agencies favor research that is based on pilot work, although a pilot study may not be warranted if the researcher has used the same techniques, instruments, and participants in the same or similar setting.

USING RESEARCH IN PRACTICE

Currently, there is extensive concern that nurses have failed to realize the potential for using research findings as a basis for making decisions and developing nursing interventions. The following case study illustrates the process of research utilization and demonstrates how useful it is to nurses in everyday practice.

CASE STUDY

Mary, a clinical nurse researcher in a medical center, asks the staff nurses on a pediatric oncology unit to identify patient care problems that need to be investigated. The nurses identify pain control as a major problem for the children admitted to the unit. In talking with the nurses on the unit, Mary discovers that the nurses routinely use physiologic measures such as heart rate and blood pressure as indicators of pain. Occasionally, the nurses rely on parents' reports, but rarely do they consult the child. Mary conducts a review of the literature to determine proven ways to assess pain in children. In the *Western Journal of Nursing Research,* Mary discovers a meta-analysis of pediatric pain assessment techniques. Findings from this study indicate that self-report tools are appropriate for most children 4 years and

CASE STUDY — Cont'd

older and provide the most accurate measure of children's pain. Mary discovers a pediatric pain interview tool in the literature that she thinks would be practical and feasible for use on the unit. She then writes a utilization memo to the nurse manager citing the problem (inadequate pain control), the research findings documented in the literature, and a suggestion for change in practice (use of the self-report pain assessment) on the pediatric oncology unit. Next, Mary organizes a meeting with the nurses to discuss conducting a pilot study on the unit for the purpose of comparing the effectiveness of the pediatric pain assessment interview tool and their usual procedures for assessing pain in the pediatric oncology patients. Findings from this study are incorporated into practice by documenting the preferred method of pain assessment in the unit's protocol. The change instituted by the pediatric oncology unit is cited in the medical center's accreditation report as an example of how the medical center is meeting standards of care in pain management.

Barriers related to research use include quality of research findings, the characteristics of nurses who need to use the findings in practice, and the characteristics of organizations in which the research should be used (Burns and Grove, 2003). Barriers related to the quality of the research findings include the following:

- Studies are not focused on clinical problems.
- Studies are not replicated.
- Findings are not stated in terms that are understood by most practicing nurses.

Evidence suggests that nurses are not always aware of research results and do not effectively incorporate these results into their practice (Polit, Beck, and Hungler, 2001). Major barriers related to nurses include the following:

- Nurses do not value research.
- Nurses are unaware or unwilling to read research reports.
- Nurses lack the ability to access research findings.
- Nurses do not know how to apply research findings in practice.

Fortunately, these barriers are slowly giving way as research findings are making their way into nursing curricula and as practicing nurses are collaborating in research efforts. Still, opinions among nurses that research is not relevant to current practice and views that theory and practice are not related are common. However, even when nurses have an appreciation for research and want to incorporate findings into their practice, they are unsure of what process to use and where to find quality studies on a specific topic or practice issue.

Health care organizations also create barriers to research utilization. These barriers include:

- Desire for stability
- Cost of development and implementation
- Authoritative management style
- Organizational disarray from internal and external forces

Thus organizations create barriers to research utilization when change is resisted, authority is frankly valued over evidence, and attention to complex regulatory requirements takes the majority of the leadership's attention, time, and financial resources (Burns and Grove, 2003). Nurses can play a key role in demonstrating and convincing organizations of the value of research utilization.

In the wake of the increasingly greater amounts of research evidence, nursing and other health care professions need detailed guidance in using research and other types of evidence. Uncertainty as to how to go about the process of using research evidence in practice has spawned recent attention to this issue. Much literature has been written to inform health care professionals about the myriad of issues to be considered when seeking to make an evidence-based change in practice. Whole texts are now available that explain the process of evidence-based practice (Brown, 1999; Dawes et al, 1999; Hamer and Collinson, 1999), and various models have been proposed that more carefully detail the process of incorporating research findings into practice (Brown, 1999; Mackay, 1998; Stetler, 1994).

Brown (1999) offers a model for achieving research-based practice that incorporates three pathways:

1. Appraisal of the findings of a single study
2. Appraisal of collective evidence from two or more studies
3. Appraisal of a state-of-the-science summary

A pathway begins with the shaping of a clinical question. Next, several reports of relevant studies are obtained and evaluated. Once the research findings from the initial set of articles are understood, it is often necessary to narrow or broaden the clinical question and obtain additional reports. Narrowing may be necessary if a very large set of reports is available; broadening may be necessary if few articles are found. On occasion, a single study may be all that is available on a given topic. More often, several studies are available. If research on a topic has been particularly rich, it may be possible to locate a state-of-the-science summary. Brown suggests that appraisal of the evidence should be specific to the breadth of the research evidence and to the particular design(s) of the study (or studies) reviewed. Careful evaluation may or may not lead one to make a change in practice. If change is implemented, there is an ethical responsibility to evaluate the quality of patient outcomes derived from the change (Brown, 1999).

Rather than being a simple process of implementing the practice suggestions found at the end of a research report, use of research requires careful and complex analysis, wise implementation, and patient outcome assessment. On the way to becoming seasoned users of research evidence, novice nurses should avail themselves of expert guidance from clinical nurse researchers, clinical nurse specialists, and other experienced health care professionals. Novice nurses can also develop skill in using research by reviewing and digesting some of the various proposed models for research utilization.

Health professionals should be familiar with two major projects on research utilization that were implemented to address the problem of nurses failing to review and use research findings. These formal projects were the Western Interstate Commission for Higher Education (WICHE) regional nursing research development project and the Conduct and Utilization of Research in Nursing (CURN) project. These projects were federally funded for the purpose of designing and implementing strategies to promote research use in practice.

Western Interstate Commission for Higher Education Project

The WICHE project was a 6-year project funded by the U.S. Public Health Service's Division of Nursing and directed by Krueger and others in the mid 1970s (Krueger, 1978: Krueger, Nelson, and Wolanin, 1978). Members for the WICHE project were recruited from various clinical settings and educational institutions to participate in a workshop that focused on improving their skills in critiquing research. Participants selected research-based interventions that they were willing to implement in practice and developed detailed plans for using selected research findings in practice. Participants in the WICHE project also functioned as change agents in clinical agencies when the research was used in practice. One of the major findings of the WICHE project was that there were few well-designed clinical studies with clearly identified implications for nursing care (Burns and Grove, 2003).

Conduct and Utilization of Research in Nursing Project

The CURN project was a 5-year (1975 to 1980) project funded by the Division of Nursing and directed by Horsley (Horsley, Crane, and Bingle, 1978; Horsley et al, 1983). The major goal of the CURN project was to increase the use of research findings in nursing practice by disseminating research findings. Facilitating organizational changes necessary for implementation of findings and encouraging collaborative research (Polit, Beck, and Hungler, 2001) also were integral to this project. For this project, research utilization was considered an organizational process rather than a process that should be implemented by an individual nurse. From this perspective clinical agencies needed to make a commitment to implement research findings and then develop policies and procedures to guide the implementation process. An outcome of the CURN project was the development of clinical protocols to direct the use of selected research findings in practice. The research utilization process included the following steps:

- Synthesizing multiple studies on a selected topic
- Organizing the research knowledge into a clinical protocol for practice
- Transforming the protocol into nursing actions
- Evaluating the protocol to determine whether it produced the desired outcome

During the CURN project clinical studies were examined for scientific merit, clinical relevance, feasibility for changing practice in an agency, and cost-benefit ratio. Protocols in the following 10 areas were developed by participants in the CURN project:

1. Structured preoperative teaching
2. Reducing diarrhea in patients fed by tube
3. Sensory preparation to promote recovery
4. Preventing decubitus ulcers
5. Intravenous cannula change
6. Closed urinary drainage systems
7. Distress reduction through sensory preparation
8. Mutual goal setting in patient care
9. Clean intermittent catheterization
10. Pain: deliberate nursing interventions

Protocols were implemented in clinical trials and evaluated for effectiveness. Based on the evaluation, decisions were made by individual agencies to reject, adopt, or modify the intervention. These protocols still are available for use in practice (CURN Project, 1981, 1982).

Evolution of Evidence-Based Practice: Some Examples

Since the time of CURN and WICHE, evidence-based practice in health care and in nursing has steadily made gains. Though much work remains to be done, the potential impact of research on health care knowledge and practice can be demonstrated by three examples.

The use of heparinized saline for flushing capped peripheral intravenous catheters was compared with saline only. Saline only was found to be clinically effective in maintaining patency of peripheral catheters (Goode et al, 1991; Goode et al, 1993). As a result of this research, many acute care facilities revised their institutional policies to recommend saline only as a flush for peripheral intravenous catheters. In contrast, Shah, Ng, and Sinha (2003), in a review of heparin use in neonates with peripheral intravenous catheters, concluded that the evidence is still insufficient for making a recommendation for the neonate population.

Research on cancer-related fatigue has been ongoing for the last decade. Mock (2003), an oncology nurse, describes a set of four studies conducted to ascertain the effects of moderate exercise on individuals undergoing active cancer treatment. Results thus far indicate that the prescribed exercise has beneficial effects on fatigue, sleep, functional capacity, and activity levels. Hence a naive belief that fatigue will be remedied only by rest does not hold true. Other interventions need exploration as well. Research plays a role in supporting or refuting common and logically held notions. In this particular context, a simplified notion that rest is the remedy for fatigue is refuted.

Pressure ulcers are a significant potential problem for multiple populations. It should not be surprising that many groups are interested in their prevention and treatment. An on-line search of the National Guideline Clearinghouse yielded 45 relevant clinical guideline statements contributed by groups, public and private, nursing and medical. The national identities of those contributing were New Zealand, Singapore, the United States, and the United Kingdom. In the case of pressure ulcers, a significant amount of research evidence is available for implementing prevention and management strategies.

From the three examples, it can be seen that research evidence can play a significant role in health care practice. However, the process of spreading the "good news" about new or refined practice-related knowledge is a complex one. Researchers must make the knowledge they generate available and understandable. Practitioners must access, digest, interpret, and carefully apply research evidence to the unique contexts presented by individual patients and by patient populations. Different persons and populations need not respond similarly to interventions. Also, there can be honest disagreement among experts about the evidence required to support a practice change. The scientific process may take years to yield enough data to make clinical recommendations and more years to evaluate the impact of evidence-based changes through outcomes research. Although these difficulties exist, nursing and other health care disciplines will continue to be held accountable by the public for developing and utilizing the best available evidence for providing health care. A specific methodology for condensing and disseminating evidence is through the development of clinical practice guidelines.

Clinical Practice Guidelines

In 1992 the federal government demonstrated support for research utilization activities when the AHCPR within the Department of Health and Human Services (DHHSs) convened panels of experts to summarize research and develop clinical practice guidelines. These panels summarized research findings and developed practice guidelines in the following three areas:

1. Acute pain care management in infants, children, and adolescents
2. Prediction and prevention of pressure ulcers in adults
3. Identification and treatment of urinary incontinence in adults

Under the reauthorization of 1999, the AHRQ (formerly AHCPR) continues to support research utilization through its oversight of the National Guideline Clearinghouse. Although

AHRQ is no longer mandated to directly develop practice guidelines, the agency continues to make guidelines available to health care professionals and to the public.

In the United Kingdom, which played a major role in the development of evidence based practice, the Cochrane Center (www.cochrane.org) has published hundreds of intervention guidelines based on meta-analyses and research reviews of important health care practice areas. These guidelines are mainly medical in nature, but not exclusively so. For example, in a review of 16 studies comparing nursing intervention for smoking cessation to comparison groups, nurse counseling on smoking cessation significantly increased the likelihood of quitting (Rice & Stead, 2001). Also, Gray and Flenady (2001) reviewed clinical trials which compared modified open cot-nursing for pre-term infants to incubator care. The review concluded that there was not enough information to recommend cot nursing as an alternative to incubator care. Therefore, research reviews do not automatically yield consensus or recommendations for a practice guideline. In the health care environment, where costs are an important factor, care alternatives are likely to be suggested and subsequently undergo trial and evaluation. Research reviews may then have a role in preventing scientifically unfounded alternatives from being promoted in clinical care.

Strategies to Promote Research

Strategies for Administrators. Burns and Grove (2003) predict that in the future accrediting agencies will require health care agencies to have protocols that are documented with research. Therefore procedure manuals, standards of care, and nursing care plans will need to reflect current nursing research. Progressive nurse executives are fostering a positive environment for conducting research and implementing findings into practice. To challenge traditional practice, an attitude of openness and intellectual curiosity must exist. Administrators should use the following strategies suggested by Polit, Beck, and Hungler (2001):

- Foster a climate of intellectual curiosity by making staff aware that their experiences and problems are important.
- Offer support in the way of encouraging individual staff members.
- Establish research utilization committees.
- Establish journal clubs.
- Serve as a role model for staff nurses.
- Offer financial and resource support for research utilization.
- Include research utilization as a criterion in performance evaluation.

Individual nurses must be empowered to be self-directed and encouraged to initiate innovative care based on research findings from sound, well-designed studies. It is important to determine the effectiveness and overall cost-benefit of implementing findings from research into practice before incorporating new techniques.

Strategies for Practicing Nurses. Strategies suggested by Polit, Beck, and Hungler (2001) for practicing nurses to promote research utilization are:

- Read widely and critically.
- Attend professional conferences.
- Expect evidence that a procedure is effective.
- Seek environments that support research utilization.
- Become involved in a journal club.
- Collaborate with nurse researchers.

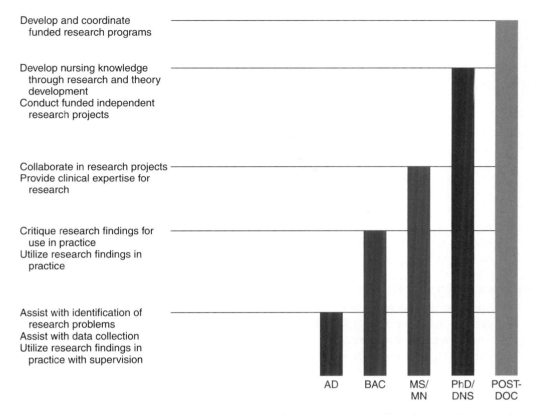

FIG. 21–1 Research participation at various levels of education preparation. (From American Nurses Association: *Education for participation in nursing research,* Kansas City, Mo, 1989, ANA.)

- Participate in institutional research utilization projects.
- Pursue appropriate personal utilization projects.

All nurses should participate in nursing research at some level, depending on the level of educational preparation (Fig. 21-1). The researcher role expands with advanced educational preparation, although nurses at all levels of preparation should at least be consumers of research (Burns and Grove, 2003).

Nurse Researcher Roles

Two nursing roles are specifically focused on research: the clinical nurse specialist (CNS) and the clinical nurse researcher (CNR).

Clinical Nurse Specialist. The CNS is a registered nurse with graduate preparation in a specialized area of nursing practice. A CNS is an expert clinician with additional responsibility for education and research. A CNS is in an ideal position to link research to practice by assessing an agency's readiness for research utilization, consulting with staff to identify clinical problems, and helping staff to discover, implement, and evaluate findings that improve health care delivery (National Association of Clinical Nurse Specialists, 1998, 2003). CNSs are educated in the research process and can conduct their own investigations and collaborate with doctorally prepared nurses.

Clinical Nurse Researcher. The CNR should be a doctorally prepared nurse with clinical and research experience. Terminology used to refer to this type of position tends to vary among countries, settings, and agencies. One might see position postings for clinical nurse scientist, nurse scientist, director of nursing research, and others. A CNR can focus either on the conduct or facilitation of research and should possess knowledge of statistics, grantsmanship, evaluation research, and administration. Interpersonal skills such as patience, flexibility, and approachability are imperative. A CNR employed by a hospital or home health agency must develop relationships with staff nurses to identify the research questions that staff nurses see as most significant in the particular setting. The CNR would be responsible for designing studies and assisting staff nurses with understanding the implications of the study. In addition, the CNR would provide guidance to the staff regarding their role in the research process. This role could involve patient recruitment for studies or actual data collection. The CNR also would be responsible for disseminating findings of the research not only to staff nurses, but also to administrators of the agency so that findings would be incorporated into practice. The CNR also may need to communicate results to legislators if the results potentially affect health policy. An example of findings that could affect health policy is the findings related to the efficacy of hospice bereavement intervention. Currently legislation mandates that hospice programs provide bereavement services, although there is no reimbursement for bereavement by Medicare. When hospice Medicare legislation was enacted in 1986, there were no well-designed studies documenting the effectiveness of bereavement programs. Therefore bereavement was not included in the funding to hospice programs provided by Medicare. If bereavement intervention studies are conducted and bereavement is found to have a positive effect on morbidity, mortality, and health care costs, legislation could be changed to include reimbursement for bereavement services.

If agencies do not have a CNR, they should be encouraged to develop relationships with researchers in university settings or other agencies. Professors in academic settings are expected to conduct research and often are interested in collaborating with health care agencies that might serve as a site. These agencies often have the patient population that can serve as a study sample. For example, a university professor interested in home health care issues might collaborate with an agency to examine the efficacy of various health care delivery models for patients with congestive heart failure. In a managed care environment it would be essential for the agency to offer care that is the most effective and efficient. Therefore this collaborative relationship would have benefits for the researcher and the health care agency.

Researchers have an obligation to take steps to ensure use of findings. Polit, Beck, and Hungler (2001) suggest the following steps:

- Conduct high-quality research.
- Replicate studies.
- Collaborate with practitioners.
- Disseminate findings aggressively.
- Communicate clearly, eliminating jargon.
- Provide nursing implications as a standard section of research reports and articles.

Locating Published Research

Many health care practitioners may routinely read clinical practice journals but are unfamiliar with research journals. Other than reading the occasional research report that may be disseminated through a practice journal, busy clinicians may not spend time browsing the library for research. Computerized databases have aided the process of locating research relevant to current practice. The Cumulative Index to Nursing and Allied Health Literature (CINAHL), available in print and electronic database versions, indexes 1695 journal titles (December 2003) categorized as follows: 520 nursing; 380 allied health; 91 consumer health; 624 biomedicine; and 82 alternative/complementary therapies, education, health services, and administration (www.cinahl.com/prodsvcs/cinahldb). MEDLINE (Medical Literature Analysis, and Retrieval System Online) is the most comprehensive on-line resource for national and international medical literature. MEDLINE includes about 12 million articles from approximately 4600 life science and biomedical journals in 30 languages (*www.nlm.nih.gov/pubs/factsheets/medline.html*) (U.S. National Library of Medicine, 2002). Computerized literature databases may simply list article information, include short summaries of the article contents, or provide access to full-text articles.

Traditionally, printed journal articles have been available on the shelves of libraries in paper or microfiche format. If articles not available locally, users may request that their library acquire the articles from another library (interlibrary loan). Increasingly in the last few years, university and public libraries have been able to enhance collections by purchasing electronic databases of full-text on-line articles. Although it greatly reduces the time required to access certain articles, this feature is initially expensive for libraries to obtain. In addition, there is a temptation to novice users to limit searches to only those articles that are available as full-text. This is a serious mistake that any student or researcher should avoid. Literature searches should be conducted with the intent of procuring all or most of the current articles appropriate to the topic of interest, regardless of the ease of obtaining sources. A truly comprehensive reading of the literature may include all articles of current and historical relevance to the topic. Therefore a relatively comprehensive literature search must anticipate by many weeks the time when the searcher needs the articles in hand.

Even though nurses may have access to computerized databases to assist with a literature search, they often are unaware of the journals that are devoted entirely to the publication of research studies. Box 21-3 contains a list of research journals and other health-related journals that publish research.

Another important publication is the *Annual Review of Nursing Research*. As of 2003 the book was in its twenty-first volume. The purpose of this annual publication is to conduct systematic reviews of nursing literature, to provide guidance to graduate students and faculty in specific fields for research, and to provide critical evaluations for health policy makers (Abdellah and Levine, 1994). These volumes are an excellent resource for nurses involved in the development and use of research. For example, if a nurse wanted to study children's responses to cancer, a good starting point in the literature review stage would be to read the review of "Symptom Experiences of Children and Adolescents with Cancer" studies published in the *Annual Review of Nursing Research* (Fitzpatrick, Miles, and Holditch-Davis, 2003). This review would give a summary of published studies focusing on symptoms experienced by children living with cancer. Important information would include study designs, variables considered, instruments, important findings from each of the reviewed studies, and gaps that exist in the body of research that has already been conducted. Reviews usually include suggestions for further study on the particular topic reviewed.

Critical Appraisal of Nursing Research

Nurses of all levels of educational preparation should read research journal articles critically. A journal article is a summary of a research study. Research reports are published in research

BOX 21-3   Nursing and Health-Related Research Journals

Nursing

Advances in Nursing Science
Applied Nursing Research
Clinical Nursing Research
Clinical Effectiveness in Nursing
International Journal of Nursing Studies
Journal of Nursing Scholarship
Journal of Advanced Nursing
Journal of Transcultural Nursing
Nursing Clinics of North America
Nursing Economics
Nursing Policy Forum
Nursing Research
Nursing Science Quarterly
Online Journal of Knowledge Synthesis for Nursing
(www.stti.iupui.edu/VirginiaHendersonLibrary/OJ
    KSNMenu.aspx)
Qualitative Health Research

Research in Nursing and Health
Scholarly Inquiry in Nursing Practice
Western Journal of Nursing Research

Health

American Journal of Public Health
Hastings Report
Health Affairs
Healthcare Management Review
Health Services Research
Heart and Lung
Hospice Journal
Journal of Health Economics
Journal of the American Medical Association
New England Journal of Medicine
Oncology Nursing Forum
Social Science and Medicine

or specialty clinical journals. These articles are accepted on a competitive basis and are peer-reviewed. Researchers who are doing work in the particular field of study are asked to review the article and recommend whether the journal should publish the article. The review is called a blind review because the reviewers are unaware of who wrote the article. Therefore readers generally can assume that experts have scrutinized it for merit and relevance to nursing. If the article is reporting the results of a study that has been funded by a grant, this is acknowledged in the credits of the article. This is added verification for the reader that the study has gone through review and probably is valid. However, readers cannot assume that findings are valid; therefore articles must be critically appraised. Critical appraisal of the validity of research findings through detailed analysis of study design and measurement strategies is another layer of evaluation that must be incorporated into appraisal of research evidence for possible use in practice. The abstract section of the article gives an overview of the study, and the discussion section offers suggestions for nursing practice based on the findings of the research study. These two sections often are the easiest for the novice to interpret. If sections on methods or statistics are confusing, the reader should consult a CNR to help interpret results.

ETHICAL ISSUES RELATED TO RESEARCH

Institutional Review

In institutional review a committee called an institutional review board (IRB) or Human Subjects Committee examines research proposals to make sure that the ethical rights of those individuals participating in the research study are protected. Persons participating in research must be assured that their right to privacy, confidentiality, fair treatment, and freedom from harm is protected. They must sign an informed consent that explains the study and assures them of their rights, including their right to refuse to participate or to withdraw from the study. Institutions that receive federal funding or conduct drug or medical device research regulated by the Food and Drug Administration (FDA) are required by federal regulations to establish an IRB. Studies that are funded federally have to meet strict guidelines to ensure the protection of the human rights of subjects such as self-determination, privacy, anonymity and confidentiality, fair treatment, and protection from discomfort and harm. The IRB is responsible for reviewing the study procedures and process of informed consent to ensure the protection of subjects. The informed consent must include essential study information and statements about potential risks and benefits, protection of anonymity and confidentiality, voluntary participation, compensation, alternative treatment, and specific information on how to contact the investigator (Polit and Beck, 2004).

Historical Examples of Unethical Research

In addition to the institutional review process, a number of codes and regulations have been implemented to ensure ethical conduct in research. The two historical documents are the Nuremberg Code and the Declaration of Helsinki, which were developed in response to unethical acts such as the Nazi experiments. These experiments occurred in the 1930s and 1940s and included experiments with untested drugs, sterilization, and euthanasia on prisoners of war. These experiments were unethical not only because they caused harm to the subjects, but also because the subjects were not given the opportunity to refuse participation (Polit, Beck, and Hungler, 2001).

Another famous incident of unethical research that prompted the need to oversee the conduct of research is the famous Tuskegee syphilis study. This study, which was initiated by the U.S. Public Health Service, continued for 40 years. The study was conducted to determine the natural course of syphilis in African-American men. Many participants were not adequately informed about the purpose and procedures of the study. The subjects were examined periodically but did not receive treatment for syphilis, even after penicillin was determined to be effective. The study was not stopped until 1972, when public outrage was sparked by published reports of the study (www.cdc.gov/nchstp/od/tuskegee/time.htm, 2003).

As late as the 1960s another famous study that violated human rights took place. The Jewish Chronic Disease Hospital in New York was the setting for a study to determine patients' rejection of liver cancer cells. Twenty-two patients were injected with liver cancer cells without being informed that they were taking part in the research. In addition, the physician directing the study did not have institutional approval for a study that had the potential to cause the subjects harm or even death (Polit, Beck, and Hungler, 2001).

In institutions where IRB approval is not required for nonfederally funded programs, the researcher should seek external advice regarding ethical considerations. When IRB approval is an option, researchers should seek it, because IRB approval demonstrates scientific rigor to the audience when the research is disseminated either through presentation or publication.

S U M M A R Y

Educators must prepare health care professionals to have an appreciation of research and to participate in research design implementation and evaluation at the level of their preparation. Practicing nurses of various educational levels must actively seek, develop, and adopt evidence-based practice protocols while encouraging affiliated institutions to support this effort. Health care administrators must facilitate an environment that fosters intellectual curiosity and supports research efforts. Collaborative arrangements between health care agencies and universities must be developed for such activities as student projects, continuing education, development of clinical practice guidelines, and research endeavors. Consumers must be educated about the value of health care research, and policy makers must be informed of pertinent findings so that results can be translated into health policy.

CRITICAL THINKING ACTIVITIES

1. Identify a research study in the literature and evaluate the findings for application to your practice in a particular clinical setting.
2. As a critical care nurse, you learn that there have been several research studies about open visitation in the critical care area. How would you find this information and use it in your practice?
3. As a home health nurse, you learn that there have been several studies on long-term caregiving and caregiver burden. What strategies could you use to facilitate staff involvement in reviewing and critiquing the literature related to this problem?
4. As a hospice nurse, you learn that there have been reports demonstrating the effectiveness of two different alternative methods of pain control: relaxation techniques and music therapy. How would you compare the effectiveness of these two methods in controlling the pain of hospice patients?

Additional resources are available on-line at: http://evolve.elsevier.com/Cherry/

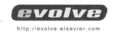

http://evolve.elsevier.com

REFERENCES

Abdellah F, Levine E: *Preparing nursing research for the 21st century,* New York, 1994, Springer.

Agency for Healthcare Research and Quality: *Budget and mission, 2003* (www.ahcpr.gov/about/budgtix.htm).

Brown S: *Knowledge for health care practice: a guide to using research evidence,* Philadelphia, 1999, WB Saunders.

Burns N, Grove S: *Understanding nursing research,* ed 3, Philadelphia, 2003, WB Saunders.

Centers for Disease Control and Prevention: National Center for HIV, STD, and TB Prevention: *The Tuskegee Syphilis Study: a hard lesson learned, 2003* (www.cdc.gov/nchstp/od/tuskegee/time.htm).

Cumulative Index to Nursing and Allied Health Literature: *The CINAHL Database, 2003* (www.cinahl.com/prodsvcs/cinahldb).

CURN Project: *Using research to improve nursing practice, series of clinical protocols: Clean intermittent catheterization (1982), Closed urinary drainage patient care (1982), Pain: deliberative nursing interventions (1982), Preventing decubitus ulcers (1982), Reducing diarrhea in tube-fed patients (1981), Structured preoperative teaching (1981),* New York, 1981, 1982, Grune and Stratton.

Dawes M et al: *Evidence-based practice: a primer for health care professionals,* Edinburgh, 1999, Churchill Livingstone.

Fain JA: *Reading, understanding, and applying nursing research,* ed 2, Philadelphia, 2004, FA Davis.

Fitzpatrick JJ, Miles MS, Holditch-Davis D: *Annual review of nursing research: research on child health and pediatric issues,* New York, 2003, Springer.

Goode CJ et al: Improving practice through research: the case of heparin vs. saline for peripheral intermittent infusion devices, *MEDSURG Nurs* 2(1):23-27, 1993.

Goode CJ et al: A meta-analysis of effects of heparin flush and saline flush: quality and cost implications, *Nurs Res* 40:324-330, 1991.

Gray PH, Flenady V: Cot-nursing versus incubator care for preterm infants *(Cochrane Methodology Review).* In *The Cochrane Library,* Issue 4, 2003. Last updated Feb 22, 2001. Chichester, UK, John Wiley & Sons, Ltd.

Hamer S, Collinson G: *Achieving evidence-based practice: a handbook for practitioners,* Edinburgh, 1999, Ballière Tindall.

Horsley JA, Crane J, Bingle JD: Research utilization as an organizational process, *J Nurs Admin* 8(7):4-6, 1978.

Horsley JA et al: *Using research to improve nursing practice: a guide, CURN project,* New York, 1983, Grune and Stratton.

Jacob S: *Outcomes of pilot work with bereaved older adults,* Presented at Annual Midsouth Conference for Research in Nursing and Health Care, April 8, 1997.

Krueger J: Utilization of nursing research: the planning process, *J Nurs Admin* 8(1):6-9, 1978.

Krueger JC, Nelson AH, Wolanin MO: *Nursing research: development, collaboration, and utilization,* Germantown, Md, 1978, Aspen.

Mackay M: Research utilization and the CNS: confronting the issues, *Clin Nurse Spec* 12:233-237, 1998.

Mateo M, Kirchoff K: *Using and conducting nursing research in the clinical setting,* Philadelphia, 1999, WB Saunders.

Mock V: Clinical excellence through evidence based practice: fatigue management as a model, *Oncol Nurs Forum* 30:790-796, 2003.

National Association of Clinical Nurse Specialists: *Statement on clinical nurse specialist practice and education,* Harrisburg, Pa, 1998, Author.

National Association of Clinical Nurse Specialists: *What is a clinical nurse specialist? 2003* (www.nacns.org/faq/).

National Institute of Nursing Research: *About NINR, 2003* (www.nih.gov/ninr/about.html).

O'Neil D: *Personal communication,* NINR, January 24, 2001.

Polit D, Beck C: *Nursing research: principles and methods,* ed 7, Philadelphia, 2004, Lippincott Williams & Wilkins.

Polit D, Beck C, Hungler B: *Essentials of nursing research: methods, appraisal and utilization,* ed 5, Philadelphia, 2001, JB Lippincott.

Rice VH, Stead LF: Nursing interventions for smoking cessation *(Cochrane Methodology Review).* In *The Cochrane Library,* Issue 4, 2003. Last updated May 15, 2001, Chichester, UK, John Wiley & Sons, Ltd.

Robert Wood Johnson Foundation: *About us, 2003a* (www.rwjf.org/about/index.jhtml).

Robert Wood Johnson Foundation: *What we fund, 2003b* (www.rwjf.org/applying/whatWeFund.jhtml).

Shah PS, Ng E, Sinha AK: Heparin for prolonging peripheral intravenous catheter use in neonates *(Cochrane Methodology Review).* In *The Cochrane Library,* Issue 4, 2003. Last updated June 4, 2002, Chichester, UK, John Wiley & Sons, Ltd.

Stetler CB: Refinement of the Stetler/Marram model for the application of research findings to practice, *Nurs Outlook* 42:15-25, 1994.

Streubert H, Carpenter D: *Qualitative research in nursing: advancing the humanistic imperative,* ed 2, Philadelphia, 1999, JB Lippincott.

US National Library of Medicine: *Fact sheet medline, 2002* (www.nlm.nih.gov/pubs/factsheets/medline).

WK Kellogg Foundation: *Who we are, 2001* (www.wkkf.org/WhoWeAre).

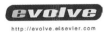

22

Making the Transition From Student to Professional Nurse

Tommie L. Norris, DNS, RN

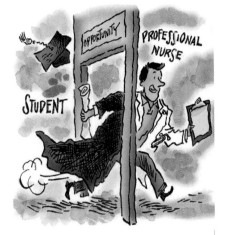

Moving from student to professional can be frightening: plan your strategies.

VIGNETTE

Moving from student to professional can be both exciting and frightening: plan your strategies. "Every nurse has experienced the transition from student to professional nurse. Why can't we learn from our experiences and help our future nurses have a positive first impression of nursing?"

Questions to consider while reading this chapter:

1. What could educators incorporate into the curriculum to decrease the "reality shock" of transition from student to professional nurse?
2. What could employers of novice nurses do during the orientation phase to help nurses "learn the ropes" of their organization, which may differ somewhat from the learning environment?
3. What strategies should novice nurses use to gain self-esteem and prove themselves capable of having the required skills while still needing help with specific tasks and skills that come with experience?
4. Should professional nurses form official task teams to look at the role of mentoring as one means of transitioning novice nurses into the profession?

Additional resources are available on-line at: http://evolve.elsevier.com/Cherry/

KEY TERMS

Biculturalism The merging of school values with those of the workplace.

Mentoring A mutual interactive method of learning in which a knowledgeable nurse inspires and encourages a novice nurse.

Novice nurse A nurse who is entering the professional workplace for the first time; usually occurs from the point of graduation until competencies required by the profession are achieved.

Preceptor An experienced professional nurse who serves as a mentor and assists with socialization of the novice nurse.

Reality shock A condition that exists when a person prepares for a profession, enters the profession, and then finds that he or she is not prepared.

Role modeling Observing experienced nurses, often in leadership positions, to internalize desired qualities during rule transition (Strader, 1995).

Socialization The nurturing, acceptance, and integration of a person into the profession of nursing; the identification of a person with the profession of nursing.

Transition Moving from one role, setting, or level of competency in nursing to another; change.

LEARNING OUTCOMES

After studying this chapter, the reader will be able to:
1. Compare and contrast the phases of reality shock.
2. Differentiate between the novice nurse and the expert professional nurse.
3. Design strategies to ease the transition from novice to professional nurse.
4. Make the transition from novice to professional nurse.

CHAPTER OVERVIEW

According to Webster, *transition* is defined as "change" or the "passage from one state, place, stage, or subject to another." As nurses prepare to enter the profession and make the transition from student to registered nurse (RN), they move not only from one role to another, but also from the school or university setting to the workplace. Transition is a complicated process during which many changes may be happening at once. The novice nurse tries to juggle all these changes while continuing his or her life outside of nursing (e.g., as mother, father, husband, wife, daughter, son, or active church leader).

To help students gain an understanding of the issues involved in the transition from the student role to that of the professional nurse, this chapter discusses the various stages of reality shock. Strategies that may alleviate this shock and ease the transition are also suggested.

REAL LIFE SCENARIO

The first impression the novice nurse has of his or her chosen profession is valuable and sets the stage for entry into nursing. This first impression occurs during the transition phase from student to professional. Consider the following scenario.

Rachel Stevens had wanted to be a nurse for as long as she could remember. As a child she donned a pretend laboratory jacket and set to work providing care to teddy bears and dolls. She softly spoke to her pretend patients, explaining that she was a nurse and would make everything better. After graduation from high school, Rachel entered nursing school and visualized her dream coming true. She was a high achiever and received comments from her instructors such as "shows evidence of applying the nursing process to the clinical environment," "psychomotor skills improving," and "becoming more autonomous." Her patients complimented her nursing abilities and caring attitude. Finally, Rachel graduated from nursing school, passed the national licensure examination, and accepted her first position as an RN. She proudly entered the hospital and felt confident that she would be a caring nurse and assist patients to achieve their highest level of health.

The hospital provided a 2-month orientation period. The first week consisted of classes to explain benefits, safety education, standard precaution protocols, and computer classes. Rachel loved her new job! The next step in her employment was orientation to the medical-surgical unit where she would be working. The nurse manager welcomed her to the unit and introduced her to the staff. Because all the seasoned nurses wanted to transfer to the day shift, Rachel was hired to work the evening shift, which had a lower nurse-patient ratio than the day shift. Rachel proudly sat through the shift report, jotting down reminders that were stressed by the previous shift, such as "The patient in Room 200 needs a blood glucose test drawn at 6:00 p.m." and "The patient in Room 215 is to receive a unit of blood." Rachel's assignment consisted of six patients. The charge nurse encouraged Rachel to ask if she had any questions. The nursing assistants hurried to complete their tasks. Rachel reread her assignment and entered the first room. "Hello, my name is Rachel Stevens, and I'll be your nurse tonight." She assessed her patients and reviewed their medication sheets. No medications were due until 6:00 p.m., so she began researching those medications with which she was not familiar. At 5:30 p.m., the charge nurse informed Rachel that the only other nurse on the floor would be going for dinner and that Rachel should respond to her patients during her absence. Rachel was a little nervous about the responsibility, but positively acknowledged the assignment.

Moments later, Rachel was paged to respond to a newly admitted patient who was assigned to the nurse on break. As soon as she entered the room, the patient complained of nausea and began vomiting. Rachel assessed and comforted the patient and reviewed the medication record for orders related to antiemetics. The physician had not ordered medication for nausea, so Rachel quickly telephoned his office to report the patient's condition. She received an order to insert a nasogastric tube and place to suction. Rachel was anxious; she had only inserted one such tube with her instructor's assistance. She gathered supplies and reentered the patient's room. She measured for correct placement and was just positioning the patient when she received a page that the blood had arrived for the other patient and the laboratory assistant could not obtain a blood culture ordered on yet another of Rachel's patients.

After numerous unsuccessful attempts to insert the nasogastric tube, Rachel became more anxious and requested assistance from the charge nurse. The charge nurse replied, "I'm admitting a new patient and can't help you. Don't you know how to insert the nasogastric tube?" Rachel explained that she had made numerous attempts, and the patient was continuing to vomit. Rachel returned to the patient's room and attempted again to insert the tube. The nurse originally assigned to the patient returned to the floor; however, neither the secretary nor the charge nurse informed her of the new admission with orders, so she proceeded to care for her other patients. Finally, Rachel again requested help, and the charge nurse inserted the tube to the relief of Rachel and the patient. Now the medications were late, she had forgotten to check the patient's blood sugar, and she had not completed the charts. "Where are my notes?" Oh well, she would just have to remember. Finally at 10 p.m., 1 hour before the shift ended, Rachel sat down to chart. She took out scrap paper and began writing her notes, but what time did she start the blood? She became more and more anxious. The clock continued to advance to 11 p.m., and Rachel was still charting. "You need to give the shift report to the oncoming shift," said the charge nurse. Rachel complied and 15 minutes later returned to her charting. At 1 a.m., Rachel left the unit feeling depressed and incompetent.

REALITY SHOCK

Nursing students are in college for several years and "learn the ropes" of that role, many of them becoming expert students (Tingle, 2000). However, when the expert student moves into the novice nurse role, uncertainty takes over, and the support of both classmates and the nursing instructors are gone. This time marks the end of one era as a student and the beginning of a new era in a nursing career.

Novice nurses often suffer what Kramer (1974) describes as reality shock, which is the result of inconsistencies between the academic world and the world of work. Reality shock occurs in novice nurses when they become aware of the inconsistency between the actual world of nursing and that of nursing school. As the novice nurse enters the new profession, reality shock begins. The excitement of passing the licensure examination quickly fades in the struggle to move from the student to the staff nurse role. Reality shock leads to stress, which can cause exacerbation of symptoms that affect health and loss of time at work (Brown, 2000). There are four phases of reality shock: honeymoon, shock or rejection, recovery, and resolution (Kramer, 1974).

Honeymoon Phase

During the honeymoon phase, everything is just as the new graduate imagined. The new nurse is in orientation with former school friends or other new graduates who often share similarities. Many novice nurses in this phase are heard making the following comments: "Just think, now I'll get paid for making all those beds" and "I'm so glad I chose nursing; I will be a part of changing the future of health care."

Shock (Rejection) Phase

Then orientation is over, and the novice nurse begins work on his or her assigned unit. This nurse receives daily assignments and begins the tasks.

"But wait! I've only observed other nurses hanging blood. Where is my instructor?"

Now the shock or rejection phase comes into play. The nurse comes into contact with conflicting viewpoints and different ways of performing skills, but lacks the security of having an expert available to explain uncertain or gray areas. The security of saying, "I am just the student nurse," is no longer valid. During this phase the novice nurse may be frightened or react by forming a hard cold shell around himself or herself. Vague feelings of discomfort are experienced, and the inexperienced nurse often wonders whether the other nurses care about the patients. After going home from a shift, the new nurse may experience feelings of rejection and a sense of lack of accomplishment. The novice nurse may reject the new environment and have a preoccupation with the past when he or she was in school. A need to contact former instructors, call schoolmates, or visit the nursing school may occur. Others may reject their school values and adopt the values of the organization. In this way, they may experience less conflict (Kramer, 1974); however, there are drawbacks to this approach as well.

During this phase, Kramer (1974) suggests that novice nurses must ask themselves two important questions:

1. What must I do to become the kind of nurse I want to be?
2. What must I do so that my nursing contributes to humankind and society?

Dealing with the shock phase can be approached in many different ways. Some common approaches for dealing with it are reviewed in the following sections. After that, each nurse must decide which method best allows the previous two questions to be answered.

Native. Many nurses choose to "go native" (Kramer, 1974). That is, they decide they cannot fight the experienced nurses or the administration; thus they adopt the ways of least resistance. These nurses may mimic other nurses on the unit and take short cuts, such as administering medications without knowing their action and side effects and the associated nursing responsibilities.

Runaways. Others choose to "run away." They find the real world too difficult. These new nurses may choose another occupation or return to graduate school to prepare for a career in nursing education to teach others their "values in nursing."

Rutters. Some adopt the attitude that, "I'll just do what I have to do to get by," or "I'm just working until I can buy some new furniture." These nurses are called "rutters." They consider nursing just a job.

Burned Out. These nurses bottle up conflict until they become burned out. Kramer (1974) describes the appearance of these nurses as having the look of being chronically constipated. In this situation, patients may feel compelled to nurse their nurse. Inexperienced nurses may become burned out because they assume too many responsibilities in a short period of time (Domrose, 2000). Some common symptoms of burnout include extreme fatigue, headaches, difficulty sleeping, mood swings, anxiety, poor work quality, depression, and anger (Larsen, 2000). The more intelligent, hard-working nurses are the most prone for burnout, but if you exhibit these symptoms, remember that they can be reduced.

Loners. These nurses create their own reality. They adopt the attitude of "just do the job and keep quiet." These nurses may prefer night shifts, during which they often are "left alone."

New Nurse on the Block. These nurses change jobs frequently. They go from the hospital setting to community health to the doctor's office. They are always new in their setting and therefore adopt the attitude of "teach me what you want; I'm new here."

Change Agents. These are the nurses who care enough to work within the system to elicit change. They frequently visit the nurse manager or head nurse to suggest change or a better way. They keep the welfare of the patient at the forefront. Unfortunately, Kramer refers to these nurses as "bicultural troublemakers" (1974).

Recovery Phase

The return of humor usually is the first sign of the recovery phase. The novice nurse begins to understand the new culture to a certain degree. There is less tension and anxiety, and healing begins. The nurse in this phase may comment, "I'll hang that blood, and I'll bet I can infuse it before 8 hours this time."

Resolution Phase

The resolution phase is the result of the shock phase combined with the novice nurse's ability to adjust to the new environment. If the nurse is able to positively work through the rejection phase, he or she grows more fully as a person and a professional nurse during the resolution phase. Work expectations are more easily met, and the nurse will have developed the ability to elicit change.

Most novice nurses experience each phase of reality shock (honeymoon, shock or rejection, recovery, and resolution); however, the degree of shock is individualized. For example, the new graduates who complete their clinical rotation during school in the same institution as they choose to begin their career may suffer reality shock to a much lesser degree because they already may be familiar with the environment, staff, and overall personality of the nursing unit. However, many students choose another institution for various reasons, such as better hours, better pay, or less travel time to work. Nurses who choose to work in an institution different from the one in which they worked as student nurses may experience a higher degree of shock. This does not imply that all nurses should work in the institution where they received their clinical educational experience. The staff in the institution where novice nurses were educated may continue to see them as only "student nurses," which simply presents another barrier for novice nurses to overcome.

Zerwekh and Claborn (2000) suggest completing a reality shock inventory to make nurses more aware of how they feel about themselves and the situation at present. The higher the score, the better the attitude. It might be helpful to take the test at different times throughout one's career or when trying to decide whether a career change would be advantageous (Box 22-1).

CAUSES OF REALITY SHOCK

Many nurses are familiar with the term *culture shock*. Culture shock occurs when people are immersed into a culture different from their own with norms that are unfamiliar and uncomfortable. This is exactly what happens in reality shock. Colleges stress patient-centered nursing, whereas the workforce stresses management of tasks, which may lead to feelings of failure because of the inability to provide holistic care (Charnley, 1999). First, consider how students were taught to think in nursing school. When they prepared a care plan that took all night to complete, how were they to view the patient? Nursing schools teach holistic nursing, or rather, "wholistic" nursing, in which students are taught to look at the patient as a whole and even incorporate the family and significant other into the care plan. However, in the real world nurses may function with a partial-person approach. Different members of the health care team divide the patient care into parts.

Partial-Task Versus Whole-Task System

This type of health care, in which different members of the health care team divide the patient care into parts, is termed the partial-task system and only requires partial knowledge (Kramer, 1974). For instance, one nurse may be assigned to administer all medications, whereas another may be assigned to dressing changes. The nursing assistant aids with personal hygiene and grooming, the physical therapist provides range-of-motion exercises, and the respiratory therapist teaches pulmonary hygiene techniques. There are many other nursing care delivery models in which the role of the RN varies considerably. The partial-task system just described is also congruent with the model known as "functional nursing," which places a high emphasis on completion of tasks. It is an efficient method when working with large numbers of patients, but the nurse cannot provide holistic care within such a system (Huber, 2000). With functional nursing and the partial-task system, the nurse is seen as only part of the care picture, but the RN is the central organizer and responsible for follow-through on all care given by other members. This type of system is popular because fewer professional staff members are required, and it is frequently used on the evening and night shifts when staffing is considerably less. This type of partial-task system encourages loyalty to the organization

BOX 22-1   *Reality Shock Inventory*

Respond to the Following Statements with the Appropriate Number.

1-strongly agree	4-slightly disagree
2-agree	5-disagree
3-slightly agree	6-strongly disagree

____ I think often about what I really want from life.
____ Nursing school and/or my work has brought stresses for which I was unprepared.
____ I would like the opportunity to start anew, knowing what I know now.
____ I drink more than I should.
____ I often feel that I still belong in the place where I grew up.
____ Much of the time my mind is not as clear as it used to be.
____ I am experiencing what would be called a crisis in my personal or work setting.
____ I can't see myself as a nurse.
____ I must remain loyal to commitments, even if they have not proven as rewarding as I had expected.
____ I wish I were different in many ways.
____ The way I present myself to the world is not the way I really am.
____ I often feel agitated or restless.
____ I have become more aware of my inadequacies and faults.
____ I often think about students or friends who have dropped out of school or work.
____ I am still finding new challenges and interest in my work.
____ My own personal future seems promising.
____ There's no sense of regret concerning my major life decision of becoming a nurse.
____ My views on nursing are as positive as they ever were.
____ I have a strong sense of my own worth.
____ My sex life is as satisfactory as it has ever been.

Scoring

To compute your score, reverse the number you assigned to statements 1, 3, 9, 10, 11, and 19. For example, if you responded to a statement with a 1, your score for that statement would be a 6. Likewise, 2 would become a 5; 3 would become a 4; 4 would become a 3; 5 would become a 2; and 6 would become a 1 Total the numbers. The higher your score, the better your attitude. The range is 20 to 120.

From Zerwekh J, Claborn JC: *Nursing today: transition and trends*, ed 3, Philadelphia, 2000, WB Saunders.

because it forces the nurse to focus on task completion and productivity. The nurse ensures that all tasks are carried out but is not the sole provider of care. A simple check mark often assesses quality, with initials being placed by completed tasks (Box 22-2).

Most novice nurses are more comfortable with the whole-task system because it is more consistent with what they were taught in school. The whole-task system requires complete knowledge and encourages loyalty to the profession. The nurse provides total patient care, which incorporates physical, emotional, spiritual, and cultural components. The model of nursing care consistent with the whole-task system is primary nursing, in which the nurse is responsible for all the needs of the patient (Huber, 2000). This model provides increased satisfaction for the patient, as well as the nurse. However, because of the need to use an increasing number of lower-salaried employees and the shortage of RNs, few institutions continue to use this model.

BOX 22–2   Whole-Task and Partial-Task Check List

Whole-Task Check List (completed by same nurse)			Partial-Task Check List (completed by different members of the health care team)		
Initials		**Task**	**Initials**		**Task**
TN	✓	Nursing history	SJ	✓	Nursing history
TN	✓	Nursing assessment	TN	✓	Nursing assessment
TN	✓	Patient education	BC	✓	Patient education
TN	✓	Medication teaching	CS	✓	Medication teaching
TN	✓	Bed made	CS	✓	Bed made
TN	✓	Intake and output recorded	SJ	✓	Intake and output recorded
TN	✓	Dressing changed	SJ	✓	Dressing changed
TN	✓	IV fluids hung	CS	✓	IV fluids hung
TN	✓	Patient turned	BC	✓	Patient turned

Evaluation Methods

Another inconsistency between the school and work environment is the means of evaluation (Kramer, 1974). The school environment evaluates care from the "correct step" aspect, whereas the evaluation phase in the work environment is based on whether components of care were completed according to established policies and procedures. Were all the steps carried out in a logical, correct, and efficient way? This is exemplified in the following scenario.

CASE STUDY

A graduate nurse was involved in a resuscitation effort. After the incident she exclaimed, "I remembered to keep the time recorded and even had all the equipment needed on hand. I did everything right." But what about the patient? This nurse may have enacted all the steps correctly but not have completed the components of care according to policies and procedures.

Think back to your first few weeks in school. Can you remember the hours of practice you spent in learning how to correctly make a patient's bed? Remember the stress you felt when the instructor observed you making your first patient bed? How much error did the instructor allow? Probably not much. This is not to say that you should become "lax" in your tolerance for error. For example, it is never acceptable to have errors in the five rights of medication administration. You must and will develop your own system and quality check for performing nursing care. Nursing texts often list supplies followed by a flow diagram for procedures in which each step is listed. Let's go back to the resuscitation scenario: even basic and advanced life support courses focus on algorithms that direct, step by step, the care of the patient. Always remember that patient safety comes first.

The transition from student to professional nurse is difficult, and changes in the health care environment have only added to the strain. Nursing as a profession is thought to be based on how novice nurses are socialized (Boyle and Taunton, 1996). Often new nurses are greeted with open hostility rather than open arms (Meissner, 1999). Nursing administrators may not support the novices' need to learn and may expect them to perform at the same level as experienced nurses. Unfortunately, the novice nurse may become bewildered and discouraged.

FROM NOVICE TO EXPERT

Benner (1984) described the following five stages through which novice nurses proceed to become clinically competent:

- *Stage 1:* The nurse has few experiences with clinical expectations, and skills are learned by rote; this stage usually occurs while completing the nursing educational requirements.
- *Stage 2:* Exemplifies advanced beginners who are able to perform adequately and make some judgment calls based on experience; most novice nurses enter the workforce during this stage.
- *Stage 3:* Includes competent nurses who are able to foresee long-range goals and are mastering skills.
- *Stage 4:* Includes proficient nurses who view whole situations rather than parts and are able to develop a solution.
- *Stage 5:* Includes expert nurses for whom intuition and decision making are instantaneous.

During these five stages of transition from novice to expert, nurses are most likely to experience stress. Charnley (1999) identified four categories that lead to stress in novice nurses: (1) reality of practice: novice nurses think that they are supposed to have all the answers, are overwhelmed by the volume of work, and feel guilty because they cannot spend more time with patients; (2) unfamiliar with the structure of the organization: valuable time is spent looking for supplies; (3) lack of professional relationships: lack of understanding roles of health care providers and being dependent on other staff may cause anxiety; and (4) lack of clinical judgment: decreased confidence in skills and decision-making abilities leads to apprehension.

SPECIAL NEEDS OF NOVICE NURSES

The following skills have been identified as needing further refinement in novice nurses. Discussion about each of these areas follows.

- Interpersonal skills/communication skills (Brown, 2000; Tingle, 2000)
- Clinical skills (Charnley, 1999; Gries, 2000)
- Organizational skills (Charnley, 1999; Tingle, 2000)
- Delegation skills (Huber, 2000; Tingle, 2000)
- Priority setting skills (Gries, 2000; Huber, 2000)
- Assertiveness skills

Interpersonal Skills

Most physicians, administrators, and nurse managers expect the novice nurse to immediately develop interpersonal skills that they take for granted. These feelings probably are rooted in the past when nurses in training spent most of their time on units caring for patients and received little theoretic information or content in the classroom setting. They had time to get to know the members of the health care team and felt comfortable interacting with them. It is difficult for many people, including novice nurses, to be comfortable with interpersonal skills at work when they feel incompetent and inadequate as a member of the interdisciplinary health care team. They are often uncomfortable making rounds, clarifying orders, and participating in interdisciplinary team conferences. However, effective communication is critical. For example, the novice nurse receives the following order from the patient's physician: "Give Tylenol as needed for pain." The unit secretary transcribes the order and hands the chart to the new nurse, stating, "You will need to clarify this order: I can't take the new order." Feelings of fear and uncertainty invade the novice nurse as he or she practices what to say to the physician.

"Can you clarify the Tylenol order on your patient?" Or possibly, "How much Tylenol did you want your patient to have" or maybe "Hey stupid, can't you write your orders using the five rights?"

Well, perhaps the conversation would go as follows:

"Dr. Jones, this is the student nurse, I mean the nurse taking care of your patient. I don't understand your order, I mean, can you clarify how much Tylenol you want me to take, I mean how much Tylenol do you want the patient to have?" The inexperienced nurse hangs up feeling ineffective, and the physician questions the nursing care the patient is being given.

Before asking the physician to clarify the order, it is a good idea to practice what will be said and even write it down so as not to forget. Then, when face-to-face with the person, state the facts simply and allow time to consider the correct answer. A smile during the exchange in conversation might provide the receiver with a little more patience. Gaps in communication may also occur between the experienced staff and the novice nurse because staff are so familiar with the routines that they may leave out information, making the novice unable to complete the task. Novice nurses must listen, ask the appropriate person, and avoid distractions when communicating (Tingle, 2000).

Clinical Skills

The novice nurse has a basic knowledge of how to perform nursing skills. However, doubt in his or her own ability to perform skills without instructor supervision becomes a reality. In other words, the knowledge is there, but the experience is not (Charnley, 1999). Practice increases the effectiveness, efficiency, and correctness of performing skills. However, until the nurse has experience, there are actions the novice nurse can take. For example, it is wise to be familiar with the procedure manual on the unit. Also, during the orientation phase the novice nurse should ask to observe or assist an experienced nurse with procedures for which there is a lower comfort level or a lesser degree of experience. It is important to remember that no skill is "basic" and step-by-step instructions such as those found in procedure manuals are helpful (Gries, 2000). Remember that everyone had to learn these skills. No one was born with a Foley catheter in one hand and the set of directions engraved in memory.

Organizational Skills

The novice nurse may lack organizational skills. This lack of proficiency may be exaggerated by feelings of being "overwhelmed" by the new environment. Typically student nurses are responsible for a limited number of patients, and although they must answer for their care, they typically are not responsible for as many patients as they will be assigned as new nurses. Someone is usually with students to offer suggestions on how to organize their time. The instructor might question: "Now what do you plan to do, and what supplies will you need to accomplish the task?" New nurses might consider asking these same questions. If unsure, the procedure book not only lists the steps to follow but also the supplies that will be needed. List specific time-limited tasks. Avoid scheduling time so tightly that a slight delay causes chaos. Charnley (1999) describes the novice nurse as lacking general organizational and prioritizing skills. Chapter 23 offers valuable tips on getting organized, setting priorities, and managing time.

Delegation Skills

Most students have limited exposure to delegation. Uncertainty or feeling uncomfortable with delegation may be a result of the characteristics of the personnel to whom one is delegating. Consider the licensed practical nurse, the nursing assistant, or other nonlicensed staff. Often these personnel are older and more experienced; therefore the new nurse might feel intimidated when delegating to these individuals. Novice nurses should familiarize themselves with policies concerning which tasks can be performed by which category or level of health care provider. The question, "Who can perform this task other than myself?" should be considered. Because of the broad span of responsibility for most nursing jobs, it is impossible for one person to complete all the work alone (Huber, 2000). Delegation relies on trust and leadership skills, both of which may be deficient in the novice nurse. Chapter 18 presents a comprehensive overview of delegation.

There are also times when the novice nurse should decline to accept a delegated responsibility because he or she may not be competent to perform the task even though it is within his or her scope of practice. Remember, patient safety is always the priority! Show your willingness to learn and ask someone to demonstrate the task. Tingle (2000, p. 3) suggests simply stating, "I haven't done this; who can talk me through it?" or "I don't know how to do that, but I am willing to help with it."

Priority-Setting Skills

Priority setting is a skill that all nursing students must demonstrate. The difference between nursing school and the real world is that serious consequences occur if prioritizing is not done effectively in the real world. Flanagan (1995) suggests asking the following questions when prioritizing:

- Will patients be jeopardized if this task is not done?
- Is this task a priority because of time deadlines?
- What other personnel can perform this task?
- Do safety concerns make this task a priority?
- What will be the consequences if this task is postponed?
- What are the legal issues related to the priority of the task?

Many novice nurses need help in organization skills, and saying "no" is difficult (Gries, 2000). Novice nurses may derive more satisfaction from performing technical skills such as starting an intravenous (IV) drip than from cognitive skills such as developing a plan of care. Once they are comfortable with basic skills, they move on to critical thinking skills. Gries (2000) stresses that with the loss of the graduate nurse role, novice nurses are propelled into practice, where they focus on what they do not know and are seemingly blind to their accomplishments. For further exploration, you can visit an on-line scenario by Gries of how this can happen to a novice nurse (http://community.nursingspectrum.com/MagazineArticles/article.cfm?AID=800).

Gries also supports the idea of nurses using an organization sheet to facilitate prioritization and completion. How many people make To-Do lists? Many make grocery lists, lists of bills to be paid, or lists of important dates. The same should be done for work, and tasks crossed off as they are completed. At the end of the day, consider what time was spent in unproductive ways, what caused interruptions, and what could have been done to save time. Huber (2000) also suggests determining the urgency of the problem, which allows for prioritization.

Assertiveness Skills

Students are often very gullible when they are told by recruiters, "Come work for us; we offer a 6-month orientation and you can ask for an extension if you feel uncomfortable. You will not be placed in charge, and only after a full year's experience will you be allowed to independently care for patients requiring advanced technology such as ventricular assist devices." Students may be mislead into feeling that they are "advanced" in their learning and moving ahead of all the others if they agree to shorten their orientation or if, after only 6 months, they take on the responsibility of caring for patients with special equipment. However, after 6 months, even though novice nurses are becoming more competent and confident, they lack the experience to make instantaneous decisions based on intuition. Unfortunately, novice nurses are often employed on the night shift working with nurses with the same or less experience. As "newer novice nurses" (those who graduated the following semester) are hired, the "more experienced novice nurses" may even be expected to serve as a preceptor. Faculty should invite recent graduates to speak to classes concerning expectations after employment. Faculty should also inform the students that they will move through many stages during the next year and they should take full advantage of this learning opportunity.

STRATEGIES TO EASE TRANSITION

When interviewing for their first positions, novice nurses should determine philosophies of the agencies and how orientation programs assist new nurses to enter the profession. There are many opinions on the best way to accomplish a smooth transition, and each nurse should evaluate orientation options available.

Novice nurses are even chatting on the Internet about their frustrations with the transition from student to professional nurse. One such novice nurse described herself as in a race, having only 5 minutes for meals, and having to stay overtime (Cybernurse, 2000). She searches the Internet for "words of encouragement for a novice" and to learn how others have dealt with the period of change.

Biculturalism

Biculturalism is the joining of two contradictory value systems, in this context, those of school values with those of the workplace. Biculturalism is designed to enhance a positive self-image and help novice nurses set realistic goals for practice. This strategy, if accepted in the workplace, allows the new nurse to introduce ideas or values brought from nursing school and integrate them into the work environment. Kramer suggests that the novice nurse appraise both sides of an issue, determine how his or her behavior will have an effect on other members of the interdisciplinary health care team, and single out accessible objectives.

Role Models and Mentors

Mentoring and role modeling are often considered to be the same, but in fact they are different. Mentoring is an interactive, mutual, and personal experience (Klein and Dickenson-Hazard,

2000; Sullivan and Decker, 1997), whereas role modeling is usually not an interactive process (Stone, 2000). A staff nurse can be a role model for a novice nurse but have no interaction with the novice. This can often be distressing for the novice (Meissner, 1999).

Mentors are experienced nurses who must be willing to commit to a 6-month relationship with novice nurses (Bozell, 2000). They help novice nurses to recognize both their limitations and assets and raise their confidence (Klein and Dickenson-Hazard, 2000). Mentors help novice nurses set and reach realistic goals by reinforcing and recommending appropriate courses of action. Mentors help novice nurses build self-confidence and gain professional satisfaction. They also serve in shorter-term arrangements such as preceptorships. The benefactor of mentoring is termed the *protégé*. Vance (2000) lists the characteristics of both the mentor and protégé in Box 22-3.

Recruitment and retention efforts are often supplemented with mentoring programs, which have become especially important in light of the current nursing shortage (Childers, 2003). Some mentoring programs are aimed specifically at pairing male students and male novice nurses with male mentors. Just as females face special challenges when entering a predominantly male profession, so do males entering the predominantly female profession of nursing. Networking with other male nurses helps with the socialization and integration of males into the profession.

Preceptorships

Another popular orientation program is the use of preceptors during the final semester of nursing school and on entering the workforce. Preceptor programs have gained popularity as a means to socialize the novice nurse into the profession and to ease the tension of transition from student to nurse. Preceptor programs often are incorporated during the senior nursing student's final practicum, but they also may be used as part of the orientation program in the first work experience. Preceptorship is often viewed as one method of orientation, which usually lasts about 3 weeks (Sullivan and Decker, 1997). Preceptors orient the novice nurse to the specific nursing area, aid in socialization, and teach skills that are deemed necessary. Preceptor programs reduce economic cost by reducing turnover of new graduates and assisting novice nurses in meeting the expectations of their employers and peers.

Self-Mentoring

Ultimately, no one is as responsible for the transition into the nursing profession as the novice nurses themselves. Mentors and preceptors can ease the transition, but novice nurses can also help by using self-mentoring when preceptors or mentors are not available. Novice nurses

BOX 22–3	*Characteristics of Mentor and Protégé*

Mentor	Protégé
Generosity	Takes initiative
Competence	Career commitment
Self-confidence	Self-identity
Openness to mutuality	Openness to mutuality

From Vance C: Discovering the riches in mentor connections, *Reflect Nurs* 26(3):24-25, 2000.

must be willing to learn appropriate references, develop problem-solving skills, and ask questions. Novices should reflect back over times when they were self-reliant and believed in themselves.

Preprofessional and Professional Organizations

Students who join preprofessional organizations such as the National Student Nurses Association (NSNA) gain leadership opportunities and meet not only other students from across the nation and internationally but also leaders in nursing, whom they thought they would only read about. Students participating in the NSNA Leadership University network learn how to "work in cooperative relationships with peers, faculty, students in other disciplines, community service organizations, and the public in a service learning environment" (www.nsnaleadershipu.org). These organizations provide another avenue for socialization and a sense of "belonging to an important profession" (Domrose, 2003). The NSNA publishes a magazine with information on job opportunities and legislative issues that affect nursing practice. Participation in preprofessional organizations develops leadership skills that will be useful in professional organizations and for potential employers after graduation. The American Nurses Association (ANA) and some state specialty organizations offer reduced rates for new graduates and student nurses and continue with the above mentioned benefits after graduation. In addition to lobbying efforts, access to up-to-date information on standards of practice, certification, and networking opportunities are also benefits of involvement in ANA.

Self-Confidence and Self-Esteem

"Even though this is my dream, I can still get discouraged. I can still forget that this is what I want to do" (Klein and Dickenson-Hazard, 2000, p. 21).

A relationship woven with encouragement can inspire self-esteem and self-confidence. It is easy to become discouraged and disillusioned when reality doesn't quite match our dreams and fantasy. Self-esteem, or belief in oneself, comes as the novice nurse passes through the stages of reality shock and into a career in nursing.

Self-esteem = Self-confidence + Self-respect

Individuals with high self-esteem can critically problem solve, tackle obstacles, take sensible risks, believe in themselves, and take care of themselves (Positive Way, 2000). Nurses with self-esteem are effective and respond to themselves and others in healthy ways (Fig. 22-1). They can accomplish more because they feel comfortable with themselves.

Take the self-esteem questionnaire in Box 22-4; then go to the Create Positive Relationships website. If your score is low, visit the Positive Way website to learn how to stop the inner critic (http://positive-way.com/stopping%20your%20inner%20critic.htm).

So far, we have discussed ways that the employer and novice nurse can use to ease the transition period—implementing biculturalism, preceptorships, mentoring, and self-mentoring. However, each new nurse must begin by evaluating his or her own self-esteem. In addition, the novice nurse must realize his or her uniqueness and rely on instinct and past experiences when maturing and moving to a higher level of responsibility. The new nurse should remember to seek a role model or mentor for guidance through the transition. It is important to remember that it is difficult to be successful if personal and social life are not kept in balance (e.g., in high school it was great to solve all the chemistry equations on an examination,

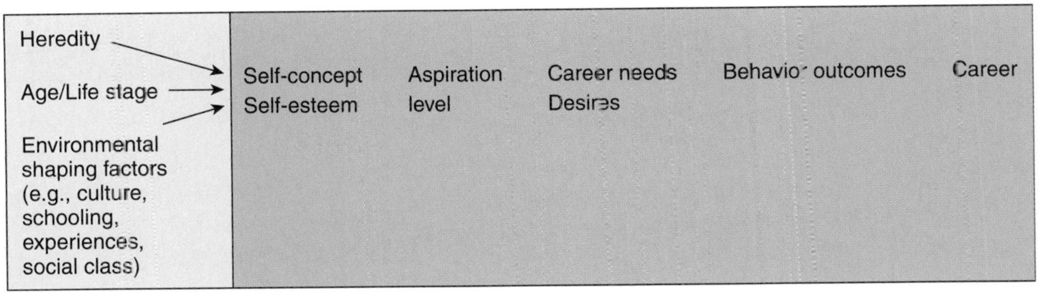

FIG. 22–1 Behavior model. (From Schutz C, Decker PJ, Sullivan EJ. *Effective management in nursing: an experiential/skill building workbook,* Menlo Park, 1992, Addison-Wesley Nursing, A Division of Benjamin Cummings Publishing Co.)

but if "personal chemistry" was neglected, a void was felt that could plague future attempts at maturing).

KEYS TO SURVIVAL DURING TRANSITION

Tingle (2000) suggests a transition strategy using the analogy NURSES (Box 22-5).

Melissa Groggin (2000) suggests 10 ways to help nurses cope and reduce stress:

1. Think before answering—take a few minutes before you answer and decide what is best for you.
2. Take vacations—what can seem like a crisis before the break may become manageable with distance.
3. Get rid of minor things that drain your energy—bring your lunch and eat in a quiet space rather than spending most of your break waiting in line, only to "swallow your lunch whole" or, even worse, eat on the unit.
4. Support your co-workers—be a good listener.
5. Wear comfortable uniforms and shoes—you can't think if your feet hurt and your pants are too tight.
6. Treat yourself—do something nice for yourself every week.
7. Avoid people who irritate or hassle you—pessimistic people can bring you down.
8. Keep in touch with yourself—don't take on everyone else's responsibilities.
9. Say NO—and don't feel guilty.
10. Remember, nursing is a noble profession.

MEETING SPECIAL NEEDS OF THE NOVICE NURSE

It is important to review some common problems perceived by novice nurses and to offer suggestions to ease the transition period.

Organizational Skills

Lack of organization is common when the novice nurse's assignment becomes much heavier than that of a student nurse. The use of a report sheet can enable the novice nurse to note

BOX 22-4 *Self-Esteem Questionnaire*

Answer *Yes* or *No* to the following questions:

_____ Do you have a hard time nurturing yourself?
_____ Have you ever turned down an invitation to a party or function because of the way you felt about yourself?
_____ Do you get your sense of self-worth from the approval of others?
_____ Are you supportive of others who berate you?
_____ When things go wrong in life, do you blame yourself?
_____ Do you react to disappointment by blaming others?
_____ Do you begin each day with a negative attitude?
_____ Do you feel underserving?
_____ Do you ever feel like an impostor and that soon your deficiencies will be exposed?
_____ Do you have an inner critic who is disparaging or demeaning?
_____ Do you believe that being hard on yourself is the best motivation for change?
_____ Do your good points seem ordinary and your failings all important?
_____ Do you feel unattractive?
_____ Have you ever felt that your accomplishments are due to luck, but that your failures are due to incompetence or inadequacy?
_____ Have you ever felt that, if you are not a total success, then you are a failure, and that there is no middle ground and no points for effort?
_____ Do you feel unappreciated?
_____ Do you feel lonely?
_____ Do you struggle with feelings of inferiority?
_____ Do other people's opinions count more to you than your own?
_____ Do you criticize yourself often?
_____ Do others criticize you often?
_____ Do you hesitate to do things because of what others might think?
The more *Yes* answers you have, the greater the opportunity exists for improving your self-esteem.

Positive Way, 2000, PO Box 1703, Williamsville, NY 14231-1703 (mailto:positive-way@positive-way.com).

important information received during the shift report and from other members of the interdisciplinary health care team as the day progresses. The report sheet can also be used to document occurrences during the shift. Another suggestion for the novice nurse is to contact a former nursing instructor. Most students have developed a special rapport with one or two instructors. Novice nurses might telephone one of their former instructors to discuss the challenges they face during transition so that the instructor can help with problem solving.

The basic report sheet (Box 22-6) also can be transformed into a unit-specific sheet. For instance, if the novice nurse is on a telemetry floor, there might be a section for "Rhythms." The orthopedic nurse could include "Traction." This form also can be used to establish and set priorities. Once the care has been prioritized, the nurse can begin those critical interventions. However, it also may be possible to delegate tasks to ancillary staff if the tasks are within their scope of practice. This requires the novice nurse to become familiar with the job descriptions of other nursing personnel, such as licensed professional nurses, nursing assistants, or unlicensed personnel, so delegation will be within their defined roles. Remember that the RN cannot do everything.

BOX 22–5 *Nurses*

Never Fail to Ask for Help.
If you don't ask, you may never receive help. The best way to get help is to ask.

Use Available Facility Resources.
Use other experienced staff, policy and procedure manuals, and staff development personnel.

Reenergize With Professional Associations.
This helps to keep the novice nurse from losing sight of the profession in favor of the job.

Stay in Contact With Friends.
Join the alumni association at your nursing school and find out what your peers are doing.

Evaluate Your Growth Realistically.
Develop short-term goals (e.g., open all charts by 9:00 a.m.), then long-term goals (e.g., gain certification in field).

Stay Focused on Your Goals.
Remember, climbing the hill of professionalism is hard, but the pure "pride" becomes your armor.

Tingle CA: *Workplace advocacy as a transition tool*, June 2000 (http://www.lsna.org/newpage12.htm).

Clinical Skills

Based on Benner's model, the graduate nurse must be allowed to develop clinical skills based on experiences. The novice nurse can develop competence with clinical skills during the orientation phase by asking to observe an experienced nurse perform those skills with which the novice nurse is less familiar. The novice nurse also can provide the nurse manager and mentor with a list of skills that need further practice. The unit's policy and procedure book is a valuable asset. It should describe in detail the steps to follow when performing a procedure. Spend time reviewing the manual before observing the procedure being performed and then ask questions. Take into consideration that there is more than one correct way to perform a skill; remember, though, it is not acceptable to take shortcuts that jeopardize the safety of the patient.

Interpersonal Skills

Developing interpersonal skills may be achieved by attending unit meetings, volunteering to serve on committees on the unit or within the agency, and taking an active interest in the nursing unit. These activities aid in socialization into the unit and profession. It is important for all nurses, regardless of their experience, to take part in professional organizations at the local, regional, state, or national level. Specialty organizations often provide valuable information and continuing education pertinent to the nurse's area of practice.

As the nurse becomes more confident in his or her nursing abilities and is less stressed by performing tasks, positive relationships with physicians and other members of the interdisciplinary health care team can be developed. Various methods that may be used to develop professional relationships should be emphasized during the orientation period. Nurses in staff development positions can be key players in assisting the novice nurse in developing

---

BOX 22–6 Worksheet

Patient's name _____	Patient's name _____
Room # _____	Room # _____
Diagnosis _____	Diagnosis _____
Diet _____	Diet _____
Activity status _____	Activity status _____
Lab ordered/time _____	Lab ordered/time _____
IV fluids _____	IV fluids _____
Intake/output	Intake/output
Urine _____ Stools _____	Urine _____ Stools _____
Other _____	Other _____
IV primary _____	IV primary _____
IV secondary _____	IV secondary _____
Other _____	Other _____
Patient's name _____	Patient's name _____
Room # _____	Room # _____
Diagnosis _____	Diagnosis _____
Diet _____	Diet _____
Activity status _____	Activity status _____
Lab ordered/time _____	Lab ordered/time _____
IV fluids _____	IV fluids _____
Intake/output	Intake/output
Urine _____ Stools _____	Urine _____ Stools _____
Other _____	Other _____
IV primary _____	IV primary _____
IV secondary _____	IV secondary _____
Other _____	Other _____

professional communication skills. Making rounds with physicians and assisting them with procedures opens the door for communication. Asking pertinent and relevant questions ensures that the door remains open.

Delegation Skills

Another important skill that novice nurses need to learn is delegating. First, nurses should consider how others have delegated to them. Body language is important when delegating. Look at the person, be pleasant, and leave room for suggestions from the delegate; however, do not allow the delegate to resist or intimidate you so that you end up completing the task yourself. After communicating face-to-face, give a list of tasks in writing or post it at the nurse's station.

This leaves little room for misunderstanding. Be willing to change the assignment if there are changes in a patient's condition, new patients are admitted, or you realize that the time needed to perform a task was underestimated. If time allows, it is always good to help those to whom you have delegated tasks. For example, if a nurse passes by a door and the attendant is trying to turn a very large patient, enter the room and ask, "How can I best help you turn the patient?" Always take time to give sincere positive reinforcement and say "Thank you."

Priority-Setting Skills

Now consider the best way to prioritize. How did you prioritize in nursing school? What worked then will probably work now with a few modifications. Remember, if it is not written down, it probably will be forgotten. Keep a notepad and pen in your pocket. Jot down reminders of things to be done, and place a number indicating their importance. For example, assume that you have already written the following list.

____ Start the IV for Mr. B in Room 211.
____ Check the IV site for Mrs. C in Room 300.
____ Call the laboratory and check on blood sugar for Mrs. M in Room 215.

Now a call is received from the licensed practical nurse that Mr. T's IV line is not dripping in Room 212. Next, the dietary worker calls to say that when she brought the patient in Room 217 her food tray, the patient vomited. Then the emergency light goes off in the bathroom of an elderly, confused patient. Now prioritize! What needs to be done first? First, answer the emergency light; don't even take time to write down this one. Now, it's time to reprioritize. The new tasks have been added to the bottom of your previous list. Look over your list below. How would you prioritize these tasks?

____ Start the IV for Mr. B in Room 211.
____ Check the IV site for Mrs. C in Room 300.
____ Call the laboratory and check the blood sugar for Mrs. M in Room 215.
____ Check Mr. T's IV line that is not dripping.
____ Assist the patient in Room 217 who is vomiting.

Now try out your delegating skills. Place a D next to any tasks that can be delegated in the list below.

____ Start the IV for Mr. B in Room 211.
____ Check the IV site for Mrs. C in Room 300.
____ Call the laboratory and check on blood sugar for Mrs. M in Room 215.
____ Check Mr. T's IV in Room 212 that is not dripping.
____ Assist the patient in Room 217 who is vomiting.

What had to be considered when you prioritized the tasks? First, you needed to consider how much time was required for each task. It usually takes longer to start a new IV line than to check an existing IV site. It also requires less time to determine why an IV is not dripping. However, this is insignificant if the patient needing the IV line started is critical and needs the medication to reduce his or her blood pressure. Delegation may be needed. What tasks can other members perform? The unit secretary can call the lab to check on lab results and a licensed practical nurse or nursing assistant can assist the patient who is vomiting, provided that you follow up very soon to assess the patient's condition. A nurse must know how to prioritize. Think through each situation. Change the priority as needed or as situations change throughout the shift.

Now that you know ways to develop organization skills, refine clinical and interpersonal skills, delegate, and set priorities; take time to remember other important areas of your life. Remember the people you may have neglected during school and make it a priority to reestablish special relationships with friends, family, and loved ones.

Try the following; these activities show appreciation for yourself and your significant others for all they have endured during your education.

- Reintroduce yourself to your spouse and close friends. You might even treat them to a special dinner at your favorite restaurant.
- Participate in your children's activities at school.
- Read a romance, mystery, or war novel, depending on your taste or mood at the time.
- Clean your house or apartment. There really is furniture under all those papers.
- Get a cookbook and try those recipes you haven't had time to prepare.
- Call old friends whom you knew before nursing school.
- Participate in a health club, learn aerobic exercise, or just walk to improve your health.
- Enjoy the nursing profession—it really is the best.

Experienced RNs should consider the following to help ease the transition of the novice nurse to the profession of nursing: The novice nurse should not be expected to enter the work environment and be as productive as experienced staff members. It is important for experienced nurses serving on agency committees to serve as advocates for novice nurses by reminding nurse managers and administrators that it is not possible for nursing students to learn everything necessary for professional practice during school. Also, remind other members of the nursing unit about this fact. If a novice nurse develops initiative, autonomy, and a desire to become a team member, he or she will succeed.

SUMMARY

The period of transition from novice to competent practitioner is critical. New skills must be learned and refined, professional relationships established, and autonomy in nursing practice gained. Knowledge and skills must be refined over time. The transition from student to RN can be compared with that of butterflies as they emerge from the cocoon. It is unfair to judge them while still nymphs; therefore the nursing profession must withhold scrutiny until novice nurses fly with their beautiful wings spread.

CRITICAL THINKING ACTIVITIES

1. What kind of nurse do I want to become?
2. What are the roles of the professional nurse as seen by the student compared with those as seen by the experienced nurse?
3. What type of nursing environment eases transition from student to professional nurse?
4. What are the important factors affecting transition from novice to experienced nurse?

Additional resources are available on-line at: http://evolve.elsevier.com/Cherry/

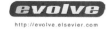

http://evolve.elsevier.com

REFERENCES

Benner P: *From novice to expert,* Menlo Park, 1984, Addison-Wesley.

Boyle DK, Taunton RL: Socialization of new graduate nurses in critical care, *Heart Lung* 25(2):141-153, 1996.

Bozell J: *Career path, Nursing Library, August 2000* (www.findarticles.com/cf_0/m3231/8_30/64427504/pl/article.jhtml).

Brown S: Shock of the new, *Nurs Times* 96(38):27, 2000.

Charnley E: Occupational stress in the newly qualified staff nurse, *Nurs Standard* 13(29):32-37, 1999 (www.nursing-standard.co.uk/archives/vol13-29/research.htm).

Childers L: Big brothers, *Future Nurse,* Fall, 37-40, 2003.

Cybernurse: *Reality shock, 2000* (http://www.cybernurse.com/wwwboard/messages/1173.html).

Domrose C: The "in" crowd, *Future Nurse,* Fall, pp. 42-45, 2003.

Domrose C: *Staying power: keeping nurses isn't about showing them the money, July 24, 2000* (http://www.nurseweek.com/news/Feature/00-07/retain.htm).

Flanagan L, editor: *What you need to know about today's workplace: a survival guide for nurses,* Washington, DC, 1995, American Nurses Publishing.

Gries M: Don't leave grads lost at sea, *Nurs Spectrum,* March 6, 2000 (http://community.nursingspectrum.com/MagazineArticles/article.cfm?AID=800).

Groggin M: Managing your career, *Nurs Spectrum,* 2000 (www.nsweb.nursingspectrum.com/Articles/CalmWithinStrm.htm).

Huber D: *Leadership and nursing care management,* ed 2, Philadelphia, 2000, WB Saunders.

Klein E, Dickerson-Hazard N: The spirit of mentoring, *Reflect Nurs* 26(3):18-22, 2000.

Kramer M: *Reality shock: why nurses leave nursing,* St Louis, 1974, Mosby.

Larsen C: *Reality shock and preventing burnout in nursing, 2000* (http://www4.allencol.edu/~lmh0/CindyL/Burnout.html).

Meissner JE: Nurses, are we still eating our young? *Nursing* 29(2):42, 1999.

NSNA Leadership University: *Welcome to Leadership University, 2003* (http://www.nsnaleadershipu.org).

Positive Way: *Self-esteem questionnaire, 2000* (www.positive-way.com/self-est1.htm).

Stone S: *Mentoring and modeling for the millennium, 2000* (www.ajj.com/jpi/deannote/backissu/mar2000/mentor.htm).

Strader MK: Role transition to the workplace. In Strader MK, Decker PJ, editors: *Role transition to patient care management,* Norwalk, Conn, 1995, Appleton & Lange.

Sullivan EJ, Decker PJ: *Effective leadership and management,* ed 4, Menlo Park, 1997, Addison-Wesley.

Tingle CA: *Workplace advocacy as a transition tool, June 2000* (http://www.lsna.org/newpage12.htm).

Vance C: Discovering the riches in mentor connections, *Reflect Nurs* 26(3):24-25, 2000.

Zerwekh J, Claborn JC: Reality shock. In Zerwekh J, Claborn JC, editors: *Nursing today: transition and trends,* ed 2, Philadelphia, 2000, WB Saunders.

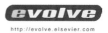

23

Managing Time: The Path to High Self-Performance

Patricia Reid Ponte, DNSc, RN, FAAN, and
Genevieve J. Conlin, MS, MBA, MEd, RN, CRRN

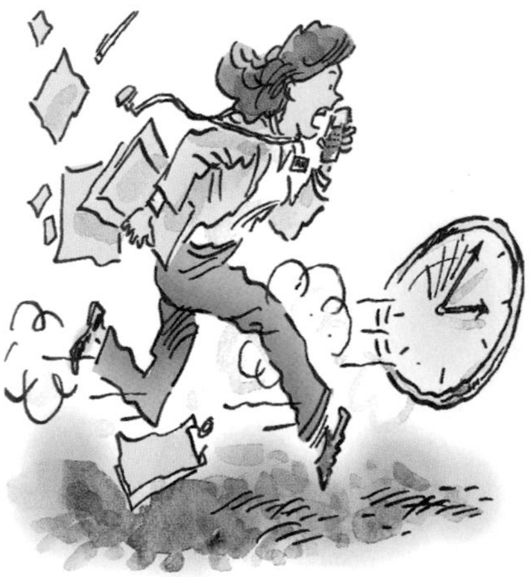

Our lives revolve around time: use it as a way to ensure high performance, positive energy, and focus in all aspects of your life.

VIGNETTE

Approximately 4 months ago, Susan Kenny transferred to a position as a staff RN at an ambulatory cancer treatment center. Today, Susan arrived at the chemotherapy infusion room 15 minutes before the start of her shift. She knew it was going to be a busy day, and given her lack of experience in this work setting, she thought she should get a head start on her assignment. She was heading towards the workstation when one of her colleagues from another unit stopped her. The colleague invited her to a holiday party, and then they both spoke fervently about how much fun it would be.

Ten minutes later, Susan resumed her trek to the workstation. Just as she arrived, the phone rang and Susan answered it. A patient was seeking information about her appointment time. It took Susan quite a while to open up the computer screen, log in, and find the information, which she communicated to the patient. By now, many of her colleagues were on site, already starting to work on their assignments.

Susan looked at her assignment and realized that in addition to her other assigned patients, one of her patients would be receiving her first treatment of a new high-dose chemotherapy protocol. She knew that given the time necessary to work with the patient and family, triple-check orders with her physician and pharmacist colleagues, and administer the premedications and chemotherapy, all while monitoring this very ill patient, she would be very busy all day.

Additional resources are available on-line at: http://evolve.elsevier.com/Cherry/

While waiting for the arrival of this patient, one of her primary patients came in unexpectedly, needing hydration and platelets. The patient also had a fever, and her pressure was low. The covering physician gave Susan orders to stabilize the patient and also asked her to arrange to transfer the patient to the inpatient unit. The hospital was full so the transfer would take some time. Susan began to get very anxious about being able to complete all of her assigned duties while giving her patients the specialized care and attention they needed. Unfortunately, this anxious feeling was becoming a common occurrence in Susan's workday.

Meanwhile, Maura Callahan, a staff RN who had been working on the inpatient oncology floor for just less than a year, was passing out 10 a.m. meds when she received a call from Susan to take report before accepting the patient later in the day when a room became available on the unit. The new bar coding system for medication administration was underway, and despite the fact that this new system would be safer and more efficient, using the new application took more time in the first few weeks. The training was great, but nonetheless, medication administration took longer. Maura asked the charge nurse if she could take report for her, but the charge nurse said she was in the midst of transferring another patient to the medical intensive care unit. "Yes," Maura said to herself, "that clearly was a priority."

Maura took the report from Susan and agreed to accept the patient at 1 p.m., when another patient's discharge would be completed and the room cleaned. Maura thought, "How will I ever get finished in time to pick up my daughter from day care by 4 p.m.?" Her day was lining up like so many before, not being able to finish her work before the end of the shift. She'd have to call her mother to help out again by picking up her daughter.

Both Susan and Maura were working frantically to ensure that the patient's needs were met in a timely way. It seemed impossible to both of them for a few moments before they decided to call their respective managers and seek assistance.

Questions to consider while reading this chapter:

1. When Susan arrived on duty, what are some of the strategies she could have employed to be sure she made the most of her early arrival?
2. What factors should Susan and Maura consider when deciding how to prioritize their patient care assignment?
3. What strategies could both Maura and Susan consider when deciding how to manage their learning needs and the need to be patient- and family-focused?
4. What are some strategies that both Maura and Susan can employ to ensure balance between their work and personal lives?

KEY TERMS

Energy management Ensuring that the right amount of effort matches the right task in order to optimize an outcome while gauging the amount of personal energy expended/taxed to achieve the desired result.

Goal A tangible, measurable, and attainable act in a specific period of time. It has broad-term results, experiences, or achievements toward which someone is willing to work.

Milieu The physical or social setting in which something occurs or develops

Novice to expert Five stages of proficiency in the development of skill acquisition and performance within the domain of clinical nursing practice that frames a transition from reliance on abstract principles of the new learner to becoming an involved performer who is engaged in a situation—the expert performer (Benner, 2001).

Objective An identifiable, measurable act that implements one's goal and is typically short-termed.

Priority setting Establishing superiority in rank, a preferential rating, or the state of "coming first" in order or ahead of others in a process by which that order will represent the execution of the ranked items.

Procrastination The act of intentionally and/or habitually putting off doing something that should be done.

Technology management Application of information systems and equipment to enhance work and life activities to maximum benefit.

Time management The development of processes and tools that increase efficiency and productivity within the set standard of time.

L E A R N I N G   O U T C O M E S

After studying this chapter, the reader will be able to:

1. Understand the unique demands of complex health care environments in today's fast-paced world of high technology and communication transfer and its effects on personal time management.
2. Understand the relationship between personal performance and time management.
3. Understand one's own time management preferences and style.
4. Create an action plan to manage procrastination, distraction, and anxiety.
5. Describe how individual learning and communication styles interact with the ability to manage time effectively.
6. Adopt into daily practice a time management strategy plan unique to one's own style to ensure high-level personal performance in work and home life.

CHAPTER   O V E R V I E W

The previous scenarios are typical of what happens daily in the lives of busy professionals. Managing multiple priorities during a particular workday, as well as integrating personal and work-related demands, is the constant dilemma of so many men and women today. Additionally, performing well in both arenas is a goal of most working professionals. To accomplish the important goals in life, it is necessary to understand your own preferred style of managing priorities, recognize your typical distracters, identify a personal performance approach, and consistently use strategies and tools to make the most of every minute. This chapter is designed to assist students and busy professionals in implementing self-management strategies to better use their time and energy to ensure a highly productive, focused life.

HEALTH CARE TODAY

Health care environments today are fraught with incredible complexities: high-acuity patients, vigilant and knowledgeable family members, ever growing information technology geared toward supporting clinicians and support staff in the care of patients, often tight quarters in which to deliver high-tech care, and little time to interact with patients on an interpersonal therapeutic level. Interdisciplinary practice models demand collaborative teamwork, when in reality disciplines often function in parallel work processes. The need to move patients quickly from one site of care to another on an ever-growing continuum that reaches into patients' homes is the norm in today's health care environment. Fast-paced clinics, high-tech ambulatory care practice settings, and quaternary care in high-intensity critical care units and operating rooms are typical. The nature of the intimate human element inherent in the delivery of health care makes it like no other work. Managing time, organizing care, and maintaining personal health and balance between work and home settings become much more demanding—and essential. Therefore it becomes critical for each professional working in these dynamic settings to receive education and coaching in managing time, energy, balance, and focus to ensure high performance.

PERSPECTIVES ON TIME

Each person has a specific perspective of time, which is based on his or her own experiences, values, education, socioeconomic factors, age, personality, culture, and genetic make up. In order to understand an individual's own perspective on time and the resulting behaviors, it is necessary to create opportunities to think introspectively and examine personal preferences, traits, habits, and tendencies. This is the critical first step in achieving an individualized time management strategy and plan.

In her book *Time Management From the Inside Out,* Julie Morgenstern (2000) presents "ten psychologic obstacles" that influence one's ability to create and sustain focused and productive work habits. As the following ten obstacles are reviewed, carefully consider how they might affect your own personal ability to develop productive, energetic work habits.

Unclear Goals and Priorities. Within a particular work shift or within your life as a whole, if you lack clarity about purpose and expected outcomes, the ability to manage time to meet your desires becomes a futile task.

Conquistador of Chaos. If you are constantly overburdened with tasks, events, urgent requests, and last-minute cancellations, you are a better crisis manager than manager of time.

Fear of Downtime. Some individuals fear the possibility of standing still too long. They feel guilty with "time outs" or time off. Often, this is a result of not wanting to address the larger issues in life. Staying too busy to think keeps long-term planning and personal introspection at bay.

Need to be a Caretaker. In professions such as nursing, the need to be a caretaker is a common devotion and can be very gratifying. However, when this need becomes unbalanced, it can cause you to feel resentful, unappreciated, and overwhelmed.

Fear of Failure. When you are unable to get to the things that are important to you and are unable to meet your personal goals, it may mean you are afraid of failure. It can be very upsetting to go after your dreams and find out you can't reach them. Sometimes it's easier to avoid making the effort. Take time to understand what your fears are and to openly address them.

Fear of Success. You may have been given a message somewhere in your life that you do not deserve to be a success. Therefore, it can be anxiety-provoking to garner success and stand apart from others who may distance themselves from you. Take time to think through whether or not this is playing out in your life.

Fear of Disrupting the Status Quo. Not pursuing your goals for fear of the reactions of those around you is very common. Your family, co-workers, or supervisors may be critical of what you want to pursue. Gradually approaching changes gives you and those around you time to acclimate.

Fear of Completion. If you are afraid of completing a project that is creative and fun because you are fearful that another similar project will not find its way to you or the project may no longer be important to you, take the time to understand why you are not completing a routine task or a major project that has been with you for some time.

Need for Perfection. If you are a perfectionist and feel that everything should be completed with the same level of excellence, you are not keeping things in perspective. If you demand extremely high standards for every single task you undertake, you simply won't get everything done.

Fear of Losing Creativity. Many creative people think that by creating an organized time management structure or approach to life, their creative natures or tendencies will be squelched. On the other hand, creating a framework to manage priorities will allow more freedom and time to enhance one's creative juices.

Here are some of the benefits that will result if you take the time to uncover your own personal tendencies, fears, strengths, and weaknesses (Morano, 1984):

- Greater personal job satisfaction because more goals are met
- Increased productivity as a result of focusing on priorities and eliminating unnecessary tasks
- Improved interpersonal relations because of less stress and anxiety
- Better future direction because of continuous goal setting and achievement
- Reduced stress because of an increased ability to meet deadlines and accomplish established goals
- Improved personal health because of decreased anxiety and increased self-esteem from accomplishing established goals

It is now more crucial than ever before that you strive to understand what you value, recognize your purpose in life, and determine strategies to ensure that both your focus and energy are geared toward your major goals in life. Whether you are trying to organize how to approach a particular workday or you are trying to balance your personal and work life, the strategies that you will learn and integrate into your daily activities now will play out the rest of your life. Managing energy to ensure high performance is the first step.

ENERGY MANAGEMENT

According to Loehr and Schwartz (2003), "Energy, not time, is the fundamental currency of high performance" (p. 4). Striving to be more efficient and more organized or to manage time and priorities better is all in the interest of becoming a better performer either in one's work or personal life. Loehr and Schwartz also state that only when we are fully engaged do we perform our best. This requires drawing on four separate but related sources of energy:

- Physical
- Emotional
- Mental
- Spiritual

Just as we build physical capacity through disciplined training, repetition, and strengthening routines, we can also strengthen our emotional, spiritual, and mental capacities.

Consider Susan from our earlier vignette. Her decision to transfer to the chemotherapy infusion center, her third transfer in 18 months, came only after sheer frustration of not being able to feel in control of her work life and home life. At work, Susan felt overwhelmed, underappreciated, and unprepared physically for the daily challenges of 12-hour shifts. She was exhausted every morning and she fell into bed as soon as she got home. Her energy level was poor. She felt dissatisfied with her inability to spend more time with friends on weekends. Susan couldn't bear the thought of getting out of bed early another day, even if it was for something fun. Because of this, she had gained weight over the past 6 months, and the only thing that seemed to make her happy was to visit her sister on Sunday afternoons for shopping and dinner. Getting to work the next day often proved difficult because her motivation was low and her energy level even lower. With this new job, Susan was attempting to get back on track. "It's going to be different this time," she thought to herself.

Physical Energy

This scenario is not uncommon as novice professionals begin the rigors of full-time work after spending time in college and working part-time. Key components of successful transition to a productive, highly energizing experience include paying attention to physical energy through a routine of proper eating, adequate sleep and exercise, frequent breaks during long shifts (about every 90 minutes), drinking plenty of water, and focusing on one activity while collecting thoughts about what to prioritize next. Once the physical capacity of your holistic self is working well, then attention can be paid to your mental, spiritual, and emotional capacities.

Mental Energy

The mental energy that is most potent in ensuring full engagement and high performance is that of realistic optimism. Realistic optimism is seeing the world as it is, but always working toward an optimal solution or goal. Mental energy is the ability to maintain sustained concentration on a task, move flexibly between broad and narrow issues and be both internally and externally focused as needed by the situation. It includes mental preparation, visualization, positive self-talk, effective time management and creativity. Susan has begun to identify this mental energy in her desire to "get back on track." She realizes that change is necessary. To move in this direction, Susan needs to spend some time to reflect on the following two questions: (1) What are my major goals in life? and (2) What is my purpose?

Spiritual Energy

Often, in today's fast-paced world, we don't take the time to reflect about what's important to us. Being in a quiet place often helps us identify our vision of life—our purpose and direction in life. Susan has yet to determine her life vision given her frequent job changes and her lack of clarity about how she wants to spend her personal time. Having direction and purpose is the key factor in one's spiritual capacity.

Peter Senge (1999) has identified "personal mastery" as the discipline of continually clarifying and deepening one's personal vision, focusing one's energies, developing patience, and seeing reality objectively. People with a high level of personal mastery live in a continual learning mode, uncovering their personal growth areas.

Emotional Energy

Physical, mental, and spiritual energy provide fuel for building our emotional capacity. Managing emotions skillfully in the service of high, positive energy and full engagement is called *emotional intelligence*. Goleman (1999) suggests that self-confidence, self-control, and interpersonal effectiveness are all key ingredients to emotional intelligence. Striving to increase one's emotional capacity—which includes improving one's self-confidence, self-control, self-regulation, social skills, interpersonal effectiveness, empathy, patience, openness, trust, and enjoyment—will result in a more positive, invigorating work experience and personal life.

Understanding how the four energies—physical, mental, spiritual, and emotional—contribute to a fully engaged individual who is productive and happy will help you use the time management skills and strategies described in the next sections of this chapter.

TIME DISTRACTORS AND ENERGY DISTRACTORS

We are all subject to distractors in our work and personal lives that may influence our propensity to procrastinate or not reach our goals. It is important for each of us to recognize and understand the distractors that inhibit our ability to complete tasks and to meet our objectives and goals. Box 23-1 lists many common internal and external time distractors and energy distractors that each of us may experience in a typical day. It is critical to be aware of those time distractors that affect us. The next section provides specific examples of how to strategically avoid these common time distractors.

BOX 23-1 *Time and Energy Distractors*

External Time and Energy Distractors	Internal Time and Energy Distractors
Interruptions	Procrastination
Socializing or visitors	Inadequate planning
Meetings	Ineffective delegation
Excessive paperwork	Failure to set goals and priorities
Understaffing	A cluttered desk or mind
Lack of information	Personal disorganization
Ineffective communication	Inability to say "No"
Lack of feedback	Lack of self-discipline
Travel	Responding to crises
Inadequate policies and procedures	Haste
Incompetent or uncooperative co-workers	Indecisiveness
Poor filing systems	An "open door" policy
Looking for misplaced files, etc.	Shifting priorities without sound rationale
Personnel or co-workers with problems	Leaving tasks unfinished
Lack of teamwork	Not setting time limits
Duplicating efforts	Daydreaming
Confusing lines of authority, responsibility, and communication	Attempting too much at once
	Overinvolvement in routine details
Bureaucratic red tape	Making numerous errors
Junk mail	Surfing the Internet
Waiting, meeting delays	Not listening

TIME MANAGEMENT STRATEGIES

It is easy to apply the perspectives-on-time concept to nurses because many nurses have type A personalities, which means they are oriented toward high achievement. Because most nurses are high achievers, they are more likely to encounter stress when they mismanage themselves and do not use time appropriately. The reason for this phenomenon becomes clear when some of the common characteristics of high achievers are examined. High achievers are identified as those who gain satisfaction through the process of achieving a goal and not just in the goal itself. In addition, they gain intrinsic satisfaction through (1) performing a task well and meeting high standards, (2) trying to overcome difficult but not impossible obstacles, and (3) implementing novel and creative solutions to problems (Webber, 1972). Thus, as high achievers, nurses are often attracted to activities that are challenging, difficult, and even risky. In most cases the activities are complex and time-consuming, which forces the person to use self-management to meet the goals and gain internal satisfaction. When these people mismanage themselves in relation to time, it results in frustration and stress. To assist nurses in improving their self-management and time management, many different management strategies have been outlined for review including planning, implementing, and organizing.

First, there are certain truisms to consider within the concept of time management:

- "Nothing changes if nothing changes."
- "We train people how to treat us."
- "Everything you own owns you."

These are powerful statements to consider when making decisions about how you manage time.

"*Nothing changes if nothing changes*" means that a person cannot effect a change on an experience if he/she is not willing to do something differently that could adjust the outcome. This can be meaningful to both Susan and Maura in the opening vignette. Each works in an environment where the milieu may and often does change in an instant. Although it is unlikely that either nurse may be able to change their overall work environment, they both own the ability to effect small, gradual changes within themselves that will ultimately affect their work environments. For example, Susan and Maura appreciated the importance of getting Susan's sick patient transferred to Maura's unit, but the priority of that situation was not to give report at that time. There is always an underlying sense of urgency when caring for compromised patients. As Susan and Maura continue to work in their respective settings, each will become more attuned to the "true" priorities that await them. As they move through the stages of novice to expert nurse, they will be able to build on past experiences in order to make future ones more successful. The next time Susan has a patient who needs to be transferred to the inpatient unit, she will know that she must first stabilize the patient then prepare to give report to the inpatient staff nurse.

A key factor in understanding time management is understanding the behavioral style one possesses—or in other words, "*we train people how to treat us.*" It is helpful to determine your own behavior style, as well as the behavior styles of those who work closely with you. There are four common behavioral types (Skillpath, 2001):

- *Self-contained:* Manages self evenly and will express concerns with a situation in a thoughtful, reasonable manner. This person is approachable and fair in decision making.

- *Open/accepting:* Always willing to help and say yes to requests. This person likely overextends himself or herself and does not share opinions or feedback. This person has the potential to become extremely stressed.
- *Indirect:* Avoids conflict and will not challenge authority. This person may express concerns to peers but does not address them with management.
- *Direct:* Clear and concise about requests; sometimes perceived as curt. This person may be perceived as difficult to approach and/or intimidating.

When you can appreciate the behaviors and personalities of those with whom you work, you are more likely to use this knowledge to your advantage to evoke the responses needed to reach your goals. When you relay a clear message about yourself—how you conduct yourself, manage your time, and interact with others—you set the tone for future interactions and your colleagues will know what to expect of you. Looking back at the vignette, Susan could have been more direct when talking with her colleague about the upcoming party and asked whether they could talk about the topic more at lunch. This would have allowed her to begin her daily planning sooner. When you are clear and constant in your work, those around you learn to respond to the tone you set.

The last truism—*"everything you own owns you"*—simply means that those tasks you assume as your responsibility have also assumed your time and energy, thus in turn "owning" you. This implies a deeper meaning than simply "having things to do"—that is, you cannot assume more tasks until you complete the ones you are already committed to. We need to be cognizant of how the demands we place on ourselves affect our time.

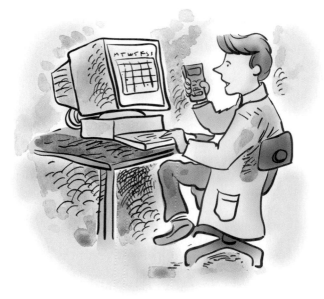

Planning is the most important step in time management.

Planning, Organizing, and Implementing to Control the Use of Time

Planning, organizing, and implementing are the key actions a person can carry out in order to best strategize and optimize the use of his or her time. Each of these three actions are sequential and build upon each other for successful time management.

Planning for Control

Planning is the *most* important step in time management. Unfortunately, few people expend as much energy planning as they should. Some shy away from planning because they believe it is too time-consuming and never leads to closure. In reality, planning allows people to better use their time and can lead to closure in relation to those goals that will produce the most internal satisfaction. For example, 1 minute of planning can transfer to at least 10 minutes of productivity, proving to be a great return on the investment of taking the time to review and plan for the day. If you arrive 10 to 15 minutes early for your scheduled shift and map out the day's priorities, your likelihood of executing those priorities is far greater than had you not taken the time to plan up front. Having that priority-planning list with you as you work is useful in keeping you on track to accomplish those tasks by the end of the shift or day. Those who plan well also tend to encounter fewer problems when Murphy's Laws become a reality. (Box 23-2 lists the three Murphy's Laws that always seem to be true when working on a project.) Thus it is important to plan before beginning any task, project, or day's activities. Planning involves (1) setting priorities and acknowledging goals, (2) scheduling activities, and (3) establishing "to do" lists.

Setting Priorities. The term *priority* implies a superiority in rank, a preferential rating, or the state of coming first in order or ahead of others in some process (Feldman, 1983). A major component of planning is deciding what should be done first and what activities should follow sequentially. The factors that influence how to establish priorities include the following:

- Urgency of a situation
- Demands of others
- Closeness of deadlines
- Existing time frame
- Degree of familiarity with the task
- Ease of the task
- Amount of enjoyment involved
- Consequences involved
- Size of the task
- Congruence with personal goals

Unfortunately, when considering the use of time, not all of these factors carry the same weight. Factors that are most likely to assist in meeting your goals need to be given more

---

BOX 23-2   *Murphy's Laws*

Nothing is as simple as it seems.
Everything takes longer than it should.
If anything can go wrong, it will.

consideration. Setting SMART goals (*s*pecific, *m*easurable, *a*chievable, *r*easonable, and *t*ime-based) may also provide the structure needed to manage these compounding factors we negotiate in our lives (Skillpath, 2001). Several processes have been proposed to assist people in setting priorities, including the **ABC approach**, the **Pareto Principle**, and the **continuum approach**.

The **ABC approach** is advocated by Lakein (1973). In this approach, a person lists every task that needs to be done. Next, an A is assigned to the high-value items, a B to the medium-value items, and a C to the low-value items. The A items should stand out from the other items because of their worth to the person making the list. Also, the A items are likely to require more energy and time, but they should be completed before any of the B or C items. As the A items are completed, you may find that the C items were of such low value that they did not need to be done at all. It is also possible that Monday's C item could become an A item on Friday, reflecting a change in values. Of course, this is an arbitrary system that is based on the person's estimation of the value of activities within his or her own life. It allows for reflection and change while maintaining focus.

The **Pareto Principle** is another process that is suggested for setting priorities. This principle is also referred to as the "80-20 rule," suggesting that 80% of the time expended produces 20% of the results, and 20% of the time expended produces 80% of the results (Mackenzie, 1974). The essence is in determining the "vital few" activities that should be done and eliminating the "trivial many." Focusing on one or two tasks at a time supports this concept (Skillpath, 2001). This principle emphasizes selecting the most productive activities, eliminating trivia, and learning to say "No."

The **continuum approach** to setting priorities encourages a person to select priorities by categorizing or ranking items according to four continuums. As you read about the four continuums, think about Susan's assignment in the opening vignette and consider which of her tasks would have been priorities based on this approach.

1. *Intrinsic importance*
   - Very important and must be done
   - Important and should be done
   - Not so important and may not be necessary, but may be useful
   - Unimportant and can be eliminated entirely

2. *Urgency*
   - Very urgent and must be done now
   - Urgent and should be done soon
   - Not urgent and can wait
   - Time is not a factor

3. *Delegation*
   - Must be done by me because I am the only one who can do it
   - Can be delegated to A; can be delegated to B
   - Can be dumped; task does not need to be done or delegated

4. *Visitations and conferences*
   - People I must see each day
   - People to see frequently but not daily
   - People to see regularly but not frequently
   - People to see only infrequently

Obviously these continuums have varying usefulness, depending on the activity being scrutinized.

Overall, it does not matter which method is used to establish priorities, as long as priorities are established using sound rationale. If Susan had established her priorities for the day, it is unlikely that talking about the holiday party or calling the inpatient unit to give report on a patient that would not transfer for several hours would have taken precedence over reviewing the new chemotherapy regimen protocol she would be administering to a patient. Setting priorities would have allowed Susan to better use her time and would have decreased her anxiety about not managing her assignment appropriately.

Scheduling Activities. Scheduling activities is an important component of planning. It is one way to control Parkinson's Law, which states that work will expand to fill the time that is available. By scheduling activities, a person determines how much time is spent on a specific activity. Such time delineations tend to focus attention and activity so that the task gets completed more efficiently and effectively. A schedule of activities can be constructed using a variety of different methods, including hourly time schedules. Hourly time schedules are not new to most people because they tend to be used continuously throughout life. Everyone has at some point used an hourly schedule for appointments, classes, or leisure activities. In addition, nurses become adept at using hourly time schedules to administer medications appropriately. Unfortunately, most people, including nurses, do not use time schedules frequently or consistently enough.

The process of scheduling activities is an important part of planning to use your time more efficiently. However, scheduling needs to be done appropriately to ensure adherence. Remember to schedule activities so that they coincide with your internal "prime" time, when you concentrate best, as well as your external "prime" time, when you deal best with other people. Typically, the first $2\frac{1}{2}$ hours of the workday are the most productive for people, so plan important tasks according to your most productive time in the day (Skillpath, 2001). As a general rule, 15 minutes of focused time and energy toward a project equates to 1 hour of productivity. Be sure to include some flexible time just for yourself. In addition, schedules have proven to be most useful when they are written down in ink. Having a written schedule tends to motivate people, particularly high achievers, because they are averse to deviate from whatever challenges them in black and white.

Establishing a "To Do" list. Writing something on paper often is the first step to accomplishing it. A "to do" list tends to keep people on track and focused on specific activities. Thus the list should be reflective of your priorities and goals. "To do" lists should be made and revised daily to be the most useful in managing your time. Sometimes they require revision more frequently, even hourly, when priorities shift for valid reasons. The list should be legible and easily accessible to review throughout the day. It is helpful to review the list at the end of the shift or day to assess how you achieved or did not achieve your goals. This is an opportunity to reflect on the distractors you experienced so that you can make note of what not to do when the next situation arises. This will also provide you the opportunity to reevaluate your tasks to see what needs to be carried over to the next day. Some people find it useful to construct their lists on note cards, in day-planner calendars, on pocket calendars, in electronic recall devices, on computers, and in a myriad of other ways. There is no right or wrong way to make a "to do" list, but it should always be available to you.

Organizing for Control

Organizing yourself and your environment is an important component of time management. Such organization requires that you be able to deal effectively with the following:

- The stacked desk syndrome
- No detourism
- The art of wastebasketry
- Email and memo mania

The Stacked Desk Syndrome. This syndrome is exactly what the label implies—a cluttered desk stacked with papers, books, and other things (Mackenzie, 1974; Minar-Baugh, 1998). The syndrome can also apply to the mind when it is cluttered with many thoughts and ideas. Both situations are distractors to accomplishing your goals. Both will divert your attention sufficiently so that you do not know where to begin. When you lose your concentration, you will again become distracted by the "clutter." To deal effectively with this syndrome, you must clear both your work area and your mind. To effectively organize or clear a work area, you should:

- Remove everything from the work surface that does not directly relate to the project at hand; only things you need every day should be on your desk top.
- Place the phone out of sight, but within reach.
- Remove all personal items such as calendars, clocks, or photographs, which might prove to be distractors.
- If possible, close the door to the work area (Kozoll, 1982).

For the nurse, this usually means eliminating the clutter from the patient's room so that care can be delivered more effectively and efficiently. Keep out in the open only things you need to use to carry out the specific task at hand—for example, if you are doing a dressing change, you do not need the catheter kit for your next patient in your immediate work space at that time. Another desk management strategy is to assign a work location at the nurses' station for each staff person working on a given shift. This allows the nurse to have a dedicated space to keep schedules and patient charts available if needed, as well as having computer access, a critical resource for delivery of care in today's health care environment.

No Detourism. To effectively organize, or clear the mind, you must practice the art of "no detourism." This requires complete concentration on one activity or task until—with no detours—it is completed. It mandates that only one activity at a time be undertaken and that it should be completed before moving to a different task. This method also implies that the task should be completed correctly the first time so that you do not waste time redoing it. Inherent in the concept of "no detourism" is the fact that the tasks undertaken are directly related to personal goals and objectives; thus completing them will result in internal satisfaction. Maura may have benefited from practicing "no detourism." Perhaps she would not have become distracted by the phone call from the infusion room if she had been focused on passing the medications via the bar coding system.

The Art of Wastebasketry. Perfecting the art of wastebasketry is mandatory for better use of time. The art of "physical" wastebasketry involves "circular filing" (in the trash can or with the delete key on the computer) of any documents, including e-mails, or other paperwork that have limited use or need no response. The goal is to handle a paper (or e-mail) only once, then either act on it (do it), send it along to another appropriate person (delegate it), or throw it away (dump it). Some also refer to this as the TRASH approach: T—throw it away, R—refer it to someone else, A—Act on it, S—save it, or H—halt it (e.g., stop junk mail from coming to you) (Skillpath, 2001). This art involves being sufficiently knowledgeable and skilled to ascertain which documents, e-mails, and paperwork are appropriate candidates for the "circular file" and then daring to follow through. Practicing this art daily will also help in managing the stacked desk syndrome by reducing much of the clutter.

The art of "mental" wastebasketry involves organizing your mind to deal with the established priorities. This requires using selective perception to attend only to those tasks at hand. It also assists in discarding useless information. "Mental" wastebasketry is a valuable skill to perfect in relation to effecting a better use of time.

E-mail and Memo Mania. Keep electronic mail and memos brief and to the point. Do not procrastinate in responding. Use correct form and proper etiquette and be accurate. Also, keep in mind that a phone call may be a sufficient and more efficient means of response and often more appropriate. The general consensus regarding e-mails and memos is that there are too many of them generated for unnecessary reasons, which may constitute a major time distractor. It is beneficial to allot specified periods of time throughout the workday to review, filter, and respond to e-mail, as appropriate. Taking 10 minutes every morning to review your e-mail messages will allow you to prioritize those activities that may be time-sensitive. Make sure to review your e-mail inbox at least once again around the lunch hour or midday, then ultimately one last review at the day's end to wrap up unfinished business.

Many organizations have instituted filters in their electronic communication systems to decrease the number of junk e-mails received. This has proven to alleviate some distractions staff may experience in having to screen these e-mails individually.

E-mail has become the primary method of communication for the majority of individuals in professional, health care, and academic settings. It is an expedient route to contact people, regardless of their location. It is also a useful way to conduct business with a group of people concurrently, when appropriate, because of the ability to share information with many parties at once. Keep in mind, however, that e-mail is a professional channel of communication and messages should contain a greeting, a clear body of text, specific and clear requests for information, and an acceptable closing to the message. Messages should also be free of grammatical and typographic errors. Guidelines for proper use of electronic communication are presented in Box 23-3. Chapter 17 provides additional information about how to use e-mail effectively.

Implementing for Control

Implementing for control refers to carrying out those activities that assist people in better self-management for better time use. The implementing activities include:

- Attacking the priorities
- Finding "extra" time
- Handling paperwork appropriately
- Avoiding procrastination
- Delegating appropriately
- Controlling interruptions such as phone calls, meetings, and visitors
- Learning the art of saying "No"

BOX 23–3 *Sample E-mail Use Policy*

Policy Statement

This policy sets forth the guidelines for the proper use of electronic communication vehicles including but not limited to e-mail, fax, Internet, and voice mail systems. These systems are business tools provided by the employer for use in the conduct of the institution's business or work-related matters. As such, all aspects of computer technology and communications systems including hardware, software, and all message contents are the property of the institution.

Applies to

All employees/users

Privacy

Employees should not have any expectation of privacy with respect to e-mail, voice mail, fax, or other electronic communication vehicles. Although the employer does not intend to routinely monitor such communications, it reserves the right to review or inspect, for legitimate business reasons, the product of any electronic communication vehicle.

Passwords

Passwords are intended to keep unauthorized individuals from accessing messages stored on either the computer or voice mail systems. Employees/users should not disclose their log-in password(s) to any other person.

Appropriate use of e-mail

1. When sending e-mail messages, employees/users should be aware that the "delete" command does not mean that an e-mail message is irretrievably erased from the computer system. Employees/users should use common sense and good judgment when sending messages to others.
2. E-mail messages are electronic communications that do not disappear, may be reproduced in written form, and are discoverable in litigation.
3. Users of the Internet should be aware that messages on the Internet are subject to interception by outsiders.

Personal use

The employer allows incidental and necessary personal use of its electronic communications vehicles provided use is kept to a minimum and doesn't interfere with an employee's/user's productivity or the productivity of other employees/users.

Prohibited activities

Prohibited activities may include, but are not limited to, the following:

1. Transmission of any messages that contain derogatory, inflammatory, offensive, or harassing remarks about a person's or group's sex, race, religion, national origin, disability, or sexual orientation
2. Transmitting and/or downloading of sexually explicit materials, including messages, images, and cartoons
3. Annoying or harassing other individuals
4. Solicitation of political, religious, or other personal causes or personal business ventures
5. Distributing or storing chain letters
6. Use of Internet access to visit websites that contain sexually explicit, racist, or other material that management, in its sole judgment, considers offensive; or posting messages on such sites
7. Engaging in illegal, fraudulent, or malicious activities
8. Downloading and/or transmission of software programs or any other copyrighted or trademarked materials in violation of the copyright or trademark
9. Attempting to disguise the employee's name or origin of transmission over e-mail

BOX 23–3 —cont'd

Confidential information

1. E-mail users are expected to use electronic communications in a way that respects the confidential information of others. Users must use special discretion in transmitting patient identifying information by electronic communication. Transmission must occur in a way that guarantees it will be seen only by a recipient who has a "need to know" the information.
2. If an employee is an unintended recipient of an e-mail message, the employee should contact the originator of the message without reading the content.

Adapted from the *Dana-Farber Cancer Institute Policy,* located at Dana-Farber Cancer Institute, Available on-line (intranet.http://helpdesk.partners.org/data/Policies).

- Rewarding yourself
- Using technology

Further exploration of these activities will clarify how they can be easily implemented within the context of daily life.

Attacking the Priorities. It is important to attack the priorities early to gain control of your time. Delay in beginning tasks will only result in crises when deadlines or personal goals are not met. One of the most cited reasons for delaying this process is fear. Usually it is the fear of failure, although it could be a fear of something else. In either case, it is important to analyze your fears to be able to identify the source and to determine whether the fear is valid or exaggerated.

Procrastination wears many disguises, and fear is just one of them (Lancaster, 1984). If the priority is a big project or large task, it can be successfully approached by examining how the project can be divided up into smaller, more manageable tasks.

Finding "Extra" Time. The concept of finding "extra" time seems paradoxical because, in reality, everyone has the same amount of time. The concept actually relates to how people *choose to use* their time. In some cases, a different use of time may result in additional time for accomplishing goals. Examples of different uses of time that could produce "extra" time are:

- Using commuting time and coffee breaks to relax so that designated working hours are more productive
- Instituting working lunches periodically, such as twice a week
- Planning subconsciously before sleep

Certainly there are other ways individuals might choose to alter their use of time. The key is knowing which activities can be altered without being detrimental to overall functioning. For example, perhaps giving up 30 minutes of television watching or reading each evening would work for some, but not if that is the only relaxation time that is available daily. Sacrificing "down time" for more work may decrease overall productivity. It may be a case of working longer, but not smarter, so less actually gets accomplished.

Handling E-mail and Paperwork Appropriately. The rule regarding paperwork is to handle it only once. Either decide to act on the paperwork or circular-file it. Shuffling papers/e-mails, filing, and retrieving are all time wasters. Plan to avoid becoming mired in paperwork. Perfecting the art of wastebasketry will assist in handling paperwork and e-mails appropriately. Another tip is to set aside a specific time each day for dealing with all e-mail and paperwork.

Avoiding Procrastination. Procrastination is a bad habit that ranks high on the list of time wasters. It has been referred to as an obstacle to success, a "close relative of incompetency," and a "handmaiden of inefficiency" (Mackenzie, 1974). It can wear many disguises, including fear, laziness, indifference, overwork, and forgetfulness. Procrastination most frequently is evident when a person is faced with an unpleasant task, a difficult task or a difficult decision. Usually procrastination is easily recognizable because it involves doing low-priority tasks rather than high-priority ones, and it always welcomes interruptions. Procrastination is the art of "never doing today what can be put off until tomorrow." The result is less productivity, less internal satisfaction, and more stress.

The first step in avoiding procrastination is being able to recognize when it is occurring. The second step is being able to admit that what is occurring is procrastination. Once those two steps are accomplished, the work of overcoming procrastination can begin. The following have been proposed as mechanisms for overcoming procrastination:

- Identify the tasks that are being put off.
- Ask why the task is being avoided.
- Determine whether the task could or should be done by someone else.
- Identify consequences of the procrastination.
- Set priorities in relation to the task.
- Establish deadlines and adhere to them.
- Focus on one aspect at a time.
- Do not strive for perfection if 95% or 98% will be just as effective (Lancaster, 1982).

It also helps if you can eliminate those tasks that comprise the procrastination. For example, if rearranging the desk, the furniture, or even the med cart is part of how a person procrastinates, then eliminate that activity by changing the work location or environment. Most important, emphasize the benefits that are to be gained by completing the task and accomplishing the goals that will provide internal satisfaction.

Delegating Appropriately. Most simplistically, delegation is the art of giving other people tasks to be accomplished. In reality, however, there is nothing simple about delegation. It usually requires considerable time and energy to delegate, but the rewards are greater in the overall context of accomplishing goals. Mackenzie (1974) and Skillpath (2001) identify the following important benefits of delegation:

- Extends the results that can be accomplished from what one person can do alone to what he or she can mange through others
- Frees time for more important tasks
- Assists in developing the initiative, skills, knowledge, and competence of others
- Maintains the responsibility and decision level
- Is often more cost-effective

With these potential benefits, it would seem that everyone would want to use delegation. Unfortunately, this is not the case. There are many barriers, both internal and external, that can hinder the delegation process.

A brief exploration of those barriers may clarify why delegation is such a problem for some people. The internal barriers to delegating include the following: a personal preference for how tasks get accomplished, demanding that everyone know all the details, believing that no one else can complete the task as well, lack of experience in delegating, insecurity, fear of being disliked, lack of confidence in others, perfectionism resulting in overcontrol, lack of organizational skill, failure to delegate authority commensurate with the responsibility delegated, indecision, poor communication skills, and lack of commitment to the development of others.

The external barriers to delegating are either inherent in the situation or in the person to whom something is being delegated. External barriers within the situation may include stringent policies that mandate who can do what, low tolerance of mistakes, the criticality of the decisions, implementation of a management-by-crisis style, confusion regarding responsibilities and authority, and understaffing. External barriers to delegation that reside within the person to whom tasks are being delegated include lack of experience, lack of competence, avoidance of responsibility, overdependence on others, disorganization, procrastination, work overload, and immersion in trivia and clutter (Mackenzie, 1974). When the barriers are identified and overcome, the delegation process can proceed.

Implementing the following steps will facilitate appropriate delegation:

- Identify exactly what is to be delegated and why.
- Select the best person for the task; this may be the person most qualified, or it may be the person whose development the delegator chooses to contribute to.
- Communicate the assignment in detail, perhaps even including written instructions.
- Involve the delegatee in establishing the objectives and deadlines for the task.
- Have the delegatee repeat the details of the task.
- Give the person the authority for accomplishing the task.
- Provide adequate resources and support as needed.
- Schedule regular meetings for progress reports.
- Establish controls and monitor the results.
- Evaluate the process and progress of the delegatee.
- Let the person do the job.
- Enjoy the results of having the delegated task completed and being able to accomplish other tasks simultaneously (Volk-Tebbitt, 1978).

It is not prudent to take shortcuts when delegating tasks because the results might be different than what was originally intended. Avoiding delegation shortcuts is an important consideration because the nurse who does the delegating also retains accountability for the task.

Delegation would have been useful to Susan in the opening vignette. It could have helped her meet her patient care goals and decreased her anxiety. Unfortunately, Susan was overwhelmed, and she could not identify those things that needed to be done or direct someone else to do them. In addition, she had not established any priorities, so it was difficult for Susan to plan for appropriate delegation. Ignoring the availability and influence of other colleagues can perpetuate a rather self-critical and individualist perspective of time management (Waterworth, 2003). As seen in the vignette, this can lead to a failure to address problems in the organization of work and in the coordination of patient care within the health care team. Chapter 18 provides a more complete discussion about delegation in the clinical setting.

BOX 23–4 *Managing Effective Meetings*

Pre-Meeting Work
Step 1—Determine the purpose(s) for calling the meeting. Common meeting purposes are:

- Communicate additions or changes to policies or processes, etc.
- Receive feedback on additions or changes to policies or processes, etc.
- Brainstorm new policies or processes, etc.
- Update team members on project progress.
- Communicate information that is important to the success of the organization, department, unit, etc.

Step 2—Create a list of meeting topics, such as "Revisions to Nursing Handbook" or "New Admission Policy." Create a fact sheet related to each topic if appropriate and circulate with the agenda.

Step 3—Determine the meeting attendees. The meeting attendees are individuals, groups, or department representatives with valuable insight or who are affected by decisions made during the meeting.

Step 4—Determine the date, time, and location for the meeting and invite attendees. To maximize meeting attendance, ask attendees what date and time would work with their schedules.

Step 5—Create the meeting agenda. The meeting agenda should contain the following components:

- Title of the group meeting
- Date, time, and location of the meeting
- The purpose(s) for the meeting in sentence form
- Agenda items, time allotted for each item, and person responsible for reporting on each item

Agenda items titled "Next meeting agenda items," "Rate the meeting" and "Assign roles for next meeting" should be listed as the last three items and allotted 3 to 5 minutes each.

Step 6—Send the meeting agenda out at least 1 week before the meeting so that attendees come prepared. Send a meeting reminder 2 days before the meeting.

During the Meeting
Step 1—Ensure that the participants' comfort needs are met by arranging the seating in an oval or circular shape and preferably around a table.

Step 2—Ask for volunteers to fulfill the following roles:

- **Leader.** The leader is usually the person calling the meeting. This person is responsible for completing all six of the meeting pre-work steps.
- **Timekeeper.** The timekeeper monitors and intervenes as necessary the time allocations for each agenda item and announces the time remaining until the end of the meeting.
- **Recorder.** This person records the major points of the meeting on paper, flipchart, or board. The person records at the level of detail requested by the group and then captures major summary points, decisions, action steps, and assignments in the meeting minutes, which should be distributed with the agenda before the next meeting.

Step 3—The leader guides the meeting by:

- Processing one agenda item at a time.
- Allowing the timekeeper to do his or her job to keep the meeting on track.
- Debriefing the end of the meeting by asking these questions: "What went well with the meeting?" and "What can we improve upon for the next meeting?" These questions should be used at the end of each meeting to improve subsequent meetings.

Controlling Interruptions. In order to focus on your priorities, it is important to establish uninterrupted blocks of time. Data suggest that the most frequent causes of interruptions are telephone calls, meetings, and visitors, particularly the drop-in type. Learning how to control such interruptions will assist in accomplishing more in less time. One of the easiest ways to manage incoming calls is to not answer them during time that is scheduled for other activities. An answering machine, voice mail service, or an assistant can take the message to be responded to later. "Later" should refer to the time that was preestablished for returning telephone calls. A good example of controlling interruptions in the vignette would have been for Susan to ask the unit secretary to assist the patient requesting information about an appointment.

Most people schedule call-backs for times when their productivity level is lower or during their "down time." Also, telephone calls can be controlled by the tone and verbiage used. If a person chooses to invite conversation and ensure a longer call, using a vague, open-ended greeting will accomplish that purpose. If a person chooses to focus the call specifically on its purpose, a specific, factual, informative greeting will enhance the productivity of the call and shorten its length. For example, "Hi Bill, how are you? How are things going?" definitely invites the person to reply at length, whereas "Hi Bill, I have two questions that I need for you to answer" tends to condense the telephoning session. Also, being prepared for the conversation with all of the pertinent facts readily available helps to focus the conversation and to shorten the call.

Meetings can become a major time waster if they are poorly managed and nonproductive. The first step in controlling this interruption is deciding whether to attend. Such a decision should be based on an evaluation of the potential productivity of the meeting. For example, is the meeting absolutely necessary? Does the agenda contain items that you should be informed about? Is it necessary for you to contribute to the discussion? Will decisions be made that will affect you and your functioning? Are you conducting the meeting? These questions should guide the decision (Schwartz and Mackenzie, 1979). Once a person is committed to attending a meeting, he or she is responsible for helping to ensure that the meeting remains focused and productive so that the goals can be accomplished. The person conducting the meeting not only shares those same responsibilities but also has a more direct role in effecting the outcome. Steps for conducting a productive meeting are presented in Box 23-4.

Visitors, particularly unplanned visitors, also create interruptions. One way to decrease the number of visitors is to seclude yourself during specific times by closing the door to others, physically and mentally. Managing visitors in today's health care environment can be difficult, given the fact that family members are able and welcome to accompany their ill members for extended periods of time and in a variety of settings. Educating family members can be a time-consuming task in the nurse's day. It is important to ensure that this time is factored into one's schedule because it is an inevitable—and important—occurrence.

Learning the Art of Saying "No." "No" is such a small word, but it is sometimes more difficult to say than any 14-syllable word. The first step in learning the art of saying "No" is determining when to say it. The cost-benefit ratio of each opportunity must be evaluated in relation to the overall goals. If the activity will be a benefit overall, obviously it must be given careful consideration. If it will not be a significant benefit, decline gracefully but emphatically. Do not buffer the "No" with a plausible excuse, unless you are willing to say "Yes" when someone finds a way to dispose of the excuse (Pagana, 1994). For example, when asked to review a clinical guideline, do not refuse based on the fact that you are overworked and do not have a free minute for 3 weeks. The person requesting the review is likely to agree that the later time frame will be fine, in which case, you find yourself committed to doing something that has low benefit unless you create another excuse. Instead, be polite and gracious in the refusal but do not allow leeway to be manipulated into saying "Yes." Some busy individuals have signs posted above all of their telephones that simply say "No." This serves as a reminder to consider the opportunity that "No" offers in terms of the overall goals.

Rewarding Yourself. All people function more productively when they are motivated. The sources of motivation vary from person to person. A person needs to identify his or her motivators and use them as rewards for accomplishing goals. It is important to identify long- and short-term rewards so that they can be implemented appropriately. Most people are familiar with rewarding themselves in exchange for doing something, and they do it frequently. For some it is a way of life. It usually amounts to bargaining with yourself to facilitate the completion of a task. For example, "If I finish reading these two work-related articles, then I can read my novel for 30 minutes." Or, "If I complete this paper, I will treat myself to an ice cream cone." You should know which rewards work best and use them appropriately to accomplish long-term goals.

Using Technology. Many of today's technologic advances can be used to improve time management. Most health care settings today have adopted more uses of technologic resources to better improve the use of time and enhance patient care. Many health care organizations are now using the computerized medical record (CPR), which allows for multiple users to access a patient's record at the same time to document and to review information. There are also electronic order entry systems now in place, where clinicians enter orders and activate orders that are then transmitted to the pharmacy to fill the medication request. Patient acuity rating systems are now completed on-line and used by admitting departments to send patients to the appropriate units for care.

Just about every work place today has a professional office system that supports email and scheduling activities. The scheduling features available can be very useful for staff in the planning phase of time management. However, there are advantages and disadvantages to most of the new technologic devices. If it takes a longer period of time to look up a telephone number in a computer system than using a traditional phonebook, for example, it makes sense to review that process for efficiency before determining which system would provide a best practice.

Technologic devices may be valuable adjuncts to other time management strategies. Many people today use personal digital assistants (PDAs) to synchronize their personal and professional calendars. The PDA also becomes a valuable resource in the clinical setting when programmed with drug information and lab value databases, which allows the nurse to have a wealth of information at her or his fingertips without having to carry or look for resource manuals. However, when considering the many technologic devices available, remember that "technology is of value only when it decreases time spent on labor-intensive tasks and reduces overall effort. It's not how many technologies and techniques you use that counts, it's how you apply them to your goals and personal style" (Bergeron, 1998, p. 33). Once the strategies have been implemented, it is important to continue to use them in order to achieve your overall goals and to gain internal satisfaction.

CONTINUING TO SUCCEED

Improving time management to enhance self-performance and accomplish goals is a lifelong process. The process becomes easier the longer you engage in it, but time management still requires continuous attention and energy. Obviously, time management does not just happen. Lakein (1973) suggests that it is important to continue doing the following to succeed:

- When feeling overwhelmed, always stop and plan activities.
- Keep focused on priorities and act accordingly.
- Avoid favorite forms of procrastination.
- Maintain a positive attitude about the established goals, or revise them so that they coincide with your value system.
- Do something for yourself everyday.
- Continue to work on overcoming your fears.
- Resist doing the easy but unimportant tasks (Lakein, 1973).

In addition, delete the words "if only" from your vocabulary. Regret is a luxury and a great time waster. Significant time is expended rehashing mistakes or determining how to make something perfect when it was a one-time occurrence that is now over. Such time usually is not productive unless you will encounter similar situations in the future. It is more productive to admit mistakes, accept responsibility for them, and move on. Thus the words "if only" should be replaced with "next time," and the incident itself should be filed in the mental circular file (Lancaster, 1982, Skillpath, 2001). Douglass and Douglass (1980) and Skillpath (2001) also have a formula for continuing success in managing time, which is presented in Box 23-5.

S U M M A R Y

This chapter has focused on how to better manage your energy to control one of our most precious and seemingly scarce resources—time. Time management is important to achieving any personal or professional goals, and it helps decrease frustration and anxiety in high achievers. Without time management, most professionals could never achieve their established goals, and for nurses, many patient care activities would never get completed, perhaps resulting in poor outcomes for the patient. Susan's and Maura's experiences in the opening vignette are an example of what your life could be like in nursing, unless strategies for better self-management are implemented. Thus it is important in your professional career to initiate habits related to time management that will continue throughout the years. Start asking "Lakein's Question" frequently throughout the day: "What is the best use of my time right now?" (Lakein, 1973). You may be surprised to learn that the answer does not coincide with your current activity. When that occurs, stop and implement the strategies for self-management to better control your time. You will become more productive and gain internal satisfaction as a result.

BOX 23–5   *Tips for Successful Time Management*

---

1. Clarify objectives, put them in writing, and establish a priority list to work from.
2. Focus on objectives, not on activities.
3. Set at least one major objective for each day and achieve it.
4. Record a time log periodically to analyze how time is used and to document bad habits.
5. Analyze everything in terms of objectives.

Continued

BOX 23–5 *Tips for Successful Time Management—cont'd*

6. Eliminate at least one time waster from your life each week.
7. Plan your time.
8. Make a "to do" list every day that includes daily objectives and priorities and time estimates to accomplish them.
9. Schedule time every day to ensure that the most important things are accomplished first.
10. Make sure the first hour of every workday is productive.
11. Set time limits for every task undertaken.
12. Take the time to do the task right the first time so that time will not be wasted doing it over.
13. Eliminate recurring crises from life.
14. Institute a quiet hour of uninterrupted time each day to work on the most important tasks.
15. Develop the habit of finishing whatever task is started.
16. Conquer procrastination and learn to do tasks now.
17. Make better time management a daily habit.
18. Never spend time on less important things when it could be spent on more important things.
19. Take time for yourself—time to dream, time to relax, time to live.
20. Develop a personal philosophy of time that is consistent with your values.
21. Know how you currently spend your time.
22. Identify your "prime productive time."
23. Do tomorrow's planning tonight.
24. Ask yourself often, "Why am I doing what I am doing right now?"
25. Handle each piece of paper only once
26. Delegate whenever possible and delegate wisely.
27. Identify your high payoff items (80/20 principle).

From Douglass ME, Douglass DN: *Manage your time, manage your work, manage yourself,* New York, 1980, AMACOM; Skillpath Seminars: *Managing multiple projects, objective and deadlines,* Mission, Kans, 2001.

CRITICAL THINKING ACTIVITIES

1. Develop your own personalized time management plan by completing the following steps:
   a. Write a one-paragraph statement regarding your philosophy of time and energy management.
   b. At the end of a day, make a record of how you spent your day. Analyze the record to determine what personal objectives were attacked or accomplished and which activities could be classified as either time wasters or procrastination efforts.
   c. Analyze each hour of the day that was recorded to determine whether it was the best use of your time.
   d. For 1 day, keep a record of the number and type of interruptions you experience. Analyze the record and develop a plan to decrease that number by at least half.
   e. Identify your three favorite time wasters and devise a plan for decreasing them each day until they finally are eliminated.
   f. Identify your three favorite forms of procrastination; then create an action plan with strategies identified to eliminate them.
2. List all of the patients on your unit, their ages, diagnoses, and specific therapeutic interventions. Prioritize the patient care activities in terms of how you would plan to deliver their care.

3. Evaluate the patient care assignment that you had today and re-plan how you would deliver the care to be able to accomplish more within the same time frame.
4. Make a "to do" list for tomorrow's tasks, complete with time estimates. Analyze the list in terms of your objectives and priorities. Revise it as necessary and then implement it.
5. Identify three of your favorite short- and long-term rewards and implement one of your short-term rewards at least every day.

Additional resources are available on-line at: http://evolve.elsevier.com/Cherry/

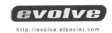

http://evolve.elsevier.com

REFERENCES

Benner P: *From novice to expert: excellence and power in clinical nursing practice*, New Jersey, 2001, Prentice Hall.

Bergeron, BP: Taming time with technology, *Postgrad Med* 103:33, 40, 1998.

Douglass ME, Douglass DN: *Manage your time, manage your work, manage yourself*, New York, 1980, AMACOM.

Feldman ES, Monicken D, Crowley MB: A systems approach to prioritizing, *Nurs Admin* Q 7:57, 1983.

Goleman D: *Emotional intelligence*, New York, Bantam Books, 1995.

Kozoll CE: *Time management for educators*, Bloomington, Ind, 1982, Phi Delta Kappa Educational Foundation.

Lakein A: *How to get control of your time and your life*, New York, 1973, Signet.

Lancaster J: Making the most of every minute: reminders for nursing leaders, *Nurs Leadership* 5:9-10, 1982.

Lancaster J: Making every minute count, *Nurs Success Today* 1:14-15, 1984.

Loehr J, Schwartz T: *The power of full engagement*, New York, Free Press, 2003.

Mackenzie RA: Myths of time management, *Notes and Quotes* 410:2, 1974.

Minar-Baugh V: Survival strategies: improving time management skills, *Ostomy/Wound Manage* 44:79 1998.

Morano VJ: Time management: from victim to victor, *Health Care Superv* 3:2, 1984.

Morgenstern J: *Time management from the inside out*, New York, 2000, Henry Holt and Co.

Pagana KD: Teaching students time management strategies, *J Nurs Educ* 33:381, 1994.

Schwartz EB, Mackenzie RA: Time-management strategy for women, *J Nurs Admin* 9:26, 1979.

Senge P: *The fifth discipline*, New York, 1990, Doubleday.

Skillpath Seminars: *Managing multiple projects, objective and deadlines* Mission, KS, 2001.

Volk-Tebbitt B: Time: who controls yours? *Supervisor Nurs* 9:19, 1978.

Waterworth S: Time management strategies in nursing practice, *J Adv Nurs* 43(5), 2003.

Webber RA: *Time and management*, New York, 1972, Van Nostrand Reinhold.

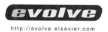
24

Contemporary Nursing Roles and Career Opportunities

Robert W. Koch, DNS, RN

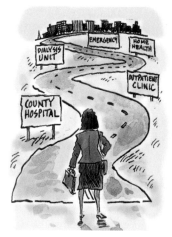

The career path for nurses is long and wide.

VIGNETTE

"When I graduated 15 years ago, I thought I would work in the hospital my entire career. However, with so many changes in the economic forces affecting health care and the resulting shift of clients outside acute care, more opportunities exist for me. I can take my skills and seek new ones to have a choice of practice roles and settings. Being a registered nurse now gives me more options for practice than I ever thought possible."

Questions to consider while reading this chapter:

1. What community-based opportunities exist for graduate nurses?
2. How can a new nurse gain knowledge about the role of the parish nurse or forensic nurse?
3. What unique skills do nurses working in community settings need?

KEY TERMS

Advanced practice nursing Defined by the National Council of State Boards of Nursing (1992) as "practice based on knowledge and skills acquired in a basic nursing education, through licensure as a registered nurse (RN), and in graduate education and experience, including advanced nursing theory, physical assessment, and psychosocial assessment and treatment of illness." Includes nurse practitioners (NPs), certified nurse midwives (CNMs), certified registered nurse anesthetists (CRNAs), and clinical nurse specialists (CNSs).

Nursing roles 1. Traditional duties and responsibilities of the professional nurse, regardless of practice area or setting, such as the roles of care provider, educator, counselor, client advocate, change agent, leader and manager, researcher, and coordinator of the transdisciplinary team. 2. Duties and responsibilities of the professional nurse that are guided by specific professional standards of practice and usually are carried out in a distinct practice area (e.g., flight nurse, forensic nurse, and occupational nurse).

LEARNING OUTCOMES

After studying this chapter, the reader will be able to:

1. Evaluate the impact of the current health care environment on the future role of nurses.
2. Analyze the influence of current demographic characteristics of RNs in the United States on contemporary nursing roles.
3. Differentiate among various innovative nursing practice roles today.
4. Differentiate between the roles of advanced practice nurses and other RNs in various settings.

CHAPTER OVERVIEW

The health care system continues to change as social and economic factors create a state of constant evolution. Professional nurses respond by creating innovative alternatives to traditional nursing practice to meet these new challenges. As nurses proactively define solutions to today's health care dilemmas, multiple career opportunities emerge.

Not long ago most nurses considered acute care hospitals the main practice setting available upon graduation. Few other career choices were available. Public health nursing was one of few exceptions providing variety in the nursing job market. With health care trends moving from inpatient treatment to outpatient and home care and acute care shifting to health promotion and disease prevention, the U.S. society is seeking alternative settings to meet this growing need. This shift in health care settings creates a variety of choices for nurses exploring career opportunities.

Nurses today have more liberty to explore and even create job opportunities. Nurses may continue to select the hospital acute care setting or may venture into less traditional nursing roles. It is imperative that nurses claim ownership of nontraditional roles as they emerge in the health care job market. As professionals, nurses should exercise their influence to develop and support new nursing roles.

This chapter presents an overview of some key opportunities available for RNs today in the United States. Included are demographics of today's nurses, as well as implications for the future. This chapter examines the traditional and less traditional options available and the current and future issues for roles in professional practice.

NURSING . . . MUCH THE SAME, BUT BIGGER AND BETTER

Not so long ago, describing the role of RNs was simple because there were few opportunities for variation. Today exploring job opportunities for RNs is more complicated as nurses are

practicing in literally hundreds of diverse settings with a broad variety of clients. The proliferation of career opportunities for nurses is growing. Although nursing roles have expanded,
the traditional functions of the nurse remain intact. Box 24-1 summarizes the roles nurses
assume in *any* employment role or setting.

Care Provider

The role of care provider is basic to the nursing profession. As the provider of care, the nurse
assesses client resources, strengths and weaknesses, coping behaviors, and the environment
to optimize the problem-solving and self-care abilities of the client and family. The nurse plans
therapeutic interventions in collaboration with the client, physician, and other health care
providers. In addition, the nurse takes responsibility for coordination of care that involves
other health professionals or resources, providing continuity and helping the client deal effectively with the health care system. As part of this role, caring is always central to nursing
interventions and an essential attribute of the expert nurse.

Educator and Counselor

Multiple factors increase the need for nurses to serve as educators. Today the new emphasis is
on health promotion and health maintenance rather than on management of disease conditions. The role of nurse counselor has been elevated to new heights. More than ever before,
nurses encourage clients to look at alternatives, recognize their choices, and develop a sense
of control in a rapidly changing health care environment.

Client Advocate

Professional nurses find that the role of client advocate is essential in various situations with
a multitude of client populations. Promoting what is best for the client, ensuring that the
client's needs are met, and protecting the client's rights remain important responsibilities of
the professional nurse.

Change Agent

When nurses first adopted the role of "change agent," few individuals anticipated to what extent
nurses would fulfill this role. However, nurses have expanded their role as change agents in
many ways. The profession continues to identify client and health care delivery problems, assess
their motivation and capacity for change, determine alternatives, explore possible outcomes of
the alternatives, and assess cost-effective resources in infinite health-related situations.

BOX 24–1 *Professional Nursing Roles*

Care provider
Educator and counselor
Client advocate
Change agent
Leader and manager
Researcher
Coordinator of the transdisciplinary health care team

Leader and Manager

The leadership role of the professional nurse is paramount to the health care system. Today nursing leadership varies according to the level of application and includes:

- Improving the health status and potential of individuals or families
- Ensuring that safe, high-quality care is provided across all health care settings
- Increasing the effectiveness and level of satisfaction among professional colleagues providing care
- Managing multiple resources in a health care facility
- Raising citizens' and legislators' attitudes toward and expectations of the nursing profession and the health care system

There is little doubt that the management role of the nurse has become more important. Nursing management includes planning, giving direction, and monitoring and evaluating nursing care of individuals, groups, families, and communities.

Researcher

During the past decades nursing has taken its place among other disciplines in the production and use of research specific to its profession. Although the majority of researchers in nursing are prepared at the doctoral and postdoctoral levels, an increasing number of clinicians with master's degrees are beginning to participate in research as part of their advanced practice role. Nurses prepared at the baccalaureate and associate degree levels are also participating in research. These nurses may be assisting with data collection, critiquing research findings, and using these findings in practice. More nursing interventions are based on nursing research than in the past.

Coordinator of the Transdisciplinary Health Care Team

Transdisciplinary teams consist of collaborative practice relationships among several disciplines of health care professionals. The disciplines include nursing, medicine, pharmacy, nutrition, social work, and other allied health professionals such as physical therapists, respiratory therapists, occupational therapists, and speech therapists. Chaplains or pastoral care representatives also serve a very valuable role on the transdisciplinary health care team. These teams are found in all health care delivery settings and function most effectively when their focus revolves around the needs of the client.

Transdisciplinary teams are valuable because professional members bring their in-depth and specialized knowledge and skills to the interaction process. In an age of exploding information, the roles of transdisciplinary team members complement one another. Through the formal and informal communication of ideas and opinions of team members, health care plans are determined. A plan of care developed by the transdisciplinary team is usually considered a valuable health management tool.

The term *transdisciplinary health care team* may not be as familiar as the terms *multidisciplinary team* or *interdisciplinary team*. Multidisciplinary health care teams consist of many disciplines involved in meeting client care needs. Interdisciplinary teams refer to coordination between and among disciplines involved in providing client care. The more global and inclusive term *transdisciplinary health care team* can be described as including multiple disciplines bonding, interacting, and uniting toward common goals of client care. The collaborative process involved in transdisciplinary health care incorporates the definitions of multidisciplinary and interdisciplinary health care and, in fact, transcends a single health profession to create comprehensive work outcomes. Studies that investigate the process of transdisciplinary health care teams in action report improved quality of care, increased client satisfaction, increased nursing satisfaction, and reduced hospital cost by decreasing hospital length of stay and increasing nurse retention (Baggs, 1989; Baggs et al, 1992; Knaus et al, 1986; Wasserman, 1997).

Successful health care team models that use concepts related to transdisciplinary health care include pain management, nutritional support, skin care, rehabilitation, mental health, and hospice. Discharge planning, which emerged as a major focus of health care delivery in the 1980s and involves developing a plan of treatment that ultimately results in the discharge of the client from the health care facility, is built on the concept of transdisciplinary care, with each discipline involved in providing care for the client included in developing the discharge plan.

Client education is another area in which collaboration of disciplines is absolutely essential. Health care professionals must understand one another's contributions to client education and ensure that the information clients and families receive is consistent and complete. This will produce the best possible health outcomes for clients and families.

In Box 24-2 some of the more common roles of transdisciplinary health care team members are addressed, and the website of their associated professional organization is listed. These team members are involved in client care to varying degrees, depending on client needs for the specific talents and knowledge of each team member. This list contains selected

BOX 24–2   Transdisciplinary Health Care Team Members

Nurse (RN): Often the coordinator of the team. RNs take licensure examinations after completing associate degree, diploma, or baccalaureate degree preparation from an accredited school of nursing. RNs are able to obtain specialty certification for advanced skills and/or advanced degrees. RNs use the nursing process in client care in any health care setting.
American Nursing Association: www.nursingworld.org/

Physician (MD or DO): Often the leader of the team, the physician diagnoses and prescribes treatment interventions for clients. Medical doctors (MDs) or doctors of osteopathy (DOs) complete 4 years of medical school and board examinations. Physicians can complete postgraduate training, including internship, residency, and fellowship training in a specialty area. Physicians also complete state licensing examinations and function in all health care arenas.
American Medical Association: www.ama-assn.org

Pharmacist (RPh or PharmD): Responsible for providing drug therapy for positive client outcomes; activities include drug information services, client and health care staff education, dispensing medications and client monitoring, adverse drug reaction reporting, research, concurrent drug use evaluation, and consultative services in areas such as pain management and nutritional support. Pharmacists complete baccalaureate preparation, an internship period, and licensing board examinations. Pharmacists can complete additional specialized training, certifications, and/or advanced degrees. In some states the PharmD, or doctor of pharmacy degree, is now the educational requirement for entering practice.
American Pharmaceutical Association www.aphanet.org/

Physician Assistant (PA): Works under the supervision of the MD or DO and performs assessments, procedures, or protocols approved by the physician. PAs complete a baccalaureate degree with specialized PA training (usually 2 years) and state licensure.
American Academy of Physician Assistants, www.aapa.org

BOX 24-2 —cont'd

Dietitian (RD/LD): Provides nutritional therapy and support to ensure that the nutritional needs of the client are met. Activities include involving both client and family in dietary assessment and teaching, identifying resources for food purchase and preparation, and identifying areas of food-drug interactions. Dietitians complete a baccalaureate degree from an accredited nutrition or food service administration program and national board examinations and may also complete state licensure and advanced educational preparation.
American Dietetic Association www.eatright.org/public

Physical Therapist (PT): Attends to the client's needs for movement. Activities include assessing physical strength and mobility needs and developing a plan of strengthening exercises for the client with movement dysfunction, maintaining range of motion and muscle tone, and identifying assistive devices that may be needed. A physical therapist may also be expert in the area of wound care. The basic educational requirement is a baccalaureate degree in a physical therapy program and completion of a national certifying examination. Advanced degrees are available.
American Physical Therapy Association: www.apta.org/

Speech Language Pathologist (SLP): Assists clients who are communicatively impaired by intervening in speech, language, and/or swallowing disorders related to receptive language, expressive language, speech intelligibility, voice disorders, alaryngeal speech, or prosody and cognitive impairments; plays an important role in evaluation and treatment of swallowing disorders. Therapists complete a master's degree from an accredited school, a 1-year fellowship, and a national certifying examination.
American Speech-Language-Hearing Association: www.asha.org/

Occupational Therapist (OT): Plans activities that assist and teach clients with physical disabilities to become independent in activities of daily living such as dressing, grooming, bathing, and eating. Once self-care goals have been met, the occupational therapist can help the client perform daily responsibilities of caring for a home and/or returning to work. Educational requirements include completion of an occupational therapy program of study at the baccalaureate, graduate certification, or master's degree level. Graduates must complete a period of supervised clinical experience and state licensure examinations.
American Occupational Therapy Association: www.aota.org/

Respiratory Therapist (RT): Responsible for assessment and maintenance of the client's airway and respiratory equipment used for diagnosis and therapy of respiratory disorders. Activities include client assessment, aerosolized medication administration, sputum sampling, arterial and mixed venous blood sampling, pulmonary function testing, cardiopulmonary stress testing, and sleep studies; may also be involved in conducting pulmonary rehabilitation programs. Respiratory therapists complete a program of study and take a national certifying examination. If the program of study is completed in an associate or bachelor's degree program, the level of credentialing examination is different.
American Association for Respiratory Care: www.aarc.org/

Social Worker: Uses skills to help clients, families, and communities address psychosocial needs. Activities include educating clients, families, and staff about community resources, discharge planning, financial counseling and identifying financial resources, crisis intervention, referring to community resources, abuse and neglect reporting, completing advanced directives, assisting with resolving ethical dilemmas, evaluating behavior and mental disorders, and conducting support groups. Social workers complete a minimum of baccalaureate preparation in the field and may pursue advanced degrees.
National Association of Social Workers: www.naswdc.org/

Chaplain or Pastoral Representative: Attends to the spiritual and emotional needs of the client and family. Activities include providing pastoral counseling and support and sacramental ministry and liturgical celebrations; not all pastoral representatives share the same religion as the client or family members but must able to acknowledge the differences among religions and help to assist the person with spirituality needs. Basic education requirements vary based on the setting and religious affiliation. The Association for Clinical Pastoral Education is a multicultural, multifaith organization devoted to improving the quality of ministry and pastoral care offered by spiritual caregivers of all faiths.
Association for Clinical Pastoral Education: www.acpe.edu

professional roles contributing to the transdisciplinary health care team approach, but there may be more in a given team.

The following case study provides an excellent example of the role of various members of the transdisciplinary health care team. Multiple professional caregivers provide health care within the limits of each provider's expertise. The joint efforts of all professionals provide the opportunity for a better overall outcome.

CASE STUDY

John was discussing a problem with a co-worker over his cell phone as he approached the intersection. He did not notice the truck approaching on his left side, and he did not see the STOP sign. After evaluation in the emergency department, John's status was diagnosed as postmotor vehicle accident with multiple trauma, closed head injury, several rib and leg fractures, lacerations, and internal injuries. His physician ordered multiple diagnostic tests, laboratory tests, medications, and treatments. His nurse monitored his physical status and carried out the orders written by the physician. The nurse organized the tests and procedures and managed his pain. The pharmacist reviewed and supplied the medications ordered and analyzed potential interaction effects of the multiple pharmaceutical agents. A respiratory therapist was consulted to perform breathing treatments to facilitate lung expansion and prevent respiratory complications. After surgical repair of his fractured leg, physical therapy was consulted to assess John's condition and his need for physical reconditioning. A plan of care was determined to enhance his mobility. His long recuperation led to mild depression and spiritual distress. The nurse who assessed these symptoms made arrangements for the chaplain to visit John. Throughout John's period of care, all involved practitioners communicated their assessments and worked together to provide collaborative interventions for holistic care. In addition, all transdisciplinary team members collaborated in medical rounds and discharge planning meetings to plan and coordinate John's care.

NURSES TODAY: WHO ARE THEY, AND WHAT ARE THEY DOING?

The phrase "a typical nurse" has become a misnomer as the profession enters the twenty-first century. Nursing roles are so diverse that there literally is no typical role or practice setting. Surveys conducted by the Division of Nursing—Bureau of Health Professions document characteristics of the people comprising nursing today (Division of Nursing—Bureau of Health Professions, 2001).

Registered Nurse Demographics

Preliminary findings indicated that there were an estimated 2,696,540 RNs in the United States as of March 2000. This represented a 5.4% increase from the 1996 survey, the smallest increase reported in previous surveys. Of these RNs, 81% held active licenses and were employed in nursing. Approximately 58.5% of this group were employed full-time in the profession, with 23.3% of nurses working part-time. In 2000, the average age of the RN population was 45.2 years, compared with 44.3 in the 1996 survey report. In 2000, 31.7% were under 40 years of age, 18.3% under 35 years, and 9.1% under 30 years. Some speculate that the increase in the average age of RNs represents the aging of society as well as the proliferation of "second-career" nurses, while more younger persons are choosing other professions.

Although the nursing profession continues to be predominantly female, the number of men working as RNs significantly increased in the past decade. The 2000 report indicates that the number of male RNs increased to 5.9%, up from 5.4% in 1996 data (Division of Nursing—Bureau of Health Professions, 2001).

Changes in racial/ethnic backgrounds were reported as well. The March 2000 survey reports that 86.6% of RNs were Caucasian/non-Hispanic; whereas 12.3% reported being from one or more racial and/or ethnic backgrounds.

Changes also are occurring in the educational preparation of RNs. There has been a substantial increase in the number of nurses graduating from associate degree nursing programs during the past decade. Although not as dramatic an increase, baccalaureate-prepared nurses also are increasing in number. In 2000 graduates from basic nursing programs were 40.3% associate degree, 29.6% baccalaureate degree, and 29.3% diploma graduates. In March 2000 nurses reported their highest degree as 22.3% diploma, 34.3% associate degree, 7% baccalaureate degree, and 10.2% master's or doctoral degree (Division of Nursing—Bureau of Health Professions, 2001).

Advanced practice nurses now comprise 7.3% of the RN population, up from 6.3% in 1996. Nurse practitioners lead this group in numbers, followed by CNSs, nurse anesthetists, and nurse midwives. Nurse practitioners and CNSs make up 80% of the advance practice group. (Division of Nursing—Bureau of Health Professions, 2001).

Acute care hospitals remain the common worksite for RNs, although there has been a trend toward the outpatient settings. In 2000 59.1% of RNs reported working in hospitals. However, the area with the largest increase in employment was in community and public health settings—a total of 18.3%. About 10% work in physician-based practices, nurse-based practices, or health maintenance organizations (HMOs). Other worksites include educational settings, occupational health settings, nursing management, prisons and jails, and insurance companies (Division of Nursing—Bureau of Health Professions, 2001).

The Health Resources and Services Administration (HRSA) is part of the U.S. Department of Health and Human Services. The Bureau of Health Professions, a division of HRSA, provides national information on the health professions workforce in this country. You can explore demographic changes in nursing on-line (www.bhpr.hrsa.gov/nursing/sampsurvpre.htm).

Hospital Opportunities

Despite enormous changes in hospital care, it seems evident that there will be jobs in the hospital environment for a long time. In the hospital the nurse provides direct care for people who are ill and unable to care for themselves. A function of the direct-care role also is to help the client and family in managing the illness event. Hospital positions can range from staff nurse to administrator and, in a general hospital, entail any of the clinical specialties and most of the target populations identified in Table 24-1. Determining the area of clinical interest depends mainly on personal preferences.

Depending on the region of the United States, the new graduate's degree of choice in the clinical setting is highly variable. However, if the desired arena for work in hospital-based acute care is not available, it may be wise to accept an alternate position, watchful of an opportunity to transfer when a position becomes available in an area of clinical preference. Such an approach is perceived as a willingness to be flexible and to learn. Accepting assignments in an open, cooperative spirit provides more opportunities for the beginning nurse to learn about the organization and gain important experiences. Furthermore, working as a staff nurse offers many learning opportunities in addition to the immediate client-centered ones.

If the choice of the clinical setting has been based on experiences as a student, the new graduate needs to be prepared to have different perceptions in a new role. At a minimum, experiences that are highly enjoyable on the limited-time basis of a student schedule may feel

Table 24-1	Trends in Health Care Delivery Systems	
FROM		**TO**
Acute inpatient care	→	Lifespan care
Treating illness	→	Maintaining health
Focus on the individual	→	Focus on aggregates/populations
Product of care orientation	→	Value of care orientation
Number of hospital admissions	→	Number of lives covered (capitation)
Managing organizations	→	Managing networks
Managing departments	→	Managing markets
Coordinating services	→	Documenting quality and outcomes

different when the new graduate functions in that role full time. It also is good to have a mix of experiences and learning opportunities before making a definitive decision.

Misleading perceptions about functioning in various clinical arenas are not limited to new graduates. Often a person perceives or believes that one clinical area is the ideal choice, only to find that it is not what he or she wanted. For example, Jane Patrick, RN, wanted to work with sick children and successfully landed a position on the pediatric unit after a couple of years' experience as a staff nurse on an adult surgical wing. Despite her eagerness for the position, Jane found it difficult to adjust to the unit. The distress of the children in the unit was painful to her, and she found herself depressed and unhappy. She began to dream about the children for whom she was caring and was increasingly unable to provide nursing intervention that entailed discomfort for the child. Jane was not in the right place.

It is critical that nurses stay attuned to their reactions and respond in a constructive manner to self-discovery such as Jane's. Internal transfers in large hospitals and health care organizations that offer a continuum of care are common; the probability is high that Jane will find a position that is deeply satisfying in another area.

In addition to clinical emphasis, nursing within hospitals offers almost endless opportunities for diversity. Staff level positions in a hospital can be on many different units, and working different shifts on those units presents different work environments, approaches to work, and priorities for client care. Some examples follow.

Infection Control. The infection control nurse assesses the total incidence of infections within the hospital. Clients who suffer an infection while in the hospital are comprehensively reviewed to ensure prompt and accurate treatment and timely containment of the client's infection so that it is not passed to other clients or staff. The infection control nurse must also conduct a thorough analysis to determine the source of the infection and its onset. If the infection is determined to have been contracted during hospitalization, an investigation is initiated to assess the sequence of events leading up to the infection. A position such as this enables the nurse to have hospital-wide interactions and functioning. Knowledge of epidemiology and outstanding interpersonal skills foster full participation in the infection assessment process.

Quality Management. Although the parameters of a position in quality management or quality control vary from institution to institution, the basic premise is to ensure that outcomes in client care services are consistent with established standards. Benchmarking activities to establish such standards have been underway on a national level for the past few decades. Quality management nurses assess the compliance of the institution with established standards and explore variations from these established standards. Chart reviews and ongoing interaction with the staff of the agency are integral components of a quality management position.

Specific Client Services. An almost endless list of specific client services can be found in hospitals, depending on the hospital's size and function within the community. Some nursing positions might be self-evident, such as the intravenous team on which the nurse provides support and interventions with the insertion and maintenance of intravenous therapies. Other services might relate to ostomy care, counseling, support groups, or health education related to a specialty area.

Coordinator Positions. Some hospitals have various coordinator positions, such as trauma nurse coordinator. The nurse in this position is responsible for the coordination and integration of the clinical and administrative requirements of the trauma victim. Comprised of equal parts of program and case management, the trauma nurse coordinator role involves overseeing the care of the client from the point of injury through acute care to rehabilitation and back to society. Maintenance of a comprehensive database on the management of trauma victims is an important part of this position (www.adbt.govt.n2/trauma/T_guidelines/nurse-coordinator.htm).

Another example of a coordinator position for a highly specialized area is the organ donor coordinator, who procures organs and oversees the transplantation program. Coordinators require considerable experience in the specialty in which they practice.

Variations on Traditional Roles in Nursing

As clients shift from hospital to ambulatory and home care, the role of the community nurse has evolved beyond the traditional public health nurse concept. Although still based in the framework of the traditional public health nurse concept, nurses today take their critical care skills into the home, where clients recover from illness and surgery, once only seen in an acute care setting. Pharmacologic and technologic advances make the care of chronic and critically ill clients in their homes a cost-effective option. For example, therapies such as dobutamine administration or chemotherapy were once considered "too risky" for home administration. Today, adequate teaching of the client and family members and careful monitoring make these therapies a daily occurrence in clients' homes.

Clients can be monitored through home visits by RNs, expanded technology, radiographs, or telemetry at home. Uterine monitoring for high-risk obstetric clients is common as vital signs of the mother and baby are observed by telephone modem. All these changes increase the need for home care nurses who are expert clinicians and client educators.

Hospice Nurse. As more clients with terminal illness choose to stop aggressive treatment, another nursing specialty has flourished. Over 3000 hospice programs exist in the United States today. The growth of hospice is seen by the 885,000 clients receiving these services in 2002. According to the National Hospice and Palliative Care Organization (NHPCO), about 25% of all Americans who die with cancer receive hospice care (http://www.nhpco.org/files/public/facts%20figures%20Feb04.pdf).

Hospice and palliative care nurses treat the symptoms of those with progressive terminal disease. These nurses work holistically with clients and families to maximize quality of life rather than focus on the quantity of life remaining. To learn more about the hospice concept, visit the NHPCO website (Box 24-3).

Informatics Nurse Specialist. As health care systems face the inevitable need for data management for decision making, another nursing role has emerged—the informatics nurse specialist. Nursing informatics (NI) is a nursing specialty whose activities center on management and processing of health care information. The Division of Nursing—Bureau of Health Professions defines the role of nurse informatics as " ... combining nursing science, information management science, and computer science to manage and process data, information, and knowledge to deliver quality care to the public, particularly disadvantaged and underserved populations" (National Informatics Agenda, 2001, p. 5). Recommendations by the National Advisory Council on Nurse Education and Practice (NACNEP) commissioned a panel of experts to advise them in setting the direction needed for NI in this country. For the executive summary of their recommendations, visit their website (see Box 24-3).

BOX 24–3 Helpful Websites

Air and Surface Transport Nurses Association
www.astna.org

Airline nursing (flight nursing)
www.nursingnetwork.com/airline.htm

All nurses
http://allnurses.com/

American Academy of Nurse Practitioners
www.aanp.org

American College of Nurse-Midwives
www.midwife.org

American College of Nurse Practitioners
www.nurse.org/acnp

American Forensic Nurses
www.amrn.com/aboutus.htm

American Nurses Informatics Association
http://www.ania.org/

careerguide@pfizer.com
discovernursing.com

CareeRxel for Nurses
www.careerxel.com

Division of Nursing—Bureau of Health Professions
www.bhpr.hrsa.gov/nursing/sampsurvpre.htm

International Association of Forensic Nurses
www.forensicnursing.com/html/about.html

BOX 24-3 —cont'd

International Parish Nurse Resource Center
http://ipnrc.parishnurse.org/index.phtml

Johnson & Johnson
discovernursing.com

National Association for Healthcare Quality
www.nahq.org

National Association of Clinical Nurse Specialists
http://www.nacns.org

National Committee for Quality Assurance
www.ncqa.org

National Hospice and Palliative Care Organization
www.nhpco.org

2000 National Sample of Registered Nurses (NSRN)
www.bhpr.hrsa.gov (Division of Nursing)

Nelson, Valerie: *Shattering the myths about forensic nursing, 1998*
www.nurseweek.com/features/98-7/forensic.html

Nursing specialties
www.allnurses.com/Nursing_Specialties/

Pfizer Pharmaceutical Group
careerguide@pfizer.com

Quality management
www.ncqa.org and www.nahq.org

So, you wanna be a flight nurse?
www.seaox.com/wannabe.html

Travel nursing
http://www.healthcaretraveler.com/healthcaretraveler/static/staticHtml.jsp?id=40099

Trauma nursing
www.traumanurse.org

The Joint Commission on Accreditation of Healthcare Organizations (JCAHO) recognized the increased need for information management in the clinical client care settings. The 1994 JCAHO standards define information management as critical to organizational success. Nurses are well positioned to assume these roles, because they best understand client care processes. The American Nurses Credentialing Center (ANCC) has developed a certification examination for nurses who demonstrate beginning levels of competency to become certified as informatics nurses. The ANA defines informatics as "the activities involved in identifying, naming, organizing, grouping, collecting, processing, analyzing, storing, retrieving, or managing data and information" (ANA, 1994, p. 3). The ANA Informatics Association has an information website (see Box 24-3). More information on the NI specialty is also available in Chapter 14.

Occupational Health Opportunities. Nursing within the framework of specific occupational groups has long been a career option for nurses. Within these settings the nurse designs and implements a program of health promotion and disease prevention for employees and assists with immediate health needs as necessary. In this primary care milieu, the nurse assesses the need for programs about specific topics of importance to the health of the employees. Some examples of these might be breast-screening programs for female employees and information on early identification of prostate cancer for male employees. Other programs might revolve around the management of developmental events such as empty nest syndrome, menopause, caring for aging parents, or retirement.

In addition to services related to maintaining the health of employees, the occupational nurse is responsible for the assessment of the work environment to ensure the safety of the employees. Examples of significant environmental improvements in the health of U.S. workers are clean air programs, antismoking-on-the-job campaigns, and eliminating the use of asbestos in heating or insulation of buildings. All these activities pose special challenges to the occupational health nurse. The nurse in this setting develops procedures to be followed in the event of illness at work, including the management of emergencies.

Opportunities also exist in specific industries. For example, within the airline industry, it is the responsibility of the nurse to contribute to airline safety through maintaining the health of employees. Protection of the employee's health is a component of the role, and of equal concern is the impact of the health of the employee on the safety of the airline and its passengers. The nurse must be vigilant in the assessment of employee health problems that could affect overall airline safety. An obvious function is alcohol and drug screening. Protocols for the maintenance of employee health programs in the airline industry must be strictly followed and enforced, as required by government regulation.

Nonetheless, the heart of this nursing position still lies with providing care to people, which sometimes can place the nurse in a difficult position. In the ongoing monitoring of the health of the employees, the nurse often is the first to spot the development of a deviation from health that could affect the career and livelihood of an employee. Such an example is hypertension. If an employee is developing high blood pressure, which will affect his or her employment status, that employee may apply pressure on the nurse to "hear" the blood pressure in the qualifying range.

Occupational health and employment screening activities are entwined with urgent care and travel assistance for passengers. Although occasionally an emergency situation develops with a passenger or an employee, most of the client problems are travel-related. For example, international travel to some countries requires comprehensive precautions regarding immunizations and inoculations. Airport nurses were critical in screening passengers on international flights during the recent severe acute respiratory syndrome (SARS) crisis (htpp://news.bbc.co.uk/ 1/hi/health/2908021.stm.). Also, passengers may forget prescribed medications, or medications may be lost in baggage. Short-term problems such as fear of flying are also managed.

Another form of transportation provides a career opportunity: cruise ship nurse. Generally, when people think of taking a cruise, they do not plan on getting sick—nor do nurses usually consider career possibilities in the industry. However, many of the cruise ships in existence are as large as small cities. The role of the nurse in this setting is similar to that of the airline nurse with respect to the health of the employees and the safety of the passengers. The unique elements of the ship relate to special sanitation requirements, such as testing and culturing the water supply and managing the total health needs of the passengers. It also is the nurse's responsibility to instruct the staff on the basic elements of emergency care and transport. Primary patient care needs are similar to those found in an emergency department. Additional career information can be found on-line (www.medhunters.com/job/519954.html).

Quality Manager. Another role that is becoming more attractive to nurses is that of quality manager. This reflects the need for health care providers to assess opportunities for process improvement, implement changes, measure outcomes, and then start the improvement process over again. Quality management nurses research and describe findings and look for opportunities to improve care. The result of quality studies may produce critical pathways or algorithms defining care and expected client outcomes. Basic and advanced knowledge of quality management tools is essential, although practice may vary from setting to setting. For instance, in the inpatient setting the quality management nurse needs strong clinical skills, those that might be acquired in medical-surgical practice, intensive care units, or the operating room. Experience in home care would be an advantage for a quality management nurse in that setting. Interpersonal skills are important, because to be successful in this role, the nurse must build relationships and rapport. The role of quality manager is one that promotes improved care for health care recipients in a variety of settings. For more information, visit the quality management websites listed in Box 24-3 and see Chapter 20 of this text.

Case Manager. This role has had a rich tradition in community and public health nursing and now has gained more prominence in acute care. Case managers coordinate resources to achieve health care outcomes based on quality, access, and cost. The complexity of case management practice is obvious in the era of chaotic systems caused by recent changes in the health care market, in which providers, services, and coverage details are constantly changing. Case managers identify the best resources at the lowest cost to achieve the optimum health outcome for the client (Stanhope and Lancaster, 2004). More information about case management can be found in Chapter 19.

Flight Nurse. Flight nursing is a specialty for nurses who desire autonomous practice and the opportunity to use advanced clinical skills. Practice is diverse since clients are all ages and from all backgrounds with different health problems. Critical care experience, with certification in advanced cardiac life support, is necessary. Most programs prefer experienced nurses in critical care and/or emergency department nursing. The two types of flight practice available are military, such as in the Air Force Reserves or active duty, and civilian flight nursing. To learn more, visit the website "So, you wanna be a flight nurse?" (see Box 24-3). Nurses who enjoy a fast-paced diverse practice in an unstructured setting may find this role a good fit. For more information, call the Air and Surface Transport Nurses Association, formerly known as the National Flight Nurse Association, at 1-800-897-NFNA (6362) or visit their website (see Box 24-3).

Telephone Triage Nurse. Another emerging career is that of telephone triage nurse. In this practice nurses interact with clients on the telephone to assess needs, intervene, and evaluate. This position requires excellent communication and assessment skills, as well as problem-solving skills. Telephone triage is used in a variety of settings, including emergency departments and physician practices.

Forensic Nurse. Forensic nursing may well be one of the fastest-growing nursing specialties in the twenty-first century. This is likely due to the epidemic increase in violence and resulting trauma in this country. The ANA's Scope and Standards of Forensic Nursing Practice, published by American Nurses Publishing, serves as a professional guide for nurses working in or entering this evolving specialty. Forensic nursing applies nursing science to public or legal proceedings in the scientific investigation and treatment of trauma and/or death of victims of violence, abuse, criminal activity, and traumatic accidents. The forensic nurse may provide direct services to individual clients, as well as consult with and/or be an expert witness for medical and law enforcement.

To learn more about this exciting practice, visit the International Association of Forensic Nurses (IAFN) website (see Box 24-3). The American Forensic Nurses' Organization offers distance-learning programs through the Internet (see Box 24-3).

School Nurse. Most registered professional nurses employed in school health are generalists prepared at the baccalaureate level who function as consultants/coordinators. The newer role for school nurses is school health manager or coordinator and includes functions such as policy making, case management and program management activities, and health promotion and protection activities (Stanhope and Lancaster, 2004).

Travel Nurse. For the person who wants to travel and still work as a nurse, travel nursing may be an answer. This role is a expanding as the demand for nurses grows nation wide. Benefits and company programs vary, but many include travel reimbursement allowance to assignments in addition to free housing, free insurance, travel money, free phone card use, and other benefits. Sign-on bonuses may also be offered. If these benefits are not important to the nurse, higher wages may be available. Some companies allow nurses' pets to travel with them. Assignments are usually for a minimum time, such as 12 weeks, but others may last as long as a year. For more information, visit the travel nurse website (see Box 24-3).

Parish Nurse. The role of parish nurse is quickly becoming a recognized specialty in a growing professional practice. In 1998 the ANA, in collaboration with the Health Ministries Association, established the scope and standards of this professional practice. This role focuses on health promotion within the beliefs, values, and practices of various faith communities. In these contexts, health is seen as a sense of physical, psychologic, social, and spiritual well-being. Health is further viewed as being in harmony with self, others, the environment, and God. The parish nurse functions as counselor, teacher, referral agent, volunteer coordinator, and integrator of spiritual care and health. Although all communities do not have a hospital or clinic, most have a faith community, providing an exciting setting in which to teach disease prevention and health promotion.

The late Granger Westberg (1988), founder of this role in the mid-1980s, proposed that clergy can and already do more in the field of preventive medicine than traditional physicians. Westberg's efforts focused on getting the medical establishment to recognize faith communities as partners in keeping people well. He stated that churches, even though they may not realize it, are in the health business. In this role parish nurses participate in joint ministry with other staff members, helping to integrate faith and health for healing and wholeness.

For more information on this practice, visit the website of the International Parish Nurse Association (see Box 24-3).

Other Unique Roles. Career opportunities described in this chapter should not be considered an exhaustive list of possibilities. Nurses now have selections for practice areas never before considered. Nurses should adopt an attitude of openness, an attitude of creativity, and a willingness to take a chance to explore these different possibilities. Nurses can let their imaginations take them to unknown settings or explore uncharted waters. To do this, nurses must develop confidence in their abilities and talents and be willing to venture outside the norm. Recently, many websites have been developed to portray nursing as an attractive career with endless opportunities. One website lists over 50 categories of roles for nurses with links and discussions areas (see Nursing Specialties, Box 24-3). In addition to exploring pertinent websites, examine the Pfizer publication *Opportunities to Care: the Pfizer Guide to Careers in Nursing*, a "must have" guide that profiles the life and work of nurses in the field.

There are those detractors in the nursing profession who would limit the possibilities for the profession, claiming that many of the aforementioned alternatives are not really "nursing." However, this mindset severely limits the expansion of professional nursing in a changing health care environment. For nursing to thrive, new roles need to be defined and refined for future success of the discipline.

One way to settle this dispute within the nursing profession is to evaluate new nursing roles through the definition established by the ANA (2003).

> Nursing is the protection, promotion, and optimization of health and abilities, prevention of illness and injury, alleviation of suffering through the diagnosis and treatment of human response, and advocacy in the care of individuals, families, communities and population (p. 6).

Therefore evolving nursing roles should be evaluated based on the ability of the new role to fit this accepted definition. Does the newly created role require assessment, diagnosis, planning, implementation, or evaluation to human responses? Does the newly created role require the knowledge and expertise of a professional nurse? By answering these questions, nurses can see that nursing is now bigger and more encompassing than what was once termed "traditional" nursing.

ADVANCED PRACTICE NURSING

Much is written in the professional and lay literature about advanced practice nursing. Although new roles in advanced nursing may be forthcoming, the term *advanced practice nurse (APN)* is presently a descriptor that includes nurse practitioners (NPs), certified nurse midwives (CNMs), certified registered nurse anesthetists (CRNAs), and clinical nurse specialists (CNSs).

Each specialty of APN has unique differences although they share key elements. All APNs make independent and collaborative health care decisions and engage in active practice as expert clinicians. APNs are educationally prepared through master's level education to assume responsibility and accountability for the health promotion, assessment, diagnosis, and management of client problems, including the prescription of medication (AACN, 1996, p.12).

Nurse Practitioner (NP)

NPs engage in advanced practice in a variety of specialty areas such as family, adult, pediatric, geriatric, women's health, school health, occupational health, mental health, emergency, and acute care. Typically, NPs assess and manage medical and nursing problems. Health promotion and maintenance, as well as disease prevention, are the emphases of their practice. Some NPs diagnose and manage acute and chronic diseases of their selected population.

Job responsibilities of NPs include taking client histories; conducting physical examinations; ordering, performing, and interpreting diagnostic tests; and prescribing pharmacologic agents, treatments, and therapies for the management of client conditions. Frequently, the NP serves as a primary care provider and consultant for individuals, families, or communities.

NPs have advanced education, with specific emphasis on pathophysiology and pharmacology. Certification is achieved via written examination after the completion of a master's level program. Several professional organizations offer certification for NPs. For example, the National Certification Board of Pediatric Nurse Practitioners certifies pediatric NPs; adult NPs or family NPs may be certified by the American Academy of Nurse Practitioners. For more information, visit their websites (see Box 24-3).

NPs achieve registration and licensure by state boards of nursing or other designated agencies. The state boards of nursing regulate NP practice and prescriptive authority.

The National Advisory Council on Nurse Education and Practice (NACNEP), established by Title VIII of the Public Health Service, provides a Nurse Practitioner Workforce report (see Box 24-3). The American College of Nurse Practitioners' website offers further professional information (see Box 24-3).

Clinical Nurse Specialist (CNS)

CNSs are APNs who possess clinical expertise in a defined area of nursing practice for a selected client population or clinical setting. This practice specialty emphasizes the diagnosis and management of human responses to actual or potential health problems.

The CNS functions as an expert clinician, educator, consultant, researcher, and administrator. The CNS monitors the care of clients and collaborates with physicians, nurses, and other members of the transdisciplinary health care team. The emphasis of this advanced nursing practice is to provide clinical support that improves client care and client outcomes.

CNSs are educated in graduate nursing programs. Their expertise is acquired from combining graduate study with clinical experience. The educational program for CNSs features an intense study of nursing theories and knowledge from other disciplines. Programs emphasize advanced scientific concepts, research methodologies, and supervised clinical practice.

CNSs practice within a systems model paradigm, which means that in performing their role, CNSs evaluate each client in the context of his or her social environment. These APNs view clients as individuals who are part of a larger society entering a complex health care delivery system. This practice philosophy prompts the CNS to use a comprehensive approach to client care.

As consultants, CNSs are called on for expert clinical advice within and outside the clinical setting. Their consultation function frequently consists of problem solving with a client who may be a colleague, an individual, family, group, agency, or community. Problems may be related to provider competence, equipment, facilities, or health care delivery systems.

CNSs contribute to research in their area of specialization, generating and refining research questions, interpreting research findings, applying them to clinical practice, and educating other nurses about research findings. As teachers, CNSs educate clients, families, and communities. The CNS functions as a role model or preceptor for nurse generalists and students in a variety of clinical settings (ANA, 1986).

The National Advisory Council on Nurse Education and Practice (NACNEP), established by Title VIII of the Public Health Service, provides a CNS report (see Box 24-3).

Certified Registered Nurse Anesthetist (CRNA)

Established in the late 1800s, nurse anesthesia is recognized as the first clinical nursing specialty. Nurse anesthesia practice developed in response to requests from surgeons seeking a solution to the high morbidity and mortality attributed to anesthesia at that time. The most famous nurse anesthetist of the nineteenth century, Alice Magaw, called the "mother of anesthesia," worked at St. Mary's Hospital in Rochester, Minnesota. Magaw was instrumental in establishing a showcase of professional excellence in anesthesia and surgery. In 1909 the first formal educational programs preparing nurse anesthetists were established.

Since World War I, nurse anesthetists have been the principal anesthesia providers in combat areas of every war in which the United States has been engaged. Although nurse anesthesia educational programs existed before World War I, the war sharply increased the demand for nurse anesthetists and, consequently, the need for more educational programs.

Founded in 1931, the American Association of Nurse Anesthetists (AANA) is the professional association, representing more than 27,000 nurse anesthetists nationwide. The AANA promotes education, practice standards, and guidelines and affords consultation to both private and governmental entities regarding nurse anesthetists and their practice.

The AANA developed and implemented a certification program in 1945 and instituted mandatory recertification in 1978. The association established a mechanism for accreditation of nurse anesthesia educational programs in 1952 (Thatcher, 1973). Additional information is available at the AANA website (see Box 24-3).

The educational preparation of CRNAs occurs at the graduate level or in association with traditional institutions of higher education, most commonly in schools of nursing or health sciences. The educational curriculum in the anesthesia specialty ranges from 24 to 36 months in an integrated program of academic and clinical study. The academic curriculum consists of a minimum of 30 credit hours of formalized graduate study in courses such as advanced anatomy, physiology, pathophysiology, advanced pharmacology, principles of anesthesia practice, and research methodology and statistical analysis. All programs require approximately 1000 hours of hands-on clinical experience. Students gain experience with clients of all ages who require medical, obstetric, dental, and pediatric interventions.

Admission requirements to a nurse anesthesia educational program include a bachelor of science degree in nursing, licensure as an RN, and a minimum of 1 year of acute care nursing experience. Nurse anesthetists are required to successfully complete a written examination for certification as a CRNA.

Recertification, which includes practice and continuing education requirements, must be met every 2 years. CRNAs are qualified to make independent judgments relative to all aspects of anesthesia care based on their education, licensure, and certification. CRNAs provide anesthesia and anesthesia-related care on request, assignment, or referral by a client's physician most often to facilitate diagnostic, therapeutic, or surgical procedures. In other instances CRNAs perform consultation or assistance for management of pain associated with obstetric labor and delivery, management of acute or chronic ventilatory problems, or management of acute or chronic pain through the performance of selected diagnostic or therapeutic blocks.

The laws of every state permit CRNAs to work directly with a physician or other authorized health care professional, such as a dentist, without being supervised by an anesthesiologist.

The JCAHO does not require anesthesiologist supervision of CRNAs, nor does Medicare. In some cases a provider, payer, or medical staff bylaws may require anesthesiologist supervision. However, these decisions are not based on legal requirements (AANA, 1992).

Certified Nurse-Midwife (CNM)

According to the American College of Nurse-Midwives (ACNM, 1995), nurse midwifery practice is the independent management of women's health care, focusing particularly on pregnancy, childbirth, the postpartum period, care of the newborn, and the family planning and gynecologic needs of women. This practice occurs within a health care system that provides consultation, collaborative management, or referral, as indicated by the health status of the client.

A CNM is educated in the two disciplines of nursing and midwifery and possesses evidence of certification according to the requirements of the ACNM. A CNM has successfully completed prescribed studies in midwifery and has met the requisite qualifications to be certified. A CNM is legally qualified to practice in one or more of the 50 states. The ACNM supports educational programs for CNMs at the certificate and the degree level but opposes mandatory degree requirements for state licensure.

The ACNM claims that mandatory degree requirements would limit access to maternity and gynecologic services for women. Several national reports specifically recommend placing greater reliance on CNMs to increase access to prenatal care for underserved populations. These reports also recommend that state laws be supportive of nurse-midwifery practice.

The entry-level nurse-midwife is a primary health care professional who independently provides care during pregnancy, birth, and the postpartum period for women and newborns within their communities. Therefore the CNM is an individual who has successfully completed an ACNM-accredited educational program in nurse-midwifery and passed the national certification examination administered by the ACNM Certification Council. Additional information is available at the ACNM website (see Box 24-3).

Midwifery care occurs within a variety of settings, including homes, birthing centers, clinics, and hospitals. The nurse-midwife works with each woman and her family to identify their unique physical, social, and emotional needs. Services provided by the CNM include education and health promotion.

With additional education and experience, the nurse-midwife may provide well-woman gynecologic care, including family planning services. When the care required extends beyond the CNM's abilities, the midwife should have a mechanism for consultation and referral.

CNMs are an expanding group of professionals. Each year approximately 400 nurse-midwives pass the national certification examination. Since 1991 the number of CNMs who are certified each year has increased by 25%. Currently there are 50 accredited nurse-midwifery education programs in the United States. Approximately 68% of CNMs have a master's degree. Four percent have a doctoral degree. Nurse-midwifery practice is legal in all 50 states and the District of Columbia (Division of Nursing-Bureau of Health Professionals, 2001).

Nurse Administrator/Nurse Executive

Although not formally considered an advanced practice nurse, the nurse administrator or nurse executive has an important advanced role within nursing. It is vital that individuals be knowledgeable about the business of the health care system and the profession of nursing. Nursing administration unites the leadership perspective of professional nursing with the various aspects of business and health administration. The practice of nursing administration focuses on the administration of health care systems for the purpose of delivering services to groups of clients.

Individuals who assume a nurse executive role typically hold a master's degree. Both master's and doctoral level programs that offer degrees in nursing administration are available, although some nursing executives are educated in additional disciplines such as business.

Nursing administration research focuses on organizational factors and management practices and their impact on nurses, nursing delivery systems, and client outcomes. Nursing administration is concerned with establishing the costs of nursing care and examining relationships between nursing services and quality client care. Nurse executives are called on to view problems of nursing service delivery within a broader context of policy analysis and delivery of health care services.

Nursing administration is an integral part of any organization that provides health care. Nurse administrators lead and direct large groups of nurses and ancillary personnel. They manage large budgets and are responsible for provision of quality care at reasonable cost. They serve at all management levels in health care organizations and in the community.

WHAT ABOUT THE FUTURE?

The future of nursing is brighter than ever. Because of never-ending changes in the health care environment, many new jobs will result. Growth of the nursing profession also will be prompted by technologic advances in client care, which allow an increased number of health problems to be detected early and managed quickly. A greater number of sophisticated health-related procedures are already performed not only in hospitals but in a variety of settings such as clinics and physician's offices. Health maintenance organizations, ambulatory surgicenters, and church health centers are only a few of the places where the public will receive their health care. Nursing can be a vital component of the "alternative setting" movement that is on the forefront of health care reform.

As the focus of health care shifts to disease prevention and modification of lifestyles, the opportunities for nurses will follow. Nursing also can benefit from the increased emphasis on primary care because prevention is the only true mechanism to reduce health care expenditures. Professional nursing services should be viewed as a cost-effective way to provide disease prevention and health-promotion activities in multiple areas of the community, including industry, business, and commerce. Wellness and disease prevention, historically fundamental to the nursing profession, are now becoming more meaningful and revitalized concepts within the larger health care system.

There always will be a need for the traditional role of the hospital nurse. In fact, with a shift to more community services, the intensity of hospital nursing care is likely to increase as only those in most need are treated there. Increases in client acuity will expand the need for professional nursing within the hospital setting. However, the most rapid growth for nursing employment is expected in outpatient facilities such as same-day surgery, rehabilitation, and chemotherapy infusion centers.

Nurses also will see job opportunities continue to develop in home health care. Many factors contribute to this phenomenon. The increasing numbers of older persons with disabilities require nursing care to minimize their functional loss and optimize their quality of life. Another factor that promotes home care is the consumer's preference for care in his or her own home. Home care is a feasible option with recent technologic advances. Complex health care treatment that was once thought only possible in the hospital setting is now a reality in the home. Professional nurses who are able to perform complex procedures and comprehensive client assessments will be invaluable to the home care industry.

Financial pressures on hospitals to discharge clients as soon as possible are producing increased admissions to nursing homes, skilled nursing facilities, and long-term rehabilitation units. In addition, because more individuals are living into their ninth and tenth decades, the number of people entering nursing homes or assisted-living facilities will increase. The opportunity for nursing is tremendous in the long-term care arena because no other discipline can offer the multiple skills that nursing has to offer to the aging population.

Despite this bright outlook, the nursing profession must heed the old cliché that "opportunity only knocks once." If nurses fail to seize their opportunity, other less qualified health care providers will attempt to move into this advantageous position. It is truly up to nursing professionals to demonstrate their contribution to health care and publicly market their potential. The nursing profession historically has requested a chance to prove its worth in producing cost-effective, quality health care—now is the time.

S U M M A R Y

This chapter has explored the various roles available to professional nurses today. Social and economic trends influencing the development of new nursing roles in innovative practice settings have been discussed. Nurses who are interested in developing new roles should be encouraged by the examples provided by nurses who first envisioned and created these new roles. Traditional, nontraditional, and advanced practice nursing roles offer many exciting opportunities for professional growth and satisfaction. The diversity and challenge available to professional nurses today is unparalleled.

CRITICAL THINKING ACTIVITIES

1. Identify a setting in the community where the influences of professional nursing may be needed but do not presently exist. Develop a job description for the newly created role. What educational preparation would be required for this role? Discuss strategies to market or support the new nursing position. Evaluate the newly developed role within the context of the ANA definition of professional nursing practice.
2. Compare and contrast advanced practice roles such as clinical nurse specialist, nurse practitioner, nurse midwife, and nurse anesthetist. How would you explain the differences to a lay person?
3. Analyze the influence of current trends in health care on the development of new nursing roles.
4. Evaluate the impact of health care trends on traditional nursing roles.
5. Compare and contrast skills needed by the nurse who works in an occupational health setting and a nurse who works in a critical care unit.

Additional resources are available on-line at: http://evolve.elsevier.com/Cherry/

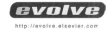

http://evolve.elsevier.com

REFERENCES

American Association of Colleges of Nursing: *The essentials of masters education for advanced practice nursing,* Washington, DC, 1996, AANA.

American Association of Nurse Anesthetists: *Qualifications and capabilities of the certified registered nurse anesthetist,* Park Ridge, Ill, 1992, AANA.

American College of Nurse Midwives: *Professional standards and practice,* Washington, DC, 1995, ACNM.

American Nurses Association: *Nursing's social policy statement,* Washington, DC, 2003, ANA.

American Nurses Association: *The role of the clinical nurse specialist,* Kansas City, Mo, 1986, ANA.

American Nurses Association: *The scope and practice of nursing informatics,* Washington, DC, 1994, ANA.

Baggs J: Intensive care unit use and collaboration between nurses and physicians, *Heart Lung* 18:332-338, 1989.

Baggs J et al: The association between interdisciplinary collaboration and patient outcomes in a medical intensive care unit, *Heart Lung* 21:18-24, 1992.

Division of Nursing—Bureau of Health Professions, Health Resources Service Administration: *The National Sample Survey of Registered Nurses, March 2000 preliminary findings,* Washington, DC, 2001, Health Resources and Service Administration (www.bhpr.hrsa.gov/nursing/sampsurvpre.htm).

Knaus W et al: An evaluation of outcomes from intensive care in major medical centers, *Ann Intern Med* 104:411-418, 1986.

National Informatics Agenda for Nursing Education and Practice (NACNEP): December 1997. Available on-line (www. bhpr.hrsa.gov/dn/nirepex.htm).

Pfizer Pharmaceuticals Group (Friedman R): *Opportunities to care: the Pfizer guide to careers in nursing,* New York, 2002, Pfizer Pharmaceuticals Group.

Stanhope M, Lancaster J: *Community and public health nursing,* ed 6, St Louis, 2004, Mosby.

Thatcher VS: *History of anesthesia with emphasis of the nurse specialist,* Philadelphia, 1973, JB Lippincott.

Wasserman K: Improving the process of care: the cost-quality value of interdisciplinary collaboration, *J Nurs Care Qual* 10(2):10-16, 1997.

Westberg GE: Parishes, nurses, and health care, *Lutheran Partners,* pp 26-29, November/December, 1988.

SUGGESTED READINGS

Cohjen SS, Juszczak L: Promoting the nurse practitioner role in managed care, *J Pediatr Health Care* 11(1):3-11, 1997.

Fitzgerald SM, Wood SH: Advanced practice nursing: back to the future, *J Gynecol Neonatal Nurs* 26(1):101-107, 1997.

Frederickson K: *Opportunities in nursing,* New York, 2003, McGraw Hill.

Hester LE, White MJ: Perception of practicing CNSs about their future role, *Clin Nurse Spec* 10(4):190-193, 1996.

Hickey JV, Quimette RM, Venegoni SL: *Advanced practice nursing—changing roles and clinical application,* Philadelphia, 1996, Lippincott-Raven.

Koch RW: Intrapreneurship: bloom where you're planted, *Tenn Nurse* 59(2):15-16, 1996.

Kupina PS: Community health CNSs and health care in the year 2000, *Clin Nurse Spec* 9(4):188-198, 1995.

O'Brien C: Sexual Assault Nurse Examiner (SANE) program coordinator, *J Emerg Nurs* 22(6):532-533, 1996.

Parker CD, Gassert C: JCAHO's management of information standards—the role of the informatics specialist, *J Nurs Admin* 26(6):13-15, 1996.

Stokes E, Whitis C, Moore-Threasher L: Characteristics of graduate adult health nursing programs, *J Nurs Educ* 36(2):54-59, 1997.

US Department of Labor, Bureau of Labor Statistics: *Occupational outlook handbook,* Washington, DC, 1996, US Department of Labor.

Watts RJ: Critical care nurse practitioner curriculum at the University of Pennsylvania: update and revision, *Am Assoc Crit Care Nurse* 8(1):116-122, 1997.

Wojner AW, Kite-Powell D: Outcomes manager: a role for the advanced practice nurse, *Crit Care Nurs Q* 19(4):16-24, 1997.

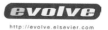
25

Job Search: Finding Your Match

Kathryn S. Skinner, MS, RN, CS, and
Laura H. Day, BSN, MS, RN

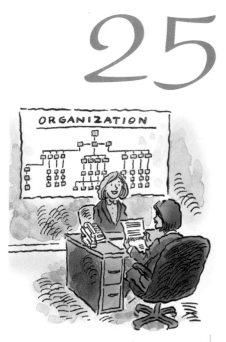

Finding the right
match can be exciting!

VIGNETTE

"For 2 years I've struggled to meet deadlines for term papers, nursing care plans, and examinations. Now that graduation is almost here, I'm scared that I don't know enough to be a 'real nurse.' And I'm confused about where to begin and what kind of nursing position I should seek. This first job seems so important."

Questions to consider while reading this chapter:
1. How should the new graduate in the scenario decide where to apply for that first position?
2. What kinds of questions should the applicant ask about a prospective position?
3. How can the applicant demonstrate knowledge, skills, and experience to the recruiter?

KEY TERMS

Orientation Activities that enhance adaptation to a new environment.
Portfolio A collection of evidence demonstrating acquisition of skills, knowledge, and achievements related to a professional career.
Professional objective Occupational position for which one aims.
Resumé Summary of a job applicant's previous work experience and education.

Additional resources are available on-line at: http://evolve.elsevier.com/Cherry/

LEARNING OUTCOMES

After studying this chapter, the reader will be able to:

1. Use the interview process to evaluate potential employment opportunities.
2. Prepare an effective resumé and nursing portfolio.
3. Compare and contrast various professional nursing employment opportunities.
4. Summarize the employment process.

CHAPTER OVERVIEW

This chapter helps student nurses prepare to successfully negotiate their first employment as professional nurses. They learn the importance of networking, researching available opportunities, and examining their personal aptitudes, interests, lifestyle priorities, and long-term goals to find the best job fit.

Readers are shown how to create and use cover letters and resumés to market themselves in written introductions and how to prepare for and actively participate in a recruitment interview. The chapter describes what can be expected from a recruiter and how to obtain the information needed to make thoughtful and rewarding job choices. Putting these recommendations into practice will ensure the new graduate of the best chance for finding a good job match as an entry-level nurse practicing in a suitable work environment.

EXPLORING OPTIONS

The job market for graduate nurses is very good. There are many opportunities in both urban and rural areas. Although health care economics ride a roller coaster from robust to lean times, with the demand and supply of nurses 1 or 2 years behind the lead, always trying to catch up, the overall need for the skills of professional registered nurses (RNs) remains constant, and the potential for finding suitable employment is excellent. Recent trends in health care dictate that today's health care providers change their orientation from disease to health and from inpatient to outpatient services. Therefore there is a growing need for professional nurses in nonacute community-based care settings such as primary care clinics, ambulatory surgery centers, and home, school, and work environments. However, although rapid changes in health care delivery systems continue to create new and varied opportunities outside the acute care settings where nurses have traditionally practiced, hospitals remain the most likely starting place for new graduates to acquire general experience helpful in opening career path doors. In fact, with the recent nursing shortage there is an increased demand for nurses to work in acute care settings.

Numerous marketing strategies have been tried in an effort to aggressively attract bright, energetic new graduates in times of demand and short supply. For some institutions cost seems irrelevant. Sign-on bonuses, expense-paid weekends to visit institutions in other parts of the United States, promises of tuition reimbursement for continued education, student loan repayment, and low-interest loans for new cars, just to name a few, have been offered as enticements. However, being aware of one's own personal qualities and taking advantage of networking opportunities are more important keys to finding just the right match in today's job market.

Knowing Oneself

The choice of a first nursing position deserves careful study. For some the opportunities seem to be a smorgasbord of possibilities, all of them attractive. The neophyte nurse should carefully explore any job under consideration and its responsibilities in light of his or her own personal qualities. Some students find it helpful to consult an instructor, job counselor, or a trusted nursing mentor for objective input and perspective. An experienced nurse can see the pros and cons that may not be visible to a new nurse. A thoughtful review of general interests, abilities, and strengths, especially those pointed out by clinical instructors, as well as attention paid to the types of patients who have provided the greatest emotional reward, is essential.

Other important considerations are one's physical and emotional stamina, energy level, and responsibilities to others-spouse, children and other family members, volunteer commitments, and social activities—all of which make legitimate demands on one's schedule. Long-term goals must be factored into the first job choice as well. Is the first job a stepping stone to an advanced degree, to a narrowly specialized area of nursing, to a traveling nurse position or to a management role? Selection of a position that fits the nurse's abilities, lifestyle, and career aspirations will affect job satisfaction, career advancement, and overall sense of success and happiness.

Finding the right practice environment is essential to long-term success and job satisfaction. The American Association of Colleges of Nursing (AACN) developed a white paper entitled *Hallmarks of the Professional Practice Environment,* which can be accessed on-line (www.aacn.nche.edu/Publications/positions/hallmarks.htm). Based on this paper, a brochure for graduates of nursing schools was developed, entitled *What Every Nursing School Graduate Should Consider When Seeking Employment.* This brochure identifies eight key characteristics or hallmarks of the professional practice setting and suggests that applicants ask the following questions about the employer they are considering—Does the potential employer:

- Manifest a philosophy of clinical care emphasizing quality, safety, interdisciplinary collaboration, continuity of care, and professional accountability?
- Recognize the value of nurses' expertise on clinical care quality and patient outcomes?
- Promote executive-level nursing leadership?
- Empower nurses' participation in clinical decision making and organization of clinical care systems?
- Demonstrate professional development support for nurses?
- Maintain clinical advancement programs based on education, certification, and advanced preparation?
- Create collaborative relationships among members of the health care team?
- Utilize technologic advances in clinical care and information systems?

Box 25-1 provides other statistics and information to request from a potential employer

The numbers of hospitals seeking and receiving "magnet" hospital credentialing are growing, and where these work environments are available, the nurse may wish to consider these organizations. Generally, hospitals with magnet status have demonstrated excellence in areas such as low RN turnover rates, adherence to standards of nursing care as defined by ANA, and mechanisms in place for staff participation in decision-making. The American Nurses Credentialing Center (AANC) lists all magnet hospitals on its website (Monarch, 2003).

BOX 25–1	Statistics and Information That Applicants May Request From a Potential Employer

- RN vacancy rate and RN turnover rate
- Patient satisfaction scores (preferably a percentile ranking)
- Employee satisfaction scores
- Average tenure of nursing staff
- Education mix of nursing staff
- Percentage of registry/travelers used
- Key human resource policies (e.g., reduction in workforce; tenure vs. performance criteria)
- Copy of the most recent JCAHO report and the number of contingencies cited
- Information about whether the nurses are unionized
- Copy of contract

From American Association of Colleges of Nursing (AACN): *What every nursing school graduate should consider when seeking employment*, Washington, DC, 2002, AACN.

Many graduate nurses have discovered that working in an environment that did not match well with their personal attributes and long-term goals not only made them miserable, but it damaged their future employment options as well. Poor job fits lead to frequent job changes, which could lead to poor references, as well as the attachment of the label "job hopper."

Ill-considered job choices obviously cost the new graduate, but they also are expensive for the employer. Some estimate the cost of recruiting, placing, and orienting a new nurse to be more than $12,000—but the costs are more than financial. Having a new nurse join a unit, start orientation, and then become disheartened and quit lowers the morale of the staff and manager and can have negative consequences on patient care, especially if turnover is repeated.

Networking

The investigative process of researching potential employers begins with networking at school, in the community, and within student nurse organizations. One may question other nurses, employees, and former employees, especially alumni of one's own school, who have worked in various settings. Faculty will have pertinent observations based on their experiences with clinical sites in the community. It is also valuable to listen to neighbors, friends and family members who have been patients.

Employment sections of newspapers, particularly Sunday editions, contain advertisements for current job openings and provide names to contact for further information. Hospital open houses and health care job fairs are also great places to pick up information about institutions. Recruitment materials and brochures often contain interesting facts about the organization, such as the mission or philosophy statement and goals, as well as available services. Such documents also often reflect the organization's attitude toward employees and patients (Zerwekh and Claborn, 2000).

The Internet offers links to actual jobs, as well as information on career planning. Most hospital and large health care systems maintain websites to post their employment needs and in many cases invite applications on-line. Some organizations view the Internet as a more

BOX 25–2 Helpful Websites

www.aacn.nche.edu/Publications/positions/hallmarks.htm
www.AirForce.com
www.careerxel.com
www.discovernursing.com
www.HospitalAmerica.com
www.nsna.org
www.medsearch.com/
www.monster.com
www.nursecredentialing.org/magnet.html
www.nursingspectrum.com
www.nursing-jobs.com/
www.wmed.com/hospdir.html
www.nursingworld.org/
www.nurse.com/
www.nursingcenter.com/
www.nursezone.com
www.rnwanted.com
www.careerbuilder.com
www.jobscout.org/

cost-effective recruiting method than advertising in newspapers. Applicants who intend to use this method to follow up on a job posting should pay particular attention to the application and resumé that is sent electronically, making sure there are no errors before submitting materials on-line. If there is no response to Internet inquiries within a week applicants should follow up with a phone call. Examples of Internet sites that would be helpful in exploring job opportunities, writing resumés, and preparing for employment interviews are provided in Box 25-2.

If a new graduate is seeking a position in a large community with multiple job choices available, this informal research will help to narrow the best place to begin the job application process. Later in the interview, the applicant may wish to describe to the recruiter how his or her search resulted in this employer being the number-one choice over others for the graduate's first job. This process of researching potential employers will continue through the interview process. Assessing the climate of the work environment is a valuable tool in "finding a match" and is discussed more thoroughly later in this chapter.

WRITTEN INTRODUCTIONS

Three of the most important steps in a job search are writing a cover letter, preparing a professional resumé, and assembling a professional portfolio. These tools introduce the applicant to a prospective employer. The first impression should be persuasive; there may not be a second chance. Presenting oneself on paper can make a difference, perhaps the difference between getting a desired interview and being passed over in favor of someone else. These written introductions should present a conscientious, mature, competent, committed professional who would be an asset to an agency that prides itself on its nursing services.

How to Write a Cover Letter

The cover letter (Box 25-3) is a chance to sell oneself and make the recruiter look forward to meeting an attractive candidate. A convincing cover letter will show how this candidate is different and will convey to the recruiter why he or she is the best fit for the position. The letter should also address why this institution is the applicant's first choice.

A cover letter should reflect the nurse's own style of writing, should never appear to have been copied from a book, and should be tailored to the particular job. Like any business document, it should be clean, direct, and letter-perfect. It should be attractive and effortless to read. There must be no obvious erasures, no typing errors, no evidence of correction fluid, and no grammar or spelling mistakes. Everything should fit on a single page of $8^{1}/_{2}$- by 11-inch white, heavyweight bond paper with ample margins on the top, bottom, and sides.

The letter should be addressed to a specific person. If the person's name or title is unknown, refer to a marketing brochure or call the recruitment office to ask for correct title and spelling of the appropriate person's first and last names.

If spelling is not your strength, use the spell-check tool on the computer. Using a dictionary and asking a competent friend to proofread the final copy is also a good idea.

BOX 25-3 *Cover Letter*

April 8, 2003

Ms. Donna Henderson, RN, MS
Director of Nurse Recruitment
Charleston Memorial Hospital
1600 Beckley Avenue
Memphis, Tennessee 38104

Dear Ms. Henderson:

I would like to apply for a new graduate position on a cardiology nursing unit at Charleston Memorial Hospital. After graduating from Smith College with a BSN on June 6, I will be ready to start work immediately. I plan to take the RN licensing examination in early July.

Through reading about your hospital and my own personal experience in a recent clinical rotation at Charleston Memorial, I have learned that your institution is a modern, professional one with an emphasis on quality patient care. For this and many other reasons, I am convinced that Charleston Memorial is where I want to work as a nurse.

I will be in Memphis on April 20-25 and will call to schedule an appointment to see you then. My phone number is (555) 912-3120.

I look forward to meeting you and discussing how I can contribute to Charleston Memorial Hospital.

Sincerely,

(Sign your name here in pen)
Bonnie McCray Pino
Enclosure

Poor typists would be well served to pay someone to type for them. A sloppy letter will cast doubt on one's abilities to practice as a professional.

The body of the letter should be single-spaced, three or four block paragraphs in length, with a blank line between paragraphs, and organized as follows:

- Paragraph 1 should be a statement of purpose that tells the recruiter what kind of position is being sought, the writer's expected date of graduation, state licensing status, and the date the writer will be ready to begin work.
- Paragraph 2 should emphasize the writer's suitability. The implied message should be, "I'm just the person for the job!" without going into all the details that will be included in the resumé. A sentence should describe past work or educational experiences that relate to the agency's particular needs and philosophy. The more homework the nurse has done in learning about the institution, the more convinced the recruiter will be. Finally, refer to the enclosed resumé.
- Paragraph 3 should request an interview appointment and give a range of dates of availability. It is a good idea for the writer to promise a telephone call "next week" or "soon" to schedule a meeting time and provide a telephone number where the writer can be reached, if the number is different from the permanent telephone number listed on the resumé.
- The letter can end with a "written handshake" such as, "I look forward to meeting with you to discuss available nursing positions in your institution"—a cautiously optimistic note.
- The letter closes with "Sincerely," and after four lines of space for a signature, the writer's name is typed. A line is skipped, and "Enclosure" is typed on the left margin to indicate that a resumé is enclosed.

The letter should be proofread carefully, signed, and copied; and the copy filed. If the nurse has chosen to use different approaches with different institutions, it would be wise to review the cover letter before the interview.

One week later, the writer should follow up by telephone to be sure the letter was received. This attention to detail and follow-through will impress the recruiter or personnel office and improve chances of getting an interview soon. These telephone calls usually become mini-interviews, and the applicant should be extra courteous, aware that it usually is the secretary who controls the interview schedule. By keeping a written list of all contacts made, the new graduate will be able to add the flattering personal touch of acknowledging previous telephone contacts when meeting them for the first time during the interview process.

The cover letter serves as the foundation on which all other follow-up is built: resumé, call for appointment, and interview. What is presented in the letter should prompt the person responsible for hiring to take a close look at the enclosed resumé.

How to Prepare a Resumé

A resumé is an opportunity to tell a condensed story of one's professional life (Box 25-4). It will complement the cover letter by filling in important details about educational and work experiences. An effective resumé should compress education and employment history into an attractive, easy-to-read, one-page summary. A wealth of valuable information can be communicated simply and straightforwardly by saying more with less. The key is writing concisely. For example, "BSN with high honors" speaks for itself. Citing exact grade point

BOX 25–4 *Resumé*

Bonnie McCray Pino
416 Melody Avenue
Bristol, Tennessee 37620
(555) 912-3720

Professional Objective:	Staff nurse position (cardiology) Anticipated date of NCLEX: July 2003
Licensure:	Eligible to take NCLEX after June 6 2003 Anticipated date of NCLEX: July 2003
Education: 1999-2003	Smith College School of Nursing Bristol, TN BSN, June 6, 2003
1995-1999	Oakview High School Nashville, TN Diploma, June 1999

Experience:
May 2002–August 2002, St. Mary's Hospital, Knoxville, TN
Patient Care Assistant: Assisted RNs in providing basic nursing care including feeding, bathing, ADLs, and patient teaching in a pediatric setting

June 2000–August 2000, Drs. Smith and Jones OB/GYN office, Bristol, TN
Office Assistant: Accompanied patients to treatment area, weighed, and recorded vital signs

Honors:	Sigma Theta Tau International, 2002 Who's Who Among American High School Students

Professional Organizations: Tennessee Student Nurses Association, 1999-2003

References: Provided on request

average or "Dean's list" standing adds little. Succinct ways to convey a message will be found by experimenting with phrases and word choices. Avoid pompous language and use of the passive voice. Instead use active verbs such as improved, established, trained, administered, prepared, wrote, and evaluated. Pepper the resumé with such words, and it will read easily.

A basic resumé contains three essential sections: identifying information, education, and work experience. In addition, optional information may include professional objectives, honors, achievements, and memberships in professional organizations. A well-designed resumé will mark the writer as a career-minded professional, just what recruiters are seeking. A succinct well-organized resumé indicates that the applicant is focused and organized in other areas as well.

The first section of the resumé, the identifying information, contains the applicant's name, address, and home and work telephone numbers, followed by licensure information.

The states of licensure and license numbers are listed. Graduating students should indicate when and where the National Council of Licensing Examination (NCLEX) was taken or will be taken.

If the resumé writer opts to include a professional objective, it should come next. Some interviewers like to see this because it shows that the nurse has put some thought into career planning. Keep in mind, though, that it is limiting to put forth a singular objective that ties the nurse to only one particular clinical area. If there is no such opening available in that department, the recruiter will consider the applicant an unlikely candidate to pursue. It is better to have an objective statement that is broad and general.

The second section should include details about education, including degrees and diplomas awarded, names and locations of schools, and graduation dates, starting with the most recent graduation and degree in reverse chronologic order.

The third section will present the information apt to be the greatest help in obtaining a job: work experience and employment history. Many recruiters are nurses themselves, so a detailed description of what a routine job entails is not needed. Instead, efforts should be directed toward illustrating any special knowledge or contributions. The new graduate's resumé might reflect student accomplishments or elaborate on jobs in which he or she has demonstrated skills also applicable to nursing responsibilities, such as organization of tasks, time management, delegation to subordinates, and ability to work well with others. Start with current or most recent position and work backward, including place of employment, job title, dates worked, and responsibilities. List accomplishments while employed, including number and type of patients cared for, any special techniques used, or any participation in the development of programs, policies, or forms pertinent to the position.

This section closes with optional information, such as seminars attended, honors received, and memberships in professional organizations. It is not advisable to list community activities or activities from more than 5 years ago unless it can be clearly shown that they are pertinent to a nursing career. Similarly, exclude personal information such as marital and health status, age, number of children, and hobbies. This information is not job-related and should not be used by the employer to screen applicants.

References do not need to be included in the resumé but should be ready for presentation in a neatly typed, photocopied list when requested from any future employer. Simply state, "References provided on request," or "References available." When someone agrees to be listed as a reference, take time to discuss what prospective employers may want to know. Former instructors or former employers may require written permission before releasing information. As the job search continues, keep references informed of the names of employers who may be inquiring.

Produce the resumé neatly and inexpensively, preferably on a computer or word processor, because a good resumé will be used repeatedly with revisions, and the nurse will want to be able to produce an up-to-date version without completely rewriting it. Production methods should be kept as simple as possible. It is not necessary to go to the added trouble and expense of having the resumé professionally typeset and printed. Having it neatly typed and reproduced using good-quality photocopying services suffices. To make the text easy to read, use one style of serif font throughout, in 11- or 12-point size. Again, have someone review the final copy for typing errors; then use a photocopying service for "quick copying" onto good-quality paper, white or ivory in color. It is important to remember that, when it comes to resumés, appearances do count. A well-formatted resumé that is properly organized and neatly typed makes a great first impression.

BOX 25-5 Documents for Professional Portfolio

Professional Credentials

Resumé

Licenses

Certifications

  Specialty practice certifications

  Basic Cardiac Life Support (BCLS)

  Advanced Cardiac Life Support (ACLS)

Educational Credentials

Diplomas

Transcripts

Continuing education certificates

Honors and awards (including program from
  awards ceremony, letters regarding awards,
  newspaper articles)

Research and Scholarly Activity

Publications

Teaching materials for patients, staff, handouts

Case studies

Photo of poster sessions, classroom presentations

PowerPoint outline of presentation

Student papers and projects

Professional Activities

Membership cards

Evidence of service as an officer or leader in student
  organizations

Community involvement and volunteer activities

Performance evaluations

Letters of recommendation

Adapted from Cardillo D: Beyond the resume: how to compile your nursing portfolio, *Crit Care Choices* 52, 54-55, 2000.

How to Prepare a Portfolio

The nursing portfolio contains more information than a resumé and provides documentation to support the resumé. The portfolio introduces the professional nurse to recruiters, employers, admissions committees, and potential supervisors in a visual and tangible way. It includes traditional documents, such as a resumé, license to practice and certifications, educational documents, (diplomas, transcripts, etc.), and examples of significant professional, community, and student activities (Box 25-5).

The simplest way to build a portfolio is to start with an attractive three-ring binder. A table of contents gives interviewers a map to guide their review of the information. Dividers can separate sections, each with its own cover page, and plastic sleeves or pocketed pages work well to hold loose items. Appropriate documents are assigned to each section. Make copies of important originals, such as diplomas, certifications, and licenses that would be difficult to replace. Include samples of letters from grateful patients, congratulations from peers, and complimentary notes from supervisors. Highlight sentences in longer letters or performance appraisals that address the information considered to be most important for the reader to note. The graduate nurse may want to include supervisor evaluations from nonnursing positions to demonstrate leadership qualities, dependability, and attention to detail, characteristics also relevant to the nursing work setting.

Graduation is the perfect time to create a career portfolio, one that will be easy to build upon and update as the nursing career evolves. If documents are created on the computer, updates and revisions will be easy when the nurse pursues new and different professional roles and responsibilities. Many baccalaureate educational programs require students to create such a portfolio as part of their preparation for graduation and entry into the first job—and increasingly, boards of nursing are making portfolios (or other methods for documenting evidence of competency) mandatory for relicensure.

Nurses who present portfolios to the recruiter may have a competitive edge over nurses who do not.

HOW TO INTERVIEW EFFECTIVELY

No matter how qualified and self-confident a person may feel, sitting across the desk from an interviewer can be intimidating. One's conduct in the recruiter's office may determine whether a job offer is made. Being a little anxious is normal, but panic is not. When the applicant has made a good first impression in the cover letter and resumé, he or she can expect to be called for an interview. The graduate's tasks then becomes to enter the interview prepared to answer and ask questions that will help determine whether this organization, with its available job opportunities, is a good match.

Every agency has its own hiring and interviewing policies. Generally, the smaller the organization and the more decentralized the nursing department, the more involved the lower-level manager is in the recruitment and hiring process. The same person who interviews nurse applicants also may be the manager, staff development instructor, quality assurance director, employee health nurse, or chair of the product standards committee. A large organization with many employees may have a separate human resources department with a nurse recruiter on staff. Within such large organizations, the hiring process becomes more complicated and more formal—applicants are more tightly screened, and the hiring decisions are farther removed from the actual work position.

Not all "nurse recruiters" are nurses themselves, which may make a difference in the kind of information exchanged in the interview. A nonnurse is not likely to be able to fully discuss questions that pertain directly to a nurse's job description, patient care workload, and nursing responsibilities. The applicant does not have to answer questions that are not job-related. In fact, some questions are not legally allowed to be asked (Box 25-6). After a job offer is made, certain non-job-related questions may be asked, but not before. They should not be a part of deciding whether the applicant is offered a position.

BOX 25–6 *Legal and Illegal Areas of Questioning*

Some questions are inappropriate to be asked of an applicant before a job offer is made.

Legal	Illegal
Educational preparation	Race
Licensure status	Creed
Work experience	Color
Reasons for leaving previous jobs	Age
Reasons for applying to this institution	Nationality
Qualifications for this job	Marital status
Strengths and weaknesses	Sexual preference
Criminal convictions	Religious beliefs
	Number of children or dependents
	Financial or credit status

How to Prepare: Planning Ahead

It is recommended that interview appointments be made as early as possible and that senior students not wait until graduation day. Job hunting takes time, and appointments are not easily scheduled near nursing school graduation dates, because these tend to be busy weeks for recruiters.

How to Prepare: Self-Talk

As the day approached, Mary obsessed about the interview, thinking to herself, "What if they ask me something I cannot answer, and I go blank like I used to do in clinicals when the instructor quizzed me about my patient's medicines. I will look like an idiot, and maybe even start to cry." The night before the appointment, Mary could not sleep.

Your thoughts dictate your reality. Nurses, especially new nurses, should be aware of what they are saying to themselves. The applicant who thinks, "Why would anyone want to hire a graduate nurse with no practical experience like me?" will project a lack of self-trust that may be interpreted by the recruiter as lack of enthusiasm or even incompetence. If instead the graduate thinks, "I have successfully completed a difficult nursing course of study. I am now ready to take on the responsibilities of a professional. With orientation, on-the-job training, and the support of experienced nurses, I can succeed as an RN. I have everything I need to begin practice." This reality-based "self-talk" is an important internal dialog for establishing feelings of confidence before the job interview.

The reality is that all graduates have met the criteria for graduation from a nursing education program and have been deemed ready by that credentialing body for an entry-level position as an RN. The final test of competence to practice, the NCLEX, will provide further proof. Graduate nurses who fear failure of this final test must remind themselves of those now successfully practicing who preceded them from the same educational program with the same preparation.

How to Prepare: Rehearse

A simple visualization of how the graduate wants to appear to the recruiter can bring about the self-assurance needed to create an attractive candidate. It is helpful to mentally review and be prepared to describe pride in any past work experiences, especially the parts of any job that relate to what is required of a nurse. Even baby-sitting jobs can validate a worker as a responsible adult if that person worked consistently for the same family and showed stability and good judgment as a trusted caretaker for children. Applicants tend to discount minimum-wage, part-time, teen-age, or summer employment, but these experiences often reveal a great deal about the applicant: Would attendance records attest to the worker's dependability? Was the worker given greater responsibility over time? Was the worker allowed to open or close the business? Handle the cash receipts? Consider the following scenario:

CASE STUDY

The only job Sam had before nursing school had been working at the customer service desk at a large children's toy store, where he scheduled and supervised the cashiers. His title was "Designated Key Carrier," which he listed on his resume. The interviewer reasonably interpreted this to be a position that demonstrated the employer's trust in Sam.

Remember, it is not only the graduate's academic standing or honors and awards that measure success as a student. Perhaps the student was not in the top 10% of the class but was active in student affairs. Perhaps the student was chair of a student government committee or a contributor to the campus newspaper. The graduate should be prepared to describe other areas of student accomplishments.

Unfortunately, many nurses are not accustomed to selling themselves and are uncomfortable in situations in which they need to be able to discuss their best attributes and market their qualifications. Therefore, after rehearsing in your own mind how to present these qualifications to interviewers, it would be wise to rehearse with another person, role-playing the expected interview dialog. Role-play with another student or an experienced nurse (even better), rehearsing answers to questions the interviewer is expected to ask. Practice descriptions of the key points of past employment. A few minutes spent in rehearsing with another will contribute to composure and self-confidence in the actual situation.

Finally, it is important for the graduate to remember that the job interview is not an examination to pass or fail, nor is it an interrogation. It is an exchange of information—the recruiter hoping to find a potential employee to fill a staff vacancy and the applicant hoping to find employment as a nurse in this organization. Each has responsibilities for informing the other, and each has rights to obtain information from the other (Box 25-7).

How to Prepare: The Interview Itself

Dress Appropriately. Business-appropriate clothing such as a neat dress, suit, or pantsuit projects a professional attitude. Casual attire projects a casual attitude. Jeans are not acceptable, nor are shorts or any clothes that are too short, too tight, or too trendy. Conservative and simple are always best. "Dressing for success" not only influences the impressions others have, but also influences the wearer's own behavior. When people are dressed to look their best, attitudes improve and levels of self-confidence increase. Facial make-up should be light, and the use of perfume or cologne should be avoided. Many institutions are fragrance-free because of patients' and employees' allergic reactions to perfumes. Large, distracting jewelry should be avoided.

Arrive on Time. Arriving late for a job interview creates a poor first impression. Be considerate of the interviewer's time and agenda. If delayed, call to reschedule. To arrive too early can make the interviewer feel rushed or the applicant appear overanxious.

BOX 25-7 Applicant's Rights

Applicants have the right to:

- Be informed of available positions at an institution and the minimum qualifications required.
- Apply for any available position for which they are qualified.
- Be seriously and fairly considered for any available position for which they are qualified.
- Be interviewed, be shown a job description, and be made aware of the requirements and expectations of the job.
- Have the work schedule discussed.
- Be informed of the benefits package.
- See the nursing unit and meet the manager if they are being seriously considered.
- Be made aware of the orientation program.
- Be given an expected time by which a decision will be made.

Bring a Resumé. Even if a resumé has already been submitted, the applicant should bring extra copies. The recruiter may have routed the mailed copy to a manager for review. Applicants probably will be asked to complete an employment application, and the resumé is a ready reference for past employers and dates of employment. Social security card, driver's license, and the nursing license, if available, also will be requested as necessary parts of the identification process. Some agencies request that a current cardiopulmonary resuscitation card be made available to photocopy. These documents will be easy to produce if the applicant has also brought a professional portfolio folder.

The Interview

The interview is the most time-consuming and subjective part of the employment process. For professionals it is appropriate for interviews to be unstructured, using open-ended questions; both recruiter and applicant will have questions. The initial interview can be expected to last 30 minutes to 1 hour. Being prepared is the key, and planning answers to the questions most likely to be asked is the best way to prepare. Eight of the most frequently asked questions follow.

What Positions Interest You? The interviewer needs to know whether there are positions available in the applicant's area of interest and whether the applicant has the required qualifications to fit the vacant positions. If there is no fit in interest or qualifications with jobs available, neither applicant nor recruiter need waste much more time in the interview.

Because titles and position names vary from organization to organization, it is better to answer the question with favorite clinical experiences. Applicants might share short- and long-term goals and how they visualize laying the groundwork today for tomorrow's professional roles. A good response might be, "I'm interested in a position that will help me grow as a professional and give me opportunities to develop greater competency as a nurse. Ultimately, I would like to work as a critical care clinical nurse specialist." If interest, qualifications, and the available positions match, the interviewer will want to start planning secondary interviews and tours.

Tell Me About Your Work History. Even if previous jobs were not nursing-related, the applicant can highlight the responsibilities carried out, the skills acquired, and how those skills can transfer to the professional nursing role. This is the point at which the interviewer will get an idea of motivation, drive, energy level, and reliability. No new graduate will be expected to have all the knowledge and skills of an experienced RN; however, when answering, the graduate may stress other aptitudes such as verbal skills or interpersonal skills. It is best to start with the current or most recent job and proceed backward. A new graduate might discuss student clinical experiences, which clinical areas were favored, and why.

How Did You Choose to Apply for a Job Here? Any previous investigative homework done on the institution is useful and helps to form honest responses. For example, an applicant might say, "This hospital has a reputation for its quality care, and I like that," or "I am interested in research and have heard you have a nursing research committee for staff nurses."

Do You Want a Full-Time or Part-Time Position, and Which Shift Do You Prefer? If there is a need or desire for a particular schedule, the nurse should be honest and ask for that schedule. If the recruiter does not have that schedule available, ask what is available, so that a decision can be made. Can the nurse be flexible to accept an undesirable shift until a preferred one becomes available? Part of one's investigation of an institution should include looking at a current list of posted positions. Particularly with smaller agencies, if what the nurse desires is not posted, it may be beneficial to ask for a particular schedule but, if willing, express an interest in working a schedule that is posted. For example, "I'm willing to work the evening shift posted for the medical-surgical unit; however, I'm most interested in moving into a day position in labor and delivery."

What Are Your Strengths and Weaknesses? Sometimes this question may be asked in less direct ways such as, "What are some of the areas you know you need to improve?" or "How have your skills developed in your advanced nursing courses?" Honesty always is best. By asking this question, the interviewer may only be trying to pinpoint the special skills and preferences of the nurse. For example, with what kind of patients has the nurse been most effective, and which ones proved most difficult? The clearer the applicant can be in articulating specific talents and deficiencies, the more closely the recruiter will be able to match the candidate to a position suited to his or her abilities. The closer this match, the more likely the employee will flourish and be able to use special talents.

It is not advisable to avoid the issue of weaknesses. Everyone has them. It is better to admit them but to present them in a positive way. In addition, it may be helpful to tell the interviewer what is being done to correct weaknesses. For example, "Sometimes I tend to see the 'big picture' and have to remind myself to pay more attention to the details. I've started keeping lists, and they seem helpful." Another suggestion might be, "I have limited bedside nursing experience, but I am excited about building on the clinical skills I have learned in school."

What Would You Do If . . . ? The recruiter probably will ask some situational questions to find out related to decision making and critical thinking skills. The nurse will be asked to explain how to assess a particular situation, set priorities, decide what should be implemented first for a patient, and what can be delegated. Rather than fabricate an answer about unfamiliar circumstances, one can honestly say, "I've never been in that situation, but I think I would . . . " or "I was in a similar situation in which . . . occurred, and this is what I did in those circumstances."

Why Should We Hire You? This is an opportunity to share the special assets that the applicant would bring to the employer's institution. Without embellishment or selling oneself short, it is important to convey pride in being a nurse and conviction that one has something special to offer.

What Questions Do You Have? Usually the interview ends with the interviewer asking whether there are any questions. This is an opportunity for the applicant to demonstrate initiative, and one should take advantage of it, although not to excess. In an effective interview with an experienced interviewer, most questions regarding salary, benefits, and human resource policies will have been addressed (Box 25-8). If not, this is the time to ask. Should a tour of the nursing unit and a meeting with the supervisor be arranged, many concerns will be answered then. Box 25-9 presents a list of suggested questions.

Mentally reviewing practiced responses to these questions will give the applicant confidence. The more information gathered, the easier it will be to make a decision, and the more likely it is that the nurse will be happy in the long term.

BOX 25–8 *What to Expect a Recruiter to Communicate*

Recruiters should inform applicants of basic human resource policies regarding job descriptions, compensation, benefits, and staff development, including:

- Conditional period
- Job descriptions
- Shift rotation
- Weekend rotation
- Salary
- Staff development
- Parking
- Security
- Health insurance and other insurance benefits
- Preemployment physical examinations

- Credit union
- Overtime
- Scheduled paydays
- Paid time off
- Leaves of absence
- Employee discounts
- Transfer and promotion policies
- Resignation policies
- Preemployment policies
- Pay increases

THE APPLICANT'S TASKS

Assess the Climate of the Work Environment

As mentioned in the previous discussion of researching potential employers, there are ways other than direct questioning to learn a lot about the institution. Every organization has its own personality and atmosphere. The first impression probably came from the secretary who answered the phone when the applicant called for an appointment with the recruiter, followed by the greeting on arrival at the recruiter's office. A tone of respect and pride in being

---

BOX 25–9 *Appropriate Questions for the Applicant to Ask*

1. May I see the job description for the position we are discussing?
2. What is the nurse-to-patient ratio?
3. What support staff are available on the unit to assist nurses?
4. What about clerical help and support services? What type of nursing is practiced here (team nursing, primary nursing, centralized, decentralized)?
5. How available are physicians? Admitting physicians and house staff?
6. How often are nursing care conferences held on this unit?
7. What type of nursing documentation is used?
8. How long is the orientation program? What does the program include? What continuing education programs are available after my initial orientation?
9. How will my performance be evaluated? How often, and by whom?
10. What exact schedule or shift will I be working in this position?
11. What will my salary be? Is there a shift differential?
12. Are there differentiated practice levels or roles and differentiated pay scales for nursing congruent with differences in educational preparation, certification, and other advanced nursing preparation?
13. How are pay increases decided?
14. What other benefits are there (health, life insurance, vacation time, retirement plan)?

associated with the organization may have been communicated in the first encounter. Every subsequent encounter builds on the first.

In the hallways of the agency, how do people acknowledge each other? A visit to the employee cafeteria to buy a cup of coffee or a sandwich at mealtime can be enlightening. Are nurses eating there? Does it seem that the staff members are enjoying themselves? Pick up for later reading any available in-house publications such as employee newsletters or bulletins.

Ask for a Tour

If the interviewer does not automatically offer a tour of the unit, the applicant can request to see it and will certainly want to meet with the person who would be the immediate supervisor. To get an accurate feel for the unit, the applicant should pay close attention to the pace, the tone of the staff interaction, and the morale. Is this a group the prospective employee would like to join? Are the manager's philosophy and management style similar to the applicant's own?

The astute applicant can get an accurate feel for the nursing unit's culture and personality if the manager's interactions with staff are observed. Is the manager accessible to the staff and supportive in response to them? How are telephone calls and other interruptions handled? How well do people seem to be getting along? Pay attention to the way people on the unit relate to each other—nurses to doctors, nurses to families, nurses to nurses. How are the patients responded to on the intercommunication system? Notice the efficiency with which staff work. How rushed are they? Also note bulletin boards and any public displays of staff recognition (e.g., "Employee of the Month" plaques or brag boards). Even a second visit to the unit might be requested before a final decision is made. The more information gathered, the easier it will be to make a decision.

Some managers offer opportunities for the applicant to meet with staff, and formal interviews with staff nurses may be scheduled as a routine part of the hiring process. This gives the applicant a closer view of the actual work organization and gives representative staff members a chance to have a voice in selecting new co-workers. Staff nurses provide bedside care to patients and best understand the qualities appreciated in a good team member. Whether the introduction to staff is a formal interview or a casual conference room encounter, the applicant can be made to feel welcome and wanted while learning about the real work and the real workers of the agency. Now that firsthand knowledge has been obtained, if the applicant confers again with these employees and former employees consulted before applying, he or she can ask more informed questions.

Follow-Up

Thank-You Letter. A follow-up letter thanking the recruiter is a courtesy and a reminder of the nurse's interest in receiving a timely response (Box 25-10). If the nurse does not hear from the employer within a reasonable length of time (1 to 2 weeks) after the interview, it is appropriate to inquire by telephone about the status of a hiring decision.

Avoid Impulse Decisions. If offered a position and time is needed to make a decision, the applicant should postpone a decision and should not feel pressured into acceptance while still unsure. An offer to telephone the recruiter with an answer within an agreed-on time is appropriate.

If there are other job opportunities, certainly comparisons need to be made by weighing the pros and cons of each position and each organization. How do benefits compare? What are the possibilities for movement within the systems laterally and vertically? How available are

BOX 25–10   *Interview Follow-Up Letter*

April 24, 2003

Ms. Donna Henderson, RN, MS
Director, Nurse Recruitment
Charleston Memorial Hospital
1265 Beckley Avenue
Memphis, Tennessee 38104

Dear Ms. Henderson:

It was a pleasure meeting with you on Monday. I now have a clear picture of what I might expect as a new graduate nurse in your hospital. Everyone on the units I visited was very friendly.

I look forward to hearing from you with good news about a position at Charleston Memorial. I can be reached in the afternoons at (555) 912-3720.

Thank you again for your time and interest.

Sincerely,

Bonnie McCray Pino

continuing education opportunities to staff nurses? How do observations of the work culture fit with the nurse's ideas of what is needed to support professional success? Does the schedule that is offered fit the applicant's lifestyle? When a decision has been reached, a telephone call should be made promptly to the recruiter, whether the answer is "yes" or "no."

Weighing Options. What questions might be asked of oneself while weighing the merits of one position against others? Remembering that no job is perfect, the following four questions should be considered.

Does the Position Match the Nurse's Qualifications? Although it is flattering to receive a job offer for a position for which a nurse has little or no preparation, one should not be influenced by such a compliment. When there is a nursing shortage, a position that is beyond an applicant's present skills and experience may sound wonderfully challenging, when in actuality it may be overwhelming and a disastrous beginning for a new graduate. Being overzealous, overconfident, and overanxious to please can only lead to feelings of guilt and inadequacy if the job is not appropriate. It is wiser to accept a position in which adequate orientation and clinical support exists, which would allow the graduate to gain the experience and preparation necessary to accept a position requiring more skills at a later time.

What Are the Actual Responsibilities of the Job? The newly hired nurse has the right to completely understand what will be expected in the position offered, including the overall and daily responsibilities and the length and nature of on-the-job training that will be provided. What will the supervisory responsibilities be? How many and what skill level employees will be under the RN's leadership? What orientation is planned to prepare the RN for practicing independently? Are there arrangements for a preceptor to guide the graduate through the difficult transition of entering a first nursing job? Reality shock can be anticipated, and the more assistance a new graduate receives in adjusting to the new role of the nurse, the more likely is the beginner to be successful and satisfied.

Does This Position Lead the Nurse in the Direction of Projected Career Goals? Is the offered job a step toward meeting long-term career objectives? For example, a graduate who wants to be a nurse midwife someday would be wiser to accept a position in postpartum if labor and delivery is not available rather than accepting a position in neurosurgery just because it offers a slightly higher salary or a few more weekends. No position or job change should be accidental or be the result of a snap decision. Wise career moves result from deliberate planning and purposeful preparation.

How Will the Work be Compensated? Experienced nurses often advise novices that money, although important, is not the only reward associated with a job. On the other hand, money does matter, especially to a new graduate who may have subsisted on a limited income while in school. It is common for loans to have accumulated, along with unpaid bills. Inadequate salary can be a real source of job dissatisfaction, of course, but with 24-hour responsibilities, nurses traditionally have basic salaries that include other income-contributing factors, such as shift differentials, weekend differentials, holiday pay, paid vacation days, and expected salary increases over time. Compensation comes in other packages besides paychecks. There are policies that allow for maternity leaves, medical leaves, tuition reimbursement, sick days, discounts on prescriptions and health insurance, retirement benefits, and malpractice insurance coverage, all of which affect income in indirect but important ways. As is true in other areas of consideration, the better the total compensation package fits one's needs, the greater the likelihood that one will remain satisfied with the job.

Well-prepared job applicants will have listed those benefits they consider essential, and these vary with individual circumstances. For example, the essentials for someone who is the sole family breadwinner probably include health insurance, paid time off, and an employer-provided retirement plan. Available childcare would be especially important for parents of preschool children. Box 25-11 further helps applicants evaluate potential employment opportunities.

THE EMPLOYER'S TASKS

In any agency providing nursing services, its nurses are the indispensable employees. The selection of new nurse employees is a critically important responsibility, and it is the recruiter's duty to make sure the best selection is made.

First, the nurse must meet the minimum requirements for the position desired. For example, 1 year of experience might be required for a nurse to work a weekender program or in a critical care area. Operating room (OR) experience may be required for OR nursing positions, and perinatal nursing experience may be required for labor and delivery positions. A secondary consideration is the nurse's suitability for contributing to the mission of the health care delivery system. The recruiter is selling the organization to the applicant and measuring the skills and aptitudes the applicant would bring to the organization.

The bottom line for any employer who provides health care services to the public is to ensure that its nursing staff practices safely. Recruiters are looking to uncover anything

BOX 25-11	*Assesment Tool for Decision Making*

When weighing options for employment, consider those measures of a professional work climate evident in written documentation and visible in the patient care areas. The following observations should guide the new graduate in making an informed decision.

- Standards of nursing practice are evident and are an integral part of patient care.
- Nurse-to-patient ratio is adequate and adjusted for patient acuity.
- Orientation is structured, individualized, and adequate for new graduates.
- Opportunities for horizontal transfer and advancement exist within the system.
- The salary is competitive and reasonable.
- Benefits are competitive.
- Continuing education is available, and staff members are encouraged to attend.
- A nurse administrator is responsible for delivery of nursing services.

that would impair a nurse applicant's ability to provide safe nursing care, such as incompetence, unprofessional conduct, unreliability in attendance, chemical dependency, or record of criminal activity. For screening, recruiters have four primary sources of information: the application, interview impressions, test results, and references.

Applications are validated. Work history and references are checked to ensure accuracy. Previous supervisors are asked about attendance, dependability, performance, attitude, ability to get along with others, integrity, and eligibility for rehire. The applicant's stated reason for termination is compared with information obtained from work references. The employer has a right to obtain reasonable information about the persons who are hired. Most employment applications ask whether the applicant has ever been convicted of a crime other than a minor traffic violation. The question is about convictions, not arrests, and the response is verified by a background or criminal record check. Response to this or any other question in the application process must be honest and truthful. Each institution has its own policies regarding convictions, but most are vitally concerned about their responsibilities regarding negligent hiring. If an applicant committed a crime that, if repeated while in the employ of the institution, would cause harm to patients, families, other employees or the institution, the applicant is rejected.

A preemployment physical examination is often required. This usually is done on site and at the employer's expense. It may involve obtaining the applicant's full medical history and vital signs, routine blood tests, a urine drug screen, and sometimes a chest radiograph. The purpose of the physical examination is to ensure protection for patients and to ensure that the caregiver can carry out the necessary physical responsibilities of the job. For example, are illegal mood-altering substances evident that would impair the nurse's abilities and judgment? Are there physical limitations the institution should know about to determine whether any special accommodations are necessary to allow the candidate to perform the usual duties associated with the position?

Even with a job offer made and a date for employment set, actual start dates are contingent on receipt of documentation of these final screenings, plus a reference check to verify the resumé; these items establish the practitioner's safety and reliability. Other parts of screening for safety might include paper-and-pencil testing, such as skills tests, pharmacology tests, and in some cases, psychologic testing for specialty areas.

A preemployment pharmacology test is common. Many institutions give such a quiz to determine basic knowledge of routinely administered medications, their purposes, and side effects. Simple dosage questions and calculation methods may be asked. Some questions may be situational ones, such as, "What would you do in this case . . . ?" or "The first nursing action in this scenario should be . . . ."

A few larger institutions also may administer a clinical skills test. This might be conducted in a simulated laboratory setting, where frequently used patient care equipment is set up. Usually a staff development instructor accompanies the nurse through a series of stations where the nurse would be asked to plan and perform the appropriate nursing actions. Examples might be starting cardiopulmonary resuscitation on a simulated patient, demonstrating the proper procedure for starting an intravenous line, or talking through an assessment of a patient.

It is far better to be prepared and even better to be proactive and offer to produce some of the documentation required. For instance, the nurse may be able to get a written reference from a former employer or a statement from a physician sooner than the institution can. The employment start date depends on the receipt of all the necessary information, so it would expedite the process if the hopeful employee volunteered to initiate some of the documentation gathering.

Once an applicant is selected, the agency has committed itself to costly training, orientation, and additional benefits that may cost as much as 30% to 40% of the employee's salary. A major element of control, which any organization possesses, is its ability to choose its employees. When the selection process is thorough, it is a sign to the committed professional that this is a reputable employer.

SUMMARY

If not offered a position, the new graduate should still feel good about himself or herself. There may have been several candidates for that same position. Perhaps it was not the best match for one's skills or preferences. There is victory in having had an opportunity to practice interview skills. Preparation, practice, and perseverance will reward the nurse with a job that is better suited to his or her personality, values, qualifications, and skills. New graduates have internalized standards of practice from their nursing education experience. On graduation they must decide where to begin to put those standards to work in real-life terms handling real responsibilities with real patients. The question becomes, "Can school and work values be reconciled in this nursing environment?" When adequate groundwork in pursuit of a job has been laid, the answer should come easy.

CRITICAL THINKING ACTIVITIES

1. In the interest of creating the right match for yourself with your first career choice as a graduate nurse, what personal qualities and professional strengths and weaknesses will you consider?
2. How would you evaluate the overall work environment of the agency you have selected for employment, other than by asking direct questions?
3. Consider the responsibility of nurse recruiters to create an environment of safe care. How thorough should preemployment examinations be? In what positions should a new graduate be allowed to function, and why? Describe what would be included in a preemployment examination.

Additional resources are available on-line at: http://evolve.elsevier.com/Cherry/

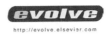

http://evolve.elsevier.com

REFERENCES

Cardillo D: Beyond the resume: how to compile your nursing portfolio, *Crit Care Choices* 52, 54-55, 2000.

Monarch K: Making informed employment decisions, *AJN* (Career Guide for 2003):29-32, 2003.

Zerwekh J, Claborn JC: *Nursing today: transition and trends,* ed 3, Philadelphia, 2000, WB Saunders.

SUGGESTED READINGS

Creating a winning resume (Editorial), *Imprint* 48(1):43, 46-48, 2001.

Meister L et al: Professional nursing portfolios: a global perspective, *MEDSURG Nurs* 11(4):177-182, 2002.

Oermann M: Developing a professional portfolio in nursing, *Orthopaedic Nurs* 21(2):73-78, 2002.

Restifo V: The successful interview, *Imprint* 49(1):37, 39-40, 2002.

Russo C: How to interview on your own terms, *AJN* (Career Guide for 2001) 101(1, Part 2):16-18, 2001.

Saver C: How to choose the right first job, *Imprint* 47(1):35-36, 2000.

Serembus J: Teaching the process of developing a professional portfolio, *Nurs Educator* 25(6):282-287, 2000.

Weinstein SM: A nursing portfolio: documenting your professional journey, *J Infus Therapy* 25(6):357-364, 2002.

Welton RH, Morton PG: Strategies for writing an effective resume, *Career Guide Critical Care Nurse,* Feb:18-23, 52, 2002.

Welton RH, Morton PG, Amig A: How to succeed in job interviewing, *Career Guide Critical Care Nurse,* Feb: 24-28, 2002.

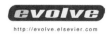

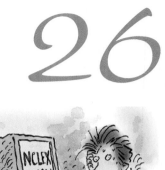

NCLEX-RN Examination

Mary Lynn Engelmann, MSN, EdD, RN

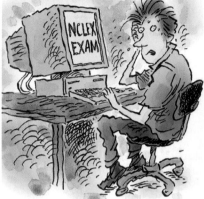

Adequate preparation for the NCLEX
can reduce panic and ensure success.

VIGNETTE

Considered for a moment how nursing and licensure examinations have changed as society has changed. Nursing is a reflection of society's values, knowledge, and needs. Test items or questions found on the NCLEX examination today have little resemblance to questions asked on state board examinations administered during the early part of the century. Questions of that era dealt with practical issues and consisted mainly of knowledge-based questions that had little to do with assessment, application, evaluation, or need. Consider, for instance, the following questions taken from the 1919 State Board Questions and Answers for Nurses (Foote, 1919):

- What are the advantages of fireplaces?
- How would you sterilize silkworm-gut and silk sutures?
- What care regarding nourishment would you give a gynaecological [sic] patient to prevent a common discomfort?
- Give some general rules for preparing meats.
- Give three common complaints that the public makes about graduate nurses.

Questions to consider while reading this chapter:
1. What is the purpose of the NCLEX-RN examination?
2. What type of questions can I expect on today's NCLEX-RN examination?
3. What is the best way to prepare for the examination?

Additional resources are available on-line at: http://evolve.elsevier.com/Cherry/

KEY TERMS

Compulsory licensure Requirement that must be met to legally practice or work as an RN. Licensure is a prerequisite to practice in each state and U.S. territory.

Computer adaptive testing (CAT) A type of testing taken on a computer, in which a person is given a test question to answer, followed by a subsequent question that is based on the answer given in the first question. CAT adapts or changes according to the answers a person gives. For example, a person missing a question dealing with assessment might be given another assessment question to determine the person's competency with assessment.

NCLEX-RN examination An examination taken by qualified graduates of approved schools of nursing. Graduates successfully taking the NCLEX are granted a license to practice as registered nurses (RNs).

LEARNING OUTCOMES

After studying this chapter, the reader will be able to:

1. Explain the purpose of the NCLEX examination.
2. Evaluate various methods of preparation for the NCLEX examination.
3. Create a personal plan for preparing for the NCLEX examination.
4. Analyze the relationship between the nursing process and client needs as they relate to NCLEX test items.
5. Compare and contrast various review courses designed to aid in review for the NCLEX examination.

ARE YOU PREPARED FOR NCLEX?

You are currently pursuing a degree in nursing, and plan to take the NCLEX licensure examination upon graduation. Do you know what to expect on the exam itself? Do you feel you have the knowledge necessary for NCLEX success? If not, you should be interested in this chapter, which offers an overview of the format and content you can expect on the test and strategies for success.

THE NCLEX EXAMINATION

The NCLEX examination and licensure to practice nursing go hand in hand. To receive a license to practice as an RN in the United States and its territories, candidates must furnish evidence of competency to provide effective nursing care by successfully completing the NCLEX examination (National Council, 2003).

Currently there are three types of registered nursing programs: (1) 2-year associate degree programs usually found in community or junior colleges, (2) hospital-based diploma programs, and (3) baccalaureate degree programs found in 4-year colleges and universities or academic health centers. Graduates from all three programs take the same NCLEX examination. The examination tests content common to all three programs, is job-related, and reflects current entry level nursing practice (National Council, 2003). Individuals taking the examination must have graduated from approved schools of nursing.

Purpose of the NCLEX Examination

All states and U.S. territories have compulsory licensure and use the NCLEX for licensure determination. The purpose of the NCLEX examination is twofold:

1. It safeguards the public from unsafe practitioners.
2. It assists state boards of nursing in determining candidates' capabilities for performing entry-level RN positions.

The National Council of State Boards of Nursing (NCSBN) periodically ascertains entry-level capabilities by investigating the jobs that entry-level nurses are performing in various health care settings in the United States (National Council, 2003).

Characteristics of the NCLEX Examination

The NCLEX is a pass-fail examination and has been computerized since 1994. Before that time the NCLEX was a paper-and-pencil examination requiring 2 days to complete. The examination was offered twice a year in selected cities in each state. Today the NCLEX is offered at more than 3400 Pearson Professional Centers throughout the country, can be taken at the candidate's convenience, and can be completed in 5 hours or less. The results of the examination are sent to candidates within a month after they have taken the examination. In some states candidates may receive unofficial results by telephone or e-mail, or they may check the state board website for licensure verification.

Computerized Adaptive Testing. The NCLEX uses computerized adaptive testing (CAT), which is a test-administering technique that uses current computer technology and measurement theory (CAT Overview, 2003). As a candidate answers questions on the examination, the CAT adapts to the level of the candidate's knowledge, skills, and ability. All examinations are consistent with the NCLEX-RN Test Plan, which controls inclusion of current nursing content. Candidates have ample opportunity to demonstrate their competence since the examination does not end until stability of the pass/fail result is certain or time runs out (CAT Overview, 2003).

A tutorial is administered before the examination actually begins, providing candidates with experience in using the computer in CAT situations (How CAT Works, 2003). Candidates should carefully read an entire question and all possible answer options before selecting an answer. Candidates may request assistance regarding the use of the computer at any point, even during the NCLEX-RN examination. In addition, candidates may find it helpful to view the PowerPoint candidate tutorial before going to the testing center. This tutorial, provided by NCSBN, may be accessed at the website listed in Box 26-1.

Skipping Questions/Changing Answers. Candidates taking the NCLEX are not allowed to skip questions and return to them at a later time or to change answers to questions once an answer has been selected and entered into the computer. These actions would defeat the purpose of adaptive testing because CAT is based on the knowledge, skills, and abilities of the examination taker and selects questions based on these three measures. Candidates are not disadvantaged using this method of testing because CAT has a built-in, self-correcting mechanism (How CAT Works, 2003).

Question Format

All of the information needed to answer a particular question appears on one computer screen, so candidates do not need to see the previous or next screen for answer determination.

Questions are presented in traditional top-down format, in which the question is presented, followed by the potential answers to it. Questions appearing on the computer screen will be either traditional multiple choice or alternate item format. These formats are discussed briefly below.

Traditional Format: Multiple Choice, One Option. With this type of format, the candidate is presented a question, followed by four possible responses. The candidate is asked to select the one option that best answers the question. Multiple choice, one option format is the style most commonly used on the examination. See the following example.

The nurse has received the following information about assigned clients. The nurse should first assess:

- 1. A 64-year-old client who had a total knee replacement 3 hours ago and has 15 ml of serosanguineous drainage in the collection device.
- 2. A 32-year-old client who had closed reduction of a fractured right malleolus 5 hours ago and has swelling of the right toes.
- 3. A 9-month-old client admitted 6 hours ago with vomiting, whose vital signs are temperature, 37.6° C (99.7° F); pulse, 124; respirations, 26.
- ● 4. A 6-week-old client who was admitted 2 hours ago with nasal flaring and has a pulse oximetry reading of 90%.

Alternate Item Format. With this type of item, the candidate uses the keyboard to select an area on the screen or to type in the correct answer. Because of the nature of CAT, the type of item presented to the candidate will depend on the content area. Consequently, candidates may or may not receive alternate item format questions on their exam. Possible alternate item formats include:

Multiple Choice–Multiple Response. The candidate is presented with a question, followed by four or more responses. The candidate is asked to check all responses that are correct. See the following example:

The nurse is caring for a 47-year-old female client who has been diagnosed with hypothyroidism. Which of the following manifestations might the nurse expect the client to report?

- 1. Intolerance to heat
- ● 2. Periorbital edema
- 3. Weight loss

- 4. Menorrhagia
- 5. Constipation
- 6. Fatigue

Fill-in-the-Blank. The candidate is presented with a question to which the answer must be typed, instead of selecting from among a set of four options. In some cases, candidates may be asked to calculate values. A drop-down calculator is available for the candidate to use. See the following example:

The nurse is completing the intake and output record for a client who had a left total knee replacement 1 day ago. The client has had the following intake and output during the shift.

Intake: 3 oz of apple juice
$\frac{1}{2}$ serving of oatmeal
8 oz of water
1 cup of fruit-flavored gelatin
$\frac{1}{2}$ cup of beef broth
800 ml of 0.45 sodium chloride (half-strength saline), IV
Output: 1200 mL of urine
50 ml from the drainage tube

How many milliliters should the nurse document as the client's intake?
Answer: <u>1490 mL</u>

Identification. The candidate is presented with a picture or a graphic image and asked to identify a particular area. See the following example:

Identify the point of maximal impulse (PMI):

- ○ 1. A
- ○ 2. B
- ○ 3. C
- ● 4. D

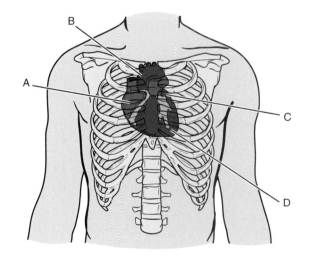

Prioritize. The candidate is presented with a set of responses to a question and asked to place them in order of priority. See the following example:

The nurse is preparing to perform a sterile dressing change. In what order would the following tasks be performed?

1. Gather supplies
2. Set up the sterile field
3. Assess the wound
4. Explain the procedure to the patient
5. Remove the soiled dressing
6. Document the dressing change

Type your answer in the box below. (Note: do not use spaces or commas between the numbers in the answer.)

145326

Any of the item formats, including standard multiple choice items may include tables, graphic images, or charts.

Cognitive Domains and NCLEX

NCLEX examination questions use Bloom's cognitive levels of knowledge, comprehension, application, and analysis (National Council, 2003). These levels may be viewed as four consecutive steps, with knowledge being the lowest, most fundamental step and analysis being the highest, most highly evolved of the steps.

Knowledge Questions. As the lowest and simplest level of learning within the cognitive domain, knowledge is remembering or recalling information. This may include knowing specific facts, common terms, methods and procedures, basic concepts, and principles (Gronlund, 1985).

Comprehension Questions. Comprehension, the second level of Bloom's cognitive domain, is the ability to grasp or understand information or material. Included in this level are the understanding of facts and principles; explaining verbal material, graphs, and charts; translating material into mathematical formulas; estimating outcomes implied in an information base; and justifying methods and procedures (Gronlund, 1985).

Application Questions. The third cognitive level, application, refers to the ability to use learned information in new situations. This level involves applying theories and principles in new or practical situations, solving mathematical problems, constructing charts and graphs, and showing accurate usage of a procedure (Gronlund, 1985).

Analysis Questions. The final and highest cognitive level, analysis, is the ability to reduce material into its elemental parts so that its design and structure may be understood. Included in this level are questions recognizing undeclared assumptions and logical inconsistencies in reasoning, discriminating between facts and deductions, and evaluating the applicability of information (Gronlund, 1985).

The majority of items are written at the application level or higher, because the practice of nursing necessitates that nurses apply knowledge, skills, and abilities to problem solve (NCLEX-RN® Test Plan, 2004). Examples of these items include making assignments for four clients, prioritizing care for four clients, and analyzing complex client data to determine an appropriate nursing action (Testing Services, 2004).

Candidates taking the examination answer a minimum of 75 questions to a maximum of 265 questions. Past candidates of the NCLEX examination have asked whether some candidates are randomly selected to receive longer versions of the examination. The National Council of State Boards of Nursing writes:

It is not true that some candidates randomly receive a maximum length examination. The length of an NCLEX examination is based on the performance of the candidate on the examination. After you have answered the minimum number of questions, the computer compares your competence level to the passing standard and makes one of three decisions:

1. If you are clearly above the passing standard, you pass and the examination ends.

2. If you are clearly below the passing standard, you fail and the examination ends.

3. If your competence level is close enough to the passing standard that it's still not clear whether you should pass or not, the computer continues to ask you questions until a clear pass or fail decision can be made, the maximum number of questions is reached, or time runs out (More untrue rumors, 2003).

COMPONENTS OF THE NCLEX TEST PLAN

The test plan for the NCLEX is based on the current nursing practice of entry-level RNs. According to NCSBN (2003):

Provision is made for an examination reflecting entry-level content and behaviors to be tested. Based on the NCLEX-RN Test Plan, each unique NCLEX-RN® examination reflects the knowledge, skills and abilities essential for the nurse to meet the needs of clients requiring the promotion, maintenance and restoration of health (p. 3).

The NCLEX test plan is framed by four major categories of client needs, which are (1) safe effective care environment, (2) health promotion and maintenance, (3) psychosocial integrity, and (4) physiologic integrity. These four categories are further subdivided into a total of six subcategories. Each of these will be examined individually, followed by a discussion of several processes which are fundamental to nursing, and integrated throughout the client needs categories and subcategories (NCLEX-RN® Test Plan, 2004, p. 4).

Client Needs

The organizing framework of the NCLEX examination is client needs. This is a broad component that "provides a universal structure for defining nursing actions and competencies across all settings for all clients" and is subdivided into four major categories (NCLEX-RN® Test Plan, 2004, p. 3).

Safe and Effective Care Environment. The first section relating to client needs is safe and effective care environment. This category is further subdivided into two categories: management of care, from which 13% to 19% of the test plan is constructed, and safety and infection control, from which 8% to 14% of the test plan is constructed (NCLEX-RN® Test Plan, 2004). Within this section the nurse should have the knowledge, skills, and ability to meet the client's needs for a safe and effective environment.

Health Promotion and Maintenance. The second section relating to client needs is health promotion and maintenance, from which 6% to 12% of NCLEX examination questions are constructed. This area "focuses on prevention and/or early detection of health problems, and strategies to achieve optimal health" (NCLEX-RN® Test Plan, 2004, p. 6).

Psychosocial Integrity. The third section dealing with client needs is psychosocial integrity. The nurse needs to "promote and support the emotional, mental, and social well-being of the client and family/significant others experiencing stressful events, and mental illness" (NCLEX-RN® Test Plan, 2004, p. 6). Psychosocial integrity is addressed in 6% to 12% of NCLEX examination questions.

Physiologic Integrity. The fourth section included in client needs is physiologic integrity. This category is further subdivided into these categories: basic care and comfort, accounting for 6% to 12% of the test plan; pharmacologic and parenteral therapies, accounting for 13% to 19% of the test plan; reduction of risk potential, accounting for 13% to 19% of the test plan; and physiologic adaptation, accounting for 11% to 17% of the test plan (NCLEX-RN® Test Plan, 2004).

Integrated Processes

Several processes that are fundamental to nursing are integrated throughout the above noted client needs categories and subcategories. These include nursing process; caring; communication and documentation; and teaching and learning (NCLEX-RN® Test Plan, 2004, p. 4). For example, a question may be a health promotion and maintenance question that has to do with assessment, or a psychosocial integrity question that also addresses implementation. All questions relate to some activity in which an entry-level nurse may engage when caring for or managing a patient. A more complete overview of these integrated processes follows.

Nursing Process. Success on the NCLEX examination relies on a sound working knowledge of the nursing process. The nursing process provides the foundation for nursing practice and is the tool that nurses use to assess, analyze, plan, implement, and evaluate the care given to their patients. The nursing process is applicable to all situations in which the nurse and patient interact and may be used with any theoretic framework. Cox et al (2000, p. 2) write:

Basically, the nursing process provides each nurse with a framework to use in working with a patient. The process begins at the time the patient needs assistance with health care through the time the patient no longer needs assistance to meet health care maintenance. The nursing process represents the cognitive (thinking and reasoning), psychomotor (physical), and affective (emotions and values) skills and abilities used by the nurse to plan care for a patient.

Assessment. Assessment is the first step of the nursing process and establishes a database for the client. Just as the nursing process provides a foundation for nursing practice, assessment provides the foundation for the nursing process. Assessment includes gathering information or data about an identified client. Depending on the nurse's focus, the client may be a person, a family, a group of people, or a community.

Information about a client will come from a variety of sources, including the client, the family and significant others, laboratory or radiographic reports, physician records, hospital or clinic records, and other caregivers. Client data are typically classified as subjective and objective. Simply put, subjective data are the client's perception or understanding of a specific event or phenomenon. It is his or her opinion, such as the degree of pain experienced during an episode of angina. Objective data are observable and measurable by the nurse and come from various patient records. Blood pressure, heart rate, and the presence or absence of edema are examples of objective data.

Cox et al (2002) suggest two additional classifications of client data—historical and current. Historical data relate to health events occurring before the current health problem or admission to the health care system. Current data include information specific to the current health problem or admission. Historical and current data may occur as subjective or objective information.

Assessment also includes verification and communication of data. Seeking additional client-related information such as laboratory work or talking with the family may confirm data. Communication of data may be accomplished by verbal report to other health care workers or by written or computerized record.

Analysis. Analysis is the second step or phase of the nursing process. Client-related data gathered during assessment provide the basis for analysis. During this phase the nurse classifies or groups assessment data and identifies actual or potential client problems. During classification, data also are validated and interpreted, and additional data may be required. Numerous frameworks exist for categorizing data. Included in the frameworks are Gordon's Functional Health Patterns, Maslow's Hierarchy of Needs, and the North American Nursing Diagnosis Association's (NANDA) Human Response Patterns (Cox et al, 2002).

Nursing diagnoses are determined based on classification of data. A working definition of nursing diagnosis is provided by NANDA:

A nursing diagnosis is a clinical judgment about individual, family, or community responses to actual or potential health problems/life processes. Nursing diagnoses provide the basis for selection of nursing interventions to achieve outcomes for which the nurse is accountable (Carroll-Johnson, 1991, p. 65).

As with assessment, nursing diagnoses must be communicated in a reliable format. It is important to remember that there must be congruency between the client's needs or problems and the nurse's ability to realistically meet those needs.

Planning. Planning is the third phase of the nursing process and includes setting realistic and measurable mutual goals, designing strategies to meet or resolve identified patient needs or problems, and modifying goals as necessary. Included in planning of care are ranking nursing diagnoses, documenting expected outcomes for each goal, and setting realistic target dates for the accomplishment of each goal. Goal setting should include the collaboration of members of the interdisciplinary health care team, the client, his or her family, and significant others as indicated.

As with the previous phases of the nursing process, the plan must be communicated to other members of the health care team to ensure continuity of care.

Implementation. The fourth phase of the nursing process is implementation. This stage includes initiating and carrying out nursing interventions or nursing actions to achieve the goals set in the planning phase of the nursing process. In discussing nursing actions, Cox et al (2002) write:

Nursing action is defined as nursing behavior that serves to help the client achieve the expected outcome. Nursing actions include both independent and collaborative activities. Independent actions are those activities the nurse performs using his or her own discretionary judgment and that require no validation or guidelines from any other health care practitioner; for example, deciding which noninvasive technique to use for pain control or deciding when to teach the patient self-care measures. Collaborative actions are those activities that involve mutual decision making between two or more health care practitioners (e.g., a physician and nurse deciding which narcotic to use when meperidine is ineffective in controlling the patient's pain) (p. 6).

Each nursing action should be geared toward achieving a particular goal of care. Included in the implementation phase are (1) organizing and managing care; (2) actually performing patient care; (3) overseeing and coordinating the delivery of care; (4) delegating nursing actions to other health care workers; (5) teaching or counseling the client, his or her family, significant others, and other caregivers; and (6) communicating and exchanging patient-related information with other health care workers (Cox et al, 2002).

Evaluation. To evaluate, data must be collected to document the progress the patient has made, or not made, in relation to the stated goal. Once data have been collected and analyzed, the nurse must decide what action to take or what modification to make regarding the goal. In all instances the nurse will make one of three choices:

1. Resolve the plan because the patient has achieved the goal
2. Continue the plan because the patient is still making satisfactory progress toward the goal but did not achieve the goal during the original time frame
3. Revise the plan because the patient is not making satisfactory progress toward the goal (Cox et al, 2002).

As with the other phases of the nursing process, evaluation involves documenting and illustrating the patient's responses to the care provided.

Caring. NCSBN defines caring as "the interaction of the nurse and client in an atmosphere of mutual respect and trust, wherein the nurse provides hope, support, and compassion, in an effort to achieve desired outcomes" (NCLEX-RN® Test Plan, 2004, p. 4).

Communication and Documentation. NCSBN defines communication and documentation as "the verbal and nonverbal interactions between the nurse and the client, the client's significant others and the other members of the health care team. Events and activities associated with client care are validated in written or electronic records that reflect quality and accountability in the provision of care" (NCLEX-RN® Test Plan, 2004, p. 4).

Teaching/Learning. NCSBN defines teaching/learning as "facilitation of the acquisition of knowledge, skills, and attitudes promoting a change in behavior" (NCLEX-RN® Test Plan, 2004, p. 4).

PREPARING FOR THE NCLEX EXAMINATION

There is no one best method for preparing to take the NCLEX examination. Success depends on a candidate's nursing knowledge and ability to use that knowledge, test-taking skills, and confidence level. The best preparation any candidate can have is what the candidate brings from his or her nursing program.

Some measure of preparation for the NCLEX examination after graduation from nursing school is a must for all candidates seeking success on the examination. Candidates should not convince themselves that they do not need to review because average or above-average grades were made in their academic and nursing course work, nor should they decide that review will serve no purpose because average or below-average grades were made in their course work.

In preparing for the NCLEX examination, it is important to remember that review is a personal undertaking. What works for one candidate may not work for another and vice versa. Use study and review methods that have proven successful in the past.

Consider the following when preparing for the NCLEX examination:

- *Perform a needs assessment.* Determine content areas of strengths and weaknesses. Look at previous academic and nursing course work, class notes and handouts, examination grades, and grades made on nursing care plans or process papers. Talk with faculty in courses in which weakness or difficulty existed. Determine where the greatest amount of review is needed. Candidates should be honest in performing the needs assessment. The foundation for success or failure on the NCLEX examination may be determined here.

- *Determine the number of days or weeks necessary for review.* Candidates with a strong nursing knowledge base may need less time than candidates with weaknesses. As with the needs assessment, candidates should be realistic in planning the amount of review time needed.

- *Decide what method of review will be used.* Individual and group study both have strong and weak points. Strong points of individual study include having total control over content and time spent in review. Weak points include having no immediate resources to explain or assist with understanding difficult concepts. Candidates with weakness in disciplining themselves may have problems sticking to review schedules and focusing on specific content with individual study. Strong points of group study include the support that members can give each other and learning from others in the group. Also, many minds working together are stronger than one working alone. Weak points of group study include a lack of preparation of some group members, weaker members of the group holding the rest back, and a tendency of the group to focus on topics that have more to do with socialization than review. Candidates using study groups should insist on members coming to sessions prepared to work.

- *Decide what materials or resources will be used during review.* Textbooks and class notes from nursing or nursing-related courses, such as anatomy and physiology, psychology, or nutrition, will prove helpful. Computer-assisted instructions used during the nursing program may be available. Numerous NCLEX review books are available. Their prices range from around $20 to $50. Many review books include a computer disk or CD-ROM to be used during review. Make sure that these computer aids are compatible with the type of computer you will be using during review.

- *Talk with nursing faculty* about using any NCLEX preparation aids the school of nursing may have available for candidates.

- *Structure review time.* Schedule review during times of peak performance. Learning is enhanced when reviewing for short blocks of time, around 50 minutes, instead of reviewing for several unbroken hours at a time. Candidates should remember that they are *reviewing* for an examination, not *cramming* for one.

- *Control the review environment.* Keep noise and distraction at a minimum. Have adequate space and lighting for review. Control the room temperature when possible; if not possible, dress for the environment. Have all materials needed for review, including soft drinks and snacks, close at hand so that time is not wasted gathering these items during review time. Make sure that friends and family know not to interrupt during review time.

- *Have a game plan for each review session.* Develop a review schedule complete with subject matter to be considered and specific tasks to be completed during each session. Stick to the schedule.
- *Learn concepts and principles, not isolated facts.* The NCLEX examination tests a candidate's ability to apply, analyze, and evaluate nursing knowledge and does not focus on isolated events. Candidates whose past test-taking success has been based on memorization rather than actual learning have an increased risk for failure on the NCLEX examination.
- *Use learning techniques that have proven successful in the past,* such as flash cards or note cards, underscoring of key points, taking notes or outlining material, or capturing pertinent information on a tape recorder for later playback. One should either quiz himself or herself or ask others to pose questions.
- *Seek qualified help* when reviewing information that is particularly difficult. Faculty members are an excellent resource. Be cautious when asking peers for assistance because they may not understand the material as well as they think they do.
- *Practice taking "NCLEX-type" examinations,* paying particular attention to the rationales or reasons provided for correct and incorrect answers. Successful test takers know why a specific option is correct or incorrect. Even though candidates may spend as much time as they want on a question when actually taking the examination, they should get into the habit of taking about 1 minute for each question. Poor time management may cause a candidate to not have enough time to complete the test and therefore be unsuccessful on the NCLEX examination. Practice also will help reduce test anxiety. NCLEX-type examinations are commonly found in NCLEX review books.
- *Use the Internet.* It provides numerous sources that may aid in preparation for the NCLEX examination. Box 26-1 provides a partial listing of available sites that might be helpful.
- *Avoid excessive stimulants* (e.g., caffeine) to increase review time. The best learning takes place when heads are clear.
- *Maintain a healthy, positive attitude* toward reviewing and taking the NCLEX examination. Have confidence in your abilities to be successful on the examination. Remember that even practicing nurses with years of experience don't know everything there is to know about every aspect of nursing and that the goal on the NCLEX examination is to demonstrate minimal competency for an entry-level RN position, not competency for an advanced RN position.

FOOD FOR THOUGHT WHEN SELECTING A NCLEX REVIEW COURSE

Just as there is no one best method for preparing to take the NCLEX examination, there is no one best review course for a candidate to take in preparation for the NCLEX examination. The most important thing to remember when considering a review course is that a review course is exactly what it says it is—a review course. Such courses are designed to reconsider or reexamine content common to the three types of nursing programs.

The purpose of a review course is to enhance or polish what candidates already know from their nursing programs. Review courses are not intended to teach totally new concepts. If candidates have an extreme weakness in one or more content areas, the review course may not provide enough content to bring the candidate up to speed on the topic.

Numerous companies and people offer review courses. Each review offering has strong and weak points, and what appeals to one candidate may not appeal to another. Some offer financial discounts or other incentives if more than one candidate from a school of nursing registers for their course.

Review courses usually are expensive and last from 1 or 2 days to a complete work week. Some courses provide books or other written materials. Others may offer additional materials for a fee. Some courses will refund a part or all of the cost of the review if a candidate takes their review course and is unsuccessful in taking the NCLEX examination.

Review courses may or may not be taught by competent people. Nurse educators who are teaching faculty at schools of nursing teach many review courses. However, people with no substantial background in nursing may teach some courses. A review course is no better than the person or people teaching it.

The decision to take a review course in preparation for taking the NCLEX examination is a personal one. Some candidates find the structure and schedule of a review course helpful in preparation. Other candidates may find the structure and schedule restrictive and overly time-consuming.

Candidates seriously interested in taking an NCLEX review course should look to the faculty at their school of nursing for guidance. Many faculty have had experience with review courses or may teach review courses. Serious candidates also should obtain written information from several different review course offerings and compare and contrast among the offerings. Selection of a review course should be based on more than the cost of the review program—it should meet the candidate's unique needs.

SUMMARY

Success on the NCLEX examination is needed to obtain a license and practice as an RN. Most candidates taking the NCLEX examination are successful. Of the 71,393 first-time, U.S.-educated candidates taking the examination during the first three quarters of 2003, approximately 88% were successful (NCLEX Results, 2003). The key to success on the NCLEX examination is sound preparation from the nursing program, adequate preparation for the examination, and confidence in oneself.

CRITICAL THINKING ACTIVITIES

1. Develop a realistic plan for reviewing for the NCLEX examination. Identify what you think is important in developing your plan and include the following:
    a. Assessment of areas of strengths and weaknesses (for example, if your school uses an exit exam, or diagnostic tool, use that feedback to design an individualized program of study)
    b. Time frame for review
    c. Methods of review

    d. Specific plans for each review session
    e. Resources
    f. Barriers to effective review
    g. Realistic solutions to barriers
2. Investigate at least two different NCLEX review courses and determine the strengths and weaknesses of each.

Additional resources are available on-line at: http://evolve.elsevier.com/Cherry/

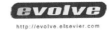

http://evolve.elsevier.com

REFERENCES

Carroll-Johnson RM: *Classification of nursing diagnoses: proceedings of the nineth conference,* Philadelphia, 1991, JB Lippincott.

Computerized adaptive testing (CAT) overview, 2003 (www.ncsbn.org).

Cox HC et al: *Clinical applications of nursing diagnosis: adult, child, women's, psychiatric, gerontic, and home health considerations,* ed 4, Philadelphia, 2002, FA Davis.

Foote J: *State board questions and answers for nurses,* Philadelphia, 1919, JB Lippincott.

Gronlund NE: *Measurement and evaluation in teaching,* New York, 1985, Macmillan Publishing.

How CAT works: a candidate primer, 2003, National Council of State Boards of Nursing Web Site (www.ncsbn.org/files/nclex/overview.asp).

More untrue rumors regarding the NCLEX examination, National Council of State Boards of Nursing Web Site, 2003 (www.ncsbn.org).

National Council of State Boards of Nursing: *NCLEX-RN examination test plan for the National Council Licensure Examination for Registered Nurses,* Chicago, 2003, Author.

NCLEX Results. Available on-line (http://www.ncsbn.org/research_stats/nclex.asp).

NCLEX-RN® Test Plan, Effective April 2004, NCSBN NCLEX® Examinations, National Council of State Boards of Nursing.

Testing Services, fact versus fiction. Retrieved February 26, 2004 (http://www.ncsbn.org/testing/generalinformation_info_fact.asp).

Index

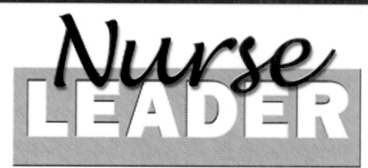
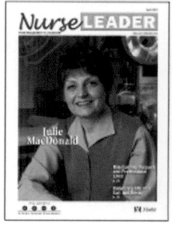
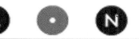
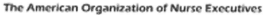